·Handbook of·
PEDIATRIC PHYSICAL AND
CLINICAL DIAGNOSIS

· Handbook of ·

PEDIATRIC PHYSICAL

AND CLINICAL

DIAGNOSIS

Lewis A. Barness, MD, DSci(hc), DPH(hc)

Distinguished University Professor Emeritus
University of South Florida College of Medicine
Department of Pediatrics
Tampa, FL

Professor Emeritus, Pediatrics
University of Wisconsin Medical School
Madison, WI

Enid Gilbert-Barness, AO, MD, MBBS, FRCPA,
FRCPath, DSci(hc), MD(hc)

Professor of Pathology and Cell Biology, Pediatrics and Obstetrics and Gynecology
University of South Florida College of Medicine
Tampa General Hospital, Tampa, FL

Professor Emeritus, Pathology, Laboratory Medicine and Pediatrics
Distinguished Medical Alumni Professor Emeritus
University of Wisconsin Medical School, Madison, WI

Dean Fauber, MD, FAAP

Pediatrician, Dunedin, FL

Foreword by
John M. Opitz, MD, MD(hc), DSci(hc), MD(hc), MD(hc)

Professor of Pediatrics (Medical Genetics), Human Genetics, Pathology,
and Obstetrics and Gynecology
University of Utah Health Sciences Center
Salt Lake City, UT

Eighth Edition

OXFORD
UNIVERSITY PRESS
2009

OXFORD
UNIVERSITY PRESS

Oxford University Press, Inc., publishes works that further
Oxford University's objective of excellence
in research, scholarship, and education.

Oxford New York
Auckland   Cape Town   Dar es Salaam   Hong Kong   Karachi
Kuala Lumpur   Madrid   Melbourne   Mexico City   Nairobi
New Delhi   Shanghai   Taipei   Toronto

With offices in
Argentina   Austria   Brazil   Chile   Czech Republic   France   Greece
Guatemala   Hungary   Italy   Japan   Poland   Portugal   Singapore
South Korea   Switzerland   Thailand   Turkey   Ukraine   Vietnam

Published by Oxford University Press, Inc.
198 Madison Avenue, New York, New York 10016
www.oup.com

Oxford is a registered trademark of Oxford University Press

Library of Congress Cataloging-in-Publication Data
Barness, Lewis A.
   Handbook of pediatric physical and clinical diagnosis / Lewis A. Barness and
Enid Gilbert-Barness. — 8th ed.
      p. ; cm.
   Rev. ed. of: Handbook of pediatric physical diagnosis / [edited by]
Lewis A. Barness. Lippincott-Raven. c1998.
   Includes bibliographical references.
   ISBN 978-0-19-537325-7
   1. Children—Medical examinations—Handbooks, manuals, etc. 2. Children—Diseases—Diagnosis—Handbooks,
manuals, etc. 3. Physical diagnosis—Handbooks, manuals, etc. I. Gilbert-Barness, Enid, 1927–   II.
Handbook of pediatric physical diagnosis. III. Title.
   [DNLM: 1. Physical Examination—Handbooks. 2. Child. 3. Infant. WS 39 B261h 2009]
   RJ50.H365 2009
   618.92'0075—dc22

                                                                            2008022054

9 8 7 6 5 4 3 2 1

Printed in the United States of America
on acid-free paper

To my wife, Mary Anne (DF), to our children, and our grandchildren who provide us joy beyond measure and to our parents whose love and strength have sustained us.
LAB, EGB, DF

Enid and Dean wish to make a special dedication to Lewis Barness—the supreme champion of children and Master of Pediatrics.

FOREWORD

I N THE INTRODUCTION to the third edition of his work on acute diseases of 1675, Thomas Sydenham, the father of modern nosology and nosography wrote: "After long deliberation and many years' close and faithful observation, I resolved (1) to communicate my thoughts relating to the manner of making further advances in physic and (2) to publish a specimen of my endeavours in this way," "physic" then referring to the science of medicine. As most advances in medicine, particularly in pediatrics, have been made through the study of sick and suffering human beings, close and faithful observation is the essential first step in making progress. Since my days as a medical student in 1957 in Iowa City, the *Handbook of Pediatric Physical and Clinical Diagnosis* by Lewis Barness has been my guide in this field. It was not just recommended by some of my greatest teachers including Hans Zellweger and Jacqueline Noonan, but required reading, and I have in the half-century since then required my students, residents, and fellows to own and to study assiduously this marvelous and extremely useful book.

Presently in its eighth edition, the *Handbook* has undergone another metamorphosis now including extensive considerations of nosology, chromosomal and genetic diseases, and separate chapters on hematologic disorders, infections, endocrine abnormalities, and child abuse. The book has been enhanced by additional tables and illustrations, many drawn by Diane Debich-Spicer. Most gratifying is the splendid collaboration between Lew Barness and his wife Dr. Enid Gilbert-Barness, which has added an important pathological perspective. As is evident throughout the book, both are experts in metabolic diseases, but even more important is the great warmth and humanity they bring to the teaching of physical examination and the evaluation of the child. I strongly suspect that this revision of the *Handbook* will be translated into more than the six languages in which this volume has appeared in the past.

As no surgeon can function without the anatomy inaugurated by Vesalius, or cardiologist without the knowledge of physiology initiated by Harvey, Malpighi, and Stensen, or developmental pathologist without a basis of embryology as founded by Aristotle, Harvey, and von Baer, so no pediatrician can function without detailed knowledge of the normal growth and developmental variability of the child. The physical examination is an essential first step in the acquisition of such knowledge. In my over fifty years in pediatrics I still find the *Handbook of Pediatric Physical and Clinical Diagnosis*, now by the Doctors Barness and Gilbert-Barness, the best resource and guide in this field.

John M. Opitz, MD

PREFACE

IN PEDIATRIC PRACTICE, there is no substitute for the physical examination. A thorough physical, along with a complete history, is still the best basis for most diagnoses. When dealing with infants, children, and adolescents, "laying on of the hands" is crucial if one is to provide effective and productive care. As the focus in the classroom, examination room, and medical literature shifts to computers, technical devices, and sophisticated laboratory tests, the importance and necessity of the comprehensive physical diagnosis and detailed history can sometimes be overlooked. This combination of incomplete physical exam and history and increased use of modern devices (along with the pressures of cost containment and shortened contact time) has led to complaints of coldness on the part of the physician. For the physician treating the pediatric patient, it is especially important to avoid this trend. The practice of laying on of the hands is a fundamental component of diagnosis. Patients and parents want a physician who can use not only the latest technological diagnostic tools but also the "old-fashioned" methods for arriving at a diagnosis. For the practicing pediatrician, physical examinations and laying on of the hands can lead to greater personal rewards and gratification.

This new edition of the *Handbook of Pediatric Physical and Clinical Diagnosis* has been expanded to include differential diagnosis. It provides the student and practitioner with an extensive review of the special methods used in pediatric physical diagnosis. The reader will find various sections that discuss the characteristics and specifics of the physical examination, including the approach to the patient, the examination of the body, the neurologic examination, and the examination of the newborn. In addition, the requests and suggestions of readers and residents have been incorporated in this edition, resulting in revisions and updates to most of the text, and more of the information (particularly diagnoses) is presented in tables and list form.

For this edition, as with the volumes in the past, I am grateful to many people for their comments and criticisms, particularly my wife, Enid. I also want to thank my grandchildren, who continue to provide new challenges in diagnosis. In part, portion of the appendix has been taken from "They Do Come with Instructions" by Ivy Faske, MD, with much gratitude.

Dr. Dean Fauber, an accomplished pediatrician, has made revisions and has reviewed the entire manuscript. Dr. Fauber deserves my appreciation and I have included him as a coauthor. My wife, Enid Gilbert-Barness, not only has contributed to making revisions but is largely responsible for much of the differential diagnosis. Her perspective as a pediatric pathologist has added another important dimension to this volume for which I am greatly indebted. She is, therefore, also a coauthor.

Many thanks to William Lamsback of Oxford University Press for his guidance and support during the preparation of this manuscript. My grandson, Christian Lawrence, provided the illustration for the cover of the book. Special thanks to Megan Klakring for proofreading some of the chapters. We also acknowledge with gratitude the superb artwork of Diane Debich-Spicer. Above all, we are indebted to Kathleen Lonkey for her timeless, diligent, meticulous, and dedicated work in the preparation of the entire manuscript, and without whom this work could not have been completed.

Lewis A. Barness, MD

CONTENTS

· Handbook of ·
PEDIATRIC PHYSICAL AND
CLINICAL DIAGNOSIS

1

APPROACH TO THE PATIENT

More is missed by not looking than not knowing.

A COMPLETE PHYSICAL EXAMINATION in a child emphasizes many characteristics that differ from those in adults. It is important to recognize these differences and also the many variations among normal children.

This is a manual of the special methods used in pediatric physical diagnosis. No extensive details are listed of the definition of a sign or of methods of eliciting a sign unless special methods are used in children. Although the material in this manual includes only the actual physical examination, diagnoses cannot be made by physical examination alone. Before the examination is started, it is important that a careful and detailed history must be taken of the patient and family and that this be made part of the patient's record. As the art of careful observation is learned, diagnosis by physical examination becomes easier. In younger children from whom no history can be directly obtained, or in the child whose parents lack the ability of accurate observation, careful physical examination is indeed necessary.

Examples of disease states are given throughout this manual. At no time are these states to be considered the complete differential diagnosis of the sign given. The examples are given only to present a better understanding of the sign under discussion. The beginner may use this manual to learn to elicit a particular sign; the disease states indicated will later have meaning.

If further examples of a sign are desired, standard references are suggested. The references used freely in the development of this manual include the easily available standard pediatric texts.

Many suggestions have been made for improvement of this manual by students, house officers, and physicians. More lists of diseases are included. We hope that this will improve readability, but it should not be construed as a complete list of differential diagnoses.

There is no "routine" physical examination of a child. Each examination is individualized. Not only are there many physical differences that an examiner accustomed to adults might consider abnormal in a child but also the variations within a group of children make the examiner more alert to the broad spectrum included in the term *normal*. The physician adept at physical diagnosis in children is one who is aware of these variants.

Most of the observed variations can best be explained by the difference in growth rates of the organ systems as they occur from infancy to maturity. For example, the lymphoid tissue is relatively well developed in infancy, becomes maximally developed during childhood, and regresses to small adult proportions at puberty. The nervous system, on the other hand, is largely developed at birth and reaches almost complete adult size by age 5 years. The genital system, however, is infantile until puberty. These and other variations will be noted throughout the discussion of the physical examination.

A mother frequently asks or silently worries: "Is my child normal?" With only a single observation of a child one is rarely able to tell whether or not the child is entirely normal, though one may frequently be able to tell that the child is abnormal. Normality in pediatrics, as in statistics, is often confused with the average, and statisticians conclude that considerable variation from the average exists in any normal static population. Normality in children includes the many differences existing at about the average age of the child being studied, with adequate consideration of the child's background and environment. Determining "normality" in an ever-changing individual is even more difficult. In conducting a physical examination, one seeks normal, variations from normal, and abnormal states. One also determines the general mental and physical state, congenital and acquired anomalies, and pathologic or disease states. One also needs to consider trends, either toward or away from perceived normal.

The record of a complete physical examination in a child has special importance not found in that of an adult. This record represents a report of one specific time in a child's life when that child is continually and rapidly changing. Therefore it will be used as a basis for determining whether that child is growing and developing normally, according to a group of standards learned from books, mothers, and patients. More important than a single observation of the child is the use made of this record in following the rate of change of the child at each subsequent examination. The rate of growth, rate of development, and, indeed, rate of progression of difficulties or anomalies far surpass for evaluation purposes the single examination. The single examination is valuable, of course, not only for determining acute illnesses but also for determining for the physician, parent, and child the gross evaluation of the potentialities and liabilities of the child. Therefore, even small and apparently insignificant variants should be noted for each child so that their importance may be adequately assessed in later examinations.

For example, if a child with nausea and vomiting was adequately examined 2 weeks before the illness and the liver was not palpable at the time but is now palpable 2 cm below the right costal margin, one should direct attention to the liver as a possible cause of the illness. In contrast, if the child's liver was palpable 2 weeks before the acute illness, the now palpable liver requires less attention. This type of notation is especially important for so-called innocent murmurs of childhood, which are notorious for their frequent change, the significance of which may take many months and many examinations to determine.

The physical examination of a child should also constitute a record that can be easily interpreted by other physicians. Appendix A contains a form for recording a physical examination. Although the method of recording the physical examination is a logical order, the examination itself is not necessarily performed in that order.

HISTORY TAKING AND APPROACH TO THE PATIENT

A complete history on a pediatric patient leads to the correct diagnosis in the majority of children. The history usually is learned from the parent, the older child, or the caretaker of a sick child. After learning the fundamentals of obtaining and recording case history data, the nuances associated with interpreting information must be learned.

For the acutely ill child, a short, rapidly obtained report of the events of the immediate past may suffice temporarily, but as soon as the crisis is stabilized, a more complete history is necessary. A convenient method of obtaining a meaningful history is to ask systematically and directly all of the questions outlined in this chapter. After confidence is gained with experience, questions can be directed at specific problems and asked in an order designed to elicit more specific information about a suspected disease state or diagnosis. More subtle details often are obtained by asking open-ended questions. Some psychosocial implications will be obvious. Those patients with organic illness usually have short histories; those with psychosomatic illness generally have a longer list of symptoms and complaints.

During the interview, it is important to convey to the parent interest in the child, as well as the illness. The parent should be allowed to talk freely at first and to express concerns in his or her own words. The interviewer should look directly either at the parent or the child intermittently. A sympathetic listener who addresses the parent and child by name frequently obtains more accurate information than does a harried, distracted interviewer. Careful observation during the interview may uncover stresses and concerns.

A well-organized record facilitates the retrieval of information and obviates problems if it is required for legal review.

The following guidelines indicate the information needed. If preferred, a number of printed forms are available that contain similar material, or forms may be modified as long as consistency is maintained.

Identifying data include the examination date; patient's name, age and birth date, gender, and race; the referral source if pertinent; the relationship of the child and informant; and some indication of the mental state or reliability of the informant. It frequently is helpful to include the ethnic or racial background, address, and telephone numbers of informants.

Chief Complaint

The chief complaint in the informant's or patient's own words is a brief statement of the reason why the patient is being seen. The stated complaint is often not the true reason for the visit. Expanding the question, "Why did you bring the child in?" to "What concerns you?" allows the informant to focus on the complaint more accurately. Carefully phrased questions can elicit information without prying.

History of Present Illness

The details of the present illness are recorded in chronologic order. For the sick child, it is helpful to begin, "The child was well until how many days before this visit?" This is followed by a daily documentation of events leading up to the present time, including signs, symptoms, and treatment, if any. Statements should be recorded in number of days before the visit or specific dates, but not by days of the week. If the child is taking medicine, the record should indicate type and brand, the amount being taken, the frequency of administration, and response.

For the well child, a simple statement such as "No complaints" or "No illness" suffices. A question about school attendance may be pertinent. If the past history is significant to the current illness, a brief summary is included. If information is obtained from old records, it should be noted.

Past Medical History

Depending on the age of the patient, some aspects of the past history that follow may not be pertinent. Obtaining the past medical history serves not only to provide a record of significant data but also provides evidence of children who are at risk for health or psychosocial problems.

Prenatal History

If a prenatal interview has been held (see section Prenatal Interview), this information may already be available. Questions to be answered include those regarding the health of the mother during the pregnancy, especially in regard to any infections, other illnesses, vaginal bleeding, toxemia, or exposure to animals, any of which can have permanent effects on the embryo and child. Inquire about the time and type of fetal movements. The record should include the number of previous pregnancies and their results; whether radiography was performed, what medications were taken, and whether the mother smoked or abused drugs or alcohol during pregnancy; whether mother's weight gain was excessive or insufficient; results of serology and blood typing of the mother and baby; and results of other tests such as amniocentesis.

Birth History

The duration of pregnancy, the ease or difficulty of labor, and the duration of labor may be important, especially if there is a question of developmental delay. The type of delivery (spontaneous, forceps assisted, or cesarean section), type of anesthesia or analgesia used during delivery, attendance by other family members at delivery, and presenting part (if known) are recorded. Note the child's birth order (if there have been multiple births) and birth weight. If born via cesarean section, stated indication should be recorded.

Neonatal History

Many informants are aware of Apgar scores at birth and at 5 minutes, any unusual appearance of the child such as cyanosis or respiratory distress, and any resuscitative efforts and their duration. If the mother was delayed in seeing the infant after birth,

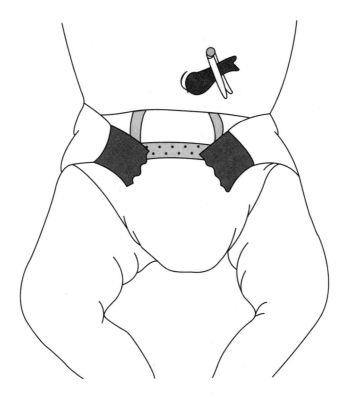

Figure 1.1
Correct position of diaper below the umbilicus.

reasons should be sought. Jaundice, anemia, convulsions, dysmorphic states, and congenital anomalies or infections in the mother or the infant are some of the reasons that viewing or handling of the newborn by the mother may be delayed. In the newborn, the diaper should be positioned such that it is below the umbilicus (Figure 1.1).

Feeding History

Note whether the baby was breast or bottle fed and how well the baby took the first feeding. Poor sucking at the first feeding may be the result of sleepiness, but also is a warning sign of neurologic abnormality, which may not become manifest until much later in life. By the second or third feeding, even brain-damaged children usually nurse well, although an otherwise normal newborn might not suckle well for 6 to 24 hours.

If the infant has been bottle fed, inquire about the type of formula used and the amount taken during a 24-hour period. Ask about the mother's initial reaction to her baby, the nature of bonding and eye-to-eye contact, and the baby's patterns of crying, sleeping, urinating, and defecating. Supplemental feeding, vomiting, regurgitation, colic, diarrhea, or other gastrointestinal or feeding problems should be noted.

Determine the ages at which solid foods were introduced and supplementation with vitamins or fluoride, the age at which baby foods, toddlers' foods, and table food were introduced, the response to these, and any evidence of food intolerance or vomiting. If feeding difficulties are present, determine the onset of the problem, methods of feeding, reasons for changes, interval between feedings, amount taken at each feeding, vomiting, crying, and weight changes. With any feeding problem, evaluate the effect on the family by asking, "How did you manage the problem?"

For an older child, ask for some breakfast, lunch, and dinner menus, likes and dislikes, and response of the family to eating problems. Toddlers frequently attempt to be quite restrictive in their dietary requests.

Development History

Estimate the physical growth rate. Attempt to ascertain the birth weight and the weight and length at 6 months, 1 year, 2 years, 5 years, and 10 years. Sudden gain or loss in physical growth should be noted, because its onset may correspond to the onset of organic or psychosocial illness. It may be helpful to compare the child's growth with the rate of growth of siblings or parents.

Ages at which major developmental milestones were met aid in indicating deviations from normal. Such milestones include following a person with the eyes, holding the head erect, smiling responsively, reaching for objects, transferring objects, sitting alone, walking with support and alone, speaking the first words and sentences, and experiencing tooth eruption. Ages of dressing self, tying own shoes, hopping, skipping, and riding a tricycle and bicycle should be noted, as well as grade in school and school performance. See Appendix E for more detailed description of normal ages of various milestones.

Note the age at which bowel and bladder control was achieved. If problems exist, the age at which toilet teaching began also may indicate reasons for problems.

Behavior History

Question the amount of sleep and sleep problems and habits such as pica and use of alcohol and drugs. The informant should state whether the child is happy or difficult to manage and should indicate the child's response to new situations, strangers, and school. Temper tantrums, excessive or unprovoked crying, nail biting, and nightmares and night terrors should be recorded. Question the child regarding masturbation, dating and dealing with the opposite sex, and parents' responses to menstruation and sexual development. Questions should be free of heterosexual assumption, direction of romantic interests, and gender of partners. Also, it is useful to ask questions concerning mood, such as anger, sadness, or anxiety.

Immunization History

The types of immunizations received, with the number, dates, sites given, and reactions should be recorded. Record these immunizations with lot numbers on the front of the chart or in a convenient obvious place.

History of Past Illnesses

A general statement should be made about the child's general health before the present encounter, such as weight change, fever, weakness, or mood alterations. Specific inquiry is helpful regarding the results of any screening tests and any history of infectious or contagious diseases, or any other illness, as well as specific treatment, result, and residua. The history of each past illness should include dates of onset, course, and termination. If hospitalization or surgery was necessary, record the diagnoses, dates, and name of the hospital. Questions concerning allergies include the occurrence and type of any drug reactions, food allergies, hay fever, asthma, accidents, injuries, and poisonings.

Review of Systems

The review of systems serves as a checklist for pertinent information that might have been omitted. If information has been obtained previously, simply state, "See history of present illness" or "See history of past illness." Questions concerning each system may be introduced with a question such as, "Are there any symptoms related to . . . ?"

- Head (e.g., injuries, headache)
- Eyes (e.g., visual changes, crossed or tendency to cross, discharge, redness, puffiness, injuries, glasses)
- Ears (e.g., difficulty with hearing, pain, discharge, ear infections, myringotomy, ventilation tubes)
- Nose (e.g., watery or purulent discharge, difficulty in breathing through nose, epistaxis)
- Mouth and throat (e.g., watery and purulent discharge, difficulty in breathing through nose, epistaxis)
- Neck (e.g., swollen glands, masses, stiffness, symmetry)
- Breasts (e.g., lumps, pain, symmetry, nipple discharge, embarrassment)
- Lungs (e.g., shortness of breath, inability to keep up with peers, timing and character of cough, hoarseness, wheezing, hemoptysis, pain in chest)
- Heart (e.g., cyanosis, edema, heart murmurs or "heart trouble," pain over heart)
- Gastrointestinal (e.g., appetite, nausea, vomiting with relation to feeding, amount, color, blood or bile stained, or projectile, number and character of bowel movements, abdominal pain or distention, jaundice)
- Genitourinary (e.g., dysuria, hematuria, frequency, oliguria, character of urinary stream, enuresis, urethral or vaginal discharge, menstrual history, attitude toward menses and opposite sex, sores, pain, sexual activity, birth control, sexually transmitted disease and protection, abortions)
- Extremities (e.g., weakness, deformities, difficulty in moving extremities or in walking, joint pain and swelling, muscle pains or cramps)
- Neurologic (e.g., headaches, fainting, dizziness, incoordination, seizures, numbness, tremors)

- Skin (e.g., rashes, hives, itching, color change, hair and nail growth, color, bruises or bleeds easily)
- Psychiatric (e.g., usual mood, nervousness, tension, drug use or abuse)

Family History

The family history provides evidence for considering familial diseases as well as infections or contagious illnesses. A genetic type chart is easy to read and should include parents, siblings, and grandparents, with their ages, health, or cause of death. If a problem with genetic implications exists, all known relatives should be inquired about. If a genetic type chart is used, pregnancies should be listed in a series and should include the health of the siblings.

Family diseases such as allergy, blood, heart, lung, venereal, or kidney disease; tuberculosis, diabetes, rheumatic fever, convulsions, skin, gastrointestinal, behavioral or mental disorders, cancer, or other disease may have a heritable or contagious effect. Pertinent negative answers should be included.

Social History

Details of the family unit include the number of people in the habitat and its size, the presence of grandparents, the marital status of the parents, the significant care-taker, the total family income and its source, and whether the mother and father work outside the home. If it is pertinent to the current problems of the child, inquire about the family's attitude toward the child and toward each other, the type of discipline used, and the major disciplinarian. If the problem is psychosocial and only one parent is the informant, it may be necessary to interview the other parent and to outline a typical day in the life of the child.

Prenatal Interview

It is desirable, if feasible, to interview the mother and father before the child is born. Not only can some necessary data be obtained, but the parents can also become acquainted with the doctor who will be seeing them shortly after the arrival of their newborn. The health of the mother, whether she will nurse or bottle-feed the baby and whether the husband supports her choice, the preparation for the baby on arrival home, and whether help will be available can be ascertained. Because the father may feel left out of the pregnancy experience, it is important to direct some questions to him (e.g., "Do you want your son circumcised?") and to get the family history of diseases from him first.

History of the Child

Even young children should be asked about their symptoms and their understanding of their problem. This also provides the opportunity to observe the child interacting with the parent. For most adolescents, it is important to take part of the history from the adolescent alone after asking for his or her approval. Regardless of your own opinion, obtain the history objectively without any moral implications, starting with open-ended questions related to the initial complaint and then directing the questions.

PHYSICAL EXAMINATION

Examination of the infant and young child begins with observing him or her and establishing rapport. The order of examination should fit the child and the circumstances. It is wise to make no sudden movements and to complete first those parts of the examination that require the child's cooperation. Painful or disagreeable procedures should be deferred to the end of the examination, and these should be explained to the child before proceeding. For the older child and adolescent, examination can begin with the head and conclude with the extremities. The approach is gentle but expeditious and complete. For the young, apprehensive child, chatter, reassurance, or other communications frequently permit an orderly examination. Some children are best held by the parent during the examination. For others, part of the examination may require restraint by the parent or assistant.

When the complaint includes a report of pain in a certain area, this area should be examined last. If the child has obvious deformities, that area should be examined in a routine fashion without undue emphasis, because extra attention may increase embarrassment or guilt.

Because the entire child is to be examined, at some time all of the clothing must be removed. This does not necessarily mean that it must be removed at the same time. Only the part that is being examined needs to be uncovered and then it can be reclothed. Except during infancy, modesty should be respected, and the child should be kept as comfortable as possible.

With practice, the examination can be completed quickly even in most critical emergency states. Only those with apnea, shock, absence of pulse, or, occasionally, seizures delay complete examination. Although the method of procedure may vary, the record of examination should be in the same format for all children. This provides easy access to information later. The description that follows is the usual way of recording the examination and not necessarily its required order. When diseases are given with a sign, these are meant as examples and not a complete differential for that sign. The significance of the record of a previous examination cannot be overstressed. A murmur that was not heard a year ago but now is easily audible has far different significance than does a similar murmur heard many years before.

Completion of the history can be accomplished during the physical examination. Talking to the parent frequently reassures the child. Praising the young child, explaining the parts of the examination to the older child, and reassuring the adolescent of normal findings facilitates the examination. Usually, if the examiner enjoys the spontaneity and responsiveness of children, the examination will be easier and more thorough.

All doctors have a series of tricks for examination that they have developed with experience. You may gain the cooperation of older children by making flattering remarks about their clothing or by holding conversations on their level and discussing mutual interests. You may reassure and distract preschool children with interesting objects. Frequently, a 2- to 4-year-old child will remain quiet and apparently interested if you start a pointless story, particularly about imaginary animals, and ask the child equally pointless questions about these animals; with infants, you must sometimes resort to physical measures such as sugar feeding to keep them quiet. Even a 2-year-old child may respond to flattery; a 3- to 6-year-old may enjoy being told he looks like a 7- to 10-year-old and, although bribery of any kind is normally deplorable, a judiciously offered lollipop may create an everlasting attachment between patient and physician.

Usually, the examination of infants or preteens is performed while the parent is present. If the child is frightened or clings to the parent, sending the parent out of the room usually serves only to frighten the child more. Failure of a child aged 4 years or more to cooperate reasonably well is evidence of something abnormal in your approach or in the child's past experience or personality. On rare occasions, you may ask the parent to leave the room, but you should do this before performing the examining. Ask adolescents if they desire a parent to be present. If not, a chaperone of the appropriate sex should be present. Before beginning the examination, always wash your hands with warm water. This serves to cleanse and warm the hands so that the patient will not be uncomfortable. The parents also become aware of your consideration and appreciate routine hand washing. If the mother stands at the examining table, she should be close to the child. Organize your approach so that each part of the body is examined only once.

In general, begin the physical examination using no instruments and gradually introduce the various necessary examining equipment. You can frequently make a tentative diagnosis by observing the young child either while the child is in the mother's arms or is walking or standing in the room. This diagnosis can be confirmed after a thorough examination is made. Usually, infants are examined in a crib or on a table. The examining table or bed should be large enough that children will have no fear of falling and high enough that the physician can examine them in comfort.

Physical examinations are performed on children by taking full advantage of opportunities as they present themselves. Physicians concerned with the physical and mental habits of children realize that they must use all their wiles to establish rapport. The order of an adequate examination is therefore determined more by the child than by the physician.

The examination is usually performed with patients in the position most suitable to them. For the most part, infants, severely ill children, or children who understand well may be conveniently examined in the supine position. However, a 6-month-old child may have just learned to sit up and may be anxious to demonstrate this ability. Therefore, the examination should be performed chiefly with the patient in the sitting position. Similarly, some children may prefer being examined while standing or in unusual positions; the physician should respect such preferences if they do not interfere with a complete examination. It is especially important that children with respiratory distress be examined in the position of most comfort that provides the best airway: usually a sitting or sometimes a prone position.

An obstreperous or frightened patient, however, may reject all attempts at examination. Frequently, even this kind of patient can be examined completely while being held in the mother's arms. This is the position of preference, especially for many children aged 1 to 3 years. Other children may have the ears or mouth examined while being held by the mother. If the patient clings to the mother, the back and extremities may be examined in this position and the remainder of the examination can be performed later with the patient supine. Examining the abdomen of a child held in the mother's lap is usually unsatisfactory. If the mother is helping restrain the patient, she should be told to hold the patient's hands rather than arms. If she holds the arms, the patient's hands are free to interfere with you.

Restraining the patient to examine such parts as the ears or mouth may occasionally be necessary. Place the infant's arms under the back so that the infant's weight rests on the palms. You or the mother can restrain the infant's head, and the examination can proceed.

Aware that the sight of many instruments may frighten the child, most pediatricians start the physical examination with observation of the hands and feet and then the chest or abdomen. They then auscultate, percuss, and palpate these areas and proceed with the remainder of the examination. The genitalia, femoral areas, and anus can be examined next in boys and younger girls, but these areas are examined last in older girls. Next, it is usually convenient to examine the head, eyes, face, and neck and then the ears, nose, and throat. In older girls, the labia and introitus are then examined. Determining blood pressure and other measurements and testing mass reflexes concludes the examination in younger children. In older children and teens, one first determines blood pressure and other measurements, and then proceeds with the examination from the head downward systematically, as in adults. While you perform the examination, it often helps if you allow the patient to play with the instruments you are going to use or have just finished using. When cooperation is desired for the difficult procedures, tell patients firmly what they are to do rather than asking them to do something.

Before you contemplate performing a frightening or painful procedure, tell patients what is to be done and what is expected of them. Reserve procedures such as examination of the head (during which instruments are inserted into the ears and mouth) and the rectum for the end of the examination in young children. Rectal examination is done whenever the patient has any symptom referable to the gastrointestinal tract. If children are old enough to understand, tell them that these procedures are "uncomfortable but not painful."

Any discomfort caused a patient should last as short a time as possible. If you feel that at any time in the examination you must hurt the patient, do not tell the patient otherwise during the visit. If the child is acutely ill or hyperirritable, take little time for the amenities and proceed rapidly with the examination.

Occasionally, especially in acutely ill patients, you may have suspicions regarding a particular diagnosis and may wish to confirm or eliminate this diagnosis before proceeding with the examination. For example, if meningitis is suspected in an infant you may palpate the fontanel first, or if acute abdomen or congenital heart disease is suspected, you may examine the abdomen or heart first. You must be cautious in following such a procedure in patients who are not as acutely ill. Too frequently, a relatively unimportant secondary diagnosis may be found, and you may forget to complete the examination that would reveal the primary diagnosis.

You must also be cautious in following this procedure in children with obvious skin blemishes or other gross deformities or in those with suspected psychiatric difficulties or mental deficiency. In such children, examining first those areas in which difficulty is not expected avoids drawing the attention of the child or parent to the obvious difficulty.

Ordinarily, an experienced physician should take no longer than 5–10 minutes to perform a complete physical examination. Speed is necessary to avoid exhausting the patient. At each visit, regardless of the patient's chief complaint or reason for the visit, you should perform a complete systematic examination and record any abnormalities. Few doctors miss diagnoses because of ignorance; errors are caused by omission of simple procedures.

During the initial interview portion of the exam, it is better to keep the patient fully dressed. This provides a more relaxed environment. During each examination, the child should be completely undressed so that the entire body may be examined. If the room is cool or if the patient is modest or frightened, one part of the child's clothing may be removed and replaced and then another. The degree of modesty varies greatly among children, and modesty should be respected in a child regardless of age.

Above all, successful doctors caring for children must obtain genuine pleasure from examining and dealing with them. They should be friendly and unharried and must proceed with the examination with interest, patience, dexterity, and confidence. Children respond well to physicians who demonstrate confidence, and parents are more likely to accept diagnoses and treatment from physicians who are thorough.

2

MEASUREMENTS, VITAL SIGNS

Let us all work with inspiration, creativity, reflection and hope . . .
for a better world in peace.

MEASURE AND RECORD the physical examination, including temperature, pulse rate, respiratory rate, height, weight, and blood pressure. For children aged less than 2 years, measure and record the circumference of the head, chest, and abdomen. Other measurements such as pelvic width, crown–rump distance, waist and hip circumference, arm span, and sitting and standing height are ordinarily not determined unless the physician suspects abnormalities. See Appendix C for normals of each for various ages.

TEMPERATURE

The patient's temperature is best taken either before the physical examination is started or after it is completed. Temperatures are probably of more value to parents than to physicians. If a patient is ill, 1 degree more or less of fever does not mean 1 degree more or less of disease. However, parents like to know how many degrees of fever their child has and are reassured if the child's temperature is normal.

Obtain a satisfactory temperature in a child aged less than 6 years by placing the thermometer in the axilla or groin, placing the arm or the leg along the patient's body, and holding the arm or leg against the thermometer for 3 minutes. Axillary or groin temperatures are about 2 degrees lower than rectal temperatures and 1 degree lower than oral temperatures, though rectal temperatures are the most accurate.

If you wish to determine an infant's temperature rectally, grease the thermometer well and insert it past the bulb. Digital rectal thermometers are the recommended device. Place the infant face down across the parent's lap with the legs dangling along the parent's leg. The parent should hold the infant's buttocks firmly with one hand and the arm of that hand should lie firmly across the infant's back. The thermometer is inserted about 2 cm and should be held by the parent or you as long as it is in place, anchoring the hand holding the thermometer against the patient's buttock. Do not attempt to take a rectal temperature in children who have rectal diseases, diarrhea, or vulvovaginitis. Rectal temperatures are more frequently elevated after exercise than are oral temperatures. Never take rectal temperatures in a child lying supine because the thermometer will be inserted at the wrong angle, increasing the chances of breaking the thermometer or perforating the rectum.

Newborns may have an axillary temperature of 33°–36°C. Only after 1 week is the temperature stabilized at 36°C axillary.

Do not take oral temperatures until children understand what is expected of them, which usually occurs after age 6 years. The newer electronic thermometers are rapid and accurate and can be used in any orifice regardless of a child's age.

Fever is a manifestation of increased metabolism and may be caused by a variety of disorders. In children, a body temperature of 40°–40.5°C corresponds approximately to a temperature of 38.5°–39°C in adults. Children normally may have elevated temperatures after eating or vigorous play, in the afternoon, or when excited.

Fever may also be evident in children who are unable to sweat because of poisoning (especially atropine) or ectodermal dysplasia. Transfusion reactions, intravascular hemolysis or inflammation, exposure to elevated ambient temperature, and sickle cell crisis may be accompanied by fever. Large daily temperature variations are sometimes noted with septicemia, liver or kidney disease, tumors, rheumatoid arthritis, Hodgkin disease, and leukemia. Persistent low-grade temperature elevations to 39°C are common but not limited to children with rheumatic fever and other collagen-vascular disorders.

Temperature elevations above 40°C (axillary), especially if the rate of elevation is rapid, are sometimes accompanied by seizures in young children with no other evidence of convulsive disorders. A temperature elevation of this degree in a child who looks well, is playing, and has no obvious disease may indicate the presence of roseola infantum.

Hypothermia is usually due to chilling but also occurs in shock states. Especially in infants, however, a normal or low body temperature is common despite overwhelming infections.

PULSE

Obtain a pulse rate in young infants by either palpation or auscultation over the heart and in older children by palpation at the wrist or at other sites (see Chapter 9). The significance of the pulse rate, rhythm, and quality is discussed in the section on examination of the heart.

RESPIRATORY RATE

Obtain the respiratory rate by watching, palpating, or auscultating the chest. A more accurate respiratory rate might be obtained if the patient is distracted into thinking the examiner is taking the pulse. In young children, accurate respiratory rates can be obtained only during sleep. The significance of the respiratory rate is discussed in the section on examination of the lungs (Chapter 6). Children with a rapid respiratory rate usually have respiratory distress or severe infection, and children with a slow respiratory rate may have increased intracranial pressure.

HEIGHT

The height or length of the child, together with the weight, is not only a good measure of overall growth but also provides a record of the rate of growth for comparison with children of similar stature and age as recorded in standard charts. One prime characteristic that distinguishes a child from an adult is increasing growth; if you note failure of growth, suspect some difficulty in the development of the child (see Appendix C).

Measure the infant supine. Hold the zero end of the tape at the infant's heel and read the marking at the infant's head to the nearest centimeter. Older children can be measured standing on the scale. Record the approximate height of parents and grandparents. The most common cause of unusual growth is genetic influence. Although height is not strictly inherited, tall parents tend to have taller children than short parents. If knowledge of true parental height is necessary, a direct measure of the parents' height by the pediatrician is recommended, as particularly fathers tend to give an inflated reading.

If broad allowances are made for normal variations and the child still appears abnormal in height, consider the variations in time of growth. Some children grow rapidly at one age and more slowly at another. The average prepubertal growth is 2–2.5 in/year. It is not unusual for growth velocity to slow significantly 6 months prior to onset of the pubertal growth spurt.

Abnormal shortness, as determined by charts with standard deviations, may be caused by any chronic disease affecting absorption or utilization of nutrients (Tables 2.1, 2.2). Dwarfism may also be due to the chondrodystrophies or other diseases involving the spine; in some cases, no cause may be found. Compare sitting height with total height in children suspected of being dwarfs. Sit the child on a hard surface with the back against the wall and measure from the top of the child's head to the surface. Sitting height accounts for approximately 70% of total height at birth and decreases to about 60% at 2 years of age and to about 52% at 10 years of age. If the sitting height is greater than half the standing height, the patient has infantile stature; if the sitting height is approximately half the standing height, the patient has adult-type stature.

Malnutrition

Deprivation	Inflammatory bowel disease, poverty
Food fads	Gastrointestinal malformation
Cystic fibrosis	Vitamin deficiencies
Food allergy	Mineral deficiencies
Celiac disease	Developmental delay
Hemolytic anemias	

TABLE 2.1
Nutritional Deficiencies With Characteristic Physical Signs

Vitamin/Mineral	Signs/Symptoms
Vitamin A	Night blindness, xerophthalmia, Bitot spots, follicular hyperkeratosis
Vitamin C	Scurvy: bone lesions, bleeding
Vitamin E	Hemolytic anemia, peripheral neuropathy
Vitamin K	Ecchymoses, petechiae
Thiamine B_1	Beriberi, heart failure, increased intracranial pressure
Niacin	Pellegra: dermatitis (sun-exposed areas), diarrhea, dementia
Riboflavin B_2	Cheilosis, angular stomatitis
B_6	Anemia, neuropathy, dermatitis
B_{12}	Neuropathy, anemia (associated with short gut syndrome)
Folate	Macrocytic anemia
Iron	Microcytic hypochromic anemia, koilonychia
Calcium phosphorus, vitamin D	Rickets/osteomalacia
Zinc	Rash (acrodermatitis, enteropathies, growth failure, delayed sexual development) (associated with total parenteral nutrition)
Copper	Bone changes, anemia, neutropenia, hypopigmentation
Selenium	Heart failure
Essential fatty acids	Rash, coagulopathy

Growth Retardation

Genetic	Russell-Silver syndrome
Chromosomal	de Lange syndrome
Familial	Prader-Willi syndrome
Chondrodystrophies	Skeletal dysplasias
Growth hormone deficiency	Hypercorticism
Thyroid deficiency	Precocious puberty
Diabetes	Hypoparathyroid

Children with sexual precocity and dwarfs with Morquio disease, mucopolysaccharidosis, or progeria attain adult body proportions early. Infantile stature persists or adult body proportions develop late in children with delayed adolescence, hypothyroidism, and some chondrodystrophies. Small children with normal body proportions for chronologic age may have genetically small stature, pituitary or primordial dwarfism, or gonadal dysgenesis. Children with sexual precocity grow rapidly before puberty and have shortened lower extremities when they are fully mature.

Abnormally large growth is rare and usually follows overfeeding or overeating, perhaps of psychologic origin. It occurs in children with mental deficiency. True gigantism caused by excess growth hormone from an overactive pituitary is rare. Measure arm span in children with unusual growth patterns by stretching their arms parallel to the floor and holding the tape measure from fingertip to fingertip (Table 2.3). The span is more than 2 cm over height in children with Marfan syndrome,

TABLE 2.2
Failure to Thrive in Infancy

Cause	Approximate Percentage of All Cases	History	System-Specific Physical Findings	System-Specific Laboratory Studies
Psychosocial	50% or >	Vague inconsistent feeding history, rumination	None. May have some neurologic signs, attachment disorder	None
Central nervous system	13%	Poor feeding, gross developmental delay, vomiting	Grossly abnormal neurologic examination, micro- or macrocephaly	Frequent gross abnormalities on EEG and CT scan or grossly abnormal neuromuscular function testing
Gastro-intestinal	10%	Chronic vomiting and/or diarrhea, abnormal stools	Often negative, may have abdominal distention	Abnormal barium studies or abnormal stool examination (pH-reducing substances, fat stain, Wright stain)
Cardiac	9%	Slow feeding, dyspnea and diaphoresis with feeding, restlessness, and diaphoresis during sleep	May have cyanosis, or signs of congestive heart failure, clubbing	Abnormal cardiac signs, EKG, catheterization
Genetic	8%	May have positive FH or developmental delay	Often have facies typical of a syndrome, skeletal abnormalities, or neurologic abnormalities, visceromegaly	May have typical radiographic findings, chromosomal abnormalities, abnormal metabolic screens
Pulmonary	3.5%	Chronic or recurrent dyspnea with feeding, tachypnea	Grossly abnormal chest examination, clubbing	Abnormal chest radiograph
Renal	3.5%	May be negative or may have history of polyuria	Often negative, may have flank masses, ↑ BP, PNE	Abnormal urinalysis, frequently elevated BUN and creatinine
Endocrine	3.5%	With hypothyroidism, constipation and decreased activity level; with diabetes, polyuria, polydipsia, history of weight loss	With hypothyroidism, no wasting but mottling, umbilical hernia, often open posterior fontanelle. With diabetes, may have signs of dehydration, ketotic breath, and hyperpnea. With hypopituitarism and isolated GH deficiency, growth normal until 9 months or later, then a plateau but normal weight for height; delayed tooth eruption	Decreased T4, increased TSH; glucosuria and hyperglycemia; abnormal pituitary function studies

Modified from Zitelli, B. J., & Davis, H. W. (2002). *Atlas of pediatric physical diagnosis* (4th ed.). St. Louis: Mosby.

TABLE 2.3
Normal Arm Span Minus Height (cm)

Age	Girls	Boys
Birth	−2.5	−2.5
10 yr	−1	0
12 yr	0	+2
15 yr	+1.2	+4.3

Klinefelter syndrome, homocystinuria, and congenital contractual arachnodactyly and is more than 2 cm less than height in children with bone or cartilage disorders or hypothyroidism.

WEIGHT

Weigh the child once a month for the first 6 months of life, once every 3 months for the next 6 months, twice a year for the next 3 years, and yearly thereafter. If you cannot weigh a child because the child is holding the scale, say, "Hold your pants." The considerations of growth and development applied to height also apply to weight. Weight will often indicate that a problem exists before height alteration. Compare child weight with standard height–weight charts with allowances for normal variations. A single measurement tells little as compared with information obtained from serial measurements.

Acute weight loss indicates acute illness, dehydration, or malnutrition. Chronic weight loss suggests chronic disease states: These include improper food or feeding, diarrhea, cystic fibrosis or other gastrointestinal disturbances, emotional difficulties, respiratory difficulty during feeding, mental deficiency, and renal, cardiac, or connective tissue diseases.

Rapid weight gain may indicate overhydration or edema, but usually indicates overfeeding or overeating. A general overweight state (true obesity) is usually due to overfeeding or overeating, generally with a discernible psychologic background, but may be due to decreased activity, mental deficiency, or intracranial disorders. Rarely, endocrine disorders such as hyperadrenalism and hypothyroidism may be associated with obesity. In contrast to the obesity of overeating, these disorders are associated with retardation of linear growth. One estimation of body bulk, body mass index (BMI), is calculated as weight (kg) divided by height (m^2).

HEAD AND CHEST CIRCUMFERENCES

In infants aged less than 2 years, determine head and chest circumferences. Measure the head at its greatest circumference and the chest at the nipple line.

At birth, the average head circumference of an infant is 34–37 cm; that of the chest is about 2 cm less. Head circumference usually approximates circumference of the chest until the child is aged 2 years, after which the chest continues to grow rapidly while head circumference increases only slightly. The significance of head and chest measurements is discussed in Chapters 5 and 6.

Body asymmetry may be noted. Such asymmetry is usually idiopathic but may be due to hemihypertrophy related to Wilms tumor or other malignancies. Hemihypertrophy may result from vascular anomalies, with increased perfusion and increased growth of the limb; it may be due to hemiatrophy and associated with cerebral cortical injuries.

BLOOD PRESSURE

Measure blood pressure either when beginning the examination or after the examination is complete. The patient should be relaxed and not crying. The proper cuff size is no less than half and no more than two thirds the length of the upper arm. Similar relative sizes are used for the thigh if leg pressures are taken. A larger cuff is difficult to apply and may give readings that are too low. A smaller cuff gives readings that are too high. Choose a rubber bag inside the cuff long enough to encircle the arm completely. For very obese patients, apply the cuff to the forearm and auscultate at the wrist.

Compare the cuff to a balloon before applying it. An automated device uses a cuff, with ultrasonic energy beamed from a transducer to a blood vessel or a recorder for systolic and diastolic pressures corresponding approximately to the first and fifth Korotkoff sounds. When using the manual device, allow the child to pump the cuff before it is wrapped. After wrapping the cuff snugly, place the manometer so that you and the child can see the silver streak of the mercury or the clock of the spring manometer. Place the bell stethoscope over the brachial artery.

Inflate the cuff higher than the expected systolic pressure and slowly deflate it. During inflation, raise the arm above the heart. The wall of the collapsed vessel suddenly distends, producing the first Korotkoff sound—the systolic pressure. Further lowering is followed by a swishing sound, then a muffling—the fourth Korotkoff sound. Sound disappears at the fifth Korotkoff sound. Record systolic and diastolic pressures at the appearance and disappearance of Korotkoff sounds, recognizing that fifth phase recordings tend to underestimate diastolic pressure. Determining the fourth phase—muffling of the heart sounds—is less consistent. Measure patients' blood pressure annually, from the time the child is about 3 years of age.

If you cannot hear the Korotkoff sounds, you can make a rough estimate by applying the cuff in the usual manner, slowly deflating it, and palpating the radial, popliteal, or dorsalis pedis arteries. The first pulsation felt is about 10 mm below the true systolic pressure. If you cannot feel these arteries, the hand, wrist, and forearm (or toes, ankle, and leg) can be elevated and tightly wrapped to exclude blood up to the place where the cuff is applied. Then inflate the cuff to a level above the suspected blood pressure. Remove the wrappings. Slowly reduce the pressure in the cuff; the first flushing noted in the hand or foot is close to the systolic pressure.

If you fail in the first attempt at obtaining the blood pressure, remove the cuff before making another attempt, since even a deflated cuff may hurt or frighten the child. If you obtain an elevated blood pressure, repeat the measurement and measure the blood pressure in the other three extremities. In any patient suspected of having heart disease, measure the blood pressure in the four extremities.

Blood pressure at birth is about 60–90 mm Hg systolic and 20–60 mm Hg diastolic. Both pressures usually increase 2–3 mm per year of age; adult levels are reached near or soon after puberty (Figure 2.1). Crying or apprehension may double these levels. Pulse pressure is normally 20–50 mm Hg throughout childhood. Systolic pressure in the arms may equal that in the legs in children until they are about 1 year of age. Thereafter the pressure in the legs is about 10–30 mm Hg higher than that in the arms. The diastolic pressure is almost equal in the arms

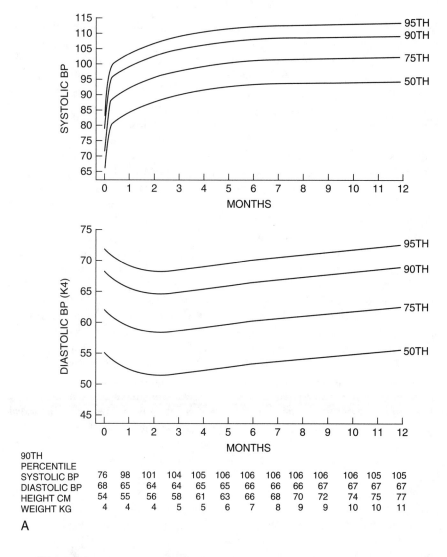

90TH PERCENTILE												
SYSTOLIC BP	76	98	101	104	105	106	106	106	106	106	106	105	105
DIASTOLIC BP	68	65	64	64	65	65	66	66	66	67	67	67	67
HEIGHT CM	54	55	56	58	61	63	66	68	70	72	74	75	77
WEIGHT KG	4	4	4	5	5	6	7	8	9	9	10	10	11

A

Figure 2.1
Age-specific percentiles of blood pressure (BP) measurements in girls from birth to 12 months of age; Korotkoff phase IV (K4) used for diastolic BP (A).
Continued

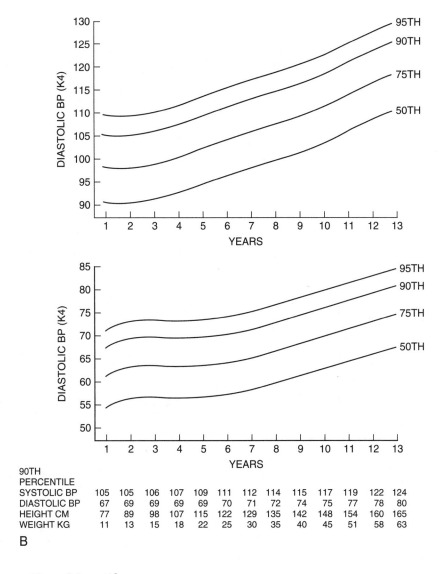

90TH PERCENTILE													
SYSTOLIC BP	105	105	106	107	109	111	112	114	115	117	119	122	124
DIASTOLIC BP	67	69	69	69	69	70	71	72	74	75	77	78	80
HEIGHT CM	77	89	98	107	115	122	129	135	142	148	154	160	165
WEIGHT KG	11	13	15	18	22	25	30	35	40	45	51	58	63

B

Figure 2.1, cont'd
(B), girls aged 1–13 years; Korotkoff phase IV (K4) used for diastolic BP.

Continued

and legs. If it is not, the cuff size is proper for the arms but too small for the legs. Very large differences in arm and leg systolic pressures (Hill's sign) suggest aortic insufficiency or coarctation of the aorta.

Elevated blood pressure values (both systolic and diastolic) may be noted. Blood pressure is usually elevated in one or both upper extremities of children with coarctation of the aorta or thoracic aortitis.

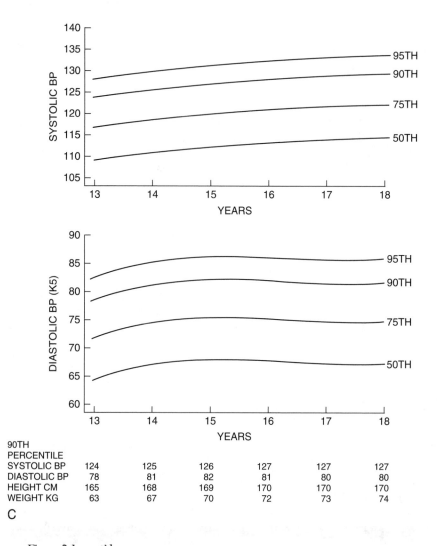

90TH PERCENTILE						
SYSTOLIC BP	124	125	126	127	127	127
DIASTOLIC BP	78	81	82	81	80	80
HEIGHT CM	165	168	169	170	170	170
WEIGHT KG	63	67	70	72	73	74

C

Figure 2.1, cont'd
(C), girls aged 13–18 years; Korotkoff phase V (K5) used for diastolic BP.

Continued

Hypertension

Causes of Hypertension

Kidney disease   Neuroblastoma
Pyelonephritis   Familial dysautonomia
Acute glomerulonephritis   Increased intracranial pressure
Chronic glomerulonephritis   Cushing disease
Renal artery stenosis   Pheochromocytoma
Nephrotic syndrome   Neurofibromatosis

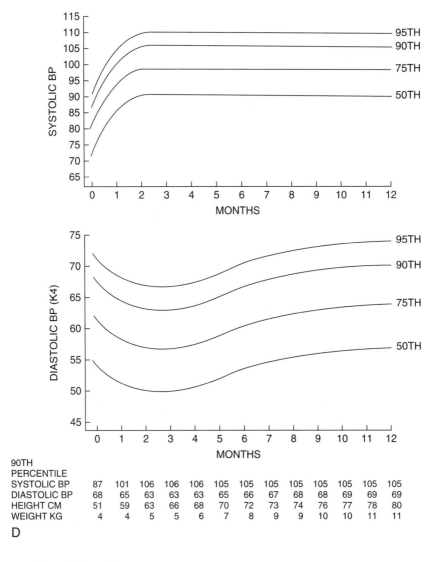

90TH PERCENTILE												
SYSTOLIC BP	87	101	106	106	106	105	105	105	105	105	105	105	105
DIASTOLIC BP	68	65	63	63	63	65	66	67	68	68	69	69	69
HEIGHT CM	51	59	63	66	68	70	72	73	74	76	77	78	80
WEIGHT KG	4	4	5	5	6	7	8	9	9	10	10	11	11

D

Figure 2.1, cont'd
(D), boys aged 1–13 years; K4 used for diastolic BP.

Continued

Renal tumors   Hyperthyroid
Renal calculi   Hypothyroid
Poisons   Vitamin A or D poisoning
Bulbar poliomyelitis   Spinal cord lesions

Children with scalenus anticus syndrome with cervical rib or with a coarctation of the aorta proximal to the left subclavian artery have unequal blood pressures in the arms. Some children with patent ductus arteriosus have unequal arm blood pressures.

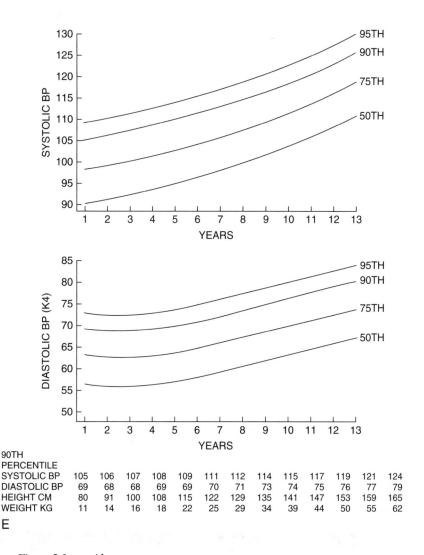

90TH PERCENTILE												
SYSTOLIC BP	105	106	107	108	109	111	112	114	115	117	119	121	124
DIASTOLIC BP	69	68	68	69	69	70	71	73	74	75	76	77	79
HEIGHT CM	80	91	100	108	115	122	129	135	141	147	153	159	165
WEIGHT KG	11	14	16	18	22	25	29	34	39	44	50	55	62

E

Figure 2.1, cont'd
(E), boys aged 1–13 years; K4 used for diastolic BP.

Continued

Variable systolic pressures are pulsus paradoxus. Inflate and lower the pressure cuff several times. Irregular or fading beats occur with inspiration. The difference between the first faint sounds and repetitive crisp regular beats (the normal systolic difference with inspiration) is about 10 mm (see Chapter 9). In certain disease states such as status asthma, this might be >10 mm Hg.

Elevated systolic pressure alone or with broadening of the pulse pressure is evident after exercise or excitement or in febrile states. It is associated with reduced

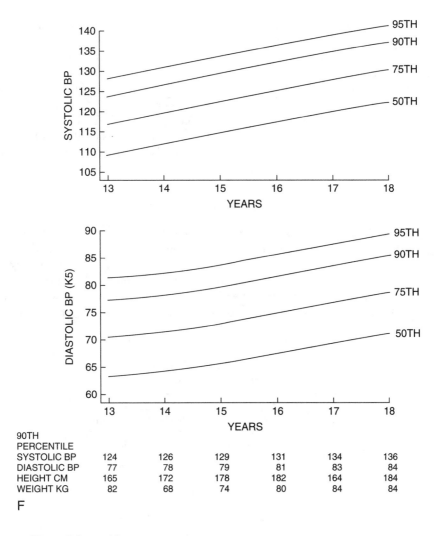

90TH PERCENTILE						
SYSTOLIC BP	124	126	129	131	134	136
DIASTOLIC BP	77	78	79	81	83	84
HEIGHT CM	165	172	178	182	164	184
WEIGHT KG	82	68	74	80	84	84

F

Figure 2.1, cont'd
(F), boys aged 13–18 years; K5 used for diastolic BP. (Courtesy of American Academy of Pediatrics.)

diastolic pressure in children with patent ductus arteriosus, arteriovenous fistula, or aortic regurgitation.

Children with aortic or subaortic stenosis or with hypothyroidism have normal or elevated diastolic pressure with a low systolic pressure, and therefore a narrow pulse pressure. Children with aortic insufficiency or hyperthyroidism have widened or elevated pulse pressure.

Children with cardiac failure and children in a state of shock from causes such as heat exhaustion, circulatory collapse, blood loss, and adrenal insufficiency have low blood pressure. Newborns with trauma in the adrenal areas, children with meningococcemia and occasionally other septicemias, and children with chronic disease states or malnutrition have low blood pressure due to adrenal insufficiency. In children with Takayasu disease, arm blood pressure is low.

Orthostatic hypotension (a decrease in blood pressure of 15 mm Hg and/or an increase in pulse rate of 15 beats/min) occurs with a 20% loss of blood volume or some reflex vasodilation or lack of vasoconstriction when an upright posture is assumed.

SKINFOLD MEASUREMENT

Place your thumb and forefinger of one hand just far enough apart so that you can pinch a full fold of the patient's skin and subcutaneous tissue firmly from the underlying tissue. Do not pick up muscle. Apply skinfold calipers just beneath your fingers. Calipers should apply a constant pressure of about 10 g/mm². Make measurements at the back of the upper arms over the triceps midway between the elbow and tip of the acromial process. Measure mid-upper arm circumference with a flexible tape.

TABLE 2.4

Approximate Limits for Mid-Upper Arm Circumference and
Triceps Skin Fold

Age	Mid-Upper Arm 3rd to 5th Percentile (cm)[a] Boys	Triceps Skin Fold 90th to 97th Percentile (mm)[b]	
		Boys	Girls
Newborn	9	10	10
3 mo	10	11	11
6 mo	11.5	12	12
9 mo	12	13	13
12 mo	13	14	14
2 yr	13	13	13
3 yr	13	13	13
4 yr	13.5	13	13
5 yr	13.5	13	13
6 yr	14	12	15
7 yr	14	13	16
8 yr	14.5	14	17
9 yr	15	14	18
10 yr	16	16	20
11 yr	16.5	17	21
12–16 yr	17–20	18–20	22–25

Modified from Zerfas, A. J., & Neumann, C. G. (1977). Office assessment of nutritional status. *Pediatric Clinics of North America, 24,* 253.
[a]A lower value suggests undernutrition.
[b]A higher value suggests obesity.

Measurements of skinfold help in identifying obesity; those of circumference help in identifying and following malnutrition as an indication of body composition. Representative values are shown in Table 2.4. In adolescents, the desirable sum of skinfold measurements of triceps and calf is 10–30 mm.

FURTHER READING

Gilbert-Barness, E. (Ed.). (2007). *Pathology of fetus, infant and child* (2nd ed., Vols. 1 and 2). New York: Elsevier.

Robertson, J., & Shilkofski, N. (Eds.). (2005). *The Harriet Lane handbook* (17th ed.). St. Louis: Elsevier Mosby.

3

GENERAL APPEARANCE, SKIN, AND LYMPH NODES

The future of a civilization may be judged by how it cares for its young.

Senator Daniel Patrick Moynihan

THE GENERAL APPEARANCE of a child may reveal much more than subtle physical findings. On first seeing the child, sit down and slowly observe the child. Does the child look well or ill? Does the child appear comfortable or uncomfortable, and if uncomfortable, in what way? Is the breathing easy or difficult? Is the child in any type of physical or emotional distress? Is the child's appearance alert or lethargic? Is the child clean or dirty? Is the child's attitude cooperative or belligerent? Does the child have any gross abnormalities or anomalies? Is the child fat or thin or tall or short? Does the child appear to be malnourished? Is the child apprehensive and, if so, is the apprehension due to new surroundings, to the parents, to the examiner, or to the disease? Is the child interested in the new instruments presented by the physician? Does the child obey the parent and the physician or fight them? If the child obeys, is the obedience due to fear? Is the child excited or calm? Does the child twitch and fidget? In essence, is the child similar to peers or different from them, and if different, in what way?

When you record the child's general features, describe the facies (facial expression and appearance) and use terms such as chronically ill, alert, comatose, lethargic, dull, responsive, hostile, and cooperative. These descriptive terms should start you on the road to proper diagnosis. Dirt, feces, or other signs of neglect alert you to possible child abuse. Also note the interaction between the patient and the parents throughout the examination. Pediatricians are fortunate because their patients, unlike adults, rarely dissimulate. Regardless of what the mother says about the patient, experienced pediatricians know that a child who does not look ill is usually not acutely ill and that a child who looks ill is usually acutely or chronically ill.

During the course of each examination, the child should be completely undressed. With infants, it is easiest to have the parent completely undress the child before the examination. In older children, respect shyness and any reticence and examine them by removing and replacing articles of their clothing as each portion of the examination is completed.

If a patient is acutely ill, try to determine the system involved and the degree of distress. For example, flaring nostrils indicate a problem in the respiratory or cardiac system, and delirium, coma, or convulsions indicate a problem in the central nervous system (CNS). Note the nature of the child's cry. A strong, loud cry may indicate that the child is in pain, is frightened, or simply wishes to cry. Even a strong cry is helpful in diagnosis because it usually indicates that the child is not weak or debilitated. In contrast, a weak cry may indicate that the child is weak, debilitated, or gravely ill. A screeching, high-pitched cry may indicate that the child has increased intracranial pressure or other CNS lesions. In infants, a hoarse, low-pitched cry may be normal or may indicate laryngeal abnormalities, tetany, or cretinism.

Normal newborns may be asleep or crying, but older children are responsive during examinations. A child who smiles, chats, and laughs is usually well or only moderately ill. A child who cries constantly may be more seriously ill.

A child who lies quietly with few movements and stares into space may be gravely ill or may have been abused. A child with paradoxical hyperirritability may lie quietly on the examining table only to scream when picked up by the parent. This is a valuable sign, since most children are calmed when picked up, and may indicate a serious disturbance in the CNS system (particularly meningitis), pain in motion (which occurs in scurvy, fracture, cortical hyperostosis, and acrodynia), or a serious disturbance in response to painful stimuli.

A child with acute illness may have parched skin and tongue, sunken dry eyes, a weak cry, and exhausted and lethargic behavior, as may children with dehydration or acute or chronic malnutrition. In patients with febrile states, the eyes may appear bright and apprehensive.

A child in pain may cry, wince, double up, rub the painful part, or display general fretfulness and other signs of discomfort. Older children can indicate the site and sometimes the cause of the pain. Painful facies may be modified in a few disease states. For example, a child with peritonitis lies ominously still, the nares flare, and respiration is entirely thoracic and very shallow. With intussusception, the child lies very still one moment and claws, twists, and screams the next moment. Watch the face of the child for apprehension as you examine other parts of the body. Palpating over a tender abdomen may elicit a grimace in a stoic child even as the child says, "It doesn't hurt." A grimace or a change in the child's cry as you palpate over the bladder or in the costovertebral angle may be a true sign of renal disease.

A dyspneic child demonstrates very rapid respiration, flaring of the nares, and possibly some cyanosis about the lips. The child may be irritable and hyperactive, possibly apprehensive, and may appear to be fighting for air. In a child with carbon dioxide retention, confusion, stupor, and finally shock may be added to these signs.

The facies of a child with nasal obstruction is characterized by mouth breathing, an open mouth, narrow pinched nose, high palate, dull appearance, and nasal voice; the sternum may be sunken. Children with hypertrophied adenoids or chronic sinusitis may exhibit this type of facies, with swelling over the cheeks.

The facies of a developmentally delayed child is sometimes diagnostic. The eyes are dull, the face is blank, and the child is unresponsive. Developmental delay in children may be due to hereditary factors, maternal infections (especially in the first trimester of pregnancy), congenital anomalies of the brain, or degenerative neurologic disorders. It is commonly due to cerebral injury, sequelae of infections, or hypoxic ischemic encephalopathy and is frequently accompanied by other signs of cerebral palsy. However, delay must not be assumed in all children who have a dull expression. Children who are deaf or blind or who have specific language difficulties and children with prolonged illness or psychologic difficulties may have a similar facies, one easily mistaken for mental deficiency.

Note the position the child assumes during the examination. Abnormal, resistant, or persistent positioning may be caused by muscular, neurologic, or emotional disorders. For example, a child with torticollis or cerebellar disease may lean the head toward the affected side; a child with appendicitis or other painful intraabdominal conditions may lie on the affected side with the leg of that side flexed at the hip and knee; and a child with unilateral labyrinthitis may insist on lying only on the affected side.

Likewise, voluntary or involuntary movement or lack of movement may direct attention to a particular system. For example, a brain-injured child with spastic paresis may keep the arm flexed at the elbow, and the wrist and fingers may be held stiffly in flexion. With extensive cerebral involvement, the child may be entirely in extensor spasticity; with cerebellar involvement, the child may be ataxic; and with basal ganglia involvement, the child may be athetoid and grimacing. Stereotaxic movements may suggest neurologic disorders.

Estimate the state of nutrition. Acute malnutrition manifests as loss of weight and skin turgor. Chronic malnutrition may be evident. Overnutrition is recognized as obesity and unusual weight gain. (Causes of weight loss and gain are discussed in Chapter 2.) Signs of chronic malnutrition:

Low weight	Bony prominences
Protuberant abdomen	Flat buttocks
Muscle wasting	Poor muscle tone
Slow response to stimuli	Prominent sucking pads in cheeks

Note development. Assess the patient's response to you and the surroundings, noting speech, action, and crying, and make a rapid estimate of mental development. Gross deviations from normal are apparent at a glance if the child appears dull or does not respond. Estimate gross physical development for the age and confirm by direct measurement.

Speech is one of the developmental signs least dependent on motor ability and should be noted in very young children. A 3-month-old infant may coo and a 7-month-old infant may say "ma-ma" and "da-da." A few more words are added at 1 year of age, and short sentences are added at 2 years of age. A 3-year-old child, even if not frightened, may stutter or stammer (see Appendix C). A child's failure to develop speech may be due to motor incoordination of the speech muscles but is commonly due to a lack of desire to speak because of adequate communication by other means. Such children respond to simple commands readily. Other causes of failure to speak include lack of stimulus by parents or environment, deafness, mental retardation, histidinemia, or psychologic disturbances. Severe dysarthria is a sign of spastic quadriplegia.

You can keep a convenient record of your patients' development by using the Denver Developmental Screening Test (Appendix B). Markedly advanced motor signs such as early rolling over, early head control with poor feeding, and decreased spontaneous muscle movements suggest spastic cerebral palsy.

ODOR

Some infants and children will have distinct body odors. A few of these odors are associated with diseases (Table 3.1).

SKIN

Although observation of the skin is essential to dermatologic diagnosis, do not neglect palpation of skin lesions. Examine the skin as a whole or examine each underlying part. Regardless of the method you adopt, note the condition of the skin

TABLE 3.1
Odors of Patient or Urine

Odors	Disease
Musty or mousy	Phenylketonuria, diphtheria
Maple syrup	Maple syrup urine disease
Sweaty sock	Isovaleric or glutaric II acidemia
Brewery, fishy	Methionine metabolism, oasthouse
Garlic	Arsenic, thallium, parathion, or phosphorus poisoning, tellurium, selenium, DMSO
Bitter almond	Cyanide poisoning
"Tomcat" urine	3-methylcrotonyl-CoA-carboxylase (biotin) deficiency
Onion	Selenium poisoning
Acetone	Isopropyl alcohol, methanol poisoning, acidosis
Wintergreen	Methyl salicylate poisoning
Violets	Turpentine poisoning
Pear	Chloral hydrate poisoning
Shoe polish	Nitrobenzene poisoning
Coal gas	Carbon monoxide poisoning
Cabbage	Tyrosinosis
Stench	Foreign body in nose, vagina, ear
Fish (spoiled)	Trimethylaminuria
Fish	Kidney failure
Fresh brown bread	Typhoid
Urine	Uremia

DMSO, dimethyl sulfoxide.

of the entire body each time you examine the patient. If skin lesions are found, note their distribution, color, and character.

Normal pigmentation is caused by melanin in the skin; depigmented areas are termed *vitiligo*. Small depigmented patches may be caused by tinea versicolor, pityriasis alba or rosea, or dermatophytosis. When they are accompanied by structural or developmental defects, chromosome abnormalities may be present. Unpigmented streaks covering large areas of the body may represent hypomelanosis of Ito, frequently associated with CNS abnormalities. In children, vitiligo in small leaf-shaped patches that may fluoresce may be the first sign of tuberous sclerosis or other neuroectodermal disease. Generalized lack of pigmentation occurs in albinism, an inborn error of tyrosine metabolism, and in the Chédiak-Steinbrinck-Higashi syndrome.

Localized areas of increased pigmentation (nevi) are common. Note the size and color and presence of hair. Various shades of red nevi are usually of vascular origin (hemangiomas). Small vascular nevi with small radiating vessels caused by capillary dilation may be easily compressed. Because of their appearance, they are termed *spider nevi* or *spider angiomas*. A few may be present on the arms or hands or high on the face of normal children. In patients with cirrhosis or hepatitis, such nevi are larger and more common on the trunk.

Port-wine stains are pink to purple with irregular borders. Where they involve the trigeminal nerve, they may cause eye and brain abnormalities (Sturge-Weber syndrome). When associated with the venous system, they cause hypertrophy of the limb (Klippel-Trenaunay-Weber syndrome). Multiple hemangiomas may cause skeletal abnormalities (Maffuci syndrome or Gorham disease); others cause intestinal bleeding (blue rubber-bleb syndrome). Any hemangioma can be associated with petechiae or bleeding because of trapping of platelets (Kasabach-Merritt syndrome).

Yellow, brown, or black nevi are usually local melanin deposits. Nevi over the lower spine may overlie spina bifida occulta or tethering of the cord. Large coarse nevi may represent the epidermal nevus syndrome, which is associated with congenital anomalies. Linear or circular sebaceous or waxy nevi and giant pigmented nevi over the buttocks may become malignant.

Multiple small pigmented spots are termed *freckles*. Multiple freckles in the axillary region are common in patients with neurofibromatosis. Multiple freckles are apparent in children with either the multiple lentigenes or Bannayan-Riley-Ruvacalba syndrome.

Pigmented Lesions

Differential Diagnosis

- Mongolian spots (dermal melanosis)
  - Present at birth; incidence 90% in black children, 80% in Asian, 65% in Latin American, 5% in white; disappears in childhood, may persist on distal extremities
  - Poorly defined, several centimeters in diameter, blue/gray macules, mostly on buttocks, back, arms, and legs; not on palms, soles, face, mucosal surfaces
- Postinflammatory hyperpigmentation
  - Follows skin inflammation, resolves within months, more common on dark skin

- Acquired melanocytic nevi (AMN, moles)
  - Benign in early childhood, darken and increase in size, can become raised during puberty, by late adolescence most people have 20–30; regress and disappear with age
  - Pink/brown/black macules or papules, <5 mm diameter, 90% flat (junctional), 10% raised, may have hair, sun-exposed skin, not on palms, soles, genitals, mucosal surfaces
- Dysplastic nevi (atypical moles)
  - Sporadic or familial (autosomal dominant, usually develops in puberty, risk of malignant change (MM) is 5%–10%
  - Pink/brown/black macules or papules, >5 mm diameter, irregular border, on sun-exposed skin
- Congenital melanocytic nevi (CMN)
  - 1%–2% of newborns
  - small CMN: malignancy risk uncertain
  - giant CMN: 2%–15% lifetime malignancy risk, <1/20,000 births; 3% of MM arise in giant CMNs
- Malignant melanoma may arise in acquired, dysplastic, or congenital nevi, on normal skin or extracutaneous
- Freckles
  - Light brown, jagged borders, darken in sun
- Lentigines
  - Dark brown, any part of skin/mucosa may be seen with syndromes (Peutz-Jeghers)
- Tinea versicolor (fungus *Malassezia furfur*)
  - Guttate pattern, can be hypopigmented
- Urticaria pigmentosa: most common form of mastocytosis; juvenile onset 7% risk of malignancy and adult onset 30% risk
  - Darier sign (pruritus/erythema upon stroking)
- Incontinentia pigmenti: streaks/whorls
- Café au lait macules: incidence 10% of children, >5 lesions of >1.5 cm diameter after puberty indicates neurofibromatosis, also in McCune-Albright, tuberous sclerosis, Bloom syndrome
- Other nevi: Ito/Ota, Blue, Spitz, Becker, halo, zosteriform, lentiginosum nevus spilus

Increased dark pigmentation, especially over the exposed areas, is most frequently due to sun or windburn.

Increased Pigment

- Mongolian spots
- Lentigenes
- Freckles
- Melanocytic lesions
- Tinea versicolor (fungus, *Malassezia* fungus)
- Addison disease
- Hemosiderosis

- Hypothyroidism
- Café au lait macules (von Recklinghausen, Albright syndrome)
- Incontinentia pigmenti
- Argyria
- Pellagra
- Lupus erythematosus

A pellagralike symmetric browning of the dorsal aspects of the hands on exposure to sunlight may be associated with cerebellar ataxia in Hartnup syndrome, a metabolic defect. Photosensitivity results from use of some drugs and is also characteristic of errors in porphyrin metabolism.

Children with polyostotic fibrous dysplasia have light brown asymmetric pigmented areas. Darker patches (café au lait spots) are evident in patients with neurofibromatosis and are a diagnostic sign of the disorder in children aged less than 5 years, especially if more than five are apparent and are more than 1 cm long. Fibromas along the course of a nerve are another sign of neurofibromatosis.

Large, flat, black or blue-black areas are frequently noted over the sacrum and buttocks. They are termed *mongolian spots* and have no pathologic significance and are more common in African American children. Bluish-black, soft, verrucous symmetric areas of the axillae, neck, and knuckles are characteristic of acanthosis nigricans and are sometimes associated with malignancies, genetic abnormalities, drug use, and endocrine diseases.

Cyanosis and Jaundice

Look for cyanosis and jaundice. Cyanosis is a bluish discoloration of a normally pink area and is most easily detected in the nail beds or in the mucous membranes of the mouth. It occurs when a minimum of 5 g/dL reduced hemoglobin is present, regardless of the total level of hemoglobin. Therefore, cyanosis develops less easily in an anemic child, more easily in a child with polycythemia, and not at all in a child with anemia with a hemoglobin content less than 5 g/dL. Visible cyanosis is not a good estimate of the degree of oxygen unsaturation except when the total amount of hemoglobin is 12–15 g/dL or more.

Central cyanosis is always a cause for concern because of its association with pulmonary, cardiovascular, CNS, and hematologic disorders.

Causes for Central Cyanosis

- Pulmonary disease
  Atelectasis
  Pneumonia
  Cystic fibrosis
  Lung anomalies

- Cyanotic congenital heart disease
  Transposition
  Tetralogy of Fallot
  Tricuspid atresia

Anomalous venous return
Truncus
Pulmonary atresia
Congestive heart failure

To recognize central cyanosis, do not look at the patient's nail beds or around the mouth. Look at the tongue. With peripheral cyanosis, the tongue is pink; with central cyanosis, the tongue is blue. Peripheral cyanosis is caused by excessive removal of oxygen from blood at the tissue level and is usually caused by slowing of blood through the capillary bed due to hypothermia, local venous obstruction, vasomotor instability, and occasionally to shock with sepsis or congestive heart failure.

Other causes of cyanosis include obstruction of the respiratory tract, prolonged crying, temper tantrums with breath holding, convulsive states, acrocyanosis, and shock. Cyanosis may occur with as little as 1–2 g/dL abnormal hemoglobin as a result of poisoning, as in methemoglobinemia and sulfhemoglobinemia.

Compare the patient's upper and lower extremities with respect to cyanosis. The lower extremities may be more cyanotic than the upper extremities in patients with coarctation of the aorta or in patients with pulmonary hypertension with patent ductus arteriosus. The lower extremities may be less cyanotic than the upper extremities in children with transposition of the great vessels with patent ductus. Acrocyanosis not caused by heart or lung disease occurs with vasospasm (Raynaud phenomenon); children with Kawasaki disease have a blue discoloration of the feet of unknown cause.

Veins are normally apparent through the thin skin of many children. Distended veins in the arms and legs are usually due to dependent position. Dilated veins elsewhere may be due to cardiac decompensation or local venous obstruction and are also evident in children with cyanosis. Collateral arterial circulation is rare in children.

Determine direction of blood flow if fistula, collateral circulation, or obstruction is suspected. First, empty the vessel by placing two fingers together and then pushing one finger along the course of the vessel for 1–2 inches. If the vessel fills before pressure is released, collateral circulation is present. Then release pressure of one finger. If the vessel fills after release of pressure, blood flows from the area of pressure release toward the area where pressure is still being applied. If the vessel does not fill, replace the first finger, release the second, and similarly observe the direction of blood flow. If the vessel still does not fill, poor circulation in the area is suggested.

The area over a vein may be tender with infection in the vein (thrombophlebitis). When thrombophlebitis becomes extensive and causes obstruction to blood flow, the veins may become tortuous, dilated, and easily palpable. Phlebitis of the deep veins of the legs can be elicited by forcibly flexing the foot and noting pain in the calf (Homan sign). In children, phlebitis usually results from infection spreading from an area near the vein or from embolism or thrombosis.

Causes for Jaundice

Hepatitis
Poisons
Leptospirosis

Infectious mononucleosis
Hemolysis
Biliary obstruction
Choledochal cyst
Hemorrhage

Jaundice can be manifest as various shades of yellow or green and is best observed by examining the patient's sclera, skin, or mucous membranes in daylight; it may be missed entirely in artificial light. It occurs in newborns when the total serum bilirubin is more than 5 mg/dL and is evident in older children when total bilirubin is more than 2 mg/dL. It is caused by cellular or obstructive liver disease or hemolysis.

In infections, especially pneumonia and congenital syphilis, jaundice may also appear anywhere in the body. Jaundice occurs in cholestasis and in prolonged parenteral alimentation. It is rarely caused by bile duct stones in childhood, although such stones sometimes occur after episodes of hemolysis. Pruritis is common in jaundice.

A pale, yellow-orange tint of the skin may be due to carotenemia and is most prominent over the palms, soles, and nasolabial folds. Carotenemia is due to excess carotene ingestion but may be an early sign of hypothyroidism. It occasionally occurs in diabetic children. Children with severe hemolytic anemias have a peculiar yellowness of the skin unrelated to jaundiced individuals.

Note pallor or paleness. In darkly pigmented children, it is most easily detected in the nail beds, conjunctivas, oral mucosa, or tongue, which are normally reddish-pink. Pallor should never be considered an accurate estimate of hemoglobin concentration. It is usually a normal complexion characteristic or sign of indoor living, but it may indicate anemia, chronic disease, edema, or shock. Plethora, due to polycythemia, is usually not easily detected in children.

Classification of Pediatric Skin Lesions

Skin Lesion	Examples
Macules	Freckles, junctional nevi, tinea versicolor
Patches	Café au lait spots, port-wine stains, vitiligo
Maculopapular rashes	Viral exanthems, drug eruptions
Papules	Warts, molluscum contagiosum, insect bites, compound nevi
Papules with burrows	Scabies
Papules with comedones	Acne
Plaques (nonscaly)	Mastocytomas, sebaceous nevus
Papulosquamous eruptions	Psoriasis, pityriasis rosea, lichen planus, fungal infections
Vesiculobullous eruptions	Friction blisters, acute contact dermatitis, herpes infections, bullous impetigo, staphylococcal, scalded skin syndrome

Eczematous eruptions	Atopic dermatitis, seborrheic dermatitis, contact dermatitis, diaper dermatitis
Nodules or tumors	Epidermoid or pilar cysts, neurofibromas, lipomas
Alopecia	Alopecia areata, trichotillomania, tinea capitis

Erythematous Rashes

Generalized erythematous rashes are common in children.

Rubeola	Toxic shock
Rubella	Toxic epidermal neurolysis
Roseola	Staphylococcal scalded skin
Parvovirus	Kawasaki disease
Scarlatina	Drug reaction

Erythematous lesions of varying types appearing simultaneously, with peripheral spreading and central clearing, are characteristic of erythema multiforme. Red patches that expand centrifugally are erythema chronicum migrans, characteristic of Lyme disease. If these lesions are 2–4 cm in diameter and are painful, tender, and nodular (especially along the shins), they are erythema nodosum. The lesions may be skin manifestations of systemic diseases.

Erythema Nodosum

Systemic	Drugs
Rheumatic fever	Sulfonamides
Streptococcosis	Oral contraceptives
Tuberculosis	Aspartame
Sarcoid	Bromides
Inflammatory bowel disease	Iodides
Behçet syndrome	
Rheumatoid arthritis	Other infections
Stevens-Johnson syndrome	Leprosy
Lupus erythematosus	Salmonellosis
Vasculitis	Yersiniosis
	Chlamydiae
	Catscratch fever
	Fungi

Erythema nodosum is more common in girls, particularly at puberty, than in boys. Similar single lesions on the hands, feet, knees, or buttocks, usually a raised circle with normal skin inside and outside the erythematous area, may be characteristic of granuloma annulare, which may be due to sensitivity to penicillin or other agents. Nontender erythematous patches on the palms and soles (Janeway lesions) occur in children with acute bacterial endocarditis. Serpiginous erythematous lines suggest cutaneous larva migrans.

A fleeting, purplish erythematous rash lasting a few minutes to a few hours and recurring at short intervals may be observed in children with rheumatoid arthritis. Erythema that is annular or circinate, 1–2 cm in diameter, serpiginous, and flat with erythematous margins surrounding intact skin over the arms, trunk, and legs but not on the face is erythema marginatum. It is characteristic of rheumatic fever. The rash may change from hour to hour.

Localized, painful, hot, erythematous, indurated areas with raised borders are characteristic of erysipelas. Erysipelas is usually caused by streptococcal infection of the skin and is accompanied by high fever. Localized, painful, hot, erythematous, indurated areas lacking raised borders are characteristic of cellulitis. A blue discoloration in the center, particularly in children aged less than 3 years, frequently indicates infection due to *Haemophilus influenzae*. Lesions of similar appearance, particularly around the face, occur with cold injury and frostbite (cold panniculitis). Cellulitis is due to infection in the subcutaneous tissues and may overlie areas of osteomyelitis of bone or thrombophlebitis.

The most common erythematous eruptions, however, are of varying extent and may be due to almost any type of irritation. In the diaper area, erythema is an early form of diaper rash—a type of contact dermatitis—and also occurs in Kawasaki disease. Wind, sun, wool, or clothing may cause erythema of the face or other exposed parts. Excoriation of the convex surfaces of the buttocks is usually due to chafing or excessive moisture. The region around the anus is usually excoriated after loose stools, whereas excoriation around the mucocutaneous area may be due to congenital syphilis. Excoriation of opposing surfaces, especially in the creases of the neck or axillae, is intertrigo and may be due to seborrheic dermatitis or to moisture, with maceration of the skin with constant irritation. In monilia infection, the excoriations are red and scaly and sharply outlined.

Pruritus

Common infections
Jaundice
Allergies
Iron deficiency
Uremia
Atopic dermatitis
Tinea dermatophytosis, ringworm
Scarlet fever
Pinworms (oral pruritis)

Group A strep
Parasites (swimmer's itch)
Scabies

Skin irritants
Drugs: opiates, barbiturates, isoniazid
Lymphoma
Diabetes
Urticaria
Xerosis (dry skin)
Contact dermatitis (soap, chemicals, metals, dyes, drugs, foods)
Herpes (varicella, zoster, herpes simplex)
Cholestasis (biliary atresia, total parenteral nutrition)
Erythema multiforme
Psoriasis
Lice and mites

Differential Diagnosis

- Urticaria
  - Hypersensitivity reaction causing edema via mast cell/basophil release of histamine, kinins, prostaglandins, and serotonin, mostly immunoglobulin E (IgE) mediated
  - Hives; subcutaneous and mucous membranes
  - Angioedema: most cases acute (resolving within 48 hours); chronic >6 weeks
  - Anaphylaxis: may be life threatening
- Atopic dermatitis
  - Incidence 2%–10% and often begins in infancy
  - Most cases improve with age
- Xerosis (dry skin)
  - Tinea (dermatophytoses, ringworm)
  - Fungal infection (*Trichophyton, Microsporum, Epidermophyton*)
  - Scalp (tinea capitis), face, trunk, extremities
  - Allergens (poison ivy, cosmetics, dyes, drugs, food, animals, jewelery/nickel)
  - Irritants (soap, chemicals, wool, fiberglass)
  - Scarlet fever (group A strep): "Sandpaper rash"
- Herpes: varicella, zoster, herpes simplex
- Lice (pediculosis): head or pubic area (Figure 3.1)
- Mites (scabies, *Sarcoptes scabiei*) (Figure 3.2)
- Pinworms (*Enterobius vermicularis*)
- Cholestasis (total parenteral nutrition, biliary atresia)
- Erythema multiforme ("bull's-eye rash"): Stevens-Johnson syndrome
- Drug induced: Opiates, barbiturates, isoniazid, phenothiazines, erythromycin

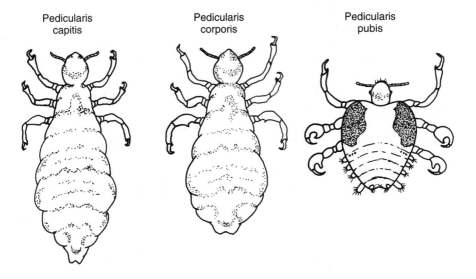

Pedicularis capitis   Pedicularis corporis   Pedicularis pubis

Figure 3.1
Lice (pediculosis): head or pubic area.

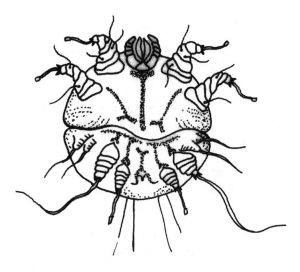

Figure 3.2
Mites (scabies, *Sarcoptes scabiei*).

- Systemic diseases: malignancies, renal failure, mastocytosis, systemic lupus erythematosus, juvenile rheumatoid arthritis (JRA), hypo- and hyperthyroidism, diabetes mellitus
- Prurigo gestations
- Parasites (swimmer's itch, trematodes)
- Chronic skin diseases (psoriasis)

Diffuse redness of the hands and feet, especially if associated with severe pain, suggests a diagnosis of acrodynia, although boric acid poisoning may cause similar signs. Intermittent pallor or cyanosis of the fingers and toes may be an early sign of Raynaud phenomenon. This condition is usually painless, may be aggravated by cold or emotion, and is due to arteriolar spasm with sympathetic nervous system overactivity. Faint erythematous streaks, especially near sites of infection or injury, which follow the course of lymphatics, are inflamed superficial lymph vessels and indicate lymphangitis. Children with fifth disease (erythema infectiosum) caused by parvovirus exhibit bright confluent warm, tender erythema of the cheeks, as though the face had been slapped, that blanches on pressure and fades in 1–4 days. Intense facial redness with pruritus occurs with rifampin toxicity. Any irritant may cause pruritus.

Discrete nonraised lesions are termed *macules*. The rapid appearance of many macules is characteristic of the exanthemata: measles, German measles, scarlet fever, roseola infantum, and typhoid fever. Distinguishing the exanthemata from drug rashes is sometimes difficult, especially when the macules are caused by penicillin or atropine. Similar eruptions may be observed in children with rickettsial diseases or infectious mononucleosis and other viral diseases, particularly the echovirus and Coxsackievirus groups and human immunodeficiency virus. Similar eruptions are apparent in fourth disease (Dukes disease or mild scarlatina) and in erythema infectiosum. A German measles–like rash was formerly evident 7 – 10 days after small-pox vaccination.

Firm skin and subcutaneous elevations with discoloration are *papules*. Papules may occur with any of the exanthemata after the macular stage and may also occur after any condition that causes the appearance of macules. Small gray or white papules are apparent in sarcoid. Red, circular, nonhemorrhagic areas 1 – 2 cm in diameter over the chest, thighs, or elsewhere on the body evidencing scratch marks may be due to ringworm. A large, purplish, maculopapular, scaly, oval area surrounded by smaller similar lesions is characteristic of pityriasis rosea. Sharply raised, red, scaly areas over the elbows and knees are characteristic of psoriasis. Erythematous papules over the finger joints suggest dermatomyositis.

Skin elevations containing serous fluid are *vesicles* or blisters. In chickenpox, lesions itch, are in varied stages, and may cover the body, including the axilla and head. In contrast to the other vesicular diseases, in herpes zoster, pain, if present, precedes the appearance of vesicles.

Important Childhood Vesicular Lesions

- Chickenpox: appear in crops
- Herpes simplex: fever blisters near mouth
- Herpes zoster: along nerves
- Insect bites: exposed areas
- Poison ivy or other poisons: exposed areas
- Molluscum: umbilicated
- Rickettsial pox: on top of maculopapules

Larger vesicles are termed *blebs* or *bullae*.

Bullae

- Burns (possibly indicating abuse)
- Scarlet fever (palms, soles)
- Congenital syphilis (palms, soles)
- Sunburn, poison ivy or oak
- Summer eruption (hydroa estivale)
- Porphyria (photosensitivity)
- Epidermolysis bullosa (irritation)
- Pemphigoid
- Dermatitis herpetiformis

Vesicular Rashes

Differential Diagnosis

- Infection
  - HSV: primary infection followed by latent infection in sensory ganglia; recurrences triggered by cold, UV light, stress, fever, HSV-2 (genital herpes)

- — Varicella (chickenpox) and herpes zoster (VZV): shingles, reactivation of latent virus in sensory ganglia
- — Coxsackievirus (CV): herpangina, hand-foot-and-mouth disease
- — Tinea (ringworm): fungal infection
- — Bullous impetigo (BI): staph, strep
- — Scabies (mites)
- — Staphylococcal scalded skin syndrome (SSSS): tender skin, generalized exfoliation
- — Contact dermatitis (CD): poison ivy, drugs, foods, jewelry, chemicals
- — Erythema multiforme (EM)/Stevens-Johnson syndrome (SJS)
- — Toxic epidermal necrolysis (TEN): same triggers as EM/SJS
- Neonatal
  - — Erythema toxicum: in up to 60% of newborns, disappears after 1 week
  - — Miliaria: obstructed sweat ducts
  - — Pustular melanosis: pustule then macule
  - — Neonatal acne
  - — Sucking blisters (bullae or hand)
  - — Acropustulosis
  - — Eosinophilic pustular folliculitis
  - — Congenital candidiasis
- Folliculitis: staph and strep infections
- Autoimmune: dermatitis herpetiformis (DH), pemphigus vulgaris (PV), linear IgA disease, bullous pemphigoid (BP)
- Hereditary: incontinentia pigmenti; epidermolysis bullosa (EB)
- Others: mastocytosis, friction, burns

Blebs or bullae occur in children with the bullous form of erythema multiforme or immune-deficient diseases. Bullae at birth followed by zebralike pigmentation are characteristic of incontinentia pigmenti or epidermolytic hyperkeratosis, which are congenital malformations of the ectoderm. Children with diarrhea who have acrodermatitis enteropathica manifest bullae of the ends of the fingers; the bullae are responsive to zinc.

Tender skin with erythema followed by bullae that may rub off is Nikolsky sign.

Nikolsky Sign

- Toxic epidermal necrolysis (TEN): drugs
- Staph-scalded skin syndrome (SSSS): staphylococcus
- Stevens-Johnson syndrome (SJS): drugs, mucosa
- Toxic shock syndrome: hands, feet
- Kawasaki disease: hands, feet

Skin elevations containing purulent fluid are *pustules*. Pustules are usually due to bacterial infection or skin abscesses. Pustules may also be evident after any of the states causing vesicles: in adolescents with acne, on the finger in herpes (herpetic whitlow), or after poisoning, such as with iodine. Groups of pustules due to staphylococci or streptococci are known as *impetigo*. Deeper infections, termed *ecthyma*, probably start as impetigo. Larger abscesses of the hair follicles or sebaceous glands are *furuncles* or *carbuncles*. Small straight lines or *burrows* associated with papules, vesicles, or pustules may be scabies, which are due to the itch mite. These lesions may appear anywhere on the body of the child (in contrast to the more localized distribution on the hands and groin of the adult) and are usually accompanied by signs of itching.

Necrotic areas of the superficial and deep layers of the skin, skin *ulcers*, are common in adults with vascular insufficiency. They occasionally occur on the legs of children with sickle cell anemia. Ulceration may occur after skin has been destroyed by burns or trauma or, as a result of hypersensitivity, after subcutaneous injection of antigens.

Petechiae are small, reddish-purple spots in the superficial layers of the skin. If palpable, they frequently indicate severe systemic disease caused by bacterial emboli or vasculitis, as occurs in meningococcemia, rickettsial diseases, leptospirosis, other overwhelming systemic infections or bacterial endocarditis, disseminated intravascular coagulation (DIC), and juvenile rheumatoid arthritis. Petechiae are not palpable in conditions in which platelets are inadequate or defective, as in thrombocytopenic or nonthrombocytopenic purpura, or when capillary permeability is increased, as in scurvy or leukemia. More frequently, they may be caused by injury or by increased capillary pressure due to severe coughing (especially pertussis), allergies in which the cause is unknown, or direct trauma. Paler red or pink areas that measure 0.5 mm may be petechiae or *rose spots*, characteristic of typhoid fever or other *Salmonella* infections.

Ecchymoses, which are evidence of blood under the skin, are usually due to bruising or other injury, but they may be a sign of increased bleeding tendency such as occurs in hemophilia, leukemia, or the purpuras. Purple-red bruises that are fresh, dark blue, or brown are 1–4 days old; greenish-yellow bruises are about 5–7 days old, and yellow bruises are more than 1 week old and healing. Multiple hematomas may indicate child abuse; such hematomas found in the genitalia may indicate sexual abuse.

Purpura

Differential Diagnosis

- Vasculitis (palpable purpura)
  - HSP: most common vasculitis
  - Polyarteritis nodosa (PAN), Wegener granulomatosis (WG): rare in children
- Hematologic
  - Idiopathic thrombocytopenic purpura: age 1–5 years, autoantibodies against platelets (platelets destroyed by splenic macrophages); usually 1–6 weeks after viral infection; 70%–80% acute self-limited; 10%–20% chronic recurrent
  - Other causes of thrombocytopenia: Wiskott-Aldrich syndrome, aplastic anemia, leukemia, disseminated intravascular coagulation (DIC), thrombocytopenia absent radius (TAR)
- Coagulation factor deficiencies
  - Hemophilia A/B (factors VIII/XI): A (1/7,500 male birth), four times more common than B; X-linked recessive

- — WD: prevalence 1%, autosomal dominant, vW factor deficiency or decreased function
  - — Liver disease: decreased production of coagulation factors
  - — Hemorrhagic disease of the newborn: decreased vitamin K–dependent coagulation factors (II, VII, IX, X)
- Infections
  - — Bacterial/rickettsial: meningococcemia (MC), Group A strep (scarlet fever), *Streptococcus viridans/Staphylococcus aureus* (endocarditis), *Gonococcus* (disseminated), *Leptospirosis*, *Rickettsia rickettsii* (Rocky Mountain spotted fever), *R. prowazekii* (epidemic typhus), *Ehrlichiosis*
  - — Viral: hepatitis B, Dengue hemorrhagic fever, atypical measles
- Drugs: coumadin, heparin, aspirin, thiazide, corticosteroids, penicillins, sulfonamides
- Others: trauma or abuse, scurvy (vitamin C deficiency)

Localized areas of swelling and scratch marks are characteristic of *hives* (urticaria or wheals), papular urticaria, insect bites, scabies, and poison ivy or sumac. Localized small swellings or excrescences without scratch marks may be warts. Scratch marks with ulcers, ecchymoses, itching, and other skin lesions may be due to neurodermatitis or may be self-inflicted dermatitis.

Urticaria

Differential Diagnosis

- Epidemiology: most cases resolve within 48 hours; chronic, more than 6 weeks
- Pathophysiology: hypersensitivity reaction allergens (IgE mediated, prior sensitization), complement, and other cytokines activate mast cells and basophils to release histamine (also kinins, prostaglandins, serotonin) with plasma extravasation
- Triggers: most are idiopathic
- IgE mediated: insects (bees, wasps, scorpions, spiders, jellyfish), foods (eggs, shellfish, tree nuts, peanuts, tomatoes), drugs (penicillins, cephalosporins, NSAIDs, barbiturates, amphetamines, insulin, blood products), pollen, dander, food additives
- Non–IgE mediated: infections (strep, Epstein-Barr virus, hepatitis A, B, and C, adenovirus, enterovirus, fleas, mites), drugs (opiates, acetylsalicylic acid, local anesthetics), physical (exercise, cold/heat, UV light, water, pressure), contrast dyes, latex uronic urticaria: associated with collagen vascular diseases (systemic lupus erythematosus, cryoglobulinemia), inflammatory bowel disease, malignancy, thyroiditis, hyperthyroidism, Behçet disease
- Anaphylaxis (IgE mediated)
  - — Most potent foods: peanuts, fish
  - — Mortality: 100–500 deaths/year in United States
- Hereditary angioedema
  - — High mortality
  - — Most cases are autosomal dominant
  - — C1 esterase inhibitor deficiency
  - — Recurrent episodes of edema (face, upper airway, extremities)
  - — Triggers: trauma, surgery
- Others: erythema multiforme, mastocytosis, guttate psoriasis, flushing, cellulitis

Increased sensitivity to skin pressure manifested by wheals or bright red lines is characteristic of *dermatographia*, a form of urticaria. Dermatographia is easily produced by lightly scratching the skin with your nail and is most easily noted over the back or upper chest. Especially persistent dermatographia (*tache cérébrale*) is a sign of CNS irritation, particularly apparent in patients with tuberculous meningitis. Large wheal formation after stroking may be a sign of generalized mast cell disease (urticaria pigmentosa) and is common in comatose patients who have taken an overdose of depressant agents.

Cutaneous Calcification (Calcinosis Cutis)

Subcutaneous nodules are usually due to absorbing or calcifying hematomas, sterile abscesses, or poorly absorbed injections:

Scleroderma	Dermatomyositis
Hyperparathyroidism	Hypervitaminosis D
Sarcoid	Excess milk ingestion
Osteomyelitis	Uremia
Leukemia	Metastatic carcinoma

Nodules over the extensor surfaces of the joints or near the occipital protuberances may aid in the diagnosis of rheumatic fever, rheumatoid arthritis, lupus erythematosus, and granuloma annulare. They may be tender. Red tender nodules on the fingertips, thumbs, or footpads (Osler nodes) are pathognomonic of subacute bacterial endocarditis. Subcutaneous nodules (blueberry muffin spots) are a characteristic of neuroblastoma.

Small yellow or orange plaques (*xanthomas*) on the skin, particularly about the nasal bridge, are usually due to local accumulations of fatty substance. Xanthomas may occur as isolated findings, particularly in infancy, or may be a manifestation of any condition causing hyperlipemia, hypercholesterolemia, or hypertriglyceridemia. The reticuloendothelioses may also cause xanthomas. Pigmented or depigmented xanthomalike lesions may be adenoma sebaceum, characteristic of tuberous sclerosis.

Cysts may be felt under the skin as superficial masses with fluid. They are usually nontender and may transilluminate light. A cyst over the dorsum of the hand or wrist is most commonly a ganglion—a degenerated cyst of the tendon sheath. Tumors of the skin may be firm or soft and are usually lipomas or fibromas. Atrophic areas of the skin may result from injury or, in diabetic patients, from use of insulin.

Skin Scaling

Feel the skin. The texture may be rough, as is common in children during the winter, especially after contact with wool or soap. In children with hyperkeratosis, the skin may be rough due to vitamin A deficiency, hypothyroidism, or hypoparathyroidism. Rough dry skin, especially over the legs, may be a manifestation of ichthyosis. Thickening of the skin in the flexor folds of the elbows and knees is characteristic of chronic eczema. The skin also hardens and thickens in sclerema, scleredema, scleroderma, and dermatomyositis.

Yellow, dirty scaling beginning on the scalp is termed *cradle cap*. Scaling beginning on the scalp and proceeding down the face and body, associated with erythema, is a self-limiting form of exfoliative seborrheic dermatitis (Leiner disease), which appears in the first 3 months of life. Scaling that begins on the cheeks and spreads to the forehead, scalp, posterior of the ears, and down the body is characteristic of infantile eczema, which begins about the second month of life and lasts 1–2 years. Eczema may occur in conditions of immunologic deficiency or in some metabolic diseases. Scaling in the diaper area, sometimes associated with vesiculation and infection, may occur with diaper rash. Scaling with plaques or vesicles on the plantar surface of the foot may occur with psoriasis, allergic contact dermatitis, or juvenile plantar dermatosis.

Seborrhea

Eczema

Histiocytosis

Contact dermatitis

Ringworm

Epidermophytoses

Dyshidrosis

Posterythematous eruptions

Congenital syphilis

Kawasaki disease

Dietary Deficiency
* Zinc
* Biotin
* Selenium
* Essential fatty acids

Other Skin Characteristics

Subcutaneous emphysema is felt as a crackling or crepitant sensation under the skin. It is most commonly associated with pneumothorax, pneumomediastinum, and gas gangrene. A similar sensation is evident if one palpates an area over a bone fracture.

Striae are usually pale white or pink lines occurring in localized areas that are growing rapidly, such as the lower abdomen or thighs of an obese child. They usually occur after overeating or during the growth spurt, but striking purple striae may indicate the presence of Cushing syndrome. Scars are red or white lines and are evidence of previous injury or operation. Scars become elevated when keloid formation occurs.

Estimate the degree of sweating. In infants sweating normally begins after the first month of life. Sweating, especially in children aged less than 1 year, may be profuse and is usually caused by exercise, crying, an overly warm atmosphere, or eating. Profuse sweating, however, may be caused by fever, hypoglycemia, hyperthyroidism, congenital heart disease, hypocalcemia, acrodynia, pneumothorax, cystic fibrosis, or fear. Night sweats may be caused by sleep apnea or spinal cord injuries. Dry skin (anhidrosis) is also normal but may be a sign of dehydration, coma, atropine poisoning, hypothyroidism, eczema, or ectodermal dysplasia.

Feel the skin for tissue turgor, elasticity, and edema. Tissue turgor is determined by pinching the skin, squeezing out the blood, and watching color change. Slow return of color denotes decreased turgor, a sign of decreased subcutaneous tissue or shock. Estimate the *capillary refill time* (return of color), which normally is less than 2 seconds. Color returns in 2–3 seconds with 50–90 ml/kg fluid depletion and in more than 3 seconds with more than 100 ml/kg, which constitutes medical shock. This test is inaccurate if heart failure or hypertonic dehydration is present. Tissue elasticity is best determined by grasping 1 or 2 inches of the patient's skin and subcutaneous tissues over the abdominal wall between the thumb and index finger, squeezing, and allowing the skin to fall back in place (Figure 3.3). It is an estimate of status of hydration and nutrition. Normally, the skin appears smooth and firm and, when grasped as described, quickly falls back in place without residual marks. The skin remains suspended and creased for a few seconds in children with poor elasticity.

The tissues feel plastic and doughy in children with chronic wasting disease, peritonitis, or hyperelectrolytemia with dehydration. Little subcutaneous tissue will be felt in malnourished children. The skin will remain suspended and in folds in dehydrated patients. This may not occur in obese infants; if dehydration is suspected in them, other signs should be sought. Poor tissue turgor may be apparent in a normal infant a few days old, especially in premature infants, but they rapidly add fat and subcutaneous tissue so that turgor is normal by body weight of 2,000 gm or more.

The skin normally feels firm, especially over the legs. Calluses occur frequently on the hands or feet following constant irritation. Thickening over the knuckles (knuckle pads) may be due to induced vomiting in patients with bulimia nervosa. The skin feels thin and loosely filled in children with chronic diseases, malnutrition, and rickets. It may feel very soft and flabby in children with flaccid paralyses and in children with muscle diseases such as myasthenia gravis or amyotonia congenita,

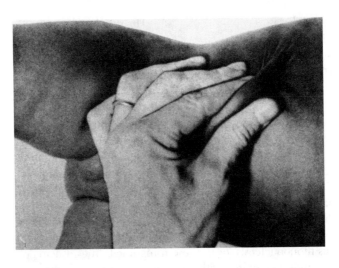

Figure 3.3
Subcutaneous turgor or elasticity. It is best demonstrated by grasping the skin and subcutaneous tissue over the abdomen and allowing it to fall back in place.

as well as in children with developmental delay. The skin may be soft and mushy in children with Down syndrome. It may feel hard and thickened in children with hypothyroidism, whether the condition is congenital or acquired.

The skin may be tender to the touch. This may indicate that the child is irritable or has CNS disease or another systemic illness. Referred pain is due particularly to intraabdominal disease. Pain elicited by light pressure is more likely due to cellulitis and deeper pressure to bone or joint infections. Painful skin over the right lower abdominal wall may signify acute appendicitis. Skin tenderness is also noted in polyneuritis, and children with ruptured spleen display tenderness over the left shoulder. Tenderness may be due to a cryptic foreign body such as a splinter. Transilluminate (particularly the fingers or toes) to help localize the object.

Edema

Impressions in the skin that remain for several seconds following finger pressure occur in patients with *pitting edema*. Edema is the presence of an abnormal amount of extracellular fluid and is caused by an increase in hydrostatic pressure, increased capillary permeability, decreased oncotic pressure, increased retention of sodium or other electrolytes, mechanical obstruction of the lymphatic channels, lymphedema, or decreased excretion of water. Puffy-appearing areas on the body that do not pit or leave marks after pressure or pinching are termed *nonpitting edema*. For example, patients with hypothyroidism manifest puffy skin with no pitting. Scleredema, a rare connective tissue disease, is a firm nonpitting edema affecting face, neck, scalp, conjunctivae, thorax, and occasionally the arms and legs but not the feet.

Edema localized in the eyelids may be the first sign of generalized edema.

Renal disease	Heart failure
Liver disease	Malnutrition
Systemic lupus erythematosus	Adrenal hormones
Hyperaldosteronism	Thyroid disease
Infectious mononucleosis	

True generalized pitting edema is found earliest over the dependent parts, especially the sacrum and ankles. Edema in the first few months of life may be seen in patients with cystic fibrosis. Adolescent girls show edema before or during menses. In warm weather, edema occasionally occurs on the skin without apparent cause.

Localized edema in the eyelids, face, or lips may be due to allergy (angioneurotic edema), sinusitis, trichiniasis (trichinosis), or insect bites in those areas. Puffiness of the eyelids may also be seen in children after a long sleep or after crying and in children with conjunctivitis, frontal or ethmoid sinusitis, cavernous sinus thrombosis, or infectious mononucleosis, or in those using illicit drugs. Edema of the face and eyelids is common in children with any of the common contagious diseases. Localized edema of the face may occur following severe cough, such as whooping cough or diphtheria. Facial edema also occurs with superior vena cava obstruction or mass lesions in the chest. Edema of the legs occurs with thrombophlebitis, deep calf vein thrombosis, inferior vena cava obstruction, cellulitis, and other lower extremity infections.

The ridges formed by the raised apertures of the sweat glands make up *dermatoglyphics*. These are best seen with adequate light and magnification or by making finger and hand prints. The otoscope without earpiece is usually adequate for both light and magnification. The ridges form arches, loops, and whorls on the fingers; three lines that meet are termed a *triradius*. The normal child usually has a triradius low on the palm, a triradius with an acute angle in the hypothenar area proximal to the midpalm, and an assortment of arches, loops, and whorls on the fingertips (Figure 3.4). Usually, approximately seven or eight fingertips will have ulnar loops and one to three will have whorls. One arch is common in normal children. Radial loops are rare in normal children. Deviations from these patterns suggest the presence of chromosome abnormalities, early intrauterine infections, gross abnormalities of growth of the extremities, or some forms of congenital heart disease. A triradius distal to the midpalm with an obtuse angle is suggestive of Down syndrome; arches on all digits suggest trisomy 18 syndrome. Radial loops may occur more commonly

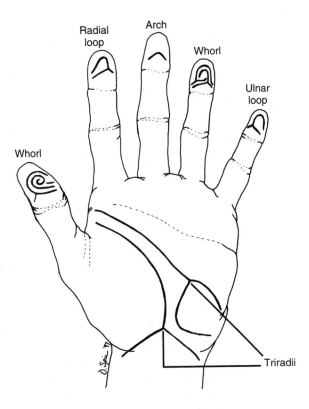

Figure 3.4
Normal hand ridges (dermatoglyphics).

in children with XXY anomaly, and large deep ridges are found in gonadal dysgenesis. Arches on the thumbs are common in children with trisomy 13 syndrome. A single flexion crease on the fifth finger suggests the presence of a chromosome abnormality.

NAILS

The nails are valuable areas for determining special disease states. The nail beds are usually the simplest site in which to determine cyanosis, pallor, capillary pulsations, and capillary refill time. In newborns, vernix can usually be found under the nails. Pitting of the nails is seen with fungal diseases of the nails and with psoriasis. Indentations (Beau lines) are markers of previous severe stress. Yellow staining of the nails is apparent in postmature infants and in the yellow nail syndrome, which is associated with lymphedema and lung disease. Darkening of the nails may be noted in children with porphyria. Nails may be absent in children with ectodermal dysplasia or fetal alcohol syndrome or in infants born to mothers receiving anticonvulsants. Infections around the nails (paronychia) are common in children, especially after desquamating skin lesions. They may be bacterial or fungal infections. Oncolysis may indicate thyroid disease.

Hemorrhage under the nails is usually due to injury, subacute bacterial endocarditis, or other diseases in which petechiae are noted. Telangiectases at the proximal nail folds occur in scleroderma, lupus erythematosus, and dermatomyositis. Redness of the half-moon (lunula) occurs in children with heart failure, corticosteroid use, pulmonary disease, or alopecia areata. Brown discoloration of the lunula may occur in children with uremia.

The nail beds are characteristically more broad than long in children with Down syndrome or pseudohypoparathyroidism or in congenital malformation syndromes characterized by broad fingers. Spoon-shaped nails with loss of the longitudinal convexity (koilonychia) may be caused by fungal infections, iron deficiency, trauma, or thyroid or intestinal diseases, or they may be congenital. White nails or paired white lines parallel to the nail base (Muehroke lines) are seen in hypoalbuminemic states, zinc and vitamin B_6 deficiencies, and other types of malnutrition. Transverse white lines (Mees lines) in the nails may occur several months after acute Kawasaki disease or other severe illnesses.

Compare the width of thumbnails, first fingernails, and great toes. These may be the easiest sites in which to detect asymmetry or hemiatrophy.

HAIR

Note hair, other than that of the head. Newborns, especially premature infants, sometimes have hair growing over their shoulders and back but it disappears at about 3 months of age. This is referred to as lanuga. Children do not usually have hair except for scalp, eyebrows, and eyelashes until near puberty. Long eyebrows and eyelashes are usually familial but occasionally appear in children with chronic or wasting diseases. Heavy facial hair occurs with de Lange and Hurler syndromes, which are associated with developmental delay, or in endocrine disorders such as virilizing tumors, polycystic ovary syndrome, arrhenoblastoma, and acromegaly. Look for nits or crab lice (a sexually transmitted disease) in these areas.

Unusual hairiness elsewhere on the body, especially over the arms and legs, may be a normal variant or familial characteristic but may be found in children with hypothyroidism, vitamin A poisoning, chronic infections, phenytoin or diazoxide use, cimetidine use, or hepatic porphyria. Those who are starving or have extreme weight loss, as with anorexia or bulimia, have lanugo-type hairiness. Hairiness of the trunk is noted in children with Cushing syndrome.

Tufts of hair anywhere over the spine and especially over the sacrum may have special significance. Although resembling a nevus, the hair may mark the site of a spina bifida occulta or spina bifida. Nevi may also be hairy.

Pubic hair begins to appear at 8–12 years of age (adrenarche), or as early as 7 years in blacks followed by axillary hair about 6 months later and by facial hair about 6 months later still in boys. Appearance of hair in these areas indicates normal adrenal and testicular function. Decrease of hair in these areas may be due to hypothyroidism, hypopituitarism, gonadal deficiency, or Addison disease. Early appearance or increase of hair in these areas may be normal, especially in obese children.

Increased Body Hair

Obese	Central nervous system lesions
Adrenal hyperplasia	Pineal hamartoma
Adrenal tumor	Testicular tumors
Acanthosis nigricans	Ovarian tumors
	Hyperinsulism
	Polyostotic fibrous dysplasia

Ingested Substances

Stilbestrol
Testosterone
Anabolic steroids

Pigmented, coarse, curly, or crinkled pubic hair indicates increased hormonal production and is believed to indicate onset of sperm formation in boys (Figure 3.5). Pubic hair without testicular growth suggests hypogonadism.

Causes of Hirsutism

- Drug induced
  - Cyclosporine, steroids, oral contraceptives, Dilantin, some diuretics (acetazolamide, hydrochlorothiazide), Minoxidil, penicillamines, cimetidine
- Syndrome associated
  - Cornelia de Lange syndrome
  - Trisomy 18
  - Bloom syndrome

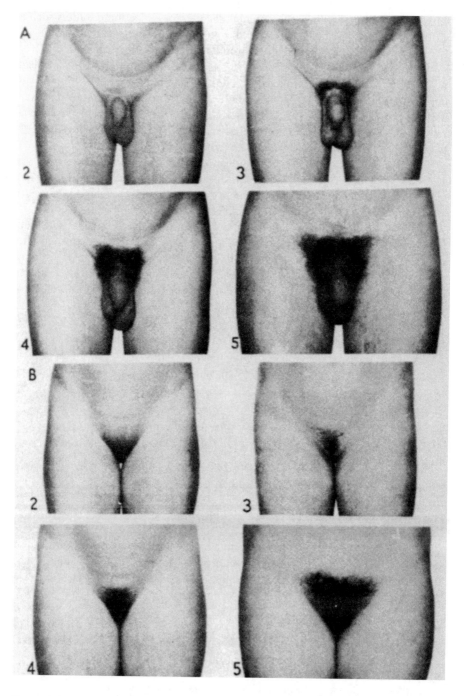

Figure 3.5
Pubic hair stages in males (A) and females (B). Stage 1 (not shown): preadolescent (no
pubic hair). Stage 2: sparse, long, slightly pigmented. Stage 3: darker, coarser, more curled.
Stage 4: adult type but smaller area. Stage 5: adult. (From Tanner, J. M., 1962. *Growth at
adolescence*. Philadelphia: F. A. Davis.).

- — Seckel syndrome
- — Marshall-Smith syndrome
- — Rubinstein-Taybi syndrome
- — Leprechaunism
- Ovarian
  - — Polycystic ovarian syndrome
  - — Gonadal dysgenesis
  - — Ovarian tumors
- Adrenal
  - — Congenital adrenal hyperplasia
    - ○ 17α-hydroxylase deficiency
    - ○ 12-hydroxylase deficiency
    - ○ Adrenal tumor
- Other causes
  - — Idiopathic
  - — 5α-reductase deficiency
  - — Hyperprolactinemia
  - — HAIR-AN syndrome (hirsutism, androgenization, insulin resistance, and acanthosis nigricans)
  - — Porphyria: congenital erythropoietic porphyria causes increased body hair, red urine, photosensitivity with bullae, and red to pink teeth

LYMPH NODES

Lymph nodes are generally examined during examination of the part of the body in which they are located. Routinely palpate occipital, postauricular, anterior and posterior cervical (Figure 3.6), parotid, submaxillary, sublingual, axillary, epitrochlear, and inguinal nodes. Note size, mobility, tenderness, and heat. Shotty, discrete, movable, cool, nontender nodes up to 3 mm in diameter are usually normal in these areas; in the cervical and inguinal regions, nodes up to 1 cm in diameter are normal until age 12 years.

Nodes that are in the anterior cervical triangle or that enlarge slowly are usually benign. Rapidly growing nodes, nodes fixed to underlying tissue, or hard, firm, or matted nodes might be malignant.

Large, warm, soft, tender nodes usually indicate acute infection. Firm, rubbery nontender nodes are more common with leukemia or sarcoid. Firm nodes that adhere to each other and the skin are found in children with tuberculosis; discrete rubbery nodes are found in Hodgkin disease, and extremely firm, hard nodes occur with metastases. Local adenopathy usually indicates local infection but may be a sign of generalized disease. Cervical nodes reflect drainage of the sinuses, ears, mouth, teeth, and pharynx (Tables 3.2, 3.3). The right supraclavicular nodes drain the lung and esophagus; the left supraclavicular nodes drain the lung, stomach, small intestine, kidney, and pancreas; and the axillary nodes drain the breasts, arms, and fingers. In children with inguinal adenopathy, investigate for sexually transmitted diseases or paragenital infections.

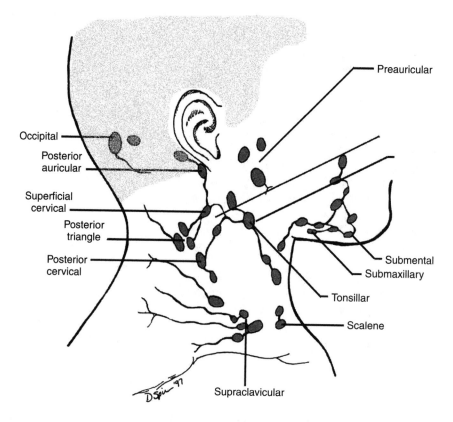

Figure 3.6
Lymph nodes of the head and neck.

Generalized Adenopathy

Generalized adenopathy with or without tenderness is seen with systemic diseases:

Bacteremia	Rheumatoid arthritis
Syphilis	Viremia
Eczema	Kawasaki disease
Infectious mononucleosis	Leukemia
Systemic fungal disease	Serum sickness
Hyperthyroid	Hodgkin disease
Chronic granulomatous disease	Sarcoid
Drug sensitivity	Hyper-IgE
Lupus erythematosus	Reticuloendothelial disease

A few isolated enlarged nodes may have special significance. Occipital or posterior auricular adenopathy is evident in local scalp infections, external otitis, German

TABLE 3.2
Common Causes of Generalized or Prominent Cervical Adenopathy Due to Infections

Infections	Site of Adenopathy	Character of Nodes	Other Features	Laboratory Findings
Herpes simplex	Anterior cervical and submandibular	Soft to mildly firm, discrete, mobile, tender	Gingival erythema and edema with discrete mucosal ulcers; high fever	+ Viral culture (diagnosis usually made on clinical grounds)
Coxsackievirus herpangina	Anterior cervical	Soft to mildly firm, discrete, mobile, slightly tender	Discrete ulcers on labial mucosa, gingival, tongue and tonsillar pillars; may have vesicles on palms and soles	+ Viral culture (diagnosis usually made on clinical grounds)
Adenovirus	Anterior cervical and preauricular	Soft to mildly firm, discrete, mobile, mildly tender	Nonspecific pharyngeal inflammation, occasionally with exudates; may have conjunctivitis	+ Viral culture
EB virus mononucleosis	Anterior and posterior cervical, or generalized	Soft to firm, discrete, mildly to moderately tender	Pharyngitis; splenomegaly (50%); rash (15%); fever, malaise, fatigue	Atypical lymphocytosis; + monospot (80% > 4 years); + EB virus titers; may have abnormal LFTs
Cytomegalovirus infection	Generalized or cervical	Soft to firm, discrete, mildly tender	Fever, malaise, fatigue; occasionally hepato-splenomegaly	Atypical lymphocytosis; abnormal LFTs; urine + for inclusions and + for CMV on culture; + CMV titers
Rubella	Anterior and posterior cervical	Soft to mildly firm, discrete, mildly tender or nontender	Fine discrete maculopapular rash; Forscheimer spots on palate	+ Rubella titer
Streptococcal pharyngitis	Anterior cervical	Soft to mildly firm, discrete, tender	Pharyngitis or nasopharyngitis headache, malaise; abdominal pain; may have palatal petechiae and/or scarlatiniform rash	+ Throat culture for group A β-hemolytic streptococcus
Toxoplasmosis	Generalized or cervical	Smooth, firm, mildly tender	Myalgias, fatigue, coryza; occasionally splenomegaly and maculopapular rash	Atypical lymphocytosis (frequent); + toxoplasma titers
Brucellosis	Generalized or cervical and axillary	Discrete, may be mildly tender or nontender	History of contact with sick farm animal or ingestion of raw milk; afternoon fever and chills; sweats, malaise, headache and backache, arthralgia; and may become chronic with metastatic abscesses	Normal or decreased WBC with lymphocytosis; + culture and serologic tests

Modified from Zitelli.

TABLE 3.3

Other Causes of Cervical Masses

Mass	Usual Site Involvement	Character	Time of Appearance
Lymphangioma	Preauricular, submental, submandibular, supraclavicular	Soft, compressible; transilluminates, margins often indistinct; may enlarge with crying or straining; nontender unless infected	Birth to 2 years
Hemangioma	Preauricular, postauricular; may occur along or under sternocleidomastoid	Soft, compressible; margins often indistinct; enlarges with crying, straining, and dependency; nontender unless infected	Birth to 1 year; gradually enlarges during first year then regresses
Branchial cleft cyst	Preauricular, at mandibular angle, along anterior border of sternocleidomastoid, suprasternal	Discrete; usually has overlying or nearby pore or fistula, which may retract with swallowing; nontender unless infected	Present at birth; often not noticed until infection produces enlargement, pain and overlying erythema with or without drainage
Thyroglossal duct cyst	Midline, often at level of hyoid or just below	Discrete; usually has overlying pore or fistula; moves with tongue movement	Present at birth; often not noticed until infection produces enlargement, pain, and overlying erythema with or without drainage
Dermoid cyst	Midline, often submental or suprasternal	Discrete, smooth; doughy or rubbery; nontender; does not retract with swallowing	Infancy/childhood
Laryngocele	Just lateral to midline along anterior border of sterno-cleidomastoid	Soft, compressible, may gurgle on compression; enlarges with straining or crying; nontender unless infected; may have associated stridor or hoarseness; air-fluid level may be seen on X-ray	Infancy/childhood
Esophageal diverticulum	Paratracheal, usually on the left	Soft, compressible; enlarges with crying or straining; nontender; may have history of dysphagia or aspiration	Infancy/childhood
Sialadenitis	Preauricular, extending under and behind ear; submandibular, submental	Firm; mildly tender when viral; exquisitely tender when suppurative, with pus exuding from orifice; pain increased with eating, especially sour foods; elevated serum or urine amylase level	Any age
Teratoma	Midline or paramedian	Solitary; firm with irregular border; rapid increase in size; calcifications may be seen on X-ray	

Condition	Location	Characteristics	Age
Thyroid goiter	Isthmus (midline) and lobes (paratracheal)	Diffuse enlargement; usually smooth contour and soft consistency, occasionally nodular; moves with swallowing	Occasionally neonatal (with maternal ingestion of iodides); childhood in endemic areas (iodine-deficient water); childhood/ adolescence in familial cases
Graves disease	Isthmus (midline) and lobes (paratrachael)	Diffuse enlargement; smooth contour and soft consistency; moves with swallowing; associated signs of thyrotoxicosis and exophthalmos	Childhood/adolescence
Hashimoto thyroiditis	Isthmus (midline) and lobes (paratrachael)	Diffuse enlargement; distinct contours; firm or rubbery; surface may be irregular; may have neck soreness and dysphagia; may have symptoms of mild hyperthyroidism	Childhood/adolescence
Thyroid carcinoma	Usually in lateral lobe or at junction of isthmus and lobe	Solitary mass; firm or hard and differs in consistency from rest of gland; may have associated adenopathy; may have past history of irradiation	Childhood/adolescence
Leukemia	Any cervical node or nodes	Firm to hard, often enlarges rapidly; may be fixed or matted; nontender; often other regions involved; often hepatosplenomegaly; may have fever, anorexia, weight loss, bone pain, pallor, petechiae	Any age
Non-Hodgkin lymphoma	Spinal accessory, supraclavicular	Firm to hard; enlarges rapidly; may be fixed or matted; nontender; often other regions are involved; may have fever, anorexia, weight loss, bone and joint pain	5–15 years
Hodgkin disease	Anterior or posterior cervical, preauricular, supraclavicular	Firm, occasionally rubbery, slow growing; may be mobile, fixed, or matted; nontender; often otherwise asymptomatic; may have fever, malaise, weight loss, night sweats, and hepatosplenomegaly	Usually >5 years
Rhabdomyosarcoma	Nasopharyngeal, parotid, anterior, or posterior cervical	When primary lesion is nasopharyngeal; symptoms of enlarged adenoids; later serosanguineous nasal discharge, weight loss, cranial nerve deficits, and secondary node enlargement When primary lesion is parotid or cervical: hard, painless, nontender mass	Any age, but more common in childhood

From Davis, H. W., & Michaels, M. G. (2002). Infectious disease. In B. J. Zitelli & H. W. Davis (Eds.), *Atlas of pediatric physical diagnosis* (4th ed.). St. Louis: Mosby.

TABLE 3.4

Mean Values for Normal Leukocyte and Differential Counts

	12 Months	4 Years	10 Years	21 Years
Leukocytes, Total	11.4	9.1	8.1	7.4
Neutrophils, Total	3.5	3.8	4.4	4.4
	(31%)	(42%)	(54%)	(59%)
Band Forms	(3.1%)	(3.0%)	(3.0%)	(3.0%)
Neutrophils, Segmented	3.2	3.5	4.2	4.2
	(28%)	(39%)	(51%)	(56%)
Eosinophils	0.30	0.25	0.20	0.20
	(2.6%)	(2.8%)	(2.4%)	(2.7%)
Basophils	0.05	0.05	0.04	0.04
	(0.4%)	(0.6%)	(0.5%)	(0.5%)
Lymphocytes	7.0	4.5	3.1	2.5
	(61%)	(50%)	(38%)	(34%)
Monocytes	0.55	0.45	0.35	0.30
	(4.8%)	(5.0%)	(4.3%)	(4.0%)

Values are expressed as cells $\times$ $10^3/\mu l$.

measles, pediculosis, varicella, tick bite, and in cases of excessive scratching. Posterior occipital nodes are frequently palpable in other viral infections but are rarely so in bacterial infections in the throat. The preauricular nodes may be enlarged in conjunctivitis (Parinaud syndrome) or in children with sties or chalazia. The "sentinel" node located near the left clavicle may be the first node enlarged in Hodgkin disease in children; in adults, this nodal enlargement may indicate gastric cancer. Cervical adenopathy usually accompanies acute infections in or around the mouth or throat, but cool, large, nontender, matted cervical glands that may suppurate (especially if unilateral) may indicate tuberculosis. Cervical or submandibular lymph node enlargement without other symptoms may herald sinus histiocytosis. When adenopathy occurs near a scratch or bite, catscratch or rat-bite fever or tularemia is suggested, as is disease resulting from tick, flea, or mite bites or local sepsis. The epitrochlear nodes in particular are enlarged in congenital syphilis and catscratch disease.

Absence of lymph nodes occurs in patients with agammaglobulinemia and in some patients with human immunodeficiency syndromes (Table 3.4).

FURTHER READING

Robertson, J., & Shilkofski, N. (Eds.). (2005). *The Harriet Lane handbook* (17th ed.). St. Louis: Elsevier Mosby.

4

NUTRITION

To laugh often and love much . . . to appreciate beauty, to find
the best in others . . . to know even one life has breathed easier
because you have lived . . . this is to have succeeded.

Ralph Waldo Emerson

THE MISSION OF this text is to describe techniques of the physical examination and the ability of the physical exam to provide accurate diagnoses. The emphasis of this chapter is more to highlight common nutrition-related states. This chapter is not intended to be a comprehensive review of childhood nutrition. This is covered more extensively in the usual pediatric textbooks and publications from the American Academy of Pediatrics (Website www.aap.org). The appendix contains various growth charts. An individual patient's growth chart in a gross manner may either suggest a healthy nutritional status or a possible nutritional disorder (Table 4.1).

FAT-SOLUBLE VITAMINS

Vitamin A (Retinol)

The usual sources of vitamin A are liver, fish-liver oils, fortified milk, egg yolks, butter, and green and deep yellow vegetables. The risk groups include children with poor dietary intake (especially in underdeveloped areas of the world) and those with fat malabsorption (e.g., patients with celiac disease and cystic fibrosis). Symptoms include irreversible cornea damage and night blindness. Worldwide, vitamin A deficiency is the most common cause of blindness in children. Deficient individuals are also at risk for an increase in morbidity and mortality from certain infections such as measles. Vitamin A administration might be lifesaving in children with chronic malnutrition during measles outbreaks. Treatment of xerophthalmia requires 5,000–10,000 IU/kg/day for 5 days. Vitamin A toxicity is manifested by anorexia, pseudotumor cerebri, painful bone lesions, precocious puberty, desquamative dermatitis, and hepatotoxicity.

Vitamin D (Calciferol)

The usual sources of vitamin D are fortified milk, egg yolks, liver, salmon, butter, and sardines. The requirement depends on the amount of exposure to sunlight. The

TABLE 4.1
Summary of Dietary Reference Intakes for Select Vitamins

	0–6 mo	7–12 mo	1–3 yr	4–8 yr	9–13 yr	14–18 yr Male	14–18 yr Female
Thiamin (mg/d)	0.2[a]	0.3[a]	0.5	0.6	0.9	1.2	1.0
Riboflavin (mg/d)	0.3[a]	0.4	0.5[a]	0.6[a]	0.9[a]	1.3[a]	1.0[a]
Pyridoxine (mg/d)	0.1[a]	0.3[a]	0.5	0.6	1.0	1.3	1.2
Niacin (mg/d)	2[a]	4[a]	6	8	12	16	14
Pantothenic acid (mg/d)	1.7[a]	1.8[a]	2[a]	3[a]	4[a]	5[a]	5[a]
Biotin (µg/d)	5[a]	6[a]	8[a]	12[a]	20[a]	25[a]	25[a]
Folic acid (µg/d)	65[a]	80[a]	150	200	300	400	400
Cobalamin (µg/d)	0.4[a]	0.5[a]	0.9	1.2	1.8	2.4	2.4
Vitamin C (mg/d)	40[a]	50[a]	15	25	45	75	65
Vitamin A (µg/d)	400[a]	500[a]	300	400	600	900	700
Vitamin D (IU/d)	200[a]	200[a]	200[a]	200[a]	200[a]	200[a]	200[a]
Vitamin E (mg/d)	4[a]	5[a]	6	7	11	15	15
Vitamin K (µg/d)	2[a]	2.5[a]	30[a]	55[a]	60[a]	75[a]	75[a]

[a] Adequate intakes (AI). All other values represent the Recommended Dietary Allowances (RDA). Both the RDA and AI may be used as goals for individual intakes.
From National Academy of Sciences, Food and Nutritional Board, Institute of Medicine. (2000). *Dietary reference intakes: Application in dietary assessment* (pp. 287–289). Washington, DC: National Academy Press, http://www.nap.edu

common risk groups for deficiency include patients with fat malabsorption, deep-pigmented breast-fed infants (especially those with inadequate sun exposure), and patients on P-450-stimulating drugs (e.g., anticonvulsant drugs). The deficiency state in adults results in osteomalacia. In children, the deficiency results in rickets. The signs of rickets include craniotabes, rachitic rosary, bowed legs, delayed teeth eruption, spinal deformities, bone pain and fractures, weakness, and failure to thrive. Treatment is with 1,600–5,000 IU/day. The toxicity results in hypercalcemia that leads to CNS depression, ectopic calcification, and nephrocalcinosis.

Vitamin E (Tocopherol)

The usual sources of vitamin E are vegetable oils, beef liver, peanuts, soybeans, milk fat, turnip greens, and butter. The deficiency state is found in prematurity, cholestatic liver disease, fat malabsorption, pancreatic insufficiency, and short bowel syndrome. The deficiency state can lead to hemolytic anemia or, if chronic, a progressive neurologic disorder with symptoms of loss of deep tendon reflexes, loss of coordination, nystagmus, weakness, brown bowel syndrome, and retinal degeneration. In premature infants, the deficiency state contributes to oxidant injury of the lungs, retina, and brain. Toxicity to excessive vitamin E might manifest itself with prolonged prothrombin time in patients on warfarin and an increased incidence of bacterial and fungal sepsis in premature infants.

Vitamin K (Phylloquinone)

The usual sources for vitamin K include live yogurt, vegetable oils, liver, pork, green leafy vegetables, and synthesis by normal intestinal flora. The deficiency occurs in newborns, especially those breast-fed and not given vitamin K prophylaxis, and those exclusively breast-fed for prolonged periods. Later deficiency may occur with malabsorption states, the use of nonabsorbed antibiotics, and with chronic diarrhea. The signs and symptoms are related to the resultant bleeding diathesis, such as hemorrhagic disease of the newborn or later bruising and bleeding in the gastrointestinal tract, gums, joints, or brain. The prophylaxis dose is 0.5–1.0 mg. For older children with active bleeding, the dose is 3–10 mg of vitamin K I.M. Toxicity of the water-soluble analog can lead to kernicterus in newborns.

WATER-SOLUBLE VITAMINS

Vitamin B₁ (Thiamine)

The usual sources for thiamine include liver, meat, milk, pork, whole grains, legumes, and nuts. The risk population includes infants breast-fed by mothers with a history of alcoholism or poor diet, as a complication of total parenteral nutrition (TPN), in the presence of kwashiorkor, and prematurity. The deficiency state is either "wet beriberi" characterized by congestive heart failure, tachycardia, and peripheral edema or "dry beriberi" characterized by neuritis, paresthesia, irritability, and anorexia. Treatment is 100 mg per day for 5 days. Toxicity to thiamine is very rare.

Vitamin B₂ (Riboflavin)

For infants, breast milk or formula is the principal source for riboflavin. Older children also receive riboflavin in milk, cheese, eggs, organ meats, fish, green leafy vegetables, and whole and enriched grains. The deficiency state exists in premature infants and if TPN is exposed to light. The deficiency may result in cheilosis, glossitis, seborrheic dermatitis, poor growth, ocular signs such as photophobia and loss of visual acuity, and psychomotor abnormalities.

Vitamin B₃ (Niacin)

The principal sources of niacin include lean meats, poultry, peanuts, organ meats, fish, green vegetables, and enriched cereals and grains. The deficiency state results in pellagra characterized by dermatitis, apathy, anorexia, dementia, and diarrhea. Toxicity can result in vasodilation. The risk population includes those on a high maize (corn) diet and premature infants.

Vitamin B₆ (Pyridoxine)

The risk factors for pyridoxine deficiency include prematurity, pyridoxine dependency syndromes, and certain drugs such as isoniazid. The usual sources include liver, meats, whole grains, potatoes, corn, soybeans, bananas, and peanuts. The clinical features of pyridoxine deficiency include intractable seizures in the newborn, listlessness, irritability, swelling of the tongue, anemia, and neuropathy. Toxicity of pyridoxine call result in neuropathy. Treatment of the deficiency state is 100 mg of pyridoxine.

Folate (Vitamin B$_9$)

The chief dietary sources of folate include liver, leafy green vegetables, legumes, asparagus, broccoli, nuts, cheese and fortified cereals. The risk populations include premature infants, infants breast-fed by folate-deficient mothers, infants fed goat's milk, those with intake of chronically overcooked food, those with celiac disease, and those on certain drugs such as phenytoin. There exists an increased demand for folate in hemolytic anemias, diarrhea, malignancies, hypermetabolic states, infection, and pregnancy. The deficiency state results in megaloblastic anemia, neutropenia, thrombocytopenia growth retardation, delayed maturation of the central nervous system in infants, diarrhea, jaundice, and mild splenomegaly. The incidence of neural tube defects has sharply declined in the presence of enhanced dietary folate intake before conception. Toxicity results in irritability. Also, if folate is given for megaloblastic anemia, a B$_{12}$ deficiency might be masked.

Vitamin B$_{12}$ (Cyanocobalamin)

The principal source of vitamin B$_{12}$ includes eggs, dairy products, liver, and meats. Plants are not a source for B$_{12}$. Colostrum contains a higher concentration of B$_{12}$. Risk groups include breast-fed infants of strict vegan mothers, bowel disease (e.g., short gut), and decreased intrinsic factor. In adults, chronic use of protein-pump inhibitors has been associated with B$_{12}$ deficiency. Vitamin B$_{12}$ has no toxicity state.

Vitamin C (Ascorbic Acid)

Vitamin C is found in fresh fruits and vegetables. The risk group includes premature infants, those with poor intake of fruits and vegetables, and infants of mothers who consumed megadoses during pregnancy. The deficiency state is scurvy. The symptoms of scurvy include diffuse tissue bleeding, easy bone fractures, poor wound healing, leg tenderness, and bleeding gums with loose teeth. Hematuria and hemocult-positive stools may also be present. Toxicity may result in nausea, diarrhea, cramps, and oxalate and cysteine nephrocalcinosis.

VARIOUS MINERAL DEFICIENCIES

Iron

Iron deficiency is the most common nutritional deficiency in the United States. The major sources in infancy include iron-fortified formulas and cereals. Also, iron from breast milk is preferentially absorbed. The risk groups include premature infants, growth-retarded infants, infants of diabetics, and adolescent females secondary to menstrual blood loss. There is an increased demand for iron during periods of growth. The last four weeks of gestation are a major time for acquiring iron stores. The characteristic symptoms of iron deficiency are growth problems, deafness, pallor, breathlessness, tiredness, edema, irritability, decreased bone density, and a heart murmur (from a high-output state). Iron deficiency can increase lead absorption. Sources of iron beyond infancy include organ meats, beans, dark chocolate, shellfish, nuts, broccoli, red meat, egg yolks, and molasses. The anemia is hypochromic/microcytic. There is a frequent associated thrombocytosis. In a classic presentation, the diagnosis is assumed if the hemoglobin increases by 1 g/dL after 3 weeks of therapeutic iron (3–6 mg/kg/day of oral elemental iron). It is recommended that all full-term infants be screened at 9–12 months. Toxicity of acute iron poisoning includes (1) hemorrhagic gastroenteritis with possible associated shock and acidosis (lasting 4–6 hours); (2) 2–12-hour period of appearing well; (3) delayed shock 12–48 hours after ingestion with metabolic acidosis, fever, and coma; (4) liver injury and hepatic failure; and (5) residual pyloric stenosis of 4 weeks gestation. Chronic iron overload is common in hemoglobinopathies.

Copper

Copper deficiency is rare. Common food sources include shellfish, meat, legumes, nuts, and cheese. The risk populations include premature infants fed formula low in copper, prolonged feeding of unmodified cow's milk, generalized malnutrition, and in children on prolonged TPN without adequate copper supplementation. Profound copper deficiency is found in Menkes syndrome, an X-linked defect in cellular metabolism of copper. Characteristics of the deficiency include osteoporosis, cartilage and metaphyseal changes, and spontaneous rib fractures. Neutropenia and hypochromic anemia unresponsive to iron are found. Treatment of the deficiency is with a 1% copper sulfate solution. The clinical condition of toxicity most commonly arises from Wilson disease, an autosomal recessive genetic disorder of copper metabolism.

Zinc

Zinc food sources include oysters, liver, meat, cheese, legumes, and whole grains. Groups at risk of developing a deficiency are patients on a diet low in zinc, patients on TPN not supplemented with zinc, patients with certain gastrointestinal disorders such as Crohn, celiac, cystic fibrosis, and chronic diarrhea, and patients with inborn errors of zinc metabolism. The signs and symptoms include anorexia, hypogeusia (loss of taste), growth retardation, failure to thrive, pubertal delay, impaired wound healing, and certain skin lesions such as acrodermatitis enteropathica. The treatment of the dietary deficiency is 1 mg/kg/day for 3 months. There are few toxic effects. It may aggravate marginal copper deficiency.

PROTEIN DEFICIENCY

Kwashiorkor

The term *kwashiorkor* comes from an African dialect, meaning "the disease of the displaced baby." This occurs in patients with inadequate protein intake in the presence of low or normal total caloric intake. It can develop quickly. Worldwide, kwashiorkor is endemic in many third world countries where the dietary staple is predominantly carbohydrate rich and protein poor (e.g., white rice, cassava, and yams). It can also develop in response to trauma, severe burns, respiratory or renal failure, and nonmalignant gastrointestinal tract disease. Symptoms include edema, red sparse hair, sluggishness, irritability, various dermatoses, and short stature. The patients appear pale, have cold extremities, manifest hepatomegaly, and demonstrate a protruding abdomen. These patients are also immunocompromised, increasing their risk for acute and chronic infections. These patients also have deficiencies in essential amino acids, vitamins, and serum minerals.

Marasmus

Marasmus is the result of a chronic deficiency in total energy and protein intake. Worldwide, it is most common in underdeveloped areas in association with social upheaval and profound poverty. In the United States, it is seen in certain wasting illnesses such as cancer. Clinically, the patients have dry skin with reduced turgor. The skin is loose and wrinkled. They have a sunken facial appearance secondary to the loss of the buccal fat pad (one of the last subcutaneous fat deposits to be mobilized during starvation). They have thin, sparse hair. Metabolically, adaptive features include hypothermia, bradycardia, and hypotension. Hypoglycemia is common. Other laboratory findings tend to reflect the underlying illness (e.g., cancer) or complications (e.g., infections).

OBESITY

Obesity is the most common nutritional disorder in the United States. The prevalence ranges are given in Table 4.2. A child who is obese at age 6 years of age has a 25% chance of being obese as an adult. This increases to 75% if the child is obese at age 12 years. Obesity is determined by using body mass index (BMI) graphs. A child greater than 3 years of age with a BMI of 85%–95% is considered at risk for obesity. A BMI greater than 95% equals by definition obesity.

Obesity is the result of a person consistently having caloric intake exceeding caloric expenditure. The parent's obesity is either due to exogenous causes (lifestyle, etc.) or endogenous (e.g., hormonal). There exists an obvious inheritable pattern

TABLE 4.2
Prevalence of Obesity in Children

| | At-Risk for Overweight (BMI 85th–95th Percentile) | | | | Overweight (BMI >95th Percentile) | | | |
| | Age 6–11 Years | | Age 12–17 Years | | Age 6–11 Years | | Age 12–17 Years | |
	Boys	Girls	Boys	Girls	Boys	Girls	Boys	Girls
All	21.6 ± 2.4	22.7 ± 2.4	22.0 ± 2.2	21.4 ± 2.7	11.3 ± 1.8	12.8 ± 1.9	10.6 ± 1.3	8.8 ± 1.4
White	20.5 ± 2.8	21.5 ± 3.7	23.1 ± 3.1	20.3 ± 3.5	10.4 ± 2.4	14.4 ± 2.7	9.8 ± 2.0	8.3 ± 1.6
African American	26.5 ± 2.7	31.4 ± 4.0	21.1 ± 3.7	29.9 ± 4.5	13.4 ± 2.3	9.3 ± 2.4	16.9 ± 2.8	14.4 ± 3.1
Hispanic American	33.3 ± 3.0	29.0 ± 2.1	26.7 ± 4.6	23.4 ± 3.0	17.7 ± 2.3	12.8 ± 3.2	14.3 ± 1.7	8.7 ± 2.5

From: Kleinman, R. E. (Ed.). (2004). *Pediatric nutrition* (5th ed.). Washington, DC: American Academy of Pediatrics, p. 553.

to obesity. If one parent is obese, the risk is increased to 40%. If both parents are obese, the risk increases to 80%. The hereditary pattern is also manifested in studies of adopted children. These children reflect a BMI more consistent with their birth parents than their adoptive parents. Environmental risk factors include lack of the family meal, excess intake of sweetened beverages and fast foods, excessive TV or video game viewing, and sedentary lifestyle.

The evaluation for obesity is recommended for children younger than 2 years with a BMI greater than 85%, for severely obese children younger than 2 years old, or for any child with rapidly increasing weight. The evaluation includes a search for a family history of obesity, lifestyle questions concerning dietary habits, TV viewing, and activity level, determining linear growth (exogenous obesity frequently results in increased stature, and endogenous obesity results in short stature), measuring blood pressure, looking for signs of hypothyroidism, observing type of fat distribution, and observing for presence of acanthosis nigricans. In the absence of other risk factors (including cigarette smoking), a fasting lipid profile is probably a sufficient lab evaluation if BMI is 85%–95%. If other risk factors exist or if the BMI is >95%, a fasting insulin and glucose, liver enzymes, serum calcium and phosphorus, and an EKG should be included.

In the treatment of obesity, first treat any underlying condition. Otherwise, treatment centers on nutritional education, encouragement of physical activity, and behavior modification. Bariatric surgery is reserved for unresponsive and severe cases of obesity. As of this writing, there are no FDA-approved medications for treatment of obesity in children. The following are suggestions to be tried in the treatment of obesity:

- Limit television time to 1 to 2 hours per day.
- Do not eat in front of the television.
- Do not use the remote while watching television.
- Exercise during television commercials instead of surfing the channels.
- Do not have TV, VCR, or video games in the child's room.
- Decrease calories being consumed from beverages (e.g., sodas, juice drinks).
- Do not use food as a reward.
- Have parents act as role models in terms of eating and exercise.
- Encourage the family to eat meals and exercise together.
- Encourage multiple types of physical activity so that the child does not get bored and take into account different times of day and weather conditions.
- Encourage daily physical activity. (From *Pediatric nutrition handbook* [5th ed.], American Academy of Pediatrics, p. 579, 2004.)

Complications of obesity include:

- Insulin resistance (type 2 diabetes mellitus)
- Hyperlipidemia
- Hypertension
- Obstructive sleep apnea

- Obesity hypoventilation syndrome (pickwickian syndrome): CO_2 retention, hypoxia, polycythemia, right ventricular hypertrophy
- Acanthosis nigricans
- Intertrigo
- Slipped capital femoral epiphysis
- Blount disease of the tibia
- Hepatic steatosis and fibrosis
- Cholelithiasis
- Gastroesophageal reflux
- Early puberty
- Advanced skeletal development: tall child, short adult
- Ovarian hyperandrogenism
- Idiopathic intracranial hypertension (Modified from Styne, D. M., & Schoenfeld-Warden, N. *Rudolph's pediatrics* [21st ed.], Appleton and Lange, 2003.)

FURTHER READING

Barness, L. A. (1997). Nutritional diseases. In E. F. Gilbert-Barness (Ed.), *Potter's pathology of the fetus and infant*. Philadelphia: Mosby Year Book.

Barness, L. A. (2007). Nutritional diseases. In E. Gilbert-Barness (Ed.), *Potter's pathology of the fetus, infant, and child*. New York: Elsevier.

Corkins, M. R. (2007). Pediatric nutrition: Growing up. *Nutrition in Clinical Practice, 22*(2), 153–154.

Crill, C. M., & Helms, R. A. (2007). The use of carnitine in pediatric nutrition. *Nutrition in Clinical Practice, 22*(2), 204–213.

Lands, L. C. (2007). Nutrition in pediatric lung disease. *Paediatric Respiratory Reviews, 8*(4), 305–312.

Rosenbaum, M., & Leibel, R. L. (1998). Pathophysiology of childhood obesity. *Advances in Pediatrics, 35*, 73–77.

Styne, D. M., & Schoenfeld-Warden, N. (2003). *Rudolph's pediatrics* (21st ed.). Philadelphia: Appleton and Lange.

Terrill, C. J. (2007). Nutrition and the pediatric patient with CKD. *Nephrology Nursing Journal, 34*(1), 89–92.

Walker, W. A., Sherman, P., Cohen, M., & Barnard, J. (2007). State of pediatric gastroenterology, hepatology, and nutrition: 2006 and beyond. *Gastroenterology, 132*(1), 434–436.

Wiskin, A. E., Wootton, S. A., & Beattie, R. M. (2007). Nutrition issues in pediatric Crohn's disease. *Nutrition in Clinical Practice, 22*, 214–222.

5

HEAD AND NECK

Friends, Romans, and countrymen, lend me your ears.

William Shakespeare, Julius Caesar, *Act III, Scene 1*

THE HEAD AND neck grow rapidly in the first few years of life and alter the appearance of the child from infancy to childhood and throughout adolescence.

HEAD

By age 1 month, the infant in a prone position will usually hold the head dorsally. At 3 months of age, the normal infant holds the head steady when held upright by the physician. Failure to hold the head up usually indicates poor motor development. Head nodding may be normal, but it is usually seen in children who have emotional issues or are mentally retarded or who have spasmus nutans.

Note the amount, color, and texture of the hair. The newborn infant usually has hair that is fully replaced beginning at about 3 months of age, though substantial new hair growth may not be observed until 9–24 months. Lack of hair (alopecia) may be a familial characteristic or a manifestation of ectodermal dysplasia, hyperthyroidism, or progeria. Localized alopecia (alopecia areata) is seen in ringworm or other infections of the scalp and in acrodynia, but in infants it is most commonly caused by rubbing of localized areas when the infant lies in one position for a long time. Rarely, alopecia areata is seen in children with syphilis or hypervitaminosis A or in children who pull out the hair or occurs after severe systemic disease (e.g., typhoid fever). Other causes include the following:

- Exposures
  X-ray
  Caustics
- Neoplasms
  Lymphoma
  Carcinoma
  Mycosis fungoides
- Skin diseases
  Bullous dermatoses

Sarcoid
Discoid lupus
Leprosy
Exfoliate dermatoses
Acrodermatitis enteropathica
• Other
Collagen diseases (such as scleroderma)
Scalp infections
After antimetabolite or heparin therapy
Arsenic or thallium poisoning
Thyroid disease
Iron deficiency
Biotin deficiency

Hair is normally smooth and of fine texture. Children with hypothyroidism, hypo-parathyroidism, ringworm of the scalp, and argininosuccinicaciduria, a rare inborn error, have brittle hair. Fine hair may be seen in any of the states causing alopecia. Fine hair distinguishes hypopituitarism from primary thyroid disease, in which the hair is coarse and brittle. Hair that is either twisted, irregularly constricted, woolly, or irregularly pigmented may be inherited as an isolated anomaly. Children with the inborn metabolic condition of Menkes kinky hair disease have steely hair. Examine the hair for the presence of pediculi or nits.

Note the shape of the head and face. Children with premature or irregular closure of the sutures exhibit marked asymmetry of the head. Flattening of part of the head or face occurs in an infant who lies in only one position (positional plagiocephaly) or who has unusually soft bones. In children with rickets or delayed physical or mental development, the back of the head is flat. One side of the head and face is also flattened in children with torticollis or may appear flattened in children with facial palsy.

Examine the scalp. Special lesions may be noted in newborns. Scaling and crusting of the scalp, if generalized, are usually due to seborrheic dermatitis or eczema; if localized, they may be caused by ringworm. Note infections of the scalp. Lymph nodes and subcutaneous nodules are identified by careful palpation, especially around the occiput. Tinea capitis can result in kerion formation with significant regional lymphadenopathy.

Palpate the sutures. Usually, they are felt as ridges until infants are about 6 months of age. Note abnormal sutures, fractures, and fontanels. The posterior fontanel closes by the fourth month; the anterior fontanel usually closes by the end of the second year (Figure 5.1), normally occurring later in breast-fed infants.

Note the size and shape of the anterior fontanel by pressing lightly in the area of the opening. Normal infants less than 6 months of age occasionally may have a large fontanel (more than 4–5 cm in diameter), but it may also be diagnostic of chronically increased intracranial pressure, subdural hematoma, rickets, hypothyroidism, and osteogenesis imperfecta.

A tenseness or bulging of the fontanel is best noted if the patient is sitting. The normal fontanel may feel questionably tense in the infant who is supine. Tenseness

Anterior

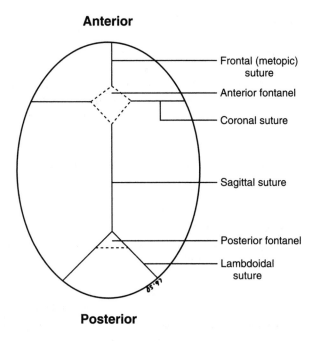

Frontal (metopic) suture

Anterior fontanel

Coronal suture

Sagittal suture

Posterior fontanel

Lambdoidal suture

Posterior

Figure 5.1
Diagram of the top of the head indicating position of fontanels and palpable sutures.

may be noted in the crying child but only during expiration; this physiologic bulging disappears when the patient relaxes or inspires. Persistent or true bulging or tenseness of the fontanel in the quiet infant in the sitting position usually accompanies an acute increase in intracranial pressure.

Bulging Fontanel—Pseudotumor Cerebri

Meningitis	Lead poisoning
Brain tumor	Retinoic acid
Pulmonary insufficiency	Tetracycline
Vitamin A excess	Nalidixic acid
Cortisone withdrawal	Subdural hematoma
Lateral sinus thrombosis	Roseola
Cardiac failure	

The fontanel is depressed in children with dehydration and malnutrition. A small fontanel is usually normal but is also an important sign of microcephaly in infants. Occasionally, the fontanel is closed with only fibrous tissue and will feel less firm than the surrounding skull. Fibrous closure should be noted, but physiologically it is comparable to an open fontanel. Bony closure usually occurs 1–2 months after fibrous closure. Closure of the fontanel may be delayed in children with hydrocephalus, rickets, or hypothyroidism. Rarely, delayed closure is due to syphilis or the osteo-chondrodystrophies.

Slight pulsations of the anterior fontanel occur in normal infants. However, marked pulsations may be a sign of increased intracranial pressure, venous sinus thrombosis, obstruction of the venous return from the head, or increased pulse pressure due to arteriovenous shunt, patent ductus arteriosus, or excitement. Aortic regurgitation is a rare cause of increased pulse pressure during the age when the fontanel is open.

Measure the circumference of the head. Until the child is 2 years of age, the circumference of the head is approximately the same as or slightly larger than that of the chest. Marked disproportions between the head and chest measurements indicate microcephaly, macrocephaly, or hydrocephaly. If the child's measurements are disproportionate, compare head and chest measurements with standards, since the chest itself may be large or small.

Microcephaly may be due to cerebral dysgenesis alone or to premature closure of the sutures (craniostenosis). Children with general growth failure rarely exhibit microcephaly.

Hydrocephalus, caused by chronic increase in intracranial pressure, is detected by noting an enlarged head, enlarged fontanel, supraorbital bulging, and open sutures. Dilated scalp veins are characteristic of early hydrocephalus. Hydrocephalus is an enlargement of the ventricular systems of the brain and may be due to blocking of the ventricular foramina (noncommunicating), blocking of the subarachnoid pathways (communicating), or, rarely, failure of the subarachnoid system to absorb cerebrospinal fluid (external).

Bulging of an area of the head occasionally occurs with brain tumors, lacunar defects of the skull, and intracranial masses. Bulging of the frontal areas (bossing) is characteristic of prematurity, rickets, and, occasionally, congenital syphilis.

Craniotabes is best detected by pressing the scalp firmly just behind and above the ears in the temporoparietal or parietooccipital region. Elicitation of a ping-pong ball-snapping sensation indicates craniotabes. It represents a softening of the outer table of the skull. Although infants with craniotabes sometimes cry, no danger is involved if the pressure is not so excessive that the inner table is pressed. Craniotabes is found in premature infants, in some normal children aged less than 6 months of age, in babies who lie constantly on one side of the head, and in children with rickets, syphilis, hypervitaminosis A, and hydrocephalus.

Macewen sign is one that many physicians like to elicit, but it usually has little significance in childhood. On percussing the skull, you hear a resonant "cracked pot" sound. As long as the fontanel is open, this type of sound is physiologic. After closure of the fontanel, the sound indicates increased intracranial pressure or a dilated ventricle.

Percuss the head in children with neurologic disorders in the indirect manner similar to that described for percussion of the heart. When the head is carefully percussed, you can occasionally elicit dullness near the sagittal sinus. This is a good sign of subdural hematoma.

Tenderness or pain over the occiput may indicate the presence of brain tumor or abscess. Pain over the scalp may accompany cerebral hemorrhage, migraine, trauma, hypertension, vascular neuralgia, anxiety, or depressive states. Press hard over the malar bones for a few seconds and then release. Functional headaches may be improved by this maneuver, but headaches with other causes will not change. Pressure over the temporomandibular joint while jaws are clenched might indicate TMJ syndrome.

In children aged more than 2–3 years of age, percuss the frontal and maxillary sinuses in the same manner or by the direct method for tenderness. Tenderness might indicate acute sinusitis. Swelling or tenderness elicited by pressure deep in the bony angle above the inner canthus of the eye is characteristic of acute ethmoiditis. It is difficult and generally unnecessary to transilluminate the sinuses in young children. The maxillary sinuses can be transilluminated after they are developed (see Table 5.1). Also observe mastoids for redness and tenderness.

Auscultation over the skull with the bell stethoscope may reveal a swishing sound (bruit) of blood flowing through dilated vascular channels. Systolic or continuous bruits may be heard normally in children until age 4 years or in children with anemia; after this age, systolic bruits suggest the presence of vascular anomalies, especially arteriovenous (A-V) malformations or increased intracranial pressure. Similar noise is sometimes heard in children with meningitis. Transmitted cardiac murmurs may sometimes be heard as bruits over the skull. Press over the carotid artery. The bruit disappears if it is not due to A-V malformation.

Determine direction of blood flow in the scalp veins in children with suspected intracranial abnormalities. You may need to shave the scalp first to determine blood flow, but this procedure occasionally reveals vascularity or vascular channels indicative of underlying abnormalities. Small ossification defects through which the dura protrudes may occur in the skull. Small defects are termed *lückenschädel*, and large defects are termed *encephaloids*. Nerve tissue protrudes in children with encephaloceles. Encephaloceles may be present anywhere in the skull and are sometimes apparent near the inner canthus of the eye. Another congenital scalp defect is cutis aplasia, a usually small area of full-thickness hair loss. On the shaved scalp, note also the presence of dimples, which may be an indication of a dermal sinus or hemangiomas. These are infrequent but sometimes remediable causes of seizures or meningitis. Scalp veins may appear dilated in very young infants; they also may indicate

TABLE 5.1
Development of Sinuses

Sinus	Present	Developed
Ethmoid	Birth	3 yr
Maxillary	Birth	3 yr
Sphenoid	3 yr	12 yr
Frontal	8 yr	12 yr
Mastoid	Birth	3 yr

the presence of hydrocephalus, tumors, subdural hematoma, or congenital vascular anomaly.

Transilluminate the skull of children suspected of having intracranial lesions. Hold the otoscope light so that a tight fit is made with the child's scalp. The room must be quite dark. A sharply delineated area of increased light transmission may be noted over a subdural hygroma. Place a bright light at the occiput of infants suspected of having anencephaly. The light is transmitted through the eyes in anencephalic infants, and you will observe this response as pinkness of the retina.

FACE

Note the shape of the face. An easy way to determine facial paralysis is to observe the child while he or she is crying, whistling, or smiling. The paralyzed or weakened side will remain immobile, and the innervated side will wrinkle. The lips will rise only on the intact side, and the angle of the mouth may droop on the paralyzed side. Wrinkling of the forehead should be noted.

Unilateral paralysis of the face excluding the muscles of the forehead indicates a central facial nerve (supranuclear) weakness and may be seen in children with cerebral palsy or other brain lesions. Unilateral paralysis of the face including the muscles of the forehead and eyelid indicates a peripheral facial nerve lesion and may be due to trauma, otitis media, viral infections, Lyme disease, or other peripheral lesions. Recovery from peripheral facial nerve palsy may occur in the upper portion of the face first and, at this point, the palsy may resemble a supranuclear weakness. Bilateral facial diplegia is a characteristic of Guillain-Barré syndrome.

Salivary flow can be measured by placing polyethylene tubes in the submaxillary ducts. Stimulate salivation by placing a slice of lemon on the tongue. Count the drops that occur in 1 minute. If measured in a child with peripheral facial palsy, salivary flow will be at least 40% of normal in those palsies that spontaneously recover.

Paralysis and asymmetry about the mouth only are usually caused by a peripheral trigeminal nerve lesion with weakness of the masseter muscles. Jaw strength can be tested by asking the child to bite on a tongue depressor on each side of the mouth. Beware of the possibility of malocclusion, which may give the impression of weakness. Isolated congenital asymmetric smile might also be the result of asymmetric development of orbicularis oris musculature.

Trismus (contracture of the facial muscles) gives the child a sardonic smile (risus sardonicus), which occurs in tetany caused by hypocalcemia, tetanus, or phenothiazine sensitivity and may occur with streptococcal pharyngitis.

Local swellings about the face are usually due to edema. Edema only in the face may be due to any of the causes of generalized edema, as well as allergy. However, enlargement of the mandible in infants may be due to infantile cortical hyperostosis (Caffey syndrome) or vitamin A poisoning and may be mistaken for parotitis. Large jaws due to fibrous swelling with upward turning of the eyes is seen in cherubism. A small mandible (micrognathia) is usually a congenital anomaly sometimes associated with certain syndromes, but may be seen in children with rheumatoid arthritis.

To determine local swelling of the parotid glands, sit the child upright, ask the child to look toward the ceiling, and note the swelling below the angle of the jaw. Next, run the flat part of your finger downward from the zygomatic arch. The swollen parotid is then felt. Confirm it by telling the child to lie supine. The parotid falls back like jelly and pushes the pinna of the ear forward. Parotid swelling has these causes:

Mumps	Allergy
Stone in parotid duct	Leukemia
Blowing balloon or wind instrument	Starch eaters
Bacterial infections in debilitated children	Persistent vomiting
Sarcoid	

Parotid swelling with lacrimal duct swelling is Mikulicz syndrome. Tumors and cysts occasionally occur in the parotid area in children. Firm swelling of the parotids (parotid sialadenitis) is usually self-limited; it may be caused by animal scratch diseases or may be seen in children who compulsively eat starch. Nontender parotid swelling may precede the onset of diabetes mellitus. Enlargement of the masseter muscles may be mistaken for parotid swelling and occurs in those who excessively chew bubble gum or binge eaters with bulimia.

Palpate the area under the jaw for glands or tenderness. Submaxillary glands are felt best by palpating lightly just below the mandible, anterior to the angle of the jaw, or by lightly rubbing this area with the fingertips. Sublingual glands are similarly palpated just behind the bony portion of the chin. These glands are ordinarily not palpable, and enlargement or tenderness usually indicates mumps, cystic fibrosis, local infection, infection in the teeth or, rarely, stones in the ducts. Recurrent swelling occurs with Sjögren syndrome. Unilateral submandibular or submaxillary swelling is more common with atypical mycobacteria, and bilateral swelling is more common with human tubercle bacilli.

Abnormal or unusual facial appearance is also seen in many children with generalized dystrophies, and some of these conditions have characteristic facies. Congenital abnormalities may be seen. Coarse facial features occur in children with mucopolysaccharidoses, hypothyroidism, multiple sulfatase deficiency, I cell disease, Job syndrome, other gangliosidoses, and Coffin-Siris syndrome.

Hypertelorism appears as a large distance between the eyes and occurs with a broadened nasal bridge. It is measured as an increased interpupillary distance and reflects the spacing of the orbits. It is due to overdevelopment of the lesser wing of the sphenoid bone. If the medial canthus is displaced laterally, telecanthus, a similar appearance, may exist. Both conditions may be normal variants. Hypertelorism with other midfacial anomalies usually occurs in children who are mentally normal. If hypertelorism is extreme or occurs with anomalies other than those of the head and face, the probability of intellectual impairment is higher (Figure 5.2).

Infants with hypotelorism and midface anomalies are almost always intellectually impaired. The normal interpupillary space is approximately 3.5–5.5 cm. For

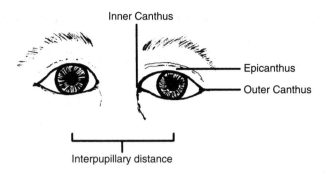

Figure 5.2
Measuring interpupillary distance.

small eyes, measure the palpebral fissure (the distance between the inner and outer canthus) with a tape. For premature infants, this fissure normally measures about 1.5 cm at 32 weeks of gestation and increases to about 1.8 cm for term infants. Infants with fetal alcohol syndrome have shortened palpebral fissures.

Twitchings of the face are usually due to tics or habit spasms, but they may be caused by muscular exhaustion or fasciculation.

To obtain Chvostek sign, tap the cheek of the child just below the zygoma with your finger. If the sign is present, that side of the face will grimace. It is difficult to elicit Chvostek sign in children under 2 weeks of age or in children who are crying. Chvostek sign may be present in normal children under 1 month or over 5 years of age. If this sign is present in children between these ages, it indicates hyperirritability and may be found with tetanus, tetany, and hyperventilation.

EARS

Except in thermolabile children, suppurative otitis media a common cause of fever without obvious reason in childhood is acute otitis. Examine the ears of all sick children.

Various anomalies of the ears occur (Figure 5.3). Obvious deformities of the auricle may be associated with other anomalies. Occasionally, a small sinus is present as a hole or pit just in front of the ear and this may be accompanied by a small swelling just inside the canal; this represents the remnant of the first brachial cleft. Large protruding auricles are a feature of children with fragile X syndrome. Lack of cartilage in the auricle may be a sign of relapsing polychondritis.

Note the position of the ears. In infants with Potter syndrome, the tops of the ears are below the level of the eye and there is congenital absence of the kidneys (as well as in children with Down syndrome). Also in Down syndrome patients, total lobe length is < 3 cm. In fragile X, the ear lobes are larger than normal. Other gross anomalies of the ears may be associated with lesser kidney anomalies and with chromosome abnormalities.

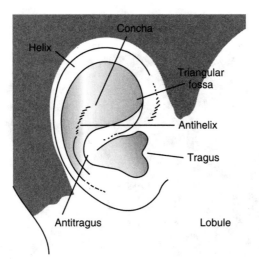

Figure 5.3
The external ear.

The auricles frequently appear to stand forward with any mass or swelling behind the ear. Important conditions causing this appearance are mastoiditis, cellulitis, mumps, and postauricular abscesses. Occasionally, enlarged postauricular nodes or external otitis with surrounding cellulitis makes the ears protrude.

Note the nature and odor of discharge from the aural canals. A greenish, foul-smelling discharge occurs with pyogenic infections. Purulent discharges are seen with any bacterial infection, particularly *Streptococcus pneumoniae* and *Mycobacterium tuberculosis*, but may also occur with fungal infections of the canal wall. Generalized eczema may cause flaking in the ears. Bloody discharge is usually due to scratching, irritation, or injury of the ear canal, but may occur with a foreign body in the canal or be a cardinal sign of basilar skull fracture. In the presence of PE tubes, ear drainage might represent an infection.

Next, use the otoscope (Figure 5.4). First, use an otoscope that is halogen illuminated and operating properly with fresh batteries, or the light will turn yellow. Second, use the largest possible speculum. The speculum should never enter the canal more than 10–15 mm. Using the 1 or 2 mm speculum, even in infants, will only cloud the field and hurt the patient. Third, examine the canal before you try to look at the drum to note the presence of a furuncle or vesicle in the outer edge of the canal. If you hit a furuncle with the otoscope, the child will feel pain and the examination will probably end. Fourth, hold the otoscope firmly with one hand and, as the speculum is inserted, rest the hand holding the otoscope firmly on the child's head or face so that any motion by the child will be accompanied by a similar movement of the otoscope. Fifth, placing the speculum just inside the canal of one ear and then the other before attempting to examine the drum is also valuable. This assures

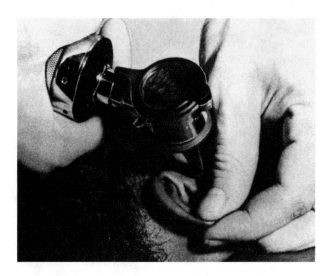

Figure 5.4
Using the otoscope. The hand holding the otoscope rests
firmly on the patient's head or face.

the child that the procedure will not hurt. Examining the child's doll or the parent's
ear first or pretending to look for an elephant in the child's ear may also reassure the
child. Finally, before using the otoscope, remember the direction of the canal. In
infants, the canal is directed upward, so the auricle should be pulled down to view
the drum. In older children, the canal faces downward and forward; therefore, pull
the tip of the auricle up and back for adequate visualization. Pulling the external ear
serves another useful purpose. Ordinarily, this movement is painless in children
with otitis media and in children without an ear infection, but it is painful in children
with a furuncle in the ear or external otitis.

Examination of the ears should be almost painless. Allow the child to play with
the otoscope, but handle the child firmly at the time of the examination. Either the
child assures you of cooperation or the parent holds the child so that the head does
not move and the hands do not interfere. The child should be placed face down and
prone with the head turned first to one side, then the other. Tell the child that the
speculum plays a song but that the child must be very quiet to hear it. After examining the first ear, ask the child if the song was heard. Then repeat the procedure in
the opposite ear.

The canal and auricle may be swollen in children with external otitis, as occurs
with seborrhea and allergic dermatitis or in children who frequently place foreign
bodies in the canal. Note any tenderness. Tenderness as the speculum is placed in the
canal may indicate disease of the canal, such as a furuncle, or disease of the middle ear
(otitis media). Vesicles in the canal may be due to viral canal infections or otitis media
caused by *Haemophilus influenzae*. If cerumen is present, a large-enough speculum
frequently allows you to look above or below the wax at the drum. If a small, easily

reached foreign body or obstructive wax is present, it is best removed with an ear spoon or wire loop. You may see ear tubes in the drum or lying free in the canal.

Discharges may arise from the canal, external otitis, otitis media with perforation of the drum, or chronic otitis media with mastoiditis. Swimmer's discharge is usually due to Gram-negative bacilli. Greenish discharge is usually from external otitis. Mucoid or mucopurulent discharge most often arises from the middle ear. Carefully wipe away discharges with a soft, cotton-tipped applicator. Be careful to blot the discharge so that nothing is pushed against the ear drum, which may be perforated. Do not use cotton-tipped applicators to remove hard wax or foreign bodies.

Rarely, you may resort to use of an ear syringe to remove adherent wax. First, soften the wax with a detergent. Fit the syringe with a narrow fistula tip to provide a thin stream. Fill the syringe with lukewarm water (cover the patient to prevent soaking), and introduce it gently into the tip of the canal, which is then flushed. In examination of children, this procedure is unpleasant and undesirable because a vestibular response, frequently with vomiting, may be induced. It should never be performed if perforation of the drum is suspected or if a foreign body is in the canal.

Pathogens of acute otitis media include the following:

S. pneumoniae (35%)
H. influenzae (23%)
M. catarrhalis (14%)
S. pyogenes (3%)
S. aureus (1%)
No growth (16%)
Ampicillin resistant (1%)

These microorganisms have been obtained in the percentages shown from aspirates of middle ear effusions of patients seen at Children's Hospital of Pittsburgh, 1979–1980. Studies at other medical centers have yielded similar findings.

The normal drum (Figure 5.5) is gray-white and translucent or opalescent. The handle of the malleus appears as a small white streak running down and back to the center of the ear and ends at the umbo. At the upper end of the malleus is a small white projection, the short process of the malleus. Below the umbo is a small circle of light, the light reflex. Even in infants, in whom the drum is almost horizontal, determine these landmarks. As the child grows older, the drum becomes vertical but points inward. The light reflex becomes cone shaped and sharply outlined, with the apex at the center and the base at the antero-inferior portion of the drum.

Acute otitis media is the term used to describe acute infection and inflammation of the middle ear with a purulent effusion in the middle ear space. Associated inflammation and edema of the mucosa of the eustachian tube appears to play a role in the pathogenesis by impeding drainage of the middle ear fluid. In some children, anatomic or chronic physiologic abnormalities of the eustachian tube predispose to infection.

The most common abnormality of the drum noted on otoscopic examination is slight redness. This may be due to crying or to manipulation. If the drum is slightly

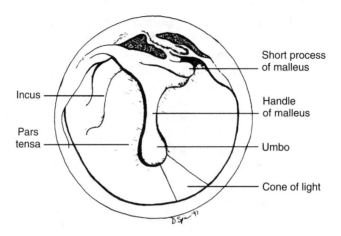

Figure 5.5
Diagram of the tympanic membrane.

to markedly reddened and retracted, as noted by the prominence of the malleus and a deeper and sharper outline of the cone of light, and if the vessels are prominent, catarrhal otitis media is present. This is usually due to any upper respiratory infection, usually viral, or to obstruction of the eustachian tube. The light reflex may appear less prominent than usual.

In acute suppurative otitis media, the light reflex is usually lost, the drum bulges outward and becomes diffusely red, the handle of the malleus is not clearly apparent, and hearing is usually decreased. Occasionally with a bulging drum, the light reflex is scattered diffusely over the drum area instead of being lost. Recognize that this reflex is coming from a convex drum, since the handle of the malleus is not observed. Otitis media in young infants may be due to congenital syphilis in addition to the usual causes of suppuration, such as *H. influenzae*, pneumococci, streptococci, staphylococci, and viruses. Otitis, sometimes with mastoiditis and abducens paralysis of the homolateral eye, occurs with petrositis (Gradenigo syndrome). Chronic otitis may be due to tuberculosis or other bacterial infections, immune defects, allergy, and histiocytosis. It may also be associated with enlarged adenoids, cleft palate, and mastoiditis. Infants who have been fed frequently with a propped bottle or in the supine position may have otitis.

Bulging may also be due to nonpurulent fluid. This occurs in children with late catarrhal otitis media or suppurative otitis in which the bacterial infection has resolved but the exudate has not yet been resorbed (serous otitis). Bulging with a bluish discoloration of the drum may be due to a collection of blood in the middle ear and occurs after trauma and sometimes after infections. Blood behind the drum suggests basilar skull fracture.

The drum may be perforated. Perforation with pus indicates acute or chronic purulent otitis media. Small perforations may be seen in the drum due to injury, insect bites, or chronic tuberculosis. You may prefer to quantitate the conducting mechanism of the ear by tympanometry, which helps document fluid in the inner ear, drum perforation, and other changes in air and sound conduction.

Myringitis may be indicated if you find varying degrees of redness of the drum, with possibly some loss of the light reflex but without bulging or retraction or evidence of fluid in the middle ear, especially if associated with exquisite pain and little hearing loss. Myringitis is a primary inflammation of the drum head without involvement of the middle ear or may be an early stage of otitis media.

Occasionally, you will see a small spherical mass (usually gray, red, or yellow) just in front of or behind the drum: a cholesteatoma (Figure 5.6). A pinpoint perforation may accompany it in the posterosuperior or central portion of the drum.

Note mobility of the drum. This requires a tight-fitting otoscope and speculum with a hole through which a puff of air can be introduced with an attached rubber bulb. Another option is to attach a tube to the otoscope, place the other end in your mouth, and blow in and suck out. The light reflex and drum will move. Acoustic reflectometry uses sound instead of air pressure to determine movement. In suppurative or serous otitis media, the drum is immovable. Serous otitis is a condition that results in conductive hearing loss. It may be caused by allergies, chronic infections, hypothyroidism, obesity, or anything that contributes to the closure of the eustachian tube. In children with osteopetrosis, the drum is also immovable.

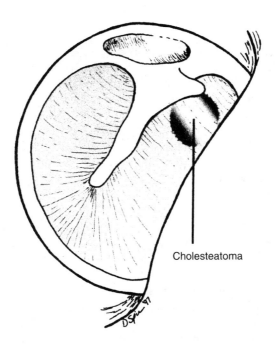

Cholesteatoma

Figure 5.6
A site for cholesteatoma.

Next, feel and tap the mastoid tip of the temporal bone. Note any fluctuation or tenderness; either may indicate mastoiditis. Just behind the mastoid, feel for the postauricular nodes. In children, these are normally about 1 or 2 mm in diameter. Enlarged nodes are characteristic of German measles (rubella), nits, or inflammation of the scalp and are usually slightly tender. They are also found in children with measles, roseola, varicella, infectious mononucleosis, leukemia, and tick bites. In this area, you may occasionally feel subcutaneous nodules about 2–5 mm in diameter. These nodules are characteristic of active rheumatic fever.

Estimate hearing. In small children, make a sharp noise at the child's ear and note a blinking of the eyes. Each ear is tested separately while you stand outside the direct line of vision of the child. In older children, testing by using the whispered voice at a distance of about 20 cm (8 inches) is sufficient. This is best done by asking the child simple questions or whispering a simple command. Nothing is quite so gratifying as diagnosing impaired hearing in a child who was believed to be intellectually delayed.

Loss of hearing can be conductive, neurosensory, or mixed. Most intellectually normal children older than 3 years are cooperative enough to be tested with a tuning fork. If your hearing is normal, press the tip of the vibrating tuning fork against the mastoid process of the child and then your own. Compare the number of seconds it is heard by both of you. If the child hears it for a shorter time than you, decreased bone conduction is indicated—a sign of neurosensory hearing loss. If the child hears it longer, conductive loss is indicated (Schwabach test). Compare air and bone conduction in the patient. First place the fork on the mastoid as before and then place it about 1 inch from the child's ear, with approximately equal vibratory stimulus. Normally, air conduction lasts twice as long as bone conduction (Rinne test). Then place the vibrating fork on the middle of the child's forehead and ask in which ear the child hears the sound better. In unilateral conductive deafness, the hearing is better in the unaffected side (Weber test). In unilateral neurosensory deafness, the hearing is better in the affected ear.

Hearing loss may be due simply to a foreign body or cerumen in the canals. Defective hearing may be noted in children with chronic catarrhal otitis media associated with enlarged adenoids or other nasal obstruction, in children who have received dihydrostreptomycin, or in children who have had meningitis, encephalitis, kernicterus, or Hunter syndrome. Congenital deafness is usually idiopathic, but may be found in children whose mothers had rubella during the first trimester of pregnancy. Unilateral deafness may be a sequela of mumps. Deafness associated with syncope may be due to congenital heart lesions (Jervell and Lange-Nielsen syndrome). Deafness may be associated with hereditary renal disease with hyperprolinemia or with a white forelock and eye abnormalities (Waardenburg syndrome). Pseudodeafness may be observed in psychotic children, especially those with autism, or in children with mental delay. Children with more complicated types of deafness should be referred to an otologist. Hyperacute hearing may occur in children with Tay-Sachs or lysosomal storage diseases or tetanus.

Children who have received amnioglycosides or who have nystagmus or an unsteady gait or dizziness (vertigo) should have their vestibular function tested. The cold caloric test usually suffices. Seat the patient and inject water of 65°F (18°C) into the ear. Nystagmus should appear within 30 seconds, with the fast movement opposite the injected ear. Fast movement toward the injection suggests CNS disease. Repeat the test in the opposite ear. Nystagmus should persist almost equally (for about 1–2 minutes) on each side. Lack of nystagmus suggests lack of labyrinth function or vestibular or brain stem disease. This may be due to amnioglycoside medication, labyrinthitis, meningitis, or brain tumor, or it may be a sign of benign paroxysmal vertigo. Vertigo with tinnitus and fluctuating hearing loss is characteristic of Ménière disease. Dizziness with progressive hearing loss and facial or corneal numbness occurs with acoustic neuroma. Acute vertigo with nausea and vomiting followed by dysarthria, dysphagia, or unilateral weakness suggests infarct in the medulla with posterior cerebellar or vertebral artery involvement (Wallenberg syndrome). Hiccups may accompany the vertigo. Vertigo with nystagmus that occurs after air pressure is exerted on the drum indicates a fistula, especially with cholesteatoma.

NOSE

Examination of the nose, even a superficial examination, is often neglected, yet it may hold the key to the proper diagnosis.

Note any unusual shape of the nose. Because the lower half of the nasal septum is cartilage, fracture or dislocation of the nose is rare in childhood. Deviation is occasionally observed in newborns, possibly due to intrauterine position. The chief cause of flattening of the nose in childhood is cleft palate. With cleft palate or injury, the nasal septum is deflected and the nose appears flattened. A saddle-shaped nose is characterized by a low bridge and broad base. This is usually a familial characteristic but also occurs in children with hypertelorism or following perforation of the septum, as in congenital syphilis.

Note flaring of the alae nasi. The alae flare with all types of respiratory obstruction or distress but particularly with pneumonia. Flaring of the alae nasi may be seen in children with fevers, acidosis, peritonitis, or any condition or illness causing anoxia.

Next, shine a light up the nose and note the color of the mucosa. If you push the tip of the nose upward with the thumb of your left hand and hold the light with your right hand, you can frequently see high into the nose. A speculum is usually not necessary for satisfactory examination of the mucosa or the ostia of the sinuses. If a nasal speculum is desired, use the spring type rather than the otoscope speculum. By placing the large otoscope speculum in the tip of the nose, you can examine the area to the middle meatus. The nasal speculum is preferably used with a head mirror, but satisfactory examination can be performed with a hand light if the patient's head is held firmly. A red, inflamed mucosa indicates infection, including sinusitis. A pale, boggy mucosa may indicate allergy. A swollen grayish mucosa may indicate chronic rhinitis.

Note the character of secretions. Purulent secretions are common with any nasal infection, even the usual upper respiratory infection in its later stages, or may be an early sign of the contagious diseases, particularly measles, pertussis, and poliomyelitis. Purulent secretions from the ostia above or below the middle turbinates indicate sinusitis; pus in the middle meatus suggests involvement of the maxillary, frontal, or anterior ethmoid sinuses; and pus in the superior meatus suggests involvement of the posterior ethmoid or sphenoid sinuses. Patients with discharge and crusting below or on the edges of the alae nasi, particularly with redness of the surrounding skin (i.e., impetigo), usually have infections with β-hemolytic streptococci. Purulent discharges may also be caused by *H. influenzae* or *S. pneumoniae*. Purulent or bloody secretions in infancy may be a sign of secondary syphilis. When due to syphilis, such secretions may occur in children until age 6 months and are usually associated with excoriations of the upper lip.

Watery nasal secretions may indicate allergy, the common cold, foreign bodies high in the nose, illicit drug use, or, rarely, skull fracture or perforated encephalocele. Unilateral possibly purulent foul-smelling secretions suggest foreign body, nasal diphtheria, nasal polyps, and sinusitis.

Note bleeding points in the nose. They are most commonly found at the lower anterior tip of the septum. Epistaxis is rare in infancy and, if present, may indicate a bleeding dyscrasia. The usual cause of epistaxis, hemoptysis, and hematemesis in children is irritation or injury of the nasal mucosa. Epistaxis is especially common in children with allergic rhinitis. Other less common causes of epistaxis include nasal infections (particularly diphtheria), typhoid fever, leukemia, rheumatic fever, foreign body, and congestion due to any cause such as congenital heart disease. Occasionally, epistaxis in childhood is caused by late syphilis, elevated blood pressure due to any cause, or any of the anemias or bleeding diseases. Bleeding after skull injury may be due to local nasal injury or to skull fracture. Rarely, a bleeding telangiectasis is noted in the mucosa and may be the cardinal sign of familial telangiectasia. Epistaxis may be the only physical sign of hereditary hemorrhagic thrombasthenia, one of the bleeding diseases. If a nasal fracture is present, need for treatment is based on degree of displacement. Also, a septal hematoma needs to be treated promptly.

Causes of Epistaxis (Nosebleed)

- Trauma
  Digital trauma (nose picking)
  Foreign body
  Air pollution
- Inflammation
  Upper respiratory infection (viral or bacterial)
  Rhinitis
- Anatomic
  Nasal septal deviation
- Platelet dysfunction
  NSAID use, especially aspirin
  Idiopathic thrombocytopenic purpura
  Leukemia
- Coagulopathy
  von Willebrand disease
  Hemophilia

Liver disease
Anticoagulants (coumadin, heparin)
- Benign masses
Nasopharyngeal angiofibroma: only in adolescent males
Pyogenic granuloma
Papilloma
- Malignant neoplasms
Rhabdomyosarcoma
Lymphoma
- Vascular abnormalities
Hemangioma

Note the child's ability to get air through the nose. A convenient test for this is to determine the child's ability to make the *m*, *n*, and *ng* sounds. Infection, foreign body, vasomotor rhinitis, tumor, polyp, or a badly deviated septum are the usual causes of inability to breathe through the nose. Newborns with bilateral choanal atresia are unable to get air through the nostrils and often appear to be choking. In the older child, large adenoids, even if uninfected, may cause nasal obstruction with a typical adenoid facies. Obstruction with recurrent epistaxis, especially in teenage boys, suggests angiofibroma.

An unusually large nasal airway with dry crusting is occasionally noted. This may be a sign of atrophic rhinitis, which occurs in older children or adults. A malodorous nasal discharge may be present. Observe for a transverse nasal crease, a good clinical sign of allergic rhinitis.

Allergic rhinitis, characterized by inflammation, edema, and weeping of the nasal mucosa, is the most common of all allergic disorders and occurs in 10%–20% of the population. Common presenting symptoms include nasal congestion and pruritus, clear rhinorrhea, and paroxysms of sneezing. Older children blow their noses frequently, younger children do not. Instead, they sniff, snort, and repetitively clear their throats.

In the older child, examine the nasal septum. Perforation may be due to injury of the nasal septum, foreign body, syphilis, tuberculosis, or sniffing of illicit drugs.

Occasionally polyps or tumors may occlude one nostril or even protrude from the nose. Polyps frequently occur with allergy but may be a manifestation of chronic infection, cystic fibrosis, or generalized polyposis. An encephalocele may protrude through the cribriform plate and appear to be a polyp. If you observe a membrane in the nose preceded by bleeding, consider diphtheria until this diagnosis can be eliminated.

Percuss the sinus areas for evidence of pain as previously described. Olfactory nerve tests are generally not performed in childhood. Anosmia is a sign of Kallmann syndrome, zinc deficiency, and chronic nasal infection.

MOUTH AND THROAT

Defer examination of the mouth and throat until the end of the examination in young children. For you to see the posterior pharynx and particularly the epiglottis during gagging, the child must be sitting and cooperative or adequately restrained when the depressor is finally placed far in the mouth. If a parent or an assistant is present, the child can sit on that person's lap. Ask the parent or assistant to hold both the child's wrists with one hand and the forehead with the other (Figure 5.7). Examine the external structures first.

Around the mouth, note circumoral pallor. With circumoral pallor, the immediate area around the mouth appears white, and the philtrum below the nose, the surface of the cheeks, and the lower chin are red. This appearance may occur with any febrile disease, but it is particularly noted in children who have just exercised or who have scarlet or rheumatic fever or hypoglycemia. Even in infants with seborrheic dermatitis and eczema, this pale area usually remains free of lesions, although the remainder of the cheeks may be covered with scales. A flattened philtrum is associated with fetal alcohol syndrome.

Inspect the lips. Asymmetry of the mouth with twisting of the lips to one side occurs with facial nerve or trigeminal nerve paralysis. Cleft lip, usually on the left side, is a congenital anomaly. Note extent and location of the cleft. Lip pits may appear as isolated deformities or may be associated with other anomalies.

Slight fissures of the lips (cheilitis) occur in children exposed to wind and sun and in children with Kawasaki disease. Rhagades are deep fissures or their resultant scars extending from the nose to the lips and extending outward from the lips. They are

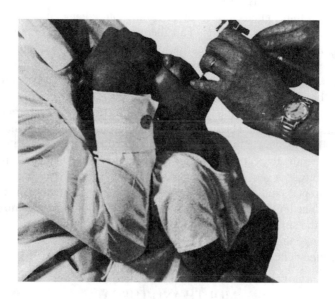

Figure 5.7
Restraint of patient in sitting position to examine posterior pharynx and epiglottis.

characteristic of congenital syphilis. Deep painful fissures radiating from the ends of the lips (cheilosis) are apparent in children with numerous nutritional disturbances, particularly riboflavin and other B vitamin, protein, or iron deficiencies, or with *Candida* and other infections. Excoriation of the upper lip is common in young children with simple upper respiratory infections. Painful ulcers on the lips and adjacent tissues are characteristic of erythema multiforme, but if chronic may be due to squamous cell carcinoma.

Vesicles and pustules appear on the lips in older children, especially after upper respiratory infections. Cold sores (herpes simplex) are vesicles at the vermillion border on an inflamed base and usually burn or itch. Bacterial infections are detected as ordinary pustules. Retention cysts, usually single, occur on the lip and appear as small protrusions containing clear fluid.

Note the color of the lips. The normal pink of white children and gray of black children is replaced by a pale mucosa when anemia is present. Gray cyanosis is seen with most congenital heart lesions, methemoglobinemia, anoxia, and bizarre poisons. Deep purple lips are seen with severe congenital heart disease. Cherry red lips are characteristically seen in infants and children with acidosis and are frequently due to aspirin poisoning or diabetes in older children and in patients with carbon monoxide poisoning. With many poisons, the child's lips may appear red although the body is pallid. Telangiectases in the lips may herald Rendu-Osler-Weber syndrome (familial telangiectasia).

The lips may be grossly swollen due to insect bites, local infection or injury, angioneurotic edema, or massive generalized edema.

Note unusual odors from the mouth, which may suggest an organic academia. The sweetish odor of acetone is common in dehydrated or malnourished children but may indicate diabetic acidosis as in adults. Children with diphtheria exude a mouselike odor. Children with typhoid fever may exude an odor similar to that of decaying tissue. An ammoniacal odor occurs in children with uremia. Halitosis (bad breath) occurs in children with many varied states, including poor local hygiene, local or systemic infections, sinusitis, and mouth breathing.

It is useless to ask a child aged less than 6 or 7 years if the throat hurts, since even with acute pharyngitis or tonsillitis, the child usually has no pain. If pain is present in younger children, it more commonly indicates the presence of epiglottitis or laryngitis or occasionally abscess, diphtheria, or scarletina.

Good lighting, preferably daylight, is necessary for further examination. Become accustomed to the use of one type of light, either daylight or electric. To grasp well what you see, develop the ability to anticipate the normal throat structures and to retain an afterimage of the abnormalities seen. With practice, you will learn to prolong the gag, so that the structures can be more carefully visualized.

Most patients will open their mouths when asked to do so. Inability of a child to open the mouth is generally only voluntary and not true inability. Ask the child to breathe rapidly through the mouth or to say "no," "ah," or "eh." If the child makes the sound loudly enough, the mouth opens wide. True inability to open the mouth occurs with tetanus (trismus), tetany, infections in the tissues surrounding the mouth, peritonsillar abscess, dislocation of the temporomandibular joint and, occasionally, parotitis.

In rheumatic fever or rheumatoid arthritis, the swollen temporomandibular joint will sometimes prevent the patient from opening the mouth. Ankylosis of the joint may occur secondary to birth injury to the joint. Temporomandibular joint involvement can frequently be recognized not only by the apparent inability to move the joint, but also by obvious asymmetry of the face. Trismus may also occur in children with infantile Gaucher disease, brain tumor, or encephalitis, and it is common in children who receive phenothiazine derivatives.

If the child does not open the mouth after suggestion, tell the child that examination of the throat is not really painful but may be uncomfortable and that the examination will take "only a second." If the child is 18 months of age or older, attempting to have the child open the mouth voluntarily is worthwhile. One device is to ask if the child would like to examine a relative (brother, sister, or cousin) after leaving. Most children say yes. Give the child a tongue blade and say: "I'll show you how to do it. First you have your brother open his mouth wide. Then you look at his teeth, then you look high, and then you look low." Even though a gag is elicited, most children are not very angry.

If this suggestion fails, tell the child to show the teeth. Then attempt to place the tongue blade on the anterior part of the tongue for a view of the tongue and palate. With the blade in this position, the child is not uncomfortable and usually does not resist patient examination. If the child resists by closing the mouth and gritting the teeth, carefully and firmly restrain the child.

Place the tongue blade gently between the lips to the posterior teeth and push the mucosa away from the teeth to obtain an adequate view of the teeth, gums, and mucosa. Use small tongue blades for small children. If mouth lesions are suspected, it is frequently less painful if the tongue blade is moistened before it is inserted. (Regardless, a moistened tongue blade makes all exams less unpleasant.) Patiently push the blade between the teeth toward the pharynx. Insert the blade with a slightly downward motion so that the tongue is pushed forward and the base of the tongue downward. Suddenly, the child will gag, the mouth will open, and in that instant, observe all the structures inside the mouth. At no time should the nose be pinched closed (see Figure 5.6). Because the child almost immediately resists further manipulation, this part of the examination should be performed expeditiously, and you should know exactly what you wish to learn before causing the gag. Remember the gag reflex can be elicted only by touching the posterior third of the tongue.

The first area that presents with the gag is the epiglottis, located at the base of the tongue. Note swelling and color. A swollen red epiglottis is apparent in some children with laryngotracheobronchitis, especially when it is due to H. influenzae, and may obstruct respiration. With viral infections and allergy, the epiglottis is swollen and pale. Either a swollen red or swollen pale epiglottis may represent a respiratory emergency. A congenitally large epiglottis or ulcers of the epiglottis may be noted. Lack of gag may be due to ninth or tenth nerve injury and is sometimes seen in patients with bulimia.

Next inspect the uvula. A very long uvula is congenital and may cause gagging or coughing. Occasionally, the uvula is congenitally bifid and may be associated with a submucous cleft of the palate. It may be absent, having been accidentally removed during tonsillectomy. Note motion of the uvula and soft palate as the patient is gagged or told to say "ah." Paralysis of the soft palate or uvula or absence of the gag reflex is an early sign of poliomyelitis and diphtheria, but is also noted in disorders involving the glossopharyngeal or vagus nerves or conditions with masses behind the palate. Limited motion of the soft palate may be caused by hypertrophied, infected adenoids. A translucent membrane in the midline of the soft palate indicates lack of continuity of muscles and may be a sign of palatopharyngeal incompetence.

Look at the posterior pharynx for lymphoid hyperplasia, color, postnasal drip, membrane, edema, exudate, abscess, and vesicles. Lymphoid hyperplasia is evident with any infection of the area. A red, inflamed pharynx is characteristic of any type of acute pharyngitis, but there are no good local signs to distinguish bacterial from nonbacterial pharyngitis. A pale, puffy mucosa indicates edema. Vesicles on the posterior pharynx, anterior pillars, or uvula surrounded by erythema of 3–6 mm are a sign of herpangina due to Coxsackievirus A infection. These vesicles ulcerate, and small ulcers may remain for 2–3 weeks. Small maculopapules on the posterior pharynx are also seen in other respiratory viral diseases.

Profuse postnasal drip indicates infection in the nose, nasopharynx, or sinuses and may cause a foul odor. A white membrane over the tonsils or posterior pharynx is evident in children with diphtheria; other bacterial infections, particularly Vincent angina and β-hemolytic streptococcal infection; infectious mononucleosis; agranulocytosis; and leukemia. In diphtheria, the mouth smells "mousy," and the membrane pulls away with bleeding. The membrane in diphtheria is usually more confluent than in the other infections and spreads to cover more of the uvula and posterior pharynx. Indeed, a confluent membrane involving the uvula or posterior pharynx should be considered diphtheritic until proved otherwise.

The pharynx or throat is separated from the mouth by the anterior and posterior pillars. The palatine (faucial) tonsils are located between these pillars. Note size of the tonsils. Like all lymphoid tissue, tonsils are much larger during early childhood than later; therefore, you should not make statements regarding enlargement of tonsils in childhood until you have examined many normal tonsils or until obstruction of the airway is obvious. Remember that with gagging, the tonsils move medially, thus giving the impression of exaggerated hypertrophy.

Crypts in the tonsillar tissue may indicate past infection; pus in the tonsils and peritonsillar abscesses indicate acute infections. The tonsils appear to be pushed backward or forward and the uvula may be displaced with peritonsillar abscesses. Peritonsillar abscesses occur more often in older children and are usually due to streptococcus infections.

In infants aged less than 2 years, erythema of the tonsils usually occurs with bacterial infections, especially streptococci, pneumococci, and H. influenzae. Purulent exudate or membrane suggests the presence of viral infections. In children aged more than 2 years, some attempt can be made to distinguish bacterial from viral tonsillitis, although obtaining cultures of the nasopharynx is usually necessary. Yellow or grayish white follicles are usually due to bacteria. Vesicles, nodules, punched-out ulcers, scanty or streaky membranes, and patchy gray, white, or yellow membranes usually indicate viral infection. A coalescent white membrane occurs with Candida infections.

A bluish gray membrane with ulceration is more common in children with agranulocytosis or other severe underlying hematologic disorders.

Tuberculosis and tumors may also cause enlargement of the tonsils. Definite unilateral enlargement of the tonsillar area is common with diseases such as Vincent infection, diphtheria, and lymphoma. Enlarged, lobulated, red orange tonsils have been reported in association with accumulation of cholesterol esters (Tangier disease).

Collections of movable mucus and pus may be noted in the posterior pharynx. This is usually postnasal drip and may be caused by sinusitis or infected adenoids.

Outpouching of the posterior pharyngeal wall is characteristic of retropharyngeal abscess. Examination of the retropharynx with a finger is usually necessary only if an abscess or submucous cleft is suspected. Retropharyngeal abscesses usually occur in children in the first 2 years of life; they are felt as unilateral soft masses in infants who are usually quite ill and have noisy respirations, that increase with upward gate and, occasionally, retracted necks. Peritonsillar abscess causes the tonsils to bulge.

Single ulcers without generalized symptoms are canker sores. A recurrent type of canker sore may occur with allergy. Sudden swelling of any part of the buccal mucosa also occurs with allergy.

Other types of stomatitis occurring on the mucosa include vesicles of chickenpox, mucous patches of early congenital syphilis, and general inflammation with vesicles of the erythroderma desquamativum syndromes.

Most children aged 2½ years or older will open the mouth, and the posterior pharynx can be visualized. Examine the throat at this time. Do not restrain patients unless they move. In older children, if you push down first one side of the tongue and then the other, visualizing all the mouth and throat is sometimes easier. Frequently, if the patient sticks the tongue out and breathes deeply, the tongue blade need not be used.

Usually, little salivary secretion is seen in infants until 3 months of age. Absence of salivation may indicate dehydration, fever, Mikulicz syndrome, botulism, atropine ingestion, or congenital ectodermal dysplasia. Drooling or collection of saliva in the mouth is normal in children until 2 years of age and persists in those with swallowing difficulty and injury to the glossopharyngeal (IX) or vagal (X) nerves or with encephalitis or myasthenia. Gag reflex may be decreased.

Thick mucoid secretions are frequently evident after tracheal irritation. Unswallowed saliva or excess mucoid secretions are noted in newborns with tracheoesophageal fistula, probably due to aspirated gastric secretions with secondary tracheal irritation.

Note excessive salivation or drooling. A child aged 2–5 years who is in respiratory distress, sitting up, and drooling should first be considered to have epiglottitis. If you do suspect epiglottitis, you must not advance the tongue blade.

Causes of Excessive Salivation

Teething	Caustic exposure
Caries	Mental delay
Mouth infection	Gingivostomatitis
Mercury poisoning	Phosphate poisoning

| Familial dysautonomia | Acrodynia |
| Salivary gland infections | Smokeless tobacco |

Note inflammation, color, swelling, and distortions of the gums. Children with gingivitis have redness, swelling, and tenderness of the gums. Inflammation of the gingiva may indicate the presence of a systemic disease or vitamin C deficiency, or it may occur in mouth breathers or in children with erupting teeth, poor mouth hygiene, or poor dental care. Swelling or small cysts on the hard palate or gums in infants may be a sign of pneumococcal sepsis.

In children with teeth, a black line along the margin of the gum may signify heavy metal poisoning. However, a melanotic line of the gums themselves is found in normal black infants. The gums near the teeth are purple and bleed easily in children with scurvy, in children with other bleeding diseases such as leukemia or chronic leukopenia, in children with poor oral hygiene, and sometimes in apparently normal children. The gums in children with herpetic stomatitis appear to be painted with a bright red pencil and are swollen and tender. Generalized hypertrophy of the gums is seen in mouth breathers, in children receiving phenytoin who have phenytoin sensitivity, in children with hereditary gingival fibromatosis, and in many vitamin deficiency states. Pinpoint inflamed elevations from which pus can be expressed with the tongue depressor are characteristic of abscess of the tooth root.

In young infants, epithelial pearls or retention cysts are found in or near the midline of the gums. These cysts have no clinical significance and usually disappear spontaneously when the infant is 2–3 months of age. Asymptomatic white patches on the cheeks or lips in older children may represent ectopic sebaceous glands (Fordyce spots).

Next, inspect the buccal mucosa. In young infants, look especially for thrush, small white patches that bleed when scraped off or rubbed. Thrush in a newborn may result from maternal infection. It also occurs in debilitated children or in children with hypoparathyroidism and after prolonged antibiotic use and HIV infections. Fixed white patches that do not rub off are leukoplakia or lichen planus. Patches that scrape off are usually due to milk or other ingested white food. Bluish white scattered spots about the size of a grain of sand on the buccal mucosa at the level of the lower teeth and within the lower lip are characteristic of Koplik spots. These spots usually indicate measles. Red spots 1–3 mm in diameter over the buccal mucosa and palate are characteristic of Forschheimer sign, frequently an early indication of rubella. Vesicles on the buccal mucosa, especially if surrounded by a red line, are usually due to herpes simplex. If on the posterior pharynx, similar vesicles usually indicate herpangina due to Coxsackievirus infection. Pale red spots may cover the buccal mucosa in measles and other viral diseases and are the enanthems of the diseases with skin exanthems. Painful mouth ulcers may be aphthous ulcers of unknown cause.

Causes of Painful Mouth Ulcers

| Unknown causes | Erythema multiforme |
| Immune deficiency | Leukemia |

Folic acid deficiency   Neutropenia

Vitamin B_{12} deficiency   Inflammatory bowel disease
                                               (e.g., Crohn disease)

Niacin or tryptophan deficiency   Diphtheria

Veins on the buccal mucosa are ordinarily not apparent. Visible or dilated veins on the buccal mucosa or tongue may be a sign of cyanosis or may indicate cardiac failure or local vascular obstruction.

View the tongue. Normally, the dorsal surface of the tongue is coated with conical filiform papillae. The circumvallate papillae form a V on the posterior third of the tongue. Coating may signify mouth breathing or lack of motion of the tongue caused by debility in severe disease. Dry tongue is a sign of general dehydration. Unilateral atrophy of the tongue may be due to injury of the hypoglossal nerve.

Large red papillae resembling a strawberry or raspberry are seen with scarlet fever. On the tip and sides are a profusion of red dots about 1 mm in diameter, the fungiform papillae. A uniformly smooth tongue with no apparent fungiform papillae is a sign of familial dysautonomia. Black tongue may be congenital but has been described as a low-grade infection subsequent to penicillin administration or chickenpox. It also occurs in mouth bleeders, as in patients with hemophilia (see Box 5.1).

Geographic tongue consists of gray, irregular areas of the tongue and usually has an unknown benign cause, but it may be related to febrile states or to allergy. Developmentally delayed children have deep furrows in the tongue due to biting of the protruding tongue. However, furrowed tongue is most commonly a congenital characteristic. Scars on the tongue may be due to previous convulsions.

BOX 5.1 TONGUE

White patches	Thrush, milk
Red, sore	Riboflavin deficiency
	Niacin deficiency
	Anemia
Melanotic pigment	Adrenal insufficiency
	Acanthosis nigricans
	Cachexia
	Neurofibromatosis
	Pellagra
Melanotic patches	Polyposis (Peutz syndrome)
Black	Congenital, oral antibiotic
	Chicken pox
	Mouth bleeders
Bright red	Kawasaki disease
Hairy	Debility, human immunodeficiency syndrome
Petechiae	Platelet abnormal
	Sexual abuse

Macroglossia (large tongue) is usually congenital and is a cardinal sign of Beckwith-Weideman syndrome. It may be an early sign of hypothyroidism or mucopolysaccharidosis or be due to a lymphangioma, cyst, or hemangioma. In patients who let the tongue protrude, the tongue may appear large. Protrusion of the tongue may also be due to a tumor or thyroglossal duct cyst at the base of the tongue.

Tongue-tie is caused by a very short frenum. If the tongue tip of an infant does not interfere with feeding or if an older child can elevate the tip to produce the sounds of *t*, *d*, *n*, and *l*, the condition does not exist. Remember, in a tongue that at birth appears to be tongue-tied, with normal growth the tip becomes more free. A torn frenum may be due to child abuse. Cysts or ranulae are occasionally seen in the floor of the mouth near the frenum.

Note tremor of the tongue as it protrudes. Fine tremor is seen with chorea, hyperthyroidism, and amyotonia congenita. Gross tremor may be seen in children with cerebral palsy. Fibrillations (slow undulating movements) indicate completely denervated muscle and may be an early sign of spinal muscular atrophy (Werdnig-Hoffmann disease).

Paralysis of the tongue may be noted. The tongue protrudes toward the involved side in patients with hypoglossal nerve lesions.

With the tongue depressor still on the anterior half of the child's tongue, inspect the hard palate. Note color of the palate. You may detect jaundice. Petechiae on the palate are usually due to any condition causing pharyngitis but may be due to other diseases that cause petechiae on the skin or elsewhere.

Look for congenital cleft palate. Note if the cleft involves only the hard palate, the soft palate, or the uvula and distinguish it from the rare condition of palatal perforation. Perforation of the palate occurs after age 2 years in those who have congenital syphilis. High, arched palates are usually seen in mouth breathers but are also seen in children with arachnodactyly and many other congenital disorders. Hypertrophy of the bone in the midline of the palate (torus palatinus) is usually an anomaly of little significance.

Inspect the teeth for number, caries, and type of occlusion. Compare the number of teeth present with the averages for age (Table 5.2). Occasionally a tooth will be seen in a newborn. Delayed appearance of the deciduous teeth (e.g., after 1 year of age) may be normal, especially in obese children, or may indicate hypothyroidism, rickets, congenital syphilis, or Down syndrome. Absence of teeth is seen with congenital ectodermal dysplasia. Loss of teeth is seen in children with metabolic diseases such as acrodynia, xanthomatosis, histiocytosis, cherubism, gingivitis, and low-phosphatase rickets. In children who grind their teeth, the edges of the teeth are usually flattened. The usual causes of tooth grinding (bruxism) are psychologic difficulties, developmental delay, tiredness, and local irritation.

Malocclusion may occur without obvious cause or after premature loss or prolonged retention of deciduous teeth. It may be a family characteristic, and it also occurs in children with mouth breathing, cleft palate, micrognathia, or prognathism. One cause of malocclusion of permanent teeth is persistent thumbsucking after 6 years of age.

Dental caries, due to bacterial decay and disintegration of tooth substance, are difficult to detect without special instruments until cavitation occurs (Tables 5.3, 5.4).

TABLE 5.2
Chronology of Tooth Eruption

Primary		Secondary	
Maxillary			
Central incisor	7½ mo	Central incisor	7–8 yr
Lateral incisor	9 mo	Lateral incisor	8–9 yr
Cuspid (canine)	18 mo	Cuspid	11–12 yr
First molar	14 mo	First bicuspid	10–11 yr
Second molar	24 mo	Second bicuspid	10–12 yr
		First molar	6–7 yr
		Second molar	12–13 yr
		Third molar	17–21 yr
Mandibular			
Central incisor	6 mo	Central incisor	6–7 yr
Lateral incisor	7 mo	Lateral incisor	7–8 yr
Cuspid	16 mo	Cuspid	9–10 yr
First molar	12 mo	First bicuspid	11–12 yr
Second molar	20 mo	Second bicuspid	11–12 yr
		First molar	6–7 yr
		Second molar	11–13 yr
		Third molar	17–21 yr

Disintegration of the enamel may be detected with a sharp instrument, especially if tooth pain is present. The number of caries is decreased in children with Down syndrome, fructose intolerance, and sucrose intolerance and is increased in children with chronic infection, including HIV.

Poor tooth formation may be evident in systemic diseases such as hypocalcemia, congenital syphilis, hypoparathyroidism, severe infections, and nutritional disturbances, including rickets and nephrosis. Enamel formation in primary teeth is defective in children with prenatal infections or cerebral palsy. Older children or adolescents with bulimia may have defective posterior incisors and enamel defects. Piercing of the tongue results in almost universal enamel defects.

Green or black teeth may be found after iron ingestion or after death of the tooth. The color change of a damaged tooth might take 3 weeks. Green teeth are also seen in children who had severe jaundice at birth. Red teeth are sometimes seen in those with porphyria. Brown teeth may be due to congenital defects in tooth formation. Mottled, pitted teeth may be seen after excess fluoride ingestion and some years after treatment with tetracycline. The back of the teeth may be eroded in those with bulimia. Centrally notched, peg-shaped permanent teeth (Hutchinson teeth) may occur in children with congenital syphilis. Mulberrylike 6-year molars occur in normal children but may also indicate congenital syphilis. Teeth may be temporarily stained by gum bleeding that can occur in normal tooth eruption.

After you examine the throat, break the tongue depressor in front of the child and throw it away so the child knows that this part of the examination has ended.

TABLE 5.3
New Approaches to Caries Prevention That Target Tooth Enamel to
Boost the Host Defense

Target	Scientific Paradigm	Technical Approach	Potential New Therapeutic
Tooth enamel	Topical fluoride-modulated calcium incorporation into tooth enamel	Increase delivery and retention of fluoride; deliver additional calcium (and phosphate)	Dual component calcium/fluoride dentifrice; slow-release fluoride systems, device, encapsulation; Ca delivery systems, protein/peptide carriers, silicate/glass carriers

From Krol, D. M., & Nedley, M. P. (2007). Dental caries: State of the science for the most common chronic disease of childhood. In M. S. Kappy, E. Gilbert-Barness, L. A. Barness, L. L. Barton, & M. Zegler (Eds.), *Advances in pediatrics*, vol. 54, p. 222.

TABLE 5.4
New Approaches to Caries Prevention That Target Bacteria to
Control Dental Plaque Formation

Target	Scientific Paradigm	Technical Approach	Potential New Therapeutic
Plaque bacteria	Infection caused by endogenous flora; specific (acid-producing, acid-tolerant) organisms that cause caries; Biofilm is a highly complex entity that behaves differently from its individual consitutents	Reduce burden of infection; eliminate causative organisms, especially *S. mutans*; prevent bacterial adhesion; modulate biofilm physiology; disrupt plaque matrix	Topical antimicrobials —Chlorhexidine, Triclosan; *S. mutans*-targeted vaccine; replacement therapy, genetically modified organism —Probiotics, targeted anti- microbial enzymes and peptides; coat enamel surface —Agents, sealants, block bacterial adhesion, bacterial surface —Glucosyltranferase and matrix formation, cell- cell signaling; control plaque pH, Xylitol —Arginine/bicarbonate buffer —Upregulate originine deaminase; glucan hydrolase enzymes

From Krol, D. M., & Nedley, M. P. (2007). Dental caries: State of the science for the most common chronic disease of childhood. In M. S. Kappy, E. Gilbert-Barness, L. A. Barness, L. L. Barton, & M. Zegler (Eds.). *Advances in pediatrics*, vol. 54, p. 223.

NECK

Examination of the neck takes 1 to 2 seconds but may help in the diagnosis of many diseases. The patient should be lying flat on the back or sitting.

First, note the size of the neck. The neck normally appears short during infancy and lengthens at about 3–4 years of age. Children with platybasia, hypothyroidism, or Morquio, Hurler, and Klippel-Feil syndromes have a short neck. Webbing of the neck is sometimes noted in children with gonadal dysgenesis or as an isolated anomaly. Marked edema of the neck is noted in children with local infections, cellulitis, diphtheria, other infections of the mouth, mumps, obstruction of the superior vena cava, and any of the causes of generalized edema.

Next, palpate the anterior and posterior cervical triangles for lymph nodes (described in Chapter 3). Observe or palpate other masses in the neck. Enlarged parotids usually extend down into the neck. Cystic masses in the midline high in the neck that are freely movable and move upward when the patient swallows may be thyroglossal duct cysts. Pulling the tongue forward causes these cystic areas to move. Fistula may accompany the cyst. Midline cystlike masses that do not move freely may be lingual thyroid cysts, sebaceous cysts, lipomas, or dermoids. Diffuse swelling of the neck with nonpitting edema (bull neck) is seen in children with severe diphtheria.

Next palpate the sternocleidomastoid muscle. A mass in the lower third of the sternocleidomastoid muscle generally indicates congenital torticollis. Torticollis without abnormality in the muscle may be associated with gastroesophageal reflux and neuroblastoma. Oval, cystic, smooth, moderately movable masses near the upper third of the muscle are usually due to branchial cysts and may be associated with fistula or may be attached to the skin, with a small dimple. These are almost always anterior to the sternocleidomastoid muscle. Cystic hygroma, which is usually posterior and above either clavicle, and hemangioma are easily compressible. Transilluminate for cystic hygroma or lymphangioma. Other masses include dermoids, neurofibroma, ectopic thyroid, and lipoma. Hard masses suggest Hodgkin disease; lymphosarcoma, rhabdomyosarcoma, or other sarcomas; and metastatic disease, neuroblastoma, and salivary or other malignancies. The callus of a fractured clavicle may be felt as a hard mass.

Next, palpate the trachea, feeling first the most anterior parts with one finger and then proceeding down both sides simultaneously with your thumb and index finger. The trachea should be slightly to the right of the midline. Any further deviation in either direction indicates mediastinal shift due to atelectasis (especially due to foreign body), effusion, pneumothorax, or tumor in the chest or neck. A palpatory thud (or audible slap) may be felt or heard over the trachea and may indicate the presence of a foreign body free in the trachea.

Next, feel just below the thyroid cartilage for the thyroid isthmus and for both lobes of the thyroid just lateral to the thyroid cartilage. The thyroid in younger children can be felt while the child is lying supine. Place your thumb on one side and your index and second fingers on the opposite side of the thyroid cartilage. In older children, it may be easier to palpate the thyroid from behind, with two fingers of each hand placed on both sides of the thyroid cartilage. The thyroid is observed or is felt to move upward when the patient swallows. Note size, shape, position, mobility, and tenderness.

Thyroid enlargement may be due to hyperactive thyroid, malignancy, or goiter. A smooth, enlarged thyroid mass indicates thyroid hyperplasia. Nodules in the thyroid are usually adenomatous and may be malignant. Enlarged tender thyroid indicates early thyroiditis. A woody feel is characteristic of Hashimoto thyroiditis. Unilateral tenderness subsequent to tonsillitis may be due to thrombophlebitis of the internal jugular vein.

Physical Findings That May Be Seen in Hypothyroidism

Short stature
Decreased height-to-weight ratio
Slow thickened speech; low croaking voice
Slow pulse
Cool, dry scaling skin with decreased body hair
Dry lifeless hair
Pale puffy face
Periorbital puffiness
Palpable stool in descending colon (constipation)
Lid lag
Enlarged calf muscles
Delay in relaxation phase of deep tendon reflexes

Goiter with hypothyroidism may be due to antithyroid drugs or foods, Hashimoto thyroiditis, enzymatic defect in hormone synthesis, or a deficit in iodine. Hypothyroidism without goiter may be hereditary, congenital, or familial or may be due to pituitary disease, sarcoid, or xanthomatosis.

Observe the vessels of the neck. Enlarged veins or abnormal venous pulsations may be due to increased venous pressure, which may be caused by heart failure, pericarditis, or masses in the mediastinum. Pulsation of the carotids may sometimes be observed in children, usually after exercise or emotional upset, but may indicate aortic insufficiency, anemia, hypertension, or patent ductus arteriosus. Venous pulsations in the neck in a child who is upright are always abnormal. In contrast to arterial pulsation, venous pulsations are obliterated by light jugular compression. Distended neck veins do not occur in patients with severe liver disease unless heart disease is also present. When heart failure is suspected, press on the liver. If the jugular veins become prominent (the hepatojugular reflex), failure is present. This sign may be misleading in very young children because they perform the Valsalva maneuver on abdominal pressure, making the jugular veins stand out. If the jugular veins do not fill on liver pressure, the venous system is not patent. This is a sign of hepatic vein thrombosis (Budd-Chiari syndrome). Unilateral distension suggests an intrathoracic abnormality. Bulging and collapse with expiration and inspiration indicate wide swings in intrathoracic pressure during respiration.

Note two small venous pulse waves: the A wave coincides with right atrial contraction, and the V wave coincides with right ventricular contraction. A prominent A wave occurs in patients with cor pulmonale, tricuspid stenosis, or atresia, and pulmonary stenosis or hypertension. Patients with auricular fibrillation do not manifest A waves. The V wave is prominent in patients with tricuspid insufficiency.

Venous pressure can be fairly accurately determined by measuring the distance from the upper border of the clavicle to the upper level of venous distention in the neck with the child in the sitting position.

The carotid sinus may be massaged in children who have histories indicative of possible heart block. Perform such massage only with the stethoscope on the chest. The carotid sinus is best reached by following the carotid artery up to the angle of the jaw and covering the whole area with your thumb. Massaging this area, one side at a time, normally slows the heart 10–20 beats per minute. A greater decrease in rate indicates abnormal carotid sensitivity, a rare cause of syncope.

Auscultate the neck with the bell stethoscope. Murmurs may be heard, particularly over the carotid area, but also elsewhere in the neck, and are frequently transmitted from the heart with organic disease. Distinguish the benign venous hum near the carotids from an organic murmur by absence of a similar sound over the heart. Also, turning the head from side to side changes intensity of venous hum. To-and-fro bruits may be heard over an enlarged thyroid. Bruits over the carotid artery may be due to increased vascular flow, as noted in persons with hyperthyroidism, anemia, or arteriovenous fistula. Bruits from aortic stenosis murmurs are heard bilaterally low in the middle part of the neck or at the angles of the jaw, which are the carotid areas. Those of vascular insufficiency are usually higher and unilateral. Other sounds in the neck may indicate other vascular anomalies. Listen on each side high along the anterior border of the sternocleidomastoid muscle, the midneck, the lower neck, and the supraclavicular space. Transmitted sounds from the trachea may obliterate these sounds, except during the clear interval between inspiration and expiration.

Finally, note motion. First ask the patient to touch the chest with the chin and to turn the head from side to side. If the patient is unable to do this, raise the head from the pillow with one hand and turn the patient's head from side to side. Resistance to flexion of the neck (stiff neck) is characteristic of meningitis or meningeal irritation; in debilitated children or infants with these diseases, the neck may remain supple.

Stiff neck may also be noted with the viral encephalitides, tetanus, lead poisoning, meningismus, and rheumatoid arthritis. It is noted in pharyngitis, cervical adenitis, retropharyngeal abscess, subluxation of the cervical vertebrae due to retropharyngeal or peritonsillar abscess, herniation of the cerebellar tonsils with increased intracranial pressure, and degenerative nervous system diseases as part of their generalized hypertonia. Brudzinski sign, obtained by flexing the neck and noting flexion at the hip, knee, or ankle, is a similar indication of CNS irritation. Episodic tonic axial extension and lateral flexion of the head may be associated with gastroesophageal reflux or hiatal hernia (Sandifer syndrome).

Hyperextension of the neck (opisthotonos) is due to any of the causes of stiff neck of a more severe degree. It occurs with respiratory tract obstruction and also in children with cerebral palsy or kernicterus. It is noted periodically in all normal infants or in infants with breath-holding spells. Recurrent hyperextension to lessen obstruction from tracheal compression strongly suggests vascular ring. True opisthotonos, which is a rigid prolonged hyperextension of the spine, usually denotes a completely decere-brate individual and is observed in those with severe developmental delay, kernicterus, CNS infections, or idiosyncratic reaction to Benadryl or phenothiazides.

Obtain the tonic neck reflex by placing the child supine and turning the head to one side. The contralateral arm and leg flex and the ipsilateral arm and leg extend. The head is turned to the opposite side, and the position of the limbs reverses. In practice, the opposite flexion and extension may occur and the test may still be positive. This reflex is present at birth and normally lasts 3–5 months. If present after this time, brain damage should be suspected.

Inability to move the neck from side to side may accompany any of the previously named states and also occurs in congenital torticollis, the Klippel-Feil syndrome, and occasionally with cervical rib. Neurologic torticollis occurs in patients with lesions of the spinal accessory nerve, causing sternocleidomastoid and trapezius muscle paralysis, or it occurs without apparent cause. Eye lesions, especially when vision is unequal, or labyrinthitis, spasmus nutans, and brain tumors may be accompanied by torticollis. If the patient cannot maintain the head elevated (head drop), consider early poliomyelitis or other causes of muscle weakness. If possibility of trauma exists, the neck should be properly restrained until cervical spine injury is ruled out.

Voluntary tilting of the neck may be seen in children with habit spasm, brain tumors, poor vision, or strabismus. Head tilting from side to side may occur in chil-dren in whom the corpus callosum is absent. Head rolling and nodding may be due to habit spasm, mental retardation, eye or ear abnormalities, or chorea.

Tongue-Tie

Tongue-tie definition:

- Inability to elevate tongue to the alveolar ridge
- Inability to touch both angles of the mouth
- Inability to achieve contact for linguadental and lingualveolar consonant
- Inability to protrude tongue beyond the lower gum
- Notching of the tongue

Ankyloglossia is a completely fused and immobile tongue. Incidence is 0.5/1,000 births. Membranous frenulum usually resolves spontaneously. Thickened fibrous frenulum may require surgery.

Thumb Sucking

The prevalence of thumb sucking is 19% of 5-year-olds. Pathophysiology consists of adaptive behavior in infants and young children, to avoid boredom, soothing during illness or other stress, associated with object attachment (the "Linus syndrome") and alopecia, and introverted children more likely to suck than extroverts. Risks and complications are harmless in infancy, psychological ostracism from parents and peers, digital complications as digital hyperextension and paronychia, and oral complications such as malocclusion, mucosal trauma, atypical root resorption, and abnormal facial growth. Avoid treatment for children in acutely stressful situations (ill parent, etc.).

FURTHER READINGS

Crutchfield, C. E. 3rd, & Lewis, E. J. (1997). The successful treatment of oral candidiasis (thrush) in a pediatric patient using itraconazole. *Pediatric Dermatology, 14*(3), 246.

Faske, I. (2007). *They do come with instructions.* Palm Beach Gardens, FL: Collier MacKenzie Davis.

Lesperance, M. M. (2007). A pediatric otolaryngologist learns to diagnose acute otitis media. *Archives of Otolaryngology—Head and Neck Surgery, 133,* 745–746.

Meltzer, E. O. (2006). Allergic rhinitis: Managing the pediatric spectrum. *Allergy and Asthma Proceedings, 27*(1), 2–8.

Prim, M. P., de Diego, J. I., Larrauri, M., Diaz, C., Sastre, N., & Gavilan, J. (2002). Spontaneous resolution of recurrent tonsillitis in pediatric patients on the surgical waiting list. *International Journal of Pediatric Otorhinolaryngology, 65*(1), 35–38.

Robertson, J., & Shilkofski, N. (Eds.). (2005). *The Harriet Lane handbook* (17th ed.). St. Louis: Elsevier Mosby.

Schraff, S. A., & Strasnick, B. (2006). Pediatric cholesteatoma: A retrospective review. *International Journal of Pediatric Otorhinolaryngology, 70*(3), 385–393.

6

THE CHEST, BREASTS, AND RESPIRATORY SYSTEM

He who has health has hope, and he who has hope has everything.

Arab Proverb

THE CHEST

Many disease states can be diagnosed by simply looking at the chest. Sometimes it is difficult to do more than observe a hyperactive or crying patient.

The order of examination of the chest in a child depends on the attitude of the child; some physicians find it easier to listen to the chest first, before a young child starts to cry, and then to proceed with the other parts of the examination; others observe and palpate first and use the stethoscope later.

Inspection

Note the general shape and circumference of the chest. Also, note respiratory rate. Obtain the chest circumference at the nipple line. It is normally the same as or slightly less than the head circumference for the first 2 years of life; it then exceeds the head circumference. In very sturdy children, the chest circumference is slightly greater than that of the head, even during the first 2 years. Marked disproportion between head and chest measurements requires comparison with standards for the child's age. Disproportions in children aged less than 2 years are usually caused by abnormal head growth rather than abnormal chest growth. When the measurements are compared with standards, however, the cause of abnormal growth can usually be determined. In children with respiratory disease, measure the chest in inspiration and expiration. The normal teenager can expand the chest at least 4–5 cm. Less expansion usually indicates intrathoracic pulmonary disease.

In premature infants, the rib cage is thin, and the chest may appear to collapse with every inspiration. In infancy, the chest is almost round, the anteroposterior diameter equaling the transverse diameter. As the child grows older, the chest normally expands in the transverse diameter. A round or emphysematous chest in a child after

6 years of age suggests a chronic pulmonary disease such as asthma. A funnel-shaped chest, pectus excavatum, characterized by sternal depression, may be a congenital anomaly or may indicate adenoid hypertrophy. A short, wide chest is noted especially in short children or in those with Morquio disease. Pigeon breast, pectus carinatum, in which the sternum protrudes, is noted as an isolated anomaly or in children with rickets or osteopetrosis. The xiphisternum may protrude and appear broken, but this condition is normal in young children and results only from a loose attachment between the xiphoid and the body of the sternum. As in adults, note is made of the rib numbers to orient the examiner. The second rib attaches at the angle of the sternum just below the clavicles.

When the patient is lying supine, swellings at the costochondral junction may be evident. These swellings or blunt knobbings form the rachitic rosary. Almost always a depression will be noted in the child in the region of the eighth to tenth ribs, and the bottom of the rib cage will appear to flare. The depression at the site of the diaphragm muscle leaving the chest wall is termed *Harrison's groove*. Although it occurs in rickets, this type of flaring is also common in many children with any pulmonary disorder, in children who were born prematurely, and in many normal young children who have no obvious pathologic disturbance. Edema of the chest wall occurs in children with superior vena cava obstruction, mediastinal compression syndrome, or mumps. Observe for congenital absence of pectoralis major (Poland).

Note the angle made by the lower rib margin with the sternum. Ordinarily this angle is about 45 degrees. You may find a larger angle in children with lung disease and a smaller angle in those with malnutrition and deficiency states. Note expansion of the chest. Most of a child's normal respiratory activity is affected by abdominal motion until age 6 or 7 years, with very little intercostal motion. Later, thoracic motion becomes responsible for air exchange. If the interspaces show much motion with intercostal muscle retraction, lung disease or peritonitis is suggested. Note whether the motion of the interspaces is restricted to one side. Less motion occurs on the involved side, and increased motion occurs on the opposite side of the chest with pneumonia, hydrothorax or pneumothorax, obstructive foreign body, or atelectasis. Expiration is normally about two thirds the length of inspiration. Expiration is increased with obstruction in the larynx or trachea or in intrinsic pulmonary disease, such as asthma, pneumonitis, or cystic fibrosis.

These disease states and paralysis of the chest musculature also produce increased motion of the diaphragm. With normal respiration the chest expands, the sternal angle increases, and the diaphragm descends on inspiration; the reverse occurs with expiration. Paradoxical respiration is noted when the diaphragm appears to rise on inspiration and to descend on expiration. Paradoxical motion of the chest and diaphragm may be produced by any of the disease states mentioned, particularly pneumothorax. The side of the chest that is involved tends to collapse on inspiration and remains stationary or appears to expand on expiration. Paradoxical respiration is also noted in children with neuromuscular diseases such as phrenic nerve paralysis or chorea.

By observation, you can sometimes determine the difference between high obstruction and low obstruction. Retraction is chiefly suprasternal and severe in high obstruction, such as laryngeal lesions, but mainly infrasternal in low obstruction, such as infantile bronchiolitis. Retractions are usually less intense in lower obstruction. Diseases such as croup, congenital laryngeal stridor, stridor resulting from injury of the laryngeal nerves, diphtheria, and bronchiolitis; diseases of the abdomen such as peritonitis and paralysis of the diaphragm also produce marked retraction above and below the sternum, with marked intercostal activity bilaterally. If patient is <2 years old, has sternal retractions at rest or stridor at rest, patient has ominous symptoms.

Note asymmetry. Precordial bulging may indicate an interatrial septal defect, other causes of right or biventricular enlargement, pneumothorax, or a chronic localized chest disease. Congenital absence of the chest muscles may cause asymmetry; however, asymmetry is most commonly found secondary to scoliosis.

Weakness or deficiency in the sternocleidomastoid or trapezoid muscles may result from injury to the spinal accessory nerve. Chest pain may be accompanied by tenderness and may be caused by extrathoracic or intrathoracic lesions or may be referred from other organs, such as the abdomen, spine, or neck. Pain over the lower ribs may follow trauma: pull the inferior rib margins anteriorly. The symptoms will be reproduced because of "slipping ribs." Two other causes of chest wall pain are costochondritis and sternal injuries from weightlifting.

Note the position of the scapulas for anomalies such as Sprengel deformity, winged scapula, and Klippel-Feil syndrome, which are described in sections on the spine (Chapters 8, 11).

Palpation

Place the palm of your hand lightly but firmly on the patient's chest and feel with the palm and fingertips. Palpate the entire chest. Palpation confirms your observation of the chest wall, such as position of the scapulas, position or fracture of the clavicles, asymmetry of the chest, and the presence of rosary, Harrison groove, breast tissue, and axillary lymph nodes. Note any masses or areas of tenderness. A thud is occasionally palpated high on the chest as the patient breathes. This is a sign of foreign body in the trachea. Palpation of the heart is discussed later in this chapter.

Tactile fremitus is easily determined by palpating the chest wall in children who are crying, who can cooperate by speaking, or who can be asked their name. Fremitus, when obtainable, is usually felt over the entire chest as a tingling sensation. Decrease in fremitus suggests the presence of airway obstruction or may indicate pleural effusion. When the patient does not make vocal sounds, fremitus is normally absent, but it is frequently felt in children who have been crying and signifies a partial movable obstruction to the passage of air. Tactile fremitus is especially valuable in distinguishing the presence of mucus high in the respiratory tract, where fremitus is very coarse, from lower respiratory tract infection, where it is absent. Fremitus is a poor sign for distinguishing pneumonia, atelectasis, or space-occupying lesions in a child.

Palpate the rib interspaces for retraction or paralysis of the intercostal muscles. Intercostal retraction is caused by increased work of breathing. Intercostal bulging during expiration indicates expiratory obstruction.

Decreased motion of the interspaces may indicate paralysis of the intercostal muscles, decreased respiratory activity, or, if unilateral, any of the causes of decreased respiration of one side of the chest. Subcostal retraction of the diaphragm with hyperinflation of the chest suggests air trapping. Pulsation of the rib vessels from coarctation of the aorta usually occurs in the teen years. Pericardial or pleural friction rubs can occasionally be palpated and feel like fine vibrations. A crackling sensation under your fingers may result from subcutaneous emphysema or a bone fracture.

The axillary lymph nodes are palpated best by bringing the palm of your hand flat into the axilla with the patient's arm hanging freely at the side. A slight rubbing motion will indicate the size of the glands. Normally, several glands as large as 3 mm in diameter will be felt in all children. Abnormalities of these nodes are described in the section on lymph nodes (Chapter 3). Normal nodes are mobile, nontender, not warm, and not red.

Percussion

Use direct and indirect methods in percussion of the chest. In the direct method (Figure 6.1), the chest wall is tapped lightly with either the index or the middle finger. Every centimeter of the chest is percussed quickly. This method is rapid, gentle, and informative but requires considerable practice.

For the indirect method of percussion, place a finger of one hand firmly on the patient's chest wall; use the index or middle finger of the other hand as the percussing hammer and cover the same areas. The bases for good indirect percussion are as follows: (a) the nonpercussing finger must be pressed firmly against the chest wall; (b) no other fingers should touch the chest wall; (c) the patient should be sitting, standing, or lying flat on the back or abdomen; and (d) the percussing finger should move like a piano hammer, with a very loose hinge-joint action at the wrist. Because the chest wall is thinner and the muscles are smaller, the chest is more resonant in children than in adults. Therefore, accurate information is much more easily obtained by examining the chest of a child. If you percuss too vigorously, however, vibrations over a large area may obscure localized areas of dullness.

Posteriorly, percuss from the shoulders down to dullness at the level of the eighth to tenth ribs, where the diaphragm causes a change in the note. It is important that the patient's head be in the midline position facing directly forward during this part of the examination. If the neck is twisted, aeration is not equal, and spurious dullness may be detected. The top of the diaphragm is usually located at about the level of the apex of the costovertebral angle. Anteriorly, tap from just below the clavicle to the level of dullness. Percuss the sides of the chest from the axillae downward. Then, starting at the lower margin of the lung fields posteriorly and the upper abdomen anteriorly, determine the lower margins and the mobility of the diaphragm. It is generally useful to begin percussing in the areas where resonance is expected and continue to where dullness is expected. This is especially important over the area of the heart. Also, comparing dullness to the contralateral side is useful.

You will find a decreased percussion note, or dullness, over the scapulas, diaphragm, liver, and heart. Demarcate these areas. Normally the top of the liver is percussed anteriorly at about the level of the sixth rib from the midaxillary line to the sternum. The lower edge of the lung or the top of the diaphragm is usually percussed

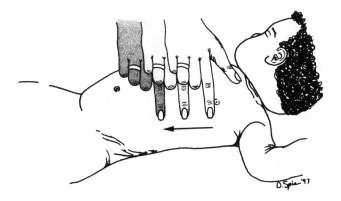

Figure 6.1
Direct percussion.

to the level of the eighth to tenth ribs posteriorly on both sides. Anteriorly, the diaphragm usually cannot be percussed below the level of the liver on the right. Occasionally, because a distended stomach will cause hyperresonance on the left, you may have difficulty delineating the level of the diaphragm. Fortunately, most children have an indentation of the ribs at the attachment of the diaphragm to help indicate where dullness is expected. Usually the diaphragm is also percussed anteriorly at the level of the eighth to the tenth rib. In all these areas, the diaphragm will usually move, as determined by changing dullness, one to two rib spaces between inspiration and expiration. In a child aged less than 2 years, this motion is very difficult to determine by percussion.

These normal areas of percussion dullness may be altered as follows: Liver dullness may be determined at a level higher than the sixth rib in conditions causing liver enlargement; in elevation of the liver, as in abdominal distention; or in atelectasis of the lobes of the right lung. The liver will be percussed at the level of the sixth rib on the left in dextrocardia with levorotation of the liver or with situs inversus. The diaphragm will be higher than normal in conditions causing collapse of the lungs or distention of the abdomen and will be lower than normal in conditions causing emphysema of the lungs with masses or space-occupying lesions in the chest.

The mediastinum in children is usually percussed as the area of cardiac dullness. Rarely, a broadened area of dullness above or at the level of the base of the heart may be caused by the thymus. Although this is without significance, note any broadening of the mediastinum, since it may indicate the presence of other masses. Heart dullness will be altered by conditions causing a shift of the heart or mediastinum. Localized areas of decreased resonance, dullness, or flatness may be found.

Areas of Dullness

Lung	Pleura
Consolidation	Effusion

Collapse (atelectasis)   Emphysema
Tumor
Edema

Left effusion more likely results from pancreatic disease. Right effusion is more likely caused by heart failure or ovarian disease. Dullness below the angle of the left scapula may occur with pericardial effusion (Ewart or Pin sign).

Hyperresonance of the chest is caused by an increase in the amount of air in the chest. It is most common in children with emphysema and asthma and is usually accompanied by a lowered diaphragm. Localized hyperresonance may also indicate the presence of free air in the chest (such as pneumothorax) or the presence of loculated air (such as lung cyst or abscess, obstructive foreign body, or diaphragmatic hernia). Increase in resonance over the area of the liver may indicate a ruptured abdominal viscus.

Auscultation

The inside of the stethoscope should be clean and the tubing intact, well fitting, and about 45 cm long. Warm the stethoscope before use and press it firmly against the chest wall, or sounds that are artifacts will be heard. A tight fit of the stethoscope with the chest is usually accomplished more easily if the bell is placed in the interspaces rather than over the ribs. If the stethoscope is not firmly placed on the chest, nothing will be heard. Auscultate the entire chest, including the axillary areas. Children's fingers must sometimes be restrained from touching the tubing during this part of the examination because touching the tubing also makes extraneous sounds. Listen for breath sounds, rales, rhonchi, and extraneous sounds (Tables 6.1, 6.2).

TABLE 6.1
Respiratory Noises

Noise	Quality	Comments
Snoring	Inspiratory noise of irregular quality	Produced by partial obstruction of the upper respiratory tract, usually in the region of the nasopharynx
Stridor	Continuous, usually harsh inspiratory sound	Caused by extrathoracic airway obstruction; may be heard on expiration if obstruction is in the subglottic area or trachea, where sound resembles a wheeze
Wheeze	Continuous sound with musical high pitched expiratory sound	Indicates intrathoracic airway obstruction; results from dynamic compression of large central airways from either peripheral or central airway obstruction
Grunting	Episodic, short expiratory sound	Caused by partial closure of glottis during expiration
Rattly breathing	Coarse, irregular sound mainly heard	Indicates secretions in trachea or major bronchi

TABLE 6.2
Breath Sounds

Sound	Quality	Comments
Tracheal	"Tubular," high-pitched	Heard during inspiration and expiration
Vesicular	Softer, lower-pitched	Heard in axillary area and lung bases; heard on inspiration and little heard on expiration
Bronchovesicular	Slightly higher pitched than vesicular breath sounds	Heard mainly on inspiration, but an early low-pitched note may be heard on expiration
Bronchial	Have a tubular quality that is less pronounced than in tracheal breath sounds	Heard on inspiration and expiration

Especially during auscultation, the child should be completely supine or totally erect, since even a slight turning of the head may decrease the breath sounds and suggest pathologic states. Because of the small size of the child's chest and the need to localize pathologic findings and to avoid the scratch sounds made by chest hair, the small bell stethoscope is most satisfactory for auscultation in children.

Breath sounds may seem much louder in children than in adults because of the thinness of the chest wall. Inspiration is three times as long as expiration with vesicular sounds, twice as long with bronchovesicular; expiration is slightly longer with bronchial sounds, and inspiration and expiration are about equal with sounds originating from the trachea. Because breath sounds in a child are almost all bronchovesicular or even bronchial, sound quality offers little help in diagnosis. Decreased breath sounds indicate decreased air flow and are noted especially in children with bronchopneumonia, atelectasis, pleural effusion, pneumothorax, and empyema. Increased breath sounds are sometimes heard with resolving pneumonia. Bronchial breath sounds may be heard over areas of consolidation in the older child. Auscultate the area over the mediastinum in the midline both anteriorly and posteriorly. Normally you will hear no breath sounds over the sternum or vertebrae. Increased breath sounds will be heard in these areas in the presence of consolidation.

Inspiratory rales are usually heard as fine crackles. They may be heard throughout the chest in infants and children with bronchiolitis, bronchopneumonia, pulmonary edema, or atelectasis. Rales heard exclusively in the upper part of the chest are more commonly associated with cystic fibrosis. Rales in the lower chest are more common in children with heart failure. Rales heard only late in inspiration are more indicative of interstitial lung disease such as fibrosing alveolitis.

The presence of fine rales may be clarified in children, as in adults, by having the patient cough at the end of expiration. Demonstrate exactly the procedure you expect the child to perform. Even young children can sometimes be induced to cough in this manner. Rales that disappear after coughing usually have no significance.

Frequently you will hear inspiratory rales only at the very end of inspiration or only after deep inspiration. Because a crying child inspires deeply before each cry, auscultation during crying may be quite informative. Instruct slightly older children to blow against your hand, or tell them to blow out the otoscope light or to blow on a pinwheel; they will usually inspire deeply before blowing. Instruct still older children to breath deeply through the mouth, especially if you demonstrate this type of breathing.

Expiratory rales or crackles are prominent in bronchiolitis, cystic fibrosis, asthma, and foreign body aspiration. Rales are mainly expiratory with intrathoracic obstruction to air flow, inspiratory with extrathoracic obstruction, or both with severe obstruction either in or outside the chest.

Pleural friction rub is a coarse grating sound heard through the stethoscope with each respiration, as though it were close to your ear, and occurs occasionally with pneumonia, lung abscess, tuberculosis, or empyema. A loud slap may be heard high on the chest in a child with a tracheal foreign body obstruction. A crunching sound near the heart and synchronous with the heartbeat occurs with left pneumothorax (Hamman sign) or with pneumomediastinum.

Rhonchi caused by crying or upper respiratory infection may be inspiratory or expiratory and are coarse sounds. You can best distinguish them from rales by tactile fremitus or by holding the bell stethoscope over the mouth and comparing the sounds from the mouth with those over the chest. If similar, the sounds are originating high in the respiratory tract near the larynx. Any sound, especially if musical, that sounds the same over different areas of the chest almost invariably arises from the larynx or high in the trachea.

Wheezes are produced by airflow through compromised larger airways and usually sound more musical or sonorous than rales or rhonchi. Wheezes are heard more commonly in expiration than in inspiration and usually indicate partial obstruction during the expiratory phase, as occurs in children with bronchospasm. Inspiratory wheezes usually are heard in children with high obstruction, such as laryngeal edema or a foreign body; expiratory wheezes are usually heard in children with low obstruction, such as asthma or bronchiolitis (Table 6.3). High-pitched wheezes are associated with severe asthma. Absence of wheezes in an asthmatic patient is a sign of a very severe disease. Crunching sounds heard during different phases of respiration may be caused by subcutaneous emphysema.

Vocal resonance can be obtained in children if they are induced to count, speak, or tell their names repeatedly. Increased resonance may indicate consolidation, and decreased resonance may indicate obstruction to flow of air.

Peristalsis is frequently heard over the left lower chest anteriorly because of the proximity of the bowel. However, peristalsis in the chest, particularly on the left side, may be a cardinal sign of diaphragmatic hernia. Murmur or bruits over the posterior lungs may be vascular or may occur with a sequestered lobe of the lung.

BREAST

Two phenomena of early breast development in girls deserve special attention. First, in many perfectly normal girls, breast development is asymmetric. A breast nodule may appear on one side months before the other. Second, it is not unusual for an early breast nodule to be a little tender or sensitive to the friction of overlying clothing.

TABLE 6.3
Differentiating Features of Asthma and Bronchiolitis in Children

	Asthma	Bronchiolitis
Etiology	Viruses, allergens, exercise, etc.	Respiratory syncytial virus, and other viruses
Age of onset	50% by 2 years of age	<24 months 80% by 5 years of age
Recurrent wheezing	Yes	70% (≤2 episodes)
Onset of wheezing	Acute if allergic or exercise-induced	Gradual
Family history of allergy and asthma	Frequent	Infrequent in children with ≤2 episodes
Concomitant symptoms of upper respiratory infection	Yes, if infectious	Yes
Nasal eosinophilia	With allergic rhinitis	Absent
Chest auscultation	If viral, as in bronchiolitis Nonviral: high-pitched expiratory wheezes	Fine, sibilant rales, and coarse inspiratory and expiratory
Concomitant allergic manifestations	If allergic asthma	Usually absent
IgE level	Elevated (if allergic)	Normal
Responsive to bronchodilator	Yes	Unresponsive or partially responsive
Steroids	Responsive	Usually nonresponsive

Note breast development (Figure 6.2). Breast development normally begins before pubic hair develops.

It may be difficult to determine whether a breast that appears large is hypertrophic or is truly developmentally enlarged. The hypertrophic breast usually has a flat nipple with a small areola, and the breast tissue feels soft. The developed breast usually has protrusion of the nipple, enlargement of the areola, and a firmness to the tissue underlying the areola. Redness, heat, and tenderness around the breast may indicate infection (mastitis). Ordinarily, do not palpate the neonatal breast, which is enlarged for about 1 or 2 months, though it may stay enlarged until 2 years old. Examine breasts during routine examinations after breast development begins, when breasts fail to develop, or when symptoms or problems occur.

In girls, normal breast is less than 2 cm in diameter and development begins between the ages of 8 and 14 years. One breast usually begins to develop before the other and is frequently tender. With the patient in the supine position with the arm under the head, palpate in concentric circles inward from the axilla and clavicle to the areola for each side. Precocious breast development in girls is usually innocuous. Complete central isosexual precocity may be caused by central nervous system (CNS) defects or precocity from any cause. With precocious thelarche, linear growth rate is normal. With precocious puberty, linear growth rate is increased. Pseudoprecocious breast enlargement occurs in corpulent children and is merely the result of adipose tissue. In such "breasts," the tissue is softer than true breast tissue and cannot be distinguished from surrounding tissue.

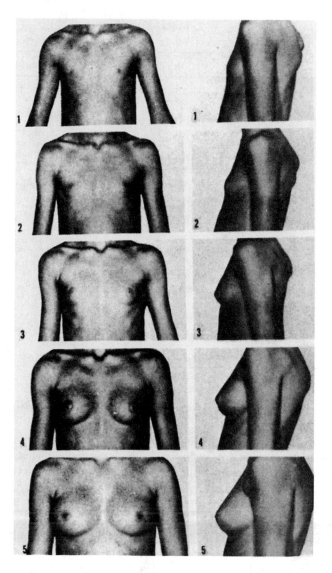

Figure 6.2
Breast development stages during adolescence. Stage 1, preadolescent (elevation of papillae). Stage 2, "bud" stage (elevation of breast and papillae with some increase in areolar diameter). Stage 3, enlargement (no separation of contours). Stage 4, projection (areolae and papillae from secondary mounds). Stage 5, mature (projection of only papillae and recession of areolae). (From Tanner, J. M., 1962. *Growth at adolescence*. Philadelphia: F. A. Davis.)

Precocious Breast Development

See Figure 6.2 for Tanner staging.

Pseudoisosexual Precocity

Granulosa cell tumor
Follicular cysts
McCune-Albright syndrome
Oral contraceptives
Adrenal feminizing tumors
Hypothyroidism
Hyperthyroidism
Marijuana, opiates, amphetamines
Stilbestrol ingestion
Prescription drugs (e.g., digitalis, cimetidine, isoniazid, phenothiazines, antidepressants)

Central Isosexual Precocity

Septooptic dysplasia
Hydrocephalus
Cysts, brain trauma, brain tumors (e.g., hamartoma, neurofibroma, optic glioma, astrocytoma, irradiation, meningitis)

Gynecomastia

Prepubertal

- Infrequent
- Asymmetrical or unilateral
- Causes
  Idiopathic
  Drugs/estrogens
  Adrenal tumor
- Investigation
  Lutein-stimulating hormone, follicle-stimulating hormone
  Testosterone, estradiol, sex hormone-binding globulin
  Human chorionic gonadotropin
  Urinary 17-ketosteroids
  Blood dehydroepiandrosterone, androstenedione

Pubertal Males

- Present in 65% of normal boys
- Incidence highest at approximately 14 years
- Uni- or bilateral
- Average duration 6–18 months

- Causes:
  Idiopathic
  Klinefelter
  Drugs (phenothiazines, marijuana)
- Follow-up
  Spontaneous remission
  Surgery

Measure and diagram any lumps and repeat the examination 1 week after menses occur. A unilateral lump immediately under the areola is normal in developing tissue. In girls 8–10 years old and in boys 13–18 years old, subareolar masses immediately behind the areola that are firm, smooth, discoid, and 2–3 cm in diameter result from hyperplasia. These masses usually regress within 1 year. Small, round, hard nodules in the breasts of children, as in adults, may be caused by cysts or tumors. These masses are usually both nontender and irregular; they may feel attached to the skin or grow out of proportion to the remainder of the breast tissue. Swelling, tenderness, heat, and redness in nodules are signs of inflammation (e.g., cellulitis or abscess) and may follow ductal obstruction, injury, or infection in a cyst; these signs occur more commonly during periods of increased hormonal secretion. Tender nodules with ecchymosis indicate trauma.

Painless, circumscribed, firm masses may result from fat necrosis after an injury. These mobile masses may be fixed to the skin and must be distinguished from those immobile and not so sharply delineated masses that result from carcinoma. Small, mobile, circumscribed, tender masses that increase in tenderness during menses may represent periductal fibrosis, cystic ductal hyperplasia, adenosis, or lobular hyperplasia. Bilateral lumpy thickening occurs with fibrocystic disease. Nodules that are nontender, firm, freely movable, and sharply demarcated are usually fibroadenomas. The long curve of breast tissue extending into the axilla enlarges with hormonal surges.

True gynecomastia in boys usually results from unknown benign factors at puberty but may be caused by tumors of the breast, severe liver disease, drug usage, and, very rarely, gonadal or adrenal lesions. Usually breast enlargement in boys is caused only by adipose tissue, but it may occur with gonadal dysgenesis, Klinefelter syndrome, or digitalis administration.

Breast development is absent in adolescent girls with pituitary failure, anorexia nervosa with onset before puberty, gonadal dysgenesis (including Turner syndrome), adrenal hyperplasia, or severe malnutrition. Record the stage of development (Figure 6.2).

Galactorrhea, a whitish discharge from the nipple, may be caused by pregnancy, hypothalamic or pituitary tumor such as prolactinoma or craniopharyngioma, or drug ingestion. A bloody discharge signals an intraductal papilloma; a purulent discharge suggests abscess; and a greenish-black discharge suggests duct ectasia.

Breast Disorders in Adolescence

Missing breast tissue: athelia (absent nipple), extremely rare; amastia (missing breast tissue). Extra breast tissue occurs in 1%–5% of the population. Polythelia (supernumerary nipples); polymastia (extra breast tissue). Juvenile (virginal) breast hypertrophy requires careful examination but no surgery because surgical excision may remove entire breast tissue. Will resolve in time. Fibroadenoma presents as a firm, discrete mobile mass (often in lateral aspect of breast). Treatment is by excision. Cysts usually are associated with fibrocystic disease and occur in later adolescence. Cysts are small, bilateral, firm, mobile masses. Rare causes of breast masses in adolescents consist of cytosarcoma phyllodes (sometimes malignant)—slow-growing, painless with shiny, taut skin, dilated veins, and superficial ulcers. Other causes include intraductal papilloma (seroanguinous discharge from duct) malignant tumors, which are very rare, fat necrosis, which is not rare, and hamartoma.

SINUSITIS IN CHILDREN

Acute sinusitis (0–3 weeks duration) is very common—5%–10% of childhood upper respiratory infections lead to sinusitis. Etiology is related to *Streptococcus pneumoniae* (40%), *M. catarrhalis* (20%), and *H. influenzae* (20%). Clinical diagnosis includes upper respiratory infection signs and symptoms present longer than 10 days and unusually severe infection (purulent rhinorrhea and fever 39.0°C). Rarely, X-rays are necessary. Approximately 40%–50% have spontaneous resolution.

Chronic sinusitis (>12 weeks duration) is much less common. Etiology is related to α-hemolytic streptococcus (23%), *Staphylococcus aureus* (19%), *Streptococcus pneumoniae* (7%), *H. influenzae* (7%), *M. catarrhalis* (7%), and anaerobes (6%).

Complications of Sinusitis

Extracranial Complications (More Common)

- Periocular
  Preseptal cellulitis
  Orbital cellulitis/abscess
- Pulmonary
  Asthma or bronchitis
  Cystic fibrosis exacerbations
  Sepsis

Cranial and Intracranial Complications

- Cranial and intracranial complications (especially from sphenoid sinusitis)
  Meningitis
  Cranial osteomyelitis
  Abscess formation (epidural, subdural, cerebral)
  Cavernous sinus thrombosis

LARYNX

Note the voice or cry for hoarseness or stridor. Stridor is due to obstruction in the airway. In the first 3 years of life, it is considered an emergency until cause is found. Inspiratory stridor generally indicates an extrathoracic lesion, and expiratory stridor occurs with an intrathoracic obstruction.

Causes of Expiratory Stridor

Subglottic edema	Asthma
Subglottic mass	Cystic fibrosis
Vascular ring	Tracheomalacia
Bronchopulmonary dysplasia	Bronchomalacia

If the obstruction is so severe that the airway cannot dilate, the stridor will be both inspiratory and expiratory. Low-pitched stridor, especially if accompanied by salivation or snoring, indicates inflammation in the supraglottic area. The cry or voice is muffled, and dysphagia may be present. Snoring indicates upper airway obstruction, such as large tonsils or adenoids, allergic rhinitis, or a mass at the base of the tongue. During inspiration with glottic obstruction, crowing is high-pitched, the voice is hoarse or aphonic, and pain is present. During inspiration with subglottic inflammation or obstruction or with vocal cord paralysis, high-pitched stridor with a weak cry and little hoarseness occurs. An easy bedside test for hyponasality is to listen to patient's pronunciation of *m*, *n*, and *ng*.

Stridor associated with wheezing occurs with intrathoracic or extrathoracic lesions such as tracheal inflammation (croup), in which it is both inspiratory and expiratory. A low-pitched fluttering sound that is best heard over the larynx is characteristic of laryngomalacia. Grunting with respiratory illness may be due to chest pain or may be a physiologic response to maintain increased airway pressure during expiration.

Causes of Hoarseness or Stridor

Laryngitis	Shouting
Tracheitis	Hypothyroid
Allergy	Tetanus
Croup	Gaucher disease
Retropharyngeal abscess	Lysosomal storage disease
Laryngeal foreign body	Vascular ring

Factors Associated With Stridor

Nasal Cavity and Nasopharynx

- Congenital
  Piriform aperture stenosis
  Choacal stenosis
  Lacrimal duct cyst
  Craniofacial anomaly
  Nasopharyngeal mass (teratoma)
- Inflammatory/infectious
  Rhinosinusitis
  Adenoid hypertrophy

Oral Cavity, Orpharynx, and Hypopharynx

- Congenital
  Macroglossia
  Glossoptosis
  Vallecular cyst
- Inflammatory/infections
  Tonsillar hypertrophy with abscess
  Retropharyngeal abscess
- Tumors
  Lingual thyroid
  Dermoid
  Lymphovascular malformation
- Foreign body

Laryngeal

- Congenital
  Laryngomalacia (number 1 cause in infants); usual onset is in the first 2 weeks of life, typically positional: most resolve spontaneously by age 1
  Saccular cyst
  Webs
  Clefts
  Vocal cord paralysis
- Inflammatory/infections
  Epiglottitis
  Laryngotracheitis (croup)
  Gastroesophageal reflux
- Tumors
  Papillomas
  Hemangiomas
- Trauma
  Subglottic stenosis
  Foreign bodies
  Laryngeal fracture
  Caustic ingestion

Tracheobronchial

- Congenital
  Tracheomalacia
  Vascular rings
  Tracheoesophageal fistula

Hoarseness

- Congenital
  Glottic webs
  Laryngeal clefts
  Laryngocele
  Tracheoesophageal fistula
  Hemangiomas
- Inflammatory/infections
  Viral/upper respiratory infection
  Diphtheria
  Laryngotracheobronchitis
  Gastroesophageal reflux disease, posterior laryngitis, vocal cord edema
  Fungal laryngitis: consider in an immunocomprised patient
  Papillomatosis secondary to human papillomavirus
- Tumors
  Traumatic birth
  Postintubation
  Laryngeal fracture
  Screamer's nodules
- Endocrine
  Hypothyroidism
- Neurogenic
  Idiopathic vocal cord paralysis
  Arnold-Chiari or Dandy-Walker malformations may lead to brainstem compression of the vagal nerve roots, leading to vocal cord paralysis
  Peripheral nerve: recurrent laryngeal nerve injury or invasion by tumor, myasthenia gravis
- Systemic disease
  Rheumatoid arthritis: fixation of the cricoarytenoid joint
  Relapsing polychondritis
- Functional
  Bacterial tracheitis, frequently caused by S. aureus

Hoarseness due to infection is more common in viral laryngitis or laryngitis due to *H. influenzae* than in infection due to streptococci. Methicillin resistant is now a more common cause of serious croup syndrome. Cretins have a low raucous cry and children with de Lange syndrome emit a growl. Infants with severe gastrointestinal disturbances such as intussusception and peritonitis have a sharp whining cry. Some children with a rare chromosome abnormality involving a deletion of material from chromosome 5 emit a catlike cry (cri-du-chat syndrome). Nasal speech may occur in children with chronic upper respiratory infection, enlarged adenoids, deafness, and neurogenic or anatomic velopharyngeal incompetence, such as in children with cleft palate.

Hoarseness in Infants and Children

- Very common.

- Numerous congenital and acquired etiologies.
- Vocal cord paralysis (idiopathic, CNS abnormality, cervical abnormality, birth trauma) is the most common congenital etiology.
- Viral laryngitis is the most common acquired etiology.
- Vocal cord nodules (voice abuse) is the second most common acquired etiology.
  Very difficult to treat
  Voice therapy if desired
  Surgical removal rarely indicated
- History and physical exam with flexible laryngoscopy in the clinic facilitates diagnosis in most cases.
- Laryngoscopy under general anesthesia rarely necessary.

Additional Acquired Etiologies of Hoarseness in Children

- Infections
  Laryngitis (viral, bacterial, other)
  Croup (viral laryngotracheobronchitis)
  Epiglottitis
  Tracheitis
- Vocal cord nodules
  Voice abuse
- Allergy
  Laryngitis
  Angioneurotic edema
  Anaphylaxis
- Trauma
  Blunt or penetrating laryngeal trauma
  Intubation injury
- Vocal cord paralysis
  Surgical injury (extracorporeal-membrane oxygenation, cervical surgery, neck surgery for thyroid)
  Neoplasm (CNS, neck, mediastinum)
- Neoplasm
  Papilloma secondary to human papilloma virus
  Hemangioma
  Lymphangioma
  Rhabdomyosarcoma
  CNS
- Gastroesophageal reflux
- Foreign body aspiration
- Others
  Voice change with puberty
  Hypothyroidism
  Tobacco use

Laryngoscopy is not performed in the routine examination. Unless good presumptive cause of hoarseness exists, laryngoscopy is necessary. It is best performed in young children with an electric laryngoscope of small or medium size with good batteries and light. The child should be placed in a supine position and should have an empty stomach to obviate aspiration of vomitus during manipulation. The head is held with the neck partly flexed by the mother. The child's tongue is held, and the laryngoscope is slowly inserted along the tongue to the base. Visualize the posterior pharynx and epiglottis and note their status. A redundant large epiglottis may be seen when it obstructs the airway. The current most common technique is nasally using a flexible nasolaryngoscope.

Pass the laryngoscope over the epiglottis and pull the handle up slightly toward the patient's head until you see the larynx. You may note laryngeal spasm, edema, paralysis, stenosis, redundancy, and tumors. You may also see thyroglossal duct cysts at the base of the tongue and the subglottic area if the larynx is normal.

In older children who can cooperate, indirect laryngoscopy is less traumatic. Seat the patient, warm the mirror, grasp the tongue, and pass the mirror back to rest on the anterior surface of the uvula, pushing it upward and backward. With good lighting, you can see the larynx. The cords are best seen if you tell the patient to say "eeee." This is the best diagnostic method for examination of the larynx when it can be used. It is particularly useful in problems of laryngeal motility and should precede direct laryngoscopy if possible.

Listen to the young child speak. The child should speak a word or two at 1 year of age, 5–6 words other than "ma-ma," "da-da" at 18 months, and should put two- to three-word sentences together at 2 years of age. At age 3 years, 75% of speech should be understood by nonfamily. Speech should be almost completely intelligible by 4 years of age. In children who are hearing or visually impaired or mentally delayed or who have neurologic or physical abnormalities of the vocalizing apparatus, speech is delayed or limited. In older children, note specific speech defects such as lisping or stuttering. Stuttering is normal at age 3 years. If stuttering does not improve after 4 years or if the child develops facial grimacing, referral is indicated. Regardless, the parents should be encouraged not to finish sentences and to give the impression of a nonhurried state. Adolescent males and children with adrenogenital syndrome and sexual precocity of other types have a deep voice. Children with large adenoids, sinusitis, or palatal paralysis have a nasal voice. Slurred indistinct speech with clicking produced by the tongue forcibly hitting the hard palate occurs in chorea. Aphonia with ability to whisper may indicate hysteria or selective mutism.

Laryngomalacia

Congenital laryngeal stridor has its onset in the first few weeks of life. Inspiratory stridor varies with changes in mental status and position. Gastroesophageal reflux noted radiographically in 80% of patients. Excessive clinical regurgitation past 3 months of age noted in 40%. Etiology is probably 2° to localized hypotonia and poor support of supraglottic structures rather than an anatomic cartilage abnormality. Patients usually outgrow by age 2.

Vocal Cord Paralysis

Vocal cord paralysis has the second most common congenital etiology. Onset occurs at birth, with inspiratory stridor. Common specific etiologies include: hydrocephalus with Arnold-Chiari malformation and meningomyelocele, other CNS diseases, and birth trauma. Idiopathic congenital paralysis is the most common diagnosis in 50% of patients.

Epiglottitis (Supraglottitis)

H. influenzae, type B is the most common agent. Epiglottitis must be distinguished from viral laryngotracheobronchitis. Treatment requires nasotracheal intubation and intravenous antibiotics. Tracheotomy is rarely indicated.

- Age 2–7 years
- Fulminant course
- No antecedent upper respiratory infection
- No cough
- High fever
- Severe toxicity
- Drooling
- Refuses to recline

Croup

- Age 3 months–5 years
- Gradual onset
- Antecedent upper respiratory infection
- Brassy cough
- Fever variable
- Toxicity varies

Bacterial Tracheitis

Always consider bacterial tracheitis in a toxic-appearing patient with signs and symptoms of croup. Diagnosis is made with bronchoscopy culture and stains. It is usually caused by S. aureus.

LUNGS

Note the type and rate of breathing. A newborn, especially a premature baby, will normally have Cheyne-Stokes respirations, characterized by periods of deep and rapid respirations alternating with periods of slow, shallow respirations or no respiratory activity (apnea); this pattern should disappear by 4 weeks of life when breathing becomes regular. Various brain or metabolic lesions that depress the central respiratory center may cause Cheyne-Stokes respirations.

The rate of respiration varies from 30 to 80 breaths per minute (bpm) at birth, 20–60 bpm in infancy, 16–20 bpm at 6 years, and 14–20 bpm at puberty.

Normal Awake Respiratory Rates in Children

Age (Years)	Respiratory Rate (breaths/min)
0–1	25–40
1–5	20–30
5–10	15–25
10–16	15–20

Because young children tend to have an abnormally high respiratory rate when even slightly excited, estimation of true respiratory rate is best obtained when the infant or young child is asleep. Children with any type of respiratory disorder almost always have a rapid respiratory rate, tachypnea; a normal respiratory rate usually indicates lack of acute pulmonary disease. Children aged less than 3 years with upper airway obstruction rarely breathe at a rate faster than 50 bpm, whereas children with lower airway obstructive disease, such as bronchiolitis, frequently breathe at rates of 80–100 bpm. In young children, tachypnea may be an early sign of heart failure.

Respiratory Distress Syndrome

Respiratory distress syndrome (RDS) is rare in full-term infants (see Chapter 20).

Transient Tachypnea of Newborn

Transient tachypnea in the newborn is caused by delayed resorption of fetal pulmonary fluid. Risk factors include prolonged labor, Cesarean section, fetal asphyxia, maternal sedation, fluid administration, and beta-agonist exposure.

Aspiration Syndromes

Aspiration syndromes consist of amniotic fluid aspiration, maternal blood aspiration, and meconium aspiration.

Meconium-Stained Amniotic Fluid

Meconium-stained amniotic fluid (MSAF) affects 12% of all deliveries and occurs predominantly in SGA, postmature, cord complications, or impaired placental circulation.

Meconium Aspiration Syndrome

Meconium aspiration syndrome affects 4% of deliveries complicated by MSAF. The infant is at risk for pulmonary hypertension and air leak, secondary pneumonitis.

Pneumonia

Bacterial (group B strep, gram-negative enterics, *Listeria*), viral (CMV, herpes simplex). Nonspecific findings; other signs of sepsis include shock, poor perfusion, and absolute neutropenia. Causes diffuse infiltrates that may appear similar to retained lung fluid or RDS; pleural effusion; rarely lobar infiltrate. Consider blood culture and broad-spectrum antibiotics until bacterial infection can be ruled out.

Persistent Pulmonary Hypertension of Newborn

Failure to transition from high pulmonary vascular resistance and low pulmonary blood flow characteristic of fetus to low pulmonary vascular resistance and high pulmonary blood flow of postnatal infant. Etiology is related to hypoxia, meconium aspiration syndrome, group B strep sepsis, RDS, total anomalous pulmonary venous return, congenital diaphragmatic hernia, pulmonary hypoplasia, polycythemia, hypoglycemia, and hypothermia. Treatment is with inhaled nitric oxide and ECMO. Rule out congenital heart disease, surfactant protein B deficiency, or alveolar capillary dysplasia.

Pulmonary Hypoplasia or Agenesis

Primary pulmonary agenesis is typically unilalteral; with or without other malformations and idiopathic pulmonary hypoplasia, basically bilateral. Secondary agenesis consists of oligohydramnios, Potter syndrome, chronic amniotic fluid leak, and renal agenesis or dysplasia.

Bronchopulmonary Malformations

Congenital Lobar Emphysema

A partial obstruction of the lobar bronchus resulting in hyperinflated lobe and 50% left upper lobe is congenital lobal emphysema; more common among males than females.

Congenital Cystic Adenomatoid Malformation

A congenital cystic adenomatoid malformation is a hamartomatous lesion characterized by overgrowth of terminal bronchioles. Multiple cysts become overdistended due to air trapping.

Pulmonary Sequestration

Pulmonary sequestration is a segment of lung parenchyma lacking connection with the tracheobronchial tree-mass of nonfunctional lung tissue supplied by anomalous systemic arteries. It is more common on the left; may be intra- or extralobar.

Bronchogenic Cyst

A bronchogenic cyst is an abnormal budding or branching of the tracheobronchial tree and is usually unilocular and has fluid-filled cyst in mediastinum.

Pulmonary Hemorrhage

Pulmonary hemorrhage is most often associated with RDS; also with hypoxia, hypervolemia, or congestive heart failure. It presents as sudden deterioration with shock, cyanosis, pallor, bradycardia, and apnea.

Mechanical Restrictive Disease

Choanal Atresia

Cyanosis is relieved with crying; inability to pass 6 Fr catheter.

Pierre-Robin Sequence

Micrognathia, cleft palate, glossoptosis.

Macroglossia

Beckwith-Wiedeman, trisomy 21. Mass effect: cyst (thyroglossal duct remnant, dermoid); lymphatic malformation, teratoma; lingual thyroid.

Vocal Cord Paralysis

Paralysis appears in 10%–15% of cases of stridor. Aphonic or weak, hoarse cry; may have coughing, choking, or cyanosis with feeds. Unilateral: damage to vagus or recurrent laryngeal nerve due to birth trauma, cardiovascular anomalies, or CT surgery; L > R; resolves spontaneously over 6–12 months.

Laryngomalacia

Most common cause of stridor in neonatal period. Usually develops at 2–4 weeks and progresses to 8 months, resolves by 2 years. Better in prone position; worsens with agitation; normal cry and no feeding difficulty. Laryngeal web, subglottic stenosis/hemangioma, tracheobronchomalacia, vascular rings, tracheoesophageal fistula, cystic hygroma, and goiter.

Congenital Diaphragmatic Hernia

This hernia occurs in 1/2,200 live births; 80% involve left hemidiaphragm with displacement of abdominal viscera into thoracic cavity through foramen of Bochdalek; 40% associated with other congenital anomalies. Mortality rate is 20%–60%. Prenatal diagnosis might permit intrauterine surgery, which might favorably affect the prognosis.

Chylothorax

May be due to traumatic injury of thoracic duct or congenital malformation of lymphatic system. Presents in the first days of life, typically lateral. Sixty percent occur on the right. Thoracentesis is diagnostic and therapeutic.

Sudden Infant Death Syndrome

Sudden infant death syndrome (SIDS) is sudden death in an infant under 1 year of age that remains unexplained after a complete postmortem examination, including an investigation of the death scene and a review of the case history. The current American Academy of Pediatrics policy of "Back to Sleep" has reduced SIDS cases in the United States by 30%–40%. Risk factors for SIDS include second-hand smoke, being small for gestational age, lower socioeconomic group, and prematurity.

Pneumonia

Nonbacterial; Viral

- Most common cause in children
- RSV, parainfluenza, influenza, adenovirus, and human metapneumovirus are most common causes
  RSV: winter and early spring, except more year round in the southern latitudes
  Parainfluenza 1: fall
  Parainfluenza 3: year round
  Influenza: winter
  Adenovirus: year round
  Human metapneumovirus: late winter and early spring
- Chest radiographs usually show patchy interstitial bronchopneumonia
- Complications unusual

Mycoplasma Pneumonia

Peak incidence is school-age children. Occasional symptomatic infections occur in children <5 years, rare in infants <6 months. Presentation is gradual with nonspecific symptoms such as cough, headache, fever, and malaise. May have crackles, wheezing, vomiting, and pharyngitis. On chest radiograph there is a nonspecific interstitial or bronchopneumonia pattern, usually in lower lobes. May have pleural effusion (20%) and/or hilar adenopathy (34%).

Chlamydia Pneumoniae (TWAR Strain)

Up to 6%–19% community acquired pneumonias, 10% of hospitalized pneumonias. Highest incidence in pediatric population is in adolescents. It should be also considered in a newborn with blepharitis. Associated with acute chest syndrome in sickle-cell disease. Nonspecific presentation. Laboratory diagnosis difficult; usually requires serologic testing. Treatment is by erythromycin and tetracycline.

Haemophilus influenzae (Rare)

Less common cause of bacterial pneumonia in children less than 5. Peak incidence 4–7 months. Decreasing incidence with vaccination. The presentation is similar to that of S. pneumonia. Chest radiograph lobar or patchy pneumonia, may have effusion. Course has more complications than with S. pneumoniae; may have extrapulmonary infection.

Uncommon Causes of Bacterial Pneumonia

- Group A Streptococcus
- Neisseriai meningitides
- Legionella pneumophilia
- Anaerobic bacteria
- Gram-negative enteric bacteria

- *Bordetella pertusis*
- Actinomycosis/*Nocardia*

Asphyxia

Seventy percent of neonatal encephalopathy is due to events before labor. Pure neonatal hypoxic-ischemic encephalopathy is rare. It occurs in 1.6 per 10,000 births.

Essential Criteria (Must Meet All Four)

Defines an acute intrapartum hypoxic event as sufficient to cause cerebral palsy.

1. Metabolic acidosis (cord pH <7.00, base deficit >12 mmol/L)
2. Early onset of severe or moderate neonatal encephalopathy in infants 34 weeks
3. Cerebral palsy (spastic quadriplegic or dyskinetic type)
4. Exclusion of other identifiable etiologies:
   Trauma
   Coagulation disorders
   Infections
   Genetic disorders

Criteria (Intrapartum Timing, 0–48 Hours)

Nonspecific to asphyxial insults.

1. Sentinel hypoxic event immediately before or during labor.
2. Sudden and sustained fetal bradycardia or absence of fetal heart rate variability with persistent, late, or variable decelerations (usually after sentinel event when pattern was previously normal).
3. Apgar scores of 0–3 beyond 5 minutes.
4. Onset of multisystem involvement within 72 hours.
5. Early imaging study showing evidence of acute nonfocal cerebral abnormality.
6. Early seizures are a worrisome prognostic event.

Nasal Flaring

You can easily overlook flaring of the alae nasi if you do not look for it specifically. It is a nonspecific but important sign of respiratory distress, probably reflecting increased work of breathing (dyspnea).

Children with generalized or localized infection, fever, poisoning, salicylism, acidosis, or shock also frequently have a rapid respiratory rate. A slow rate suggests central respiratory depression, especially that caused by increased intracranial pressure, sedatives or other drugs, alkalosis, poisons, or impeding respiratory failure. Slow, jerky respiratory movements or bursts of hyperpnea alternating with apnea (Biot breathing) may be noted in cases of CNS lesions involving the respiratory center, such as encephalitis.

Note the depth of respiration. Deep respirations are termed hyperpnea. Depth of respiration is an indication of the degree of anoxia present, the state of activity of the respiratory center, and the presence of acidosis or alkalosis.

In obstructive respiratory diseases, breathing is usually rapid and may be deep or shallow, depending on the degree and nature of the obstruction. In metabolic acidosis, breathing is deep; the respiratory rate is usually rapid but is depressed in alkalosis of long duration. Listening while holding the bell of the stethoscope over the mouth of a young child helps one estimate the rate and depth of respiration and frequently assists in diagnosing the degree of acidosis.

Establishing your own standards for depth of respiration is worthwhile. Examine a group of children aged 1, 3, 6, 9, and 12 months and 1, 2, 3, 4, 5, 6, 8, and 10 years in both the normal standing and in the supine position. During normal respiration, air from the child's nose will be felt a measurable distance from the nose. Record this distance for each age. You can then use each figure, plus or minus 2 cm, as your norm. My measurements for these ages, when the patients are supine, are 4 and 6 cm for infants aged 1 and 3 months, respectively; 10 cm for 6, 9, and 12 months; 12 and 15 cm for 1 and 2 years, respectively; 20 cm for 3 and 4 years; 22 cm for 5 and 6 years; and 25 cm for 8 and 10 years. You can determine increased depth of respiration by feeling the child's breath from a farther distance and decreased depth by feeling the child's breath closer to the child's nose.

Dyspnea

Recognize dyspnea, or distress during breathing, by observing flaring of the nares and intercostal spaces, cyanosis, suprasternal and infrasternal retraction, and rapid respiratory rate. Try to note whether the distress is mainly inspiratory or expiratory; inspiratory distress occurs more frequently with high obstructions, and expiratory distress occurs with low obstructions. Distress in tracheal obstruction is both inspiratory and expiratory. Dyspnea may also occur with pulmonary infections, pain, fright, anemia, cardiovascular disorders, and hyperthyroidism.

Dyspnea is usually increased by exercise and forms the basis of the exercise tolerance test. If limitation of exercising ability is suspected, some type of graded measurement of this ability is desirable. For infants, their highest exertion is with feeding. Dyspnea on exertion for them will be manifested as poor feeding. Usually, children of various ages can be asked to run about or up and down stairs and are then compared with their peers for the development of dyspnea. Dyspnea that occurs too soon indicates any state that may cause anoxia or causes such as lack of habit of exercise, obesity, or emotional distress. Exercise of the arms causes more dyspnea than an equivalent amount of exercise of the lower extremities.

Causes of Dyspnea

- Hypoxia
- Obstructive disease
  Upper airway: nasal congestion, choanal atresia, foreign body, tonsils, adenoids, macroglossia, decreased tone, retropharyngeal abscess, laryngomalacia, vocal cord paralysis, laryngeal web or polyp, subglottic stenosis
  Lower airway: asthma, bronchus-associated lymphoid tissue (BALT), bronchiolitis obliterans, tracheobronchomalacia, bronchial atresia, bronchiectasis, bronchitis, cystic fibrosis, primary ciliary dyskinesia (PCD), hemangioma, polyps, tracheo-esophageal fistula

- Restrictive disease
  Small or stiff lungs, obesity, kyphoscoliosis, chest deformity, respiratory muscle weakness (Duchenne muscular dystrophy, paralysis)
- Parenchymal disease
  Pneumonia, congenital lesions
- Vascular disease
  Pulmonary hypertension, sequestered lung
- Cardiac disease
  Congenital cyanotic heart disease (e.g., tetralogy of Fallot, total anomalous pulmonary venous return, transposition of great arteries)
  Pericarditis
  Myocarditis
  Cardiac tamponade
- Compression of the lung
  Pneumothorax
  Tumors (e.g., cyst, teratoma)
  Elevated diaphragm
  Effusions (e.g., empyema, hemothorax)
- Pulmonary embolism (rare)

Cough

Cough may result from intrathoracic or extrathoracic causes. Expiratory paroxysmal cough followed by an inspiratory whoop in a child more than 6 months of age or followed by vomiting in a child less than 6 months of age is characteristic of pertussis, parapertussis, and respiratory infection even months after pertussis. A loose productive cough is noted in children with bronchitis, upper respiratory infection with postnasal drip, and cystic fibrosis with pulmonary involvement. A sharp, brassy, nonproductive, barking cough, which sounds like the bark of a seal, is heard in children with laryngeal diphtheria, foreign body obstruction, croup, and, occasionally, tuberculosis. The child with croup is usually 3 months to 5 years old, is in distress, and is in the supine position. A tight, nonproductive cough is heard with pneumonia. A staccato cough suggests chlamydial infection.

Cough is usually nonproductive in children, even those with tuberculosis or bronchiectasis, and expectoration is rare. Hemoptysis may indicate foreign body obstruction, tuberculosis, other pulmonary infections, trauma, tumors, heart disease, or bleeding from high in the respiratory tract. Children with chronic pulmonary disease may have purulent sputum. Children with measles, tracheitis, or laryngitis have a dry, irritative persistent cough.

You can usually elicit the cough reflex by examining the child's throat with a tongue blade or by placing your finger in the suprasternal notch and pressing, which causes the child to gag. The cough reflex may be depressed in children with mental retardation, debilitating disease, and paralysis of the respiratory musculature and in those who have received sedatives or cough depressants.

Retropharyngeal Abscess

Always consider retropharyngeal abscess in a toxic patient with signs and symptoms of croup. Symptoms are high fever, stiff neck, and drooling. Widening of prevertebral soft tissues and/or gas in soft tissues noted on lateral neck film. Polymicrobial, *S. aureus*, Group A beta streptococcus, surgical drainage, and IV antibiotics (clindamycin or chloramphenicol and Roxacillin) are necessary.

Peritonsillar Abscess

Always consider peritonsillar abscess in a patient with severe tonsillitis and stridor. Includes high fever, stiff neck, trismus, unilateral pain, and "hot potato voice." Tonsil deviated medically, anteriorly, and inferiorly. Polymicrobial, *S. aureus*, Gr. A beta St. Needle aspirate, I and D, tonsillectomy, and IV antibiotics (penicillin G or clindamycin).

Tonsil and Adenoid Hypertrophy

History of mouth breathing, drooling, snoring, and frank obstruction. Sleep is often very restless and daytime somnolence may be noted. Parents are often frightened by apparent apneic episodes. Some children will have very poor weight gain. Children may also have enuresis or symptoms mimicking ADHD.

Causes of Cough: Acute and Chronic

- Upper airway disease
  Upper respiratory infection or common cold
  Chronic sinusitis, tonsillitis, laryngitis, and croup
  Allergic diseases
  Gastrointestinal reflux disease
  Foreign body
- Lower airway disease
  Asthma is inflammatory triad of edema, mucus, and bronchospasm
  Infectious diseases: Bronchiolitis, caused by RSV in babies; bronchitis is more common in older children and may be secondary to smoking or environmental tobacco smoke (ETS) exposure.
  Viral lower airway diseases include adenovirus, pneumonitis, influenza, and parainfluenza due to foreign body aspiration
  Chronic diseases (e.g., cystic fibrosis and bronchiectasis) and structural abnormalities (e.g., PCD, tracheoesophageal fistula (TEF), or cleft, rings, and slings) may present with intermittent rather than chronic cough
- Parenchymal and pleural disease
  Pneumonia
  Usually infectious agents include bacterial disease (e.g., streptococcal, staphylococcal) and atypical pneumonias (e.g., *Mycoplasma pneumoniae*), tuberculosis

Types of Cough

Bronchitis	Initially dry; after a few days, may become loose and rattling
Asthma	Classic cough is dry, tight; occasionally wheezy
Croup (acute laryngotracheo bronchitis)	Sounds like the bark of a seal
Pertussis	Spasmodic, choking, repetitive cough with no inspiration during coughing spasm
Chlamydia pneumoniae pneumonia	Typically paroxysmal, dry, and staccato (short inspiration between coughs), unlike pertussis
Tracheomalacia	Loud characteristic brassy or vibratory sound
Psychogenic	Sounds like a loud honk

Bronchitis

Acute: transient inflammation of trachea and major bronchi, prominent cough, resolves within two weeks. Chronic: persistent or recurrent episodes.

Differential Diagnosis of Bronchitis in Children

Chronic/Recurrent

- Cystic fibrosis
- Asthma
- Immotile cilia syndrome
- Tuberculosis
- Retained foreign body (airway, esophageal)
- Aspiration
  Anatomic abnormalities (tracheoesophageal fistula, laryngeal cleft)
  Dysfunctional swallowing with and without gastroesophageal reflux
  Gastroesophageal reflux
- Immunodeficiency
  IgA, IgG, IgG subclass, combination IgA and IgG subclass
- Inhalation injury
  Smoking: active and passive
  Indoor/outdoor pollution
  Marijuana
- Chronic airway damage
  Postinfection or traumatic airway injury with delayed or incomplete healing
- Large airway compression
  Dynamic: tracheomalacia, bronchomalacia
  Extrinsic: vascular or nodal compression

Acute

- Viral
  Parainfluenza, influenza, adenovirus, rhinovirus
- Bacterial
  Streptococcus pneumoniae, S. aureus, Hemophilus influenza (type B, nontypeable)
  Mycoplasma, chlamydia, pertussis, tuberculosis, diphtheria
  Chemical reaction, acute aspiration, smoke inhalation (Chernick & Kendig, 1990, p. 353)

Tracheomalacia

Tracheomalacia is a term used when a portion of the trachea is unusually soft. Tracheomalacia usually occurs in children with esophageal atresia and tracheoesophageal fistula, but it also can arise secondary to a vascular compression, usually by an anomalous artery. Tracheomalacia can also occur without any associated abnormality. The soft area of the trachea is more collapsible and causes a rather coarse inspiratory stridor. A viboratory expiratory stridor, or occasionally a wheeze, is often heard in these patients. When the child coughs, the more easily collapsible soft area of the trachea generates a loud, brassy sound.

Wheezing

Wheezing is defined as continuous breath sounds that are more prominent during expiration and often accompanied by expiratory prolongation. High-pitched wheezes originate from smaller airways; low-pitched wheezes (sometimes called rhonchi) originate from larger airways (Table 6.4).

Causes of Wheezing

Lower airway (expiratory polyphonic):

- Extraluminal compression of airways
  Parenchymal pneumonia, pulmonary edema, bronchogenic cyst
  Vascular ring, sling, cardiac wheeze
  Lymphatics: enlarged lymph nodes (tuberculosis, sarcoidosis, malignancy)
  Structural, congenital lobar emphysema (CLE), scoliosis, or chest wall deformity with airway kinking
- Transluminal change in airways
  Asthma: inflammation, edema, hyperemia, mucus gland hypertrophy and proliferation, smooth muscle bronchospasm
  Bronchiectasis/bronchitis
  Cystic fibrosis
  Ciliary disease: primary ciliary dyskinesia, dysfunction due to ETS or hyperoxia
  Anatomic: hemangioma, polyps, TEF, bronchial atresia, BALT, bronchiolitis obliterans, tracheobronchomalacia
  Immunologic disorders (e.g., IgA deficiency)

TABLE 6.4
Causes of Wheezing in Children

Associated Symptoms/Signs	Diseases Associated With Wheezing	
	Infants	Older Children
Failure to thrive	Cystic fibrosis, tracheo-esophageal fistula, bronchopulmonary dysplasia	Cystic fibrosis, chronic hypersensitivity pulmonary pneumonitis, alpha$_1$- antitrypsin deficiency, bronchiectasis
Associated with feeding	Tracheoesophageal fistula, gastroesophageal reflux	Gastroesophageal reflux
Positional changes	Anomalies of great vessels, gastroesophageal reflux	Gastroesophageal reflux
Environmental exposure	Allergic asthma	Allergic asthma, allergic bronchopulmonary aspergillosis, acute hypersensitivity pneumonitis
Sudden onset	Allergic asthma, croup (frequently at night)	Allergic asthma, foreign body aspiration, croup, acute hypersensitivity pneumonitis
Fever	Bronchiolitis, pneumonitis	Infectious asthma, acute hypersensitivity pneumonitis, croup, epiglottis
Rhinorrhea	Bronchiolitis, pneumonitis	Infectious or allergic asthma, croup
Stridor	Tracheal or bronchial stenosis, anomalies of the great vessels, croup	Foreign body aspiration, croup
Clubbing and/or cyanosis	Cystic fibrosis, bronchiectasis, bronchopulmonary dysplasia	

- Intraluminal change in airway
  Mucus (increased production or decreased clearance), pus (infected sputum), blood
  Foreign body
  Aspirated food or stomach contents secondary to gastroesophageal reflux

Upper airway (usually inspiratory and monophonic):

- Nasal (congestion, choanal atresia, foreign body)
- Oropharyngeal (tonsils, adenoids, macroglossia, foreign body, decreased tone, retropharyngeal abscess)
- Laryngeal (laryngomalacia, vocal cord dysfunction or paralysis, laryngeal web or polyp, subglottic stenosis)

Central nervous system:

- Structural disease (e.g., Arnold-Chiari malformation leading to vocal cord paralysis)
- Functional (e.g., vocal cord dysfunction, chronic aspiration)

REFERENCE

Chernick, V., & Kendig, E. (Eds.). (1990). *Disorders of the respiratory tract in children.* Philadelphia: WB Saunders.

FURTHER READING

Altman, R. P., & Stylianos, S. (Eds.). (1996). Pediatric surgery [Special issue]. *Pediatric Clinics of North America, 40*(6).

Avery, G. B., Fletcher, M. A., & MacDonald, M. D. (Eds.). (1999). *Neonatology: pathophysiology and management of the newborn* (5th ed., pp. 279–299, 1037–1038). Philadelphia: JB Lippincott.

Chernick, V., & Kendig, E. (Eds.). (1990). *Disorders of the respiratory tract in children* (5th ed., pp. 321–436). Philadelphia: WB Saunders.

Fanaroff, A., & Martin, R. (Eds.). (2002). *Neonatal-perinatal medicine, diseases of the fetus and infant* (7th ed., pp. 1276–1277). Philadelphia: Mosby Year Book.

Friedland, I. R., & McCracken, G. H. (1994). Management of infections caused by antibiotic-resistant *Streptocccus pneumoniae. New England Journal of Medicine, 331,* 377–382.

Hilman, B. C. (Ed.). (1993). *Pediatric respiratory disease* (pp. 185–305). Philadephia: WB Saunders.

Kattwinkel, J. (Ed.). (2000). *Textbook of neonatal resuscitation* (4th ed.). Elk Grove Village, IL: American Academy of Pediatrics.

Loughlin, G. M., & Eigen, H. (Eds.). (1994). *Respiratory disease in children* (pp. 351–372). Baltimore: Williams and Wilkins.

Overall, J. C. (1993). Is it bacterial or viral? Laboratory differentiation. *Pediatric Review, 14,* 251–261.

Panitch, H. B., Callahan, C. W., & Schidlow, D. V. (1993). Bronchiolitis in children. *Clinics in Chest Medicine, 14,* 715–731.

Stark, J. M. (1993). Lung infections in children. *Current Opinion in Pediatrics, 5,* 273–280.

Taeusch, H. W., Ballard, R. A., & Avery, M. E. (Eds.). (1998). *Schaeffer and Avery's diseases of the newborn* (7th ed., pp. 319–333, 933–937). Philadelphia: WB Saunders.

7

ABDOMEN

The true and lawful end of sciences is that human life be enriched by new discoveries and powers.

Francis Bacon

THE ABDOMEN IS frequently examined first in younger children. The examination requires few instruments, but even they may frighten the child. Warm your hands before examining the abdomen. A thorough examination is impossible if the child is afraid or crying or if the abdominal wall is taut. Examine the abdomen of a frightened child on the parent's lap. Sometimes it is necessary to examine parts of the abdomen while the child is quiet and to examine the abdomen later when the child quiets again. If the child is ticklish, have the child place a hand over your palpating hand.

When infants cry, they are often believed to have abdominal pain. When crying is recurrent, the infant is said to have colic. Although the term infantile colic was probably used because of the suspected similarity of its symptoms to symptoms of intestinal colic, it does not have any pathophysiologic implication. The cause of infantile colic is unknown. It is a syndrome of recurrent, intense, and inconsolable crying in otherwise healthy infants. Most infants with colic are free of symptoms during the day but have recurrent evening episodes of crying. However, normal, healthy infants also cry for prolonged periods, most commonly in the evening. Studies suggest that the average amount of crying in normal infants increases from 2 hours a day at 2 weeks to a maximum of 3 hours daily at 6 weeks and that by 3 months of age, normal infants cry for an hour or less each day.

INSPECTION

First, inspect the abdomen, noting its shape. Ordinarily the abdominal musculature of children is thinner than that of adults and children have a lordotic stance, giving the appearance of a potbelly. This appearance can generally be considered normal until children reach puberty.

Real distention of the abdomen is usually caused by air or fluid in the bowel or peritoneal cavity, but it may also be caused by atonic abdominal musculature, paralysis of the abdominal musculature, feces in the bowel, abnormal enlargement of organs, intestinal duplication, or tumors. Distention is frequently noted in children with cystic fibrosis, celiac disease, hypokalemia, rickets, hypothyroidism, bowel obstruction, constipation, ileus, or ascites. Transilluminate the abdomen with a strong light beam in a darkened room to differentiate cystic from solid masses in a child with an enlarged abdomen. Transillumination helps detect cystic tumors, bladder distention, and multicystic or hydronephrotic kidneys, as well as ascites.

Respiration is largely abdominal in children until age 6 or 7 years; even after this age, the abdominal wall usually moves with respiration in children lying supine and in pregnant adolescents. Peritonitis, appendicitis, other acute surgical emergencies of the abdomen, paralytic ileus, diaphragmatic paralysis, a large amount of ascitic fluid, or a large amount of abdominal air may be present if the abdominal wall fails to move with respiration. If respiration is entirely abdominal in a young child or largely abdominal in an older child, suspect emphysema, pneumonia, or other pulmonary disorders.

The abdomen is normally flat when the child is in the supine position. Occasionally, however, the abdomen will appear depressed or scaphoid. In newborns this may signify a large diaphragmatic hernia with most of the abdominal contents in the chest. In older children, scaphoid abdomen occurs in cases of marked dehydration or high intestinal obstruction. With pneumothorax, the chest is large and the abdomen, although normal, may appear to be scaphoid.

Observe the umbilicus. Normally it is closed and puckered, but hernia may be present as observed by protrusion of some abdominal contents. Retraction of the umbilicus during voiding may indicate a urachal anomaly. Umbilical hernias are common in all infants until age 2 years and in black children until age 7 years. Hernias are especially common in children with hypothyroidism, Down syndrome, or the chondrodystrophies, or in large, chronically distended abdomens. Granulomas, ulcers, and drainage of the umbilicus occur in newborns and are discussed in Chapter 20. Umbilical hernias and diastasis of the recti can become obvious when the child cries or coughs. Paradoxical motion of the umbilicus is noted in unilateral or asymmetric paralysis of the abdominal wall musculature or of one part of the diaphragm.

Diastasis of the rectus muscles may be noted as a protrusion in the midline, usually from the xiphoid to the umbilicus but occasionally down to the symphysis pubis. Ordinarily the protrusion is 1–5 cm wide; it is usually a normal variant but may be caused by a congenital weakness of the musculature or a chronically distended abdomen.

Note the veins. In infants with good subcutaneous tissue, veins are rarely visible. Visible but not distended veins are usual until puberty in healthy children and are especially noticeable in malnourished children. Veins are distended in heart failure, peritonitis, and venous obstruction. Milk a vein toward and away from the heart to determine direction of flow of blood in dilated veins. Blood flow from the veins below the umbilicus, normally downward, is usually reversed in children with obstruction of the inferior vena cava or portal hypertension (caput medusae). Diffuse epigastric pulsations may be normal or may indicate right ventricular hypertrophy with transmission of the pulsations through the diaphragm.

Next look for peristalsis, or gastric waves. Peristalsis is most easily seen if your eye is about at the level of the abdomen and a light is directed across the abdomen. Moving shadows will be noted in the presence of excessive peristalsis. Visible peristalsis is always a sign of obstruction until ruled otherwise. It may be seen normally in thin, small infants, especially premature ones. In infants aged 2 months or less, visible peristalsis may indicate pyloric stenosis or pylorospasm, but the type of obstruction cannot be distinguished by the nature of the visible peristalsis.

AUSCULTATION

Next, auscultate the abdomen and listen for peristalsis. It is better to auscultate the abdomen before proceeding, not only because you may forget to listen if this part of the examination is postponed, but also because later manipulation may so alter peristaltic sounds that appraisal becomes inaccurate.

Peristaltic sounds are normally heard as metallic short tinkling. A sound may be heard normally every 10–30 seconds. Place the stethoscope firmly over the abdomen and listen carefully because the sounds may normally be of low intensity. You may cause sounds to increase in frequency and intensity simply by stroking the abdomen with a fingernail. The sounds are high pitched and frequent in early peritonitis, diarrhea from any cause, intestinal obstruction, and gastroenteritis. Peristaltic sounds are absent in paralytic ileus. Listening to the abdomen and hearing the typical sounds of peritonitis may be the only way of detecting peritonitis in nephrosis or in other conditions in which there is free fluid in the abdomen, since free fluid may give you the impression of a nontense abdomen even though peritonitis is present. Rarely a venous hum may be heard during auscultation as a sign of portal obstruction. A murmur may be heard over the abdomen in children with coarctation of the aorta. Auscultate the area over the kidneys posteriorly with the bell stethoscope in children with hypertension. A murmur in this area may suggest constriction of one of the renal arteries.

PERCUSSION

After auscultating the abdomen, percuss by the indirect or scratch methods previously described. A tympanitic sound in a distended abdomen signifies that gas is present in the abdomen. Tympanites, or an unusually tympanitic sound, is common with low intestinal obstruction, air swallowing, and paralytic ileus.

A distended abdomen with little tympany suggests the presence of fluid or solid masses. When you suspect fluid, test for fluid wave and shifting dullness. Fluid wave may be elicited in the following manner: The edge of an aide's hand is placed firmly along the midline of the abdomen. Place one of your hands on one side of the patient's abdomen. Sharply strike the opposite side of the patient's abdomen with your other hand. A wave is felt against your first hand, as if the wave arises from deep in the abdomen. Shifting dullness is most easily obtained by percussing and delineating the area of dullness with the patient in one position. Then, change the position of the patient and elicit dullness again. Mark the area of dullness with a marker or pen. Slight shifting dullness is normal or may be found with tumors, but considerable shift usually indicates free abdominal fluid. Fluid in the abdomen (ascites) is found in children with chronic liver disease (e.g., cirrhosis), chronic kidney disease (e.g., nephrosis), tuberculous peritonitis, and, rarely, heart failure or rupture or other leak of the abdominal lymphatics (chylous ascites).

Solid masses will also be percussed. Frequently, a dull percussion note indicates a mass that cannot be felt. There is always dullness to percussion in the area of the liver unless free air is present in the abdominal cavity.

PALPATION

Several methods are satisfactory for palpating the abdomen, but in using all methods you should consider the comfort of the patient and yourself.

Distract the patient during abdominal palpation by making unrelated conversation or using other means. Palpating the abdomen with the child asleep is especially helpful if an acute abdomen is suspected. If the patient will cooperate, ask the patient to take deep breaths and to flex the knees during this part of the examination. Palpation is best performed if it can be done in inspiration and expiration. Place one hand flat on the patient's back and the other on the anterior surface of the abdomen. First, palpate gently and superficially, using the upper hand for most of the palpatory sensation. Begin in the left lower quadrant and then proceed to the left upper, right upper, and right lower quadrants, and the middle. If a localized site of pain or tenderness is found, palpate this area after the other parts of the abdomen have been palpated. Note first whether the abdomen is soft or hard. In a tense abdomen, there is a feeling of marked rigidity or resistance to pressure. A hard, tense abdomen immediately directs you to consider a surgical condition, any condition that may produce tenderness, or, rarely, tetanus and hypoparathyroidism. In a crying child, distinguish between a soft and hard abdomen by feeling immediately on inspiration when the child may relax for an instant. This act may relax the abdomen enough to allow you to feel masses or to localize tenderness or rigidity.

Note tenderness and the point of maximal tenderness. Frequently a patient will say an area is tender, and you may doubt the accuracy of the statement. In such case, it is best to touch a completely neutral area such as the thigh and ask the patient if that area is tender. Do not ask the patient, "Does this hurt?" unless the patient is old enough to give a completely reliable response. Rather, you can determine the site of tenderness by watching the patient's face, noting wincing, cry, and change in pitch of cry as the actual tender area is touched. Note the patient's pupils when you palpate. When a truly tender area is touched, the pupils will dilate. Frequently, a child with pseudopain will keep the eyes closed during the examination, but with organic pain the child will eye your hand as you palpate.

When asked where the abdomen hurts, a young child almost always points to the umbilicus. If the child points to any other part, pathology may be indicated. Tenderness can be further localized by noting pain on rebound. Place one hand deep in the abdomen, away from the suspected area of tenderness, and quickly remove your hand. The child may again complain of pain in the originally suspect area.

In general, even localized tenderness is not well correlated with underlying pathology. Tenderness in the lower quadrants may be due to such states as gastroenteritis, feces, obstruction, tumor, or, rarely, Meckel diverticulum with ulceration, torsion of the ovary, and torsion of the testes. Lower abdominal tenderness after a menstrual period may result from pelvic infection. Tenderness in the right lower quadrant with exquisite superficial skin tenderness may be caused by appendicitis or abscess; in the right upper quadrant by acutely enlarged liver, hepatitis, cholecystitis, pelvic inflammation, or intussusception; and in the left upper quadrant by acute splenic enlargement, intussusception, or splenic rupture. Midline tenderness in the upper abdomen may result from gastroenteritis, coughing, vomiting, or gastric or duodenal ulcer. In the midline of the lower abdomen, you can distinguish marked superficial tenderness from muscle tenderness by asking the child to raise the head and then palpating. Intraabdominal tenderness is lessened, whereas superficial tenderness is increased by this maneuver. Disease in or near the spinal cord can cause referred pain to the abdomen. If the abdominal wall is not tense, feel for the superficial masses.

Other masses (Figure 7.1) such as neuroblastoma, Wilms tumor, duplication of the intestinal tract and urinary bladder, circumscribed collections of blood, collection of fluid in the uterus resulting from an imperforate hymen, hydrometrocolpos, and an enlarged uterus attributed to pregnancy may be palpated superficially. Push the spleen medially, laterally, and upward if necessary to distinguish it from an enlarged left lobe of the liver. It may be felt superficial to the colon, distinguishing it from a retroperitoneal mass. Wilms tumor may be distinguished from a neuroblastoma, since Wilms tumor ordinarily does not cross the midline; however, it may be bilateral, especially in younger children. Ovarian tumors palpated in preadolescent girls may be malignant; after menarche, they are more likely to be functional.

After palpating, superficially proceed in the same manner around the quadrants of the abdomen but palpate more deeply, using the posterior hand to push masses forward. The anterior hand pushes down so that the skin of the anterior abdomen is actually indented 2–5 cm. In children with ascites, it may be difficult to feel any masses directly. However, percussion may indicate a few areas of increased dullness, and palpation by ballottement should delineate a few of the larger masses. In ballotting (Figure 7.2), place one hand lightly above and one hand firmly below the area to be balloted. With the balloting hand, quickly flick the area. If a ballottable mass is present, a rebound sensation will be felt in the flicking hand, as if a ball had been thrown forward and came back.

In addition to delineating the masses felt on light palpation, look for deeper masses. For example, the tumor of pyloric stenosis is best felt on deep palpation after an infant vomits. This mass is usually located at the end of the stomach anywhere along the edge of the liver from the costal margin in the midline to the underside of the right lobe of the liver. The sausage-shaped tender mass of intussusception can usually be palpated in the right upper quadrant. Other masses such as those caused by urinary tract anomalies (e.g., malposition, hydroureter, and hydronephrosis) and the filled bladder may be palpated. Bladder enlargement may be attributable to anatomic urinary tract obstruction, voluntary control, embarrassment of the patient, or low spinal cord lesions.

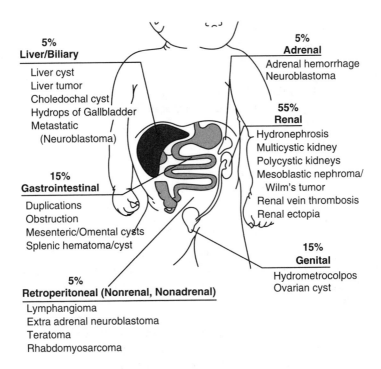

5%
Liver/Biliary

Liver cyst
Liver tumor
Choledochal cyst
Hydrops of Gallbladder
Metastatic
  (Neuroblastoma)

15%
Gastrointestinal

Duplications
Obstruction
Mesenteric/Omental cysts
Splenic hematoma/cyst

5%
Retroperitoneal (Nonrenal, Nonadrenal)

Lymphangioma
Extra adrenal neuroblastoma
Teratoma
Rhabdomyosarcoma

5%
Adrenal

Adrenal hemorrhage
Neuroblastoma

55%
Renal

Hydronephrosis
Multicystic kidney
Polycystic kidneys
Mesoblastic nephroma/
  Wilm's tumor
Renal vein thrombosis
Renal ectopia

15%
Genital

Hydrometrocolpos
Ovarian cyst

Figure 7.1
Distribution of abdominal masses in the neonate by organ system. (Data
derived from Kirks et al., 1981. *Radiologic Clinics of North America*, 19,
527–545).

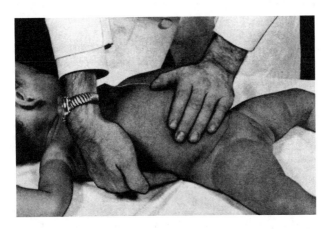

Figure 7.2
Balloting for right kidney.

By placing the index finger in the costovertebral angle and pushing up gently but sharply (as in ballottement), you can usually palpate about 1 or 2 cm of the right kidney and frequently the tip of the left kidney. The reverse procedure even more frequently allows you to feel the normal as well as the enlarged kidney: Gently elevate the abdomen of the child in the supine position with one hand, and place all the fingers of the other hand flat over the back of the elevated side so that the index finger lies in the costovertebral angle. Release the hand that is holding the abdomen forward; as the side of the abdomen falls toward the mattress, the kidney will hit the back of your hand. Enlarged kidneys usually indicate infection, congenital anomaly, tumor of the kidney, or renal vein thrombosis.

Remember that a few children have malrotation of the organs, as in situs inversus and congenital malrotation. In children who have had operations for repair of omphalocele and sometimes for diaphragmatic hernia, the organs are so displaced that it may be impossible to recognize even normal organs.

Every mass in the abdomen must be explained adequately before a patient can be considered free of disease. Occasionally, however, you may mistake feces in a child who is not even constipated for an abnormal mass or confuse the abdominal aorta with such a mass.

Palpate the umbilical hernia previously noted. Note the presence of bowel in the hernia by palpating a gas-filled loop and obtaining the feeling of silk rubbing against silk on replacing the viscus. If the hernia cannot be easily reduced, make careful note of its size. Palpate also for a diastasis between the rectus muscles.

Obtain abdominal reflexes by scratching the skin of the abdomen with four scratches to make a diamond, the points of the diamond being the midline shortly below the xiphoid and above the symphysis and both sides of the abdomen at the level of the umbilicus. The umbilicus normally moves at each scratch. The upper scratches are innervated at T 7 – T 9, and the lower at T 11 – T 12. This skin reflex is absent in normal children aged less than 1 year and in children with early poliomyelitis, multiple sclerosis, or other central or pyramidal disorders.

Next, palpate the inguinal and femoral regions for hernias, lymph nodes, and femoral pulses (Figure 7.3). Femoral pulses are best felt by placing the tips of two or three fingers along the inguinal ligament about midway between the iliac crest and symphysis pubis. With gentle pressure, you should feel definite pulsation with one of the fingers. Alternatively, pressure on the two or three fingers by the fingers of the other hand may make it easier to feel the pulse. Absent femoral pulse indicates coarctation of the aorta. Auscultation over the femoral artery may detect booming sound or "pistol shot," characteristic of aortic insufficiency (AI) or other causes of increased pulse pressure. A double sound (Traube double tone) is indicative of the same conditions. A systolic and diastolic murmur may also be heard in these conditions (Duroziez disease). Hernias are palpated as described below.

Palpate the fontanels. A sunken fontanel occurs with dehydration. One of the sites of determining dehydration in a child is over the abdomen. Pull up about 5–6 cm of the skin and subcutaneous tissue and quickly release it. If the creases formed by pulling the skin do not disappear immediately, dehydration exists.

Occasionally the wall of the abdomen feels puttylike in consistency. This may be normal, but it occurs in children who are chronically malnourished or dehydrated

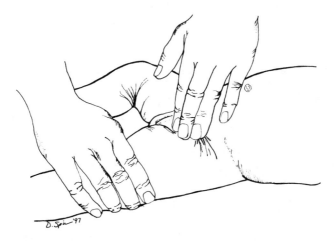

Figure 7.3
Palpating femoral area for femoral pulse.

and in children with such diseases as peritonitis, tuberculous enteritis, the lysosomal storage diseases, myxedema, and hyperelectrolytemia.

VOMITING

Vomiting is actually a symptom. However, when vomiting occurs, note the nature of the vomitus and save the vomitus if physical and chemical examinations are desired. Vomiting in newborns may have special significance.

Overfeeding, food intolerance, and improper handling of the infant are the usual causes of vomiting during infancy. However, vomiting of recently ingested food in children may be an early sign of infection in the intestinal tract or elsewhere. A common form of severe vomiting occurs in children 2–12 years of age; it occurs periodically, is probably due to a combination of psychogenic factors and lability of ketone-producing mechanisms, and is termed *cyclic vomiting*. Vomiting associated with nausea and occurring before breakfast may indicate hypoglycemia. Vomiting without nausea or vomiting of liquids but not solids, especially in the early morning, may be a sign of brain tumor.

Causes of Vomiting

Cough	Gastroesophageal reflux
Increased intracranial pressure	Migraine
Brain tumor	Poison (e.g., lead)
Food allergy	Medications
Enteritis	Parenteral infections
Chalasia	Psychogenic
Metabolic diseases	Abdominal epilepsy

In infants, forceful vomiting, especially of curdled milk free of bile staining, may be a sign of pylorospasm or pyloric stenosis but may also be the presenting sign of imperforate hymen. Vomitus containing bile may indicate duodenal or jejunal obstruction, whereas fecal vomiting is more common in children with lower intestinal obstruction, ileus, or peritonitis.

Bloody vomitus is most commonly due to swallowed blood from the nose and upper respiratory tract or from the mother's fissured nipple in a breast-fed infant. It is also seen in children with hemorrhagic diseases including Henoch-Schoenlein purpura, after the ingestion of foreign body or poisons, and after severe vomiting from any cause. Occasionally, bloody vomitus is seen in children with gastric, duodenal, or esophageal ulcers, anomalies of the portal vein, or cirrhosis of the liver with esophageal varices.

GASTROINTESTINAL BLEEDING

Blood in the GI tract of the healthy newborn is most often of maternal origin from blood swallowed during delivery or during breast-feeding (Table 7.1).

Intussusception

Acute episodes of apparent severe abdominal pain in the infant always call for urgent assessment. Middle to late infancy is the peak age for intussusception, with two thirds of all cases occurring in the first year of life. Intussusception is the telescoping of a proximal segment of bowel (usually the distal ileum) into the distal segment. The onset is sudden. Typically, the infant screams with pain, draws up both legs, and cannot be settled. Because the intussusception lodges in the distal bowel segment, the entrapment causes vascular obstruction with engorgement and mucosal swelling. Eventually, blood and mucus ooze from the entrapped bowel and are passed through the rectum. The stool may resemble currant jelly. At this stage, the bowel becomes ischemic and gangrenous if the process is not reversed. Examination of the infant is almost impossible during episodes of pain, but between episodes, the baby may sleep or become quiet enough to be examined. Typical findings in ileocolic intussusception are a flat right lower quadrant and a palpable, sausage-shaped mass in the right upper quadrant, either in the region of the hepatic flexure or more distally along the course of the colon.

TABLE 7.1
Differentiating Features of Upper and Lower Gastrointestinal Bleeding

	Upper GI	Lower GI
Presenting manifestation	Hematemesis and/or	Hematochezia
Nasogastric aspirate	Bloody	Clear
Blood urea nitrogen	Elevated	Normal
Bowel sounds	Hyperactive	Normal

Criteria for Diagnosis of Irritable Bowel Syndrome

- Abdominal pain that is relieved by defecation or is associated with a change in the consistency or frequency of stool
- A variable pattern of defecation at least 25% of the time with at least three of the following findings:
  Altered stool frequency
  Altered stool form (constipation, diarrhea)
  Straining, urgency, feeling of incomplete evacuation
  Passage of mucus with stool
  Feeling of abdominal distention, bloating

ANUS AND RECTUM

Examine the anal region; however, rectal examination is not performed in a routine examination but is reserved for children with symptoms referable to the lower gastrointestinal tract or those with abdominal pain.

Causes of Intestinal Obstruction

- Congenital lesions (atresias, bands, megacolon)
- Intussusception
- Late appendicitis
- Incarcerated hernia
- Postoperative adhesions
- Inflammatory bowel disease

Observe the buttocks for masses and firmness. The intergluteal cleft should be straight. Deviation occurs with sacrococcygeal tumor in the buttocks or hip dysplasia. Masses over the coccygeal area are usually sacrococcygeal tumors. Tufts of hair, meningocele, pilonidal dimple, and perianal abscess may be noted. If a pilonidal dimple is present, carefully inspect it for presence of a sinus. Abscesses may be caused by rectal fistula. Therefore, determine the extent of any rectal fistula by observation and probe if the full extent of the fistula cannot be visualized.

The buttocks are usually firm, even in advanced malnutrition; however, in cystic fibrosis and celiac syndrome, they are flattened. The skin creases of the buttocks are usually asymmetric but may indicate the presence of congenitally dysplastic hips. Skin creases of the buttocks are especially prominent in children with recent weight loss.

Anal fissure appears as a cut or tear in the mucosa. It is one of the most frequent causes of constipation or rectal bleeding in infants until age 2 years and may cause infantile colic (Table 7.2). Anal fissure is best detected by placing the infant on the abdomen, pulling the buttocks apart, and noting the fissure and asymmetry of mucosal folds. This maneuver may cause bleeding.

TABLE 7.2
Diagnosis of Rectal Bleeding

Condition	Symptom	Causes
Well	Bright blood around stool	Anal fissure or rectal polyp
Well	Red blood in stool	Meckel or duplication cyst
Well	Blood/mucus/diarrhea	Intussusception/gastroenteritis
Well	Melena ± hematemesis	Midgut volvulus, peptic ulceration, esophageal varices

Note prolapse of the rectal mucosa. It may be a cause of infantile colic. It may be caused by chronic constipation, straining, severe coughing, or diarrhea and may occur with cystic fibrosis or neurologic or anatomic abnormalities.

Note other protrusions from the anus. Small mucosal tabs have no significance; however, cherry red, round protrusions may be rectal polyps and cause rectal bleeding. Solid dark protrusions are hemorrhoids. They may be caused by portal hypertension, and may cause profuse bleeding. Large flat tabs of skin may be condylomas, a sign of papilloma virus infection, syphilis, or sexual abuse.

Necrotizing Enterocolitis

Necrotizing enterocolitis usually occurs in premature infants, particularly in those weighing less than 1,500 g (Table 7.3). Evidence has accumulated to support the hypothesis that an infectious agent contributes to the etiology of necrotizing enterocolitis, possibly that necrotizing enterocolitis is caused by a single, as yet unidentified, infectious agent (Figure 7.4). Other infectious diseases such as acquired immunodeficiency syndrome, bacteremia, neutropenia, disseminated intravascular coagulation, and shock develop in patients with necrotizing enterocolitis. Bowel sounds are diminished. The abdomen is distended, and there may be distended loops of bowel. The radiographic hallmark of necrotizing enterocolitis is pneumatosis intestinalis, gas trapped in small cysts within the bowel wall. Survivors of necrotizing enterocolitis are susceptible to stricture formation, which usually occurs 2 to 8 weeks after the acute onset of necrotizing enterocolitis.

Etiology of Neonatal Necrotizing Enterocolitis

- Sepsis
- Gastroenteritis
- Intestinal obstruction
  Jejunal atresia
  Malrotation
  Intestinal duplications
  Volvulus
  Meconium ileus
  Hirschsprung colitis
  Intussusception
- Milk protein intolerance
- Neonatal appendicitis

TABLE 7.3

Modified Bell's Staging Criteria for Necrotizing Enterocolitis

Stage	Systemic Signs	Intestinal Signs	Radiologic Signs	Treatment
I. Suspected				
A	Temperature instability, apnea, bradycardia	Elevated pregavage residuals, mild abdominal distention, occult blood in stool	Normal or mild ileus	NPO, antibiotics ×3 days
B	Same as IA	Same as IA, plus gross blood in stool	Same as IA	Same as IA
II. Definite				
A: Mildly ill	Same as IA	Same as above, plus absent bowel sounds, abdominal tenderness	Ileus, pneumatosis intestinalis	NPO, antibiotics ×7–10 days
B: Moderately ill	Same as I, plus mild metabolic acidosis, mild thrombocytopenia	Same as above, plus absent bowel sounds, definite abdominal tenderness, abdominal cellulites, right lower quadrant mass	Same as IIA, plus portal vein gas, ± ascites	NPO, antibiotics ×14 days
III. Advanced				
A: Severely ill, bowel intact	Same as IIB, plus hypotension, bradycardia, respiratory acidosis, metabolic acidosis, disseminated intravascular coagulation, neutropenia	Same as above, plus signs of generalized peritonitis, marked tenderness, and distention of abdomen	Same as IIB, plus definite ascites	NPO, antibiotics ×14 days, fluid resuscitation, inotropic support, ventilator therapy, paracentesis
B: Severely ill, bowel perforated	Same as IIA	Same as IIA	Same as IIB, plus pneumoperitoneum	Same as IIB, plus bowel perforated surgery

Modified from Walsh, M. C., & Kliegman, R. M. (1986). Necrotizing enterocolitis: Treatment based on staging criteria. *Pediatric Clinics of North America, 33,* 179–201.

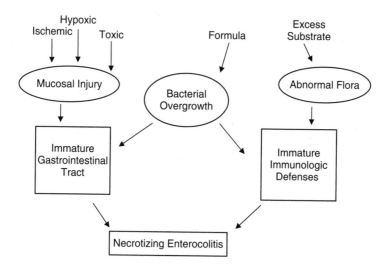

Figure 7.4
Proposed schema by which multiple factors combine to initiate necrotizing enterocolitis.

Pinworms occasionally are noted in the perianal area in the folds of rectal mucosa; these may cause rectal itching. A dark ring around the rectal mucosa may be an early sign of lead poisoning.

Most of the eruptions around the rectum in the young result from diaper rash. Usually the eruption is a generalized reddened or brawny area with vesicles or papules. However, pustules may be present and represent secondary infection of the diaper rash or perianal cellulitis resulting from streptococcus or candida.

A rectal examination is best performed with the infant or child lying supine with the legs flexed. A child who is old enough is asked to empty the bladder before this examination. Ordinarily, your fifth finger is long enough to provide the required information in infants and hurts the patient less than a larger finger. Because you may have better control and mobility of the index finger, use it for more precise information. Grease the anus and glove well before inserting your finger. Imperforate anus is evident immediately, since the finger cannot enter beyond the dimple.

Note sphincter tone. A patulous rectum is associated with sexual abuse or a low cord injury, including myelomeningocele and diastematomyelia. A tight sphincter is generally a developmental variation indicating stenosis. Anal stenosis may cause constipation and pain on defecation. A rectovaginal fistula exists if your finger enters the vagina through the rectum.

Occasionally, you will feel a shelflike protuberance 2–5 cm above the anus; this, with absence of feces in the rectum, may be a sign of aganglionic megacolon. Anterior position of the anal opening with a posterior shelf on rectal examination is a sign of anterior ectopic anus, a cause of chronic constipation. If position is uncertain, measure in girls from fourchette to anus to coccyx and in boys from the base of the scrotum. The distance of fourchette or scrotum to anus divided by four-chette or scrotum to coccyx is 0.39 or 0.56, respectively. Marked deviation indicates displacement.

The anus and rectum may be distended with feces in children with develop-mental delay, chronic constipation, or psychogenic difficulties. Absence of feces in the rectum in an acutely ill child may indicate ileus, peritonitis, or obstruction.

Note masses. Fecal masses of any consistency can be removed. A tender mass in the lower quadrants may be found with a low intussusception. A right lower quad-rant mass is occasionally noted with acute appendicitis or appendiceal abscess and sometimes with regional ileitis. Polyps may occasionally be felt in the rectum. Masses that displace the rectum forward frequently are teratomas. Other masses described under examination of the abdomen are also noted.

Palpate for the prostate, a flat mass several centimeters up and on the midline anterior wall of the rectum. Any prostate that is larger than 1 cm before age 10 years may indicate precocious puberty or congenital adrenal hyperplasia. After puberty, the prostate is 2–3 cm and is smooth. A tender prostate indicates infection; an uneven or large prostate suggests tumor.

Rectal examination is also useful in palpating the uterus. In pubertal children and occasionally in younger children, the ovaries may also be palpated. The prepu-bertal uterus is felt as a 1–2 cm oval mass anterior to the rectum and about 3 or 4 cm above the symphysis pubis. When the ovaries are palpable before puberty, they are about 0.5–1.0 cm in diameter, situated about 2–3 cm laterally and just above the uterus. Foreign bodies in the vagina or rectum can also be felt by palpation.

Even though a rectal examination is usually uncomfortable and is reserved for the last part of the physical, it can frequently localize tenderness in the abdomen. After your finger is well up in the patient's rectum, place it in the midline and press the other hand toward the finger. Note facial expression. Next, move the finger and the abdominal hand to the left, and repeat on the right. Differences in facial expres-sion or rigidity of the lower abdomen are a clue to abdominal or rectal pathology.

Sensation should be tested in children who are suspected of having a spinal cord lesion or a patulous rectal sphincter. Use a pin to touch the perineal region at closely approximated points. Twitching of the perineum normally occurs with a slight lateral movement of the anus. Absence of this reflex suggests lower motor neuron lesion.

If you wish to visualize the rectal mucosa for suspected internal rectal fissure, polyp, hemorrhoid, colitis, proctitis, or bleeding site, you may do so with relative ease with a small proctoscope or without special equipment. Grease a clean test tube and push it about 5 cm into the rectum. Place a small light just behind your shoul-der, shining into the tube. Slowly withdraw the tube, and note the mucosa as it falls back into place. Note the color of the stool (see Box 7.1).

Causes of Abdominal Distention

- Functional intestinal obstruction
  Paralytic ileus, postoperative ileus, reflux ileus (from sepsis or acute infection)
  Peritonitis or intestinal perforation
  Severe hypokalemia

Gastroparesis
Necrotizing enterocolitis
Toxic megacolon (inflammatory bowel disease)
Dysmotility (pseudo-obstruction syndrome)
- Renal enlargement
Hydronephrosis (most common cause of abdominal distention in the newborn)
Ureteropelvic junction obstruction
Bladder distention
Congenital polycystic kidney
- Ascites
- Mechanical intestinal obstruction
Incarcerated inguinal hernia
Malrotation with volvulus
Intestinal atresia (newborns)
Imperforate anus (newborns)
Intussuception
Hirschsprung disease
Meconium ileus (in newborns, due to cystic fibrosis)
Left microcolon syndrome (typically in infants of diabetic mothers)
Fecal impaction (from chronic constipation)
Bezoars: lactobezoars in premature infants
- Splenomegaly
- Hepatomegaly
Budd-Chiari or Beckwith-Wiedemann
Glycogen storage disease
Amyloidosis
Congestive heart failure
- Tumors/cysts (Wilms tumor, neuroblastoma, lymphoma, teratoma, sarcoma, ovarian cyst or tumor, omental cyst, dermoid cyst)
Pancreatic pseudocyst
Obesity: protuberant abdomen (common)
Acrophagia
Pregnancy
Hematometrocolpos
Malnutrition (e.g., kwashiorkor, celiac)
Abdominal abscess
Prune-belly syndrome
Poor posture

Differential Diagnosis of Abdominal Masses

- Wilms tumor
- Neuroblastoma
- Leukemia/lymphoma
Involvement of retroperitoneal nodes, liver, or spleen
- Germ cell tumors
Ovarian, teratoma

BOX 7.1 STOOL COLOR

Brown, yellow	Normal
White	Acholic, excess milk ingestion
Bright red (blood)	Anal fissure, lower colon
Bright red (not blood)	Foods, dyes
Black, tarry (blood)	Bleeding proximal to ileocecal valve

- Soft tissue sarcoma
  Rhabdomyosarcoma
- Benign tumors
  Adenomas (especially liver), hamartomas, pheochromocytoma
- Cystic masses
- Gynecologic
  Ovarian torsion, endometriosis, pelvic inflammatory disease
- Rare malignancy in children
  Carcinoid tumors, adrenocortical carcinoma, pancreatoblastoma, malignant rhabdoid tumor
- Gastrointestinal
  Constipation/stool impaction, intestinal obstruction (e.g., Hirschsprung), gastrointestinal duplication, incarcerated hernia
- Pancreatic pseudocyst
- Vascular lesions (e.g., hemangioma)
- Renal disorders
  Distended, nonemptying bladder, bladder outlet obstruction
  Congenital mesoblastic nephroma
  Severe hydronephrosis
- Structures normally palpable in small children are liver edge, spleen tip (especially with viral illness), aorta, sigmoid colon, and spine
- Infections
  Abscess, hepatitis, virus (EBV, CMV) causing splenomegaly or hepatomegaly

Differential Diagnosis of Ascites

- Bile ascites (bile peritonitis)
- Peritoneal dialysis
- Cardiac
  Congestive heart failure
  Chronic constrictive pericarditis
  Inferior vena cava web
  Erythroblastosis fetalis
- Renal
  Nephrotic syndrome
  Urinary ascites (due to bladder rupture)
  Obstructive uropathy: congenital ascites may be seen with bilateral hydronephrosis

- Gastrointestinal disorders
  Infracted bowel
  Bowel perforation
  Protein-losing gastroenteropathy
  Pancreatitis, ruptured pancreatic duct
- Gynecologic
  Ovarian tumors, cyst torsion or rupture
- Malignancy
  Leukemia, lymphoma, neuroblastoma
- Hepatic, resulting in portal hypertension
  Hepatic cirrhosis
  Portal vein thrombosis
  Cavernous transformation: catheterization, dehydration, clotting disorder, omphalitis
  Arteriovenous fistula
  Fulminant hepatic failure
  Congenital hepatic fibrosis
  Lysosomal storage disease
- Peritonitis
  Tuberculous peritonitis
  Schistosomiasis (Mansoni)
  Tularemia
  Abscess
- Chylous ascites
  Collection of lymph within the abdominal cavity; secondary to lymphatic obstruction from trauma, surgery, tumor, tuberculosis, or filariasis

Differential Diagnosis of Constipation

- Functional constipation
  By far the most common etiology
  Rome II criteria define chronic functional constipation in infants and young children as at least 2 weeks of scybalous, pebblelike, hard stools for the majority of stools, or firm stools two or fewer times per week
  Presents with stool withholding behavior
  Often due to inadequate fluid or fiber intake
- Drugs: antacids with aluminum and calcium, anticholinergics, antidepressants, bismuth, calcium antagonists, cough suppressants, opioid analgesics, phenobarbitol
- Endocrine disorders
  Hypercalcemia
  Hypothyroidism
  Hyperthyroidism
  Pregnancy
  Reduction of steroid hormones in luteal and follicular phases of menstrual cycle
- Irritable bowel syndrome
- Ogilvie syndrome
- Celiac disease
- Inflammatory bowel disease

- Cystic fibrosis
- Hirschsprung disease
  1/5,000 births, male-to-female ratio 4:1
  94% do not pass meconium within 24 hours of birth
  61% diagnosed by 12 months of life
- Lead toxicity
- Neurologic disease
  Myelomeningocele
  Hypotonia (e.g., Down, myopathies, prune-belly syndrome)
  Cerebral palsy
- Metabolic disorders
  Uremia
  Hypokalemia
  Amyloid neuropathy
- Structural abnormalities
  Anal disorders (imperforate anus, anteriorly displaced anus, perianal fissures, strep infection, and stenosis)
  Pelvic masses (sacral teratoma)
- Infectious disease
  Infantile botulism
  Chagas disease

Differential Diagnosis of Encopresis

- Functional constipation accounts for 66%
  Chronic constipation with fecal impaction results in a functional megacolon and overflow incontinence
  Repeated soiling of underpants
  Involuntary passage of loose feces around large balls of impacted feces
  Child is unaware of accidents and odor
- Anorectal malformations
  Incidence is 1/4,000 live births
  Anal stenosis with overflow incontinence
  Imperforate anus with perineal fistula
  Vestibular fistula: most frequent defect seen in females; rectum opens into the vaginal vestibule
  Rectovaginal fistula: can result from pressure necrosis with obstructed labor
  Persistent cloaca: the rectum, vagina, and urinary tract meet and fuse into a single common channel
- Functional nonretentive fecal soiling
  Rome II criteria: inappropriate defecation in the absence of constipation and structural or inflammatory disease
  May be the manifestation of an emotional disturbance in a child
  Affects 2% of school-age children
- Spina bifida
  Incidence is 1/1,000 live births
  Myelomeningocele is the most common

Bladder and bowel dysfunction is usual
- Spinal tumors
- Tethered cord
- Diarrheal disease: transient fecal soiling resolves with cessation of diarrhea
- Postsurgical repair
  Common sequel of the repair of high imperforate anus and Hirschsprung
- Inflammatory bowel disease
  Perianal fistulas or sinuses (Crohn disease)
- Diastematomyelia
  Difficulty in walking, dribbling of urine, and fecal incontinence
- Organic constipation
  Hypothyroidism, celiac disease, amyloid neuropathy, and endocrine disorders

Differential Diagnosis of Hematemesis

- Esophagitis
  Gastroesophageal reflux disease
  Crohn disease
  Infection (e.g., *Candida, Aspergillus,* cytomegalovirus, herpes simplex virus)
  Medications (e.g., tetracycline, aspirin, NSAIDs, potassium chloride)
- Peptic ulcer disease
- Tumors
  Polyps
  Lipomas
  Adenocarcinoma
  Lymphoma
- Traumatic
  Mallory-Weiss tear
  Prolapsing gastropathy
  Foreign body ingestion
  Direct abdominal trauma
- Gastritis
  More common than ulcers in children
  Medications (e.g., NSAIDs, aspirin)
  Infections (e.g., *Helicobacter pylori,* cytomegalovirus, herpes)
  Crohn disease
- Vascular malformations
  Hemangiomas
  Aortoenteric fistulas
  Dieulafoy lesion
  Osler-Weber-Rendu syndrome
  Watermelon stomach
  Hemorrhagic telangiectasia
  Blue rubber-bleb nevus syndrome

- Portal hypertension
  Esophageal varices
  Gastric varices
  Hypertensive gastropathy
- Eosinophilic enteropathy
- Milk protein allergy
- Zollinger-Ellison syndrome
  Gastrinoma
  Results in multiple small bowel ulcers
- Miscellaneous
  Hemosuccus pancreaticus
  Hemobilia
  Swallowed maternal blood
  Gastric duplication
  Munchausen by proxy syndrome
  Coagulopathy
  Epistaxis (initially swallowed blood)
  Hemoptysis

Hematochezia

Hematochezia refers to bright red blood per rectum (BRBPR). When the blood is maroon, the bleeding source is usually colonic. Massive upper gastrointestinal bleeding may rarely present with BRBPR because blood is a cathartic and children have a short intestinal transit time. Milk protein allergy is the common factor, followed by anorectal fissure in infants.

Differential Diagnosis

- Milk or soy protein allergy (colitis)
- Anorectal fissure: passage of hard stool causing rectal trauma
- Necrotizing enterocolitis: vast majority occur in premature infants
- Infectious colitis
  Bacterial: *Salmonella, Shigella, Campylobacter, Yersinia, Clostridium difficile,* and *E. coli* (0157:H7)
  Parasitic: Entamoeba histolytica
- AIDS
  Aphthous ulcerations of the intestine
- Inflammatory bowel disease
- Intestinal duplication
- Immunocompromised host
  Cytomegalovirus enterocolitis
  Disseminated aspergillosis
  Mycobacterium avium complex
  Typhlitis: Polymicrobial inflammation of the cecum associated with neutropenia
- Meckel diverticulum: Ectopic gastric mucosa, 2% of population

- Juvenile polyps
  Most common source of significant rectal bleeding in childhood
  Pathologically benign inflammatory polyps
- Solitary rectal ulcer
- Henoch-Schönlein purpura
- Ischemic injury
  Malrotation with volvulus
  Intussusception
  Postoperative (colonic watershed regions)
  Acute drug-induced ischemia (cocaine)
- Lymphonodular hyperplasia
- Hemorrhoids and colorectal varices from portal hypertension
  Hemorrhoids rarely bleed in children
- Hirschsprung enterocolitis
- Vascular lesions
  Hemangiomas (rare)
  Arteriovenous, venous malformations
  Klippel-Trenaunay syndrome
  Blue rubber-bleb nevus syndrome
  Hereditary hemorrhage telangiectasia
- Foreign body injury: ingested glass, broken glass thermometer, other sharp objects
- Munchausen syndrome by proxy

Nonspecific (Toddlers') Diarrhea

Symptoms

- Normal growth (unless diet restriction)
- Stools intermittently loose, increasingly watery during the day, undigested particles

Etiology

- Altered motility
- Excess fluid, fructose, sorbitol

Treatment

- Whole milk
- Fat (ileal break)
- Eliminate juices

Common Causes of Chronic Diarrhea

Infants

- Dietary protein allergy
- Protracted viral enteritis
- Zinc deficiency
- Cystic fibrosis

Toddlers

- Nonspecific diarrhea
- Giardiasis
- Celiac disease

Older Children

- Inflammatory bowel disease
- Primary acquired lactose intolerance
- Irritable bowel syndrome

Dietary Protein Allergy

Antigens

- Cow/soy protein (40%–50% cross-reactivity)
- Protein hydrolysate
- Breast milk
- Sensitization in utero

Symptoms

- Diarrhea (mucus, blood, colitis)
- Vomiting

Diagnosis

- Rule out infection

Protracted Diarrhea of Infancy

- At 5 months old, diarrhea for 4 weeks and failure to thrive (FTT)
- Initially: improvement with Pedialyte
- Relapse with cow milk formula
- Albumin 2.8 g/dL; stool pH 4.5; respiratory syncytial virus (RS2+)
- Best test: small bowel biopsy
  Partial villous atrophy
  Rule out villous atrophy
  Rule out microvillous inclusion disease
- Therapy: lactose-free formula and continued nasogastric feeding

Diarrhea: Acute

Differential Diagnosis

- Parasitic infestations
  Giardia lambia
  Cryptosporidium (severe in AIDS patients)
  Entamoeba histolytica
- Overfeeding (relative lactose deficiency)
- Bacterial overgrowth

- Antibiotics
- Adrenogenital syndrome
- Zinc deficiency
- Irritable bowel syndrome
- Constipation with encopresis
- Hirschsprung toxic colitis
- Laxative abuse
- Vitamin deficiency (e.g., niacin)
- Lactose or fructose intolerance
- Malabsorption (celiac disease, cystic fibrosis)
- Food allergies
  Cow milk and soy protein allergy are most common in infancy
- Viral gastroenteritis
  Calcivirus
  Enteric adenovirus
  Astrovirus
  Noravirus, rotavirus, most common in winter
- Bacterial gastroenteritis
  Campylobacter jejuni (associated with Guillain-Barré syndrome)
  Salmonella
  Shigella: may cause seizures (up to 30%) hemolytic uremic syndrome (HUS)
  Escherichia coli (various types): enteropathogenic, enterohemorrhagic (0157:H7)
  verotoxin can cause HUS (6%–8% of cases), enterotoxigenic (traveler's diarrhea),
  enteroinvasive
  Clostridium difficile (toxin A or B)
  Yersinia enterocolitis (mimics acute appendicitis)
  Vibrio cholerae
  Aeromonas hydrophilia
  Bacillus cereus, Staphylococcus aureus, Clostridium perfringens

Differential Diagnosis of Abdominal Pain

Epigastric Pain

- Peptic ulcer disease/gastroesophageal reflux disease
  May be due to *Helicobacter pylori* or NSAID use
- Gallbladder disease
  Most commonly with hemolytic disorders with pigment stones
- Pancreatitis
- Trauma and idiopathic are common causes

Periumbilical Pain

- Functional abdominal pain/irritable bowel syndrome
  Most common cause of nonorganic pain
  Occurs in children 3–15 years old
- Abdominal migraine
- Streptococcal pharyngitis

- Small bowel bacterial overgrowth
- Gastroenteritis (viral, bacterial, parasite)
- Appendicitis
  Periumbilical pain moves to right lower quadrant
- Carbohydrate intolerance
- Lactase, trehelase deficiency

Right Lower Quadrant Pain

- Ovarian torsion
- Appendicitis
- Pelvic inflammatory disease
- Ectopic pregnancy
- Mittelschmerz
  Pain midcycle with ovulation
- Right lower lobe pneumonia
- Inguinal hernia
- Iliopsoas abscess

Left Lower Quadrant Pain

- Constipation
- Right ovarian/testicular pain

Suprapubic Pain

- Urinary tract infection
  With dysuria, fever, foul-smelling urine
  Pyelonephritis may have costovertebral angle (CVA) tenderness
- Constipation
  Accounts for 3% of visits to pediatrician
  May have a palpable fecal mass
- Urinary retention
- Hydrometrocolpos
  Associated with imperforate hymen
  Cyclic pain with onset of menstrual cycle

Other Organic Causes of Constipation

- Anatomic
  Anterior displacement of anus
- Metabolic
  Hypothyroidism
  Hypercalcemia
- Neuropathy/myopathy
- Drugs
- Celiac disease
- Distal colitis
- Lead toxicity

Hirschsprung Disease

Red Flags Suggesting Hirschsprung Disease

- Failure to thrive
- Obstructive symptoms
- Bloody diarrhea
- Tight empty rectum
- Occult blood
- Lack of soiling

Diagnosis

- Rectal suction biopsy
  Ganglion cells
  Acetylcholine esterase stain
- Anorectal manometry
  Internal sphincter relaxation reflex
- Barium enema
  Confirmation
  Level of transition

Performance of the Slide Guaiac Test for Occult Fecal Blood

1. For 3 days before and during testing, patients should avoid:
   - Meat (rare or well done)
   - Peroxidase-containing vegetables and fruits (broccoli, turnips, cantaloupes, cauliflower, tomatoes, radishes, fresh red cherries)
   - The following medications: Iron preparations (stool pH <6.0), vitamin C, aspirin, nonsteroidal anti-inflammatory drugs, bismuth (e.g., Pepto-Bismol)
   - Other: Commercial dyes No. 2 and No. 3, licorice, beets, spinach, blueberries
2. Two samples of each of three consecutive stools should be tested. It is proper to sample areas of obvious blood.
3. Slides should be developed within 4–6 days.
4. Slides should not be rehydrated prior to developing (for average-risk screening).
5. If rehydrated, red meat must have been avoided (otherwise, too many false positives).

FURTHER READING

Baley, J. E. (1989). Neonatal candidiasis: The current challenge. *Clinics in Perinatology, 18,* 263–280.

Barnard, J. A. (2004). Gastrointestinal polyps and polyp syndromes in adolescents. *Adolescent Medical Clinics, 15,* 119–129.

Dahms, B. B., & Morrison, S. C. (1993). *Helicobacter pylori* gastritis. Pathological case of the month. *American Journal of Diseases of the Child, 147,* 315–316.

deSa, D. J. (1976). The spectrum of ischemic bowel disease in the newborn. *Perspectives in Pediatric Pathology, 3,* 273–309.

Moir, C. R. (1996). Abdominal pain in infants and children. *Mayo Clinic Proceedings, 71,* 984–989.

Orenstein, S. R., Shalaby, T. M., DiLorenzo, C., Putnam, P. E., Sigurdsson, L., Mousa, H., et al. (2000). The spectrum of pediatric eosinophilic esophagitis beyond infancy: A clinical series of 30 children. *American Journal of Gastroenterology, 95,* 1422–1430.

Rudolph, C. D., Mazur, L. J., Liptak, G. S., Baker, R. D., Boyle, J. T., Colletti, R. B., et al. (2002). Guidelines for evaluation and treatment of gastroesophageal reflux in infants and children: Recommendations of the North American Society for Pediatric Gastroenterology and Nutrition. *Journal of Pediatric Gastroenterology and Nutrition, 35,* 583.

Russo, P. (2004). Enteropathies associated with chronic diarrhea and malabsorption of infancy and childhood. In P. Russo (Ed.), *Pathology of pediatric gastrointestinal and liver disease.* New York: Springer.

Valdes-Dapena, M. (1989). Iatrogenic disease in the perinatal period. *Pediatric Clinics of North America, 36,* 67–93.

Walker, W. A., Kleinman, R. E., Sherman, P. M., Shneider, B. L., & Sanderson, I. R. (Eds.). (2000). *Pediatric gastrointestinal disease* (3rd ed.). Hamilton, Ontario: BC Decker.

8

EXTREMITIES, JOINTS, AND SPINE

Though there were many Giants of old in Physick and Philosophy,
yet I say with Didacus Stella: A dwarf standing on
the shoulders of a Giant sees farther than a Giant himself;
I may likely add, alter, and see farther than my predecessors.

Democritus Junior to the Reader, The Anatomy of Melancholy,
Robert Burton

IN PRACTICE, THE physician usually examines the extremities, bones, joints, and muscles simultaneously and then, if abnormalities are detected, examines the systems under suspicion individually and more extensively. Examination of muscles is described in Chapter 18.

Patients with muscle disorders can present with various weakness and wasting, pain, cramps, and fasciculations.

Muscle weakness can be classified anatomically as follows:

- Ocular (weakness of the eye muscles, causing double vision)
- Facial (may cause difficulties with facial expressions and eating)
- Bulbar (weakness of the muscles that control speech and swallowing)
- Neck (weakness may produce head drop)
- Truncal (can cause kyphosis and scoliosis)
- Limb (affecting the upper or lower limbs)

Typically, muscle disorders tend to cause proximal weakness, but there are rare muscle conditions that can cause a distal pattern of weakness. Patients may have either a focal weakness affecting only a few muscle groups, or generalized weakness, affecting many widespread muscle groups.

The sensory examination should be normal in patients with a muscle disorder, and reflexes are usually normal, although they may be decreased if there is significant weakness. Reflexes are also reduced in patients with neuropathies presenting

TABLE 8.1
The 2-Minute Orthopedic Examination

Instructions	Observation
Stand facing examiner	Acromioclavicular joints, general habitus
Look at ceiling, floor, over both shoulders	Cervical spine motion
Shrug shoulders (examiner resists)	Trapezius strength
Abduct shoulders 90° (examiner resists at 90°)	Deltoid strength
Full external rotation of arms	Shoulder motion
Flex and extend elbows	Elbow motion
Arms at sides, elbows 90° flexed; pronate and supinate wrists	Elbow and wrist motion
Spread fingers; make fist	Hand or finger motion and deformities
Tighten (contract) quadriceps; relax quadriceps	Symmetry and knee effusion; ankle effusion
"Duck walk" four steps (away from examiner with buttocks on heels)	Hip, knee, and ankle motion
Turn back to examiner	Shoulder symmetry, scoliosis
Keep knees straight, touch toes	Scoliosis, hip motion, hamstring tightness
Raise up on toes; raise heels	Calf symmetry, leg strength

Reproduced from American Academy of Pediatrics. (1983). *Sports medicine: Health care for young athletes.* Elk Grove, IL: Author.

with proximal weakness, including Guillain-Barré syndrome and chronic inflammatory demyelinating polyneuropathy.

The order of examination of these systems depends largely on the age, condition, and cooperation of the child. If the child walks, make preliminary observations of posture, gait, and stance immediately. Note the position the child assumes during the examination, either during this part of the examination or as part of the general appearance of the patient. For teenage athletes, a brief examination is helpful (Table 8.1).

LABORATORY INVESTIGATIONS

Measurement of Serum Enzyme Levels

Measurement of creatine kinase (CK) is very sensitive but nonspecific marker of muscle disease.

Measurement of Electrolytes (Including Potassium, Magnesium, Calcium, and Phosphate)

Abnormal electrolyte levels may be a cause of muscle weakness or provide a clue to the underlying disorder; for example, low potassium levels may occur with diuretic use and in disorders such as Cushing disease.

Autoimmune Screen

An autoimmune screen is useful to look for the inflammatory myopathies and should include the erythrocyte sedimentation rate and the antinuclear antibody level.

Measurement of the anti-double-stranded DNA antibody (anti-dsDNA) is useful if systemic lupus erythematosus is suspected. Measurement of extractable nuclear antigens is useful in further classifying the inflammatory condition. For instance, the anti-Jo1 antibody can be positive in polymyositis/dermatomyositis. Measurement of angiotensin-converting enzyme is useful if sarcoidosis is suspected.

Measurement of Vitamin D Level

A normal vitamin D level is greater than 50 nmol/L; borderline levels are between 25 and 50 nmol/L; and muscle disorders occur when the level is below 25 nmol/L.

Measurement of Lactate Level

A raised lactate level may be seen in patients with a mitochondrial disorder. Use of a tourniquet during venipuncture can lead to falsely elevated lactate levels.

NEUROPHYSIOLOGICAL INVESTIGATIONS

Two important tests to consider in the evaluation of a patient with generalized muscle weakness are:

1. The nerve conduction study to exclude neuropathy
2. Needle electromyography (EMG) to detect the presence of a muscle disorder, provide information on disease activity and the muscles involved, and select an appropriate muscle for biopsy

Further specialized neurophysiology techniques include repetitive nerve stimulation and single-fiber EMG for the investigation of myasthenia gravis and other neuromuscular transmission disorders.

Magnetic Resonance Imaging

The MRI is used to identify clinically affected muscles, including atrophic muscles or areas of significant myositis.

Other Tests

If a mitochondrial disorder is suspected, tests involve the collection of blood, hair, or urine for specialized mitochondrial DNA analyses. If sarcoidosis is considered, the patient may be sent for a chest X-ray, pulmonary CT scan, or gallium scan to look for hilar lymphadenopathy or pulmonary fibrosis.

Muscle Biopsy

Muscle biopsy is the gold standard in the investigation of muscle weakness. The muscle biopsy should be clinically affected muscle. Muscles that are often biopsied include the quadriceps, the gastrocnemius, and the deltoid muscle.

CAUSES OF ACUTE GENERALIZED MUSCLE WEAKNESS

Electrolyte Imbalance

Abnormalities in electrolyte levels, especially potassium, magnesium, calcium, and phosphate, can lead to acute generalized muscle weakness (Table 8.2).

Rhabdomyolysis and Myoglobinuria

Rhabdomyolysis and myoglobinuria may occur in individuals under the following conditions:

- Severe electrolyte imbalance
- Heatstroke
- After extreme amounts of exercise (e.g., after a marathon run)
- After excessive ingestion of alcohol (e.g., after an alcoholic binge)
- Snakebite envenomation (in addition to myotoxic effects, there may be neuro-toxic and hematologic effects)

Rhabdomyolysis and myoglobinuria may also occur in individuals with an underly-ing muscle disorder, including metabolic malignant hyperthermia associated with anesthesia and hereditary muscle disorders.

Periodic Paralysis

Patients with periodic paralysis develop bouts of generalized muscle weakness in association with an acute electrolyte abnormality (e.g., hypokalemic periodic paraly-sis). Periodic paralysis may be hereditary or acquired. Hereditary cases are usually associated with an abnormality in an electrolyte channel gene. Acquired cases are usually seen in association with thyrotoxicosis.

TABLE 8.2
Scale for Grading Muscle Strength

Grade	Percentage of Function	Activity Level
0 None	0	No evidence of muscle contractility
1 Trace	15	Evidence of slight contractility; no effective joint motion
2 Poor	25	Full range of motion without gravity
3 Fair	50	Full range of motion against gravity
4 Good	75	Complete range of motion against gravity with some resistance
5 Normal	100	Complete range of motion against gravity with full resistance

Neuromuscular Junction Disorders

Myasthenia gravis can present acutely with generalized weakness. Botulism is an important, potentially fatal, condition to consider. It may occur in infants after the ingestion of botulinum toxin in honey.

Guillain-Barré Syndrome

Guillain-Barré syndrome is an acute nerve disorder characterized by ascending muscle weakness and sensory features. It may occur after an infection (e.g., upper respiratory tract infection or gastroenteritis) or vaccination. It may progress rapidly and patients may require ventilatory support.

CAUSES OF CHRONIC AND SUBACUTE GENERALIZED MUSCLE WEAKNESS
Medicine Related

- Statins
- Other lipid-lowering medications, including gemfibrozil and ezetimibe
- Corticosteroids
- Diuretics
- Colchicines
- Some cardiac medications (e.g., amiodarone in high doses)
- Isotretinoin
- Chloroquine
- Emetine
- Antiretroviral agents (e.g., zidovudine) can cause a myopathy. HIV infection or AIDS can be associated with a myopathy.
- Penicillamine can cause a myasthenic-type state

Toxin-Related

- Alcohol: muscle weakness may occur in people with chronic alcohol use.

Inflammatory

- Polymyositis and dermatomyositis
- Inclusion body myositis, usually in older patients
- Sarcoidosis
- Connective tissue diseases
- Chronic inflammatory demyelinating polyneuropathy with mainly proximal weakness. Typically there is also distal weakness, hyporeflexia, and sensory symptoms

Infectious

- Influenza virus, coxsackieviruses and Epstein-Barr virus, may be myotoxic
- HIV infection/AIDS

HEREDITARY CAUSES OF MUSCLE WEAKNESS

Mitochondrial Myopathies

Mitochondrial myopathies may be associated with ophthalmoplegia, migraines, neuropathy, strokes, and seizures. Other nonneurological manifestations may include cardiac dysfunction and gastrointestinal symptoms. The serum and cerebrospinal fluid lactate levels tend to be elevated in patients with mitochondrial disorders.

Muscular Dystrophies

Important examples of the muscular dystrophies that may present in adulthood include:

- Myotonic dystrophy
- Facioscapulohumeral muscular dystrophy
- Limb girdle muscular dystrophy
- Becker muscular dystrophy

Central Core Disease

Central core disease is a rare but important disorder to consider as affected patients are at high risk of malignant hyperthermia and anesthetic complications. Patients may present with very minor features, such as an asymptomatic elevation of the creatine kinase level or a proximal myopathy.

FINDINGS IN JOINT HYPERMOBILITY

The diagnosis of joint hypermobility requires the presence of three of these findings:

- Passive hyperextension of fifth finger parallel to extensor aspect of forearm
- Passive opposition of thumb to flexor aspect of the forearm
- Ability to touch floor with flat of hands without bending knees
- Hyperextensions of knees to $> 10°$
- Hyperextension of elbows to $> 10°$

EXTREMITIES

In patients aged 2–6 years, you may begin the physical examination with observations of the hands and feet. Most children at this age are happy to show their hands and feet when requested and are especially happy to see no instruments present at the beginning of the examination. Persistently pink hands and feet are a sign of poor nutrition, poor hygiene, or other types of deprivation.

Infants who hold both their arms immobile in 90° flexion at the elbow when lying, sitting, or standing may be suffering from emotional deprivation. Infants who appear to look at one arm for a long time or who hold one arm in an unusual position for 1 or 2 minutes may have infantile autism. Such posturing is normal until about age

6 months. Stereotypic hand movements and hand wringing in young girls may be a sign of Rett syndrome or autism.

Note congenital anomalies of the arms, hands, legs, and feet. These include amelia (absence of the part), webbing, and extra digits.

Length and shape of the extremities are usually determined by nutritional and congenital factors. Abnormalities (e.g., long, thin extremities) are noted in children with arachnodactyly. Broad, short extremities are noted in children with Down syndrome, mucopolysaccharidoses, or chondrodystrophies. Apparent shortening of the thumb and fourth and fifth fingers occurs almost always in children with pseudohypoparathyroidism.

Shortening of an extremity is usually congenital but may result from disease of the epiphyses or cerebral palsy. Inequality of leg length may be present in children after femoral fractures or with dislocation of the hip or other hip disorders.

Lengthening of an extremity is usually congenital but may result from large hemangiomas, lymphangiomas, arteriovenous fistula, neurofibromatosis, or hemihypertrophy. Generalized enlargement of the extremities may result from any of these factors and, when unilateral, may cause hemigigantism. Enlargement may also be attributable to lymphedema praecox or congenital lymphedema (Milroy disease), or as a manifestation of ovarian dysgenesis, Turner syndrome, or edema.

Inspect fingers and toes for clubbing (hypertrophic osteoarthropathy; Figure 8.1). Elevation of the nail base is an early sign of clubbing. Later, the entire end of the finger, including the nail region, appears expanded and rounded as compared with the remainder of the finger. Ask the child to oppose both thumbnails. A small diamond-shaped opening is normally visible. With clubbing, no space is present. Clubbing may occur in any condition of reduced circulating oxygen, such as cyanotic congenital heart disease or chronic pulmonary disease, and also in patients with chronic liver disease

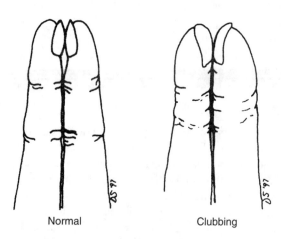

Normal   Clubbing

Figure 8.1
Clubbing (described in text).

or bacterial endocarditis. Clubbing may be a presenting sign of cystic fibrosis, Crohn disease, ulcerative colitis, celiac disease, gastroesophageal reflux, intestinal parasite infestation, and thalassemia. Unidigital clubbing may be due to phalangeal bone lesions, as in sarcoidosis.

Pain and tenderness in the extremities are usually caused by trauma or infection. Pain, especially of the legs, is noted in infants with scurvy. Infants aged less than 3 months with congenital syphilis may have pain causing pseudoparalyses. Tenderness over the sartorius muscle may be noted in children with tuberculous meningitis. Tenderness elicited at a point in the bone by sharp percussion of the distal end of the bone suggests the presence of osteomyelitis (Figure 8.2). Inability to supinate the hand with the arm held in flexion and pain in the elbow indicates subluxation of the head of the radius.

Pain in the knee or foot may result from local disease, but it also requires examination of the hips. Pain in the knee that increases with internal rotation of the tibia may be caused by osteochondritis dissecans. Pain in a bone that is worse at night and is rapidly relieved by aspirin is characteristic of osteoid osteoma. Pain and hard swelling over proximal anterior tuberosity is characteristic of Osgood-Schlatter disease. Pain over the medial and lateral aspect of the calcaneous is characteristic of Sever disease.

Note the temperature of the extremities, taking special care to note whether the temperature is equal bilaterally. Differences in temperature are usually attributed to neurologic or vascular abnormalities. Cold, pallid extremities may occur after sympathetic nervous system stimulation or may be a manifestation of venous or arterial thrombosis or embolism. With nervous system lesions, pulsations are usually present, whereas with vascular lesions pulsations are usually diminished or absent.

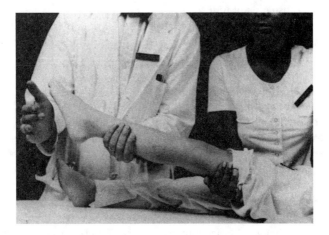

Figure 8.2
Striking the foot to elicit pain of osteomyelitis in the tibia or fibula.

Necrosis of an extremity, or gangrene, may result from obliteration of the vascular supply. The area is cold, avascular, pallid, and tender, with loss of muscle power. The area may gradually become black and less painful as necrosis proceeds. It may ooze and be moist and obviously infected or it may be dry. Gangrene may develop in infants after embolism, particularly from the umbilical venous system; after severe trauma or infection to the part; and sometimes after frostbite.

Enlargement of the bones may be caused by infection in the bone. Swelling with joint tenderness, heat, and redness near but not in the joint is characteristic of osteomyelitis. Swelling may result from periosteal hemorrhage, as in scurvy; from cortical thickening, as in congenital syphilis, vitamin A poisoning, or infantile cortical hyperostosis; from localized increased calcification, as in callus formation after fracture or in rickets; or from bone cysts or tumors. Auscultation over the area of the swelling may reveal a bruit, more common in osteomyelitis than in the other causes of increased vascularity of the bone.

Enlargement of the tibial tubercles with tenderness is characteristic of Osgood-Schlatter disease, probably from stress on the patellar tendon.

Bony, painless swelling at the epiphysis adjacent to the knee or wrist joints is one of the most definite signs of rickets. Symmetric swelling of both hands or both feet in infants may indicate the hand-foot syndrome of sickle cell anemia.

Other deformities of the bones are usually caused by fractures. Fractures are evidenced by the patient's inability to use the limb, by deformity, or by excess motion in the bone with pain and crepitation. Auscultating at the proximal epiphysis while tapping the distal end of a bone elicits a difference in sound on the nonfractured side from sound elicited on the fractured side. Fractures are almost always caused by trauma and may suggest child abuse. Multiple fractures may result from polyostotic fibrous dysplasia, bone cysts, other diseases of the parathyroid gland, prolonged bed rest, or osteogenesis imperfecta. Toddler's fracture is a midshaft tibial fracture caused by torsion and is usually not indicative of abuse.

Note shape of the bones. Lateral bowing of the tibia (genu varum) is present when the child stands with the medial malleoli in apposition, and a persistent space more than 2 cm is observed between the medial surfaces of the knees. It is physiologic for infants and children to be bowlegged past 18 months. Significant genu varum may result from anomalies of the feet or from rickets. Anterior curvature of the tibia may indicate congenital syphilis. Excess bowing just below the knee may indicate osteochondrosis deformans, Blount disease, or tibia vara.

Knock-knees (genu valgum) can be determined when, with the knees together, a child's medial malleoli persistently are separated more than 2 cm. Knock-knees are usually normal in children from about 2–3½ years of age with self-correction by age 7 years. Knock-knees may also be evident in children with pronated feet as seen in pes planus, rickets, or syphilis.

Bony hard enlargement of the medial or external aspects of the femoral or tibial epiphyses is usually a normal variant but may occur with rickets or other metabolic bone diseases or with dysgenesis of the knees such as dysplasia epiphysialis hemimelia.

Tibial torsion, a twisting of the tibia probably initiated by the intrauterine position, is best determined with the patient on the back and the knees facing upward.

Both the forefoot and the hindfoot will be held in a plane but not in line with the knees. With the tibial tubercle and the patella in a straight line, place your fingers on the malleoli. In infants, the line joining the four malleoli should be parallel to the table. In older children, as much as 20° of external torsion is normal. With any greater deviation, or if the lateral malleolus is anterior to the medial malleolus, inward tibial torsion may be present. With fixed deformities of the foot such as metatarsus varus, the forefoot will be adducted in this position but the hindfoot will be in a straight line with the patella. An alternative method of diagnosing tibial torsion is to have the patient prone, with the knees apart and flexed 90°. The longitudinal plane of the feet should be in the same plane as the femur, not inwardly deviated as in tibial torsion.

Note the feet for abnormalities. At birth, the child's feet are usually held in varus or valgus attitude—almost never straight. An easy method to determine whether this position, which is the intrauterine position, will straighten is simply to scratch first the outside and then the inside of the lower border of the foot. In self-correctable deformities, the foot will assume a right angle with the leg. More severe anomalies, such as clubfeet or metatarsus adductus, either can be straightened only by forceful manual stretching or cannot be straightened by manual means at all (Figure 8.3).

Because all children have a fat pad under the arch, the feet may appear flat until the child is approximately 2 years old. A very high-arched foot (pes cavus) may be noted in some normal children or in patients with Friedreich ataxia or in various lower motor neuron lesions. Talipes equinus, with short heel cords and weight bearing on the toes, may be characteristic of cerebral palsy or muscular diseases; it results in spasm and contracture of the muscles of the leg and may cause toe walking. Many normal children walk on their toes until age 3 years. The child with toe walking caused by cerebral palsy will have brisk deep tendon reflexes.

Toe walking may also indicate muscle imbalance, spasticity, muscular dystrophy of the Duchenne type, or disorders causing weakness of the peroneal and anterior tibial muscles. Children with septic arthritis of the hip walk on their toes to relieve strain around the hip. Some autistic and some normal children also toe walk until age 4 years (Table 8.3).

Examine the heel cords with the patient in the supine position and the knee extended. Grasp the foot by the heel (Figure 8.4), with the sole lying in your hand; slightly invert the foot to lock the heel and then dorsiflex it. Tight cords are present if dorsiflexion cannot be carried to about 20–30° beyond a right angle.

Note pronation of the feet. Pronation becomes apparent when the child stands. A pronated foot is flexible and may appear normal when the child lies on the table, but it will abduct at the forefoot when the patient stands, with obliteration of the long arch, bulging of the medial border of the foot, and outward angulation of the forefoot on the hindfoot. This is normal until age 7. Treatment of the flexible pes planus is reserved for only those with pain, usually in the anterior tibial location. The medial malleolus may appear closer to the floor than normal; there may be knock-knees; and the thighs may appear adducted. The weight-bearing line, which is the line through the middle of the patella perpendicular to the floor, will cross the inner border of the foot instead of going through the second toe as is normal. From

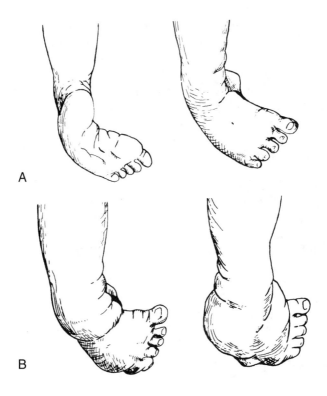

Figure 8.3
A: forefoot adduction; heel inversion. B: talipes equinovarus.

the back, the heel cord, which normally descends perpendicularly, will be noted to curve outward with eversion of the heel (valgus heel).

After examining the feet, look at the patient's shoes. Abnormal wear or misshaped shoes may help you to diagnose gait or foot disorders. Then note the patient's gait and stance. Observing the child in a room with a mirror at one end is helpful when

TABLE 8.3
Relative Frequency of Pathogens in Septic Arthritis According to Age

Neonate	1 Month–2 Years	2–5 Years	>5 Years
S. aureus	H. influenzae type B	A. aureus	A. aureus
Group B streptococci	Group A streptococci	Group A streptococci	Group A streptococci
Gram-negative enteric pathogens	S. pneumoniae	H. influenzae type B	Neisseria gonorrhea
	N. meningitides	N. meningitis	P. aeruginosa
	P. aeruginosa Salmonella species		

From: Davis, H. W., & Michaels, M. (2002). Infectious disease. In B. J. Zitelli, & H. W. Davis (Eds.), *Atlas of pediatric physical diagnosis* (4th ed.). St. Louis: Mosby, p. 442.

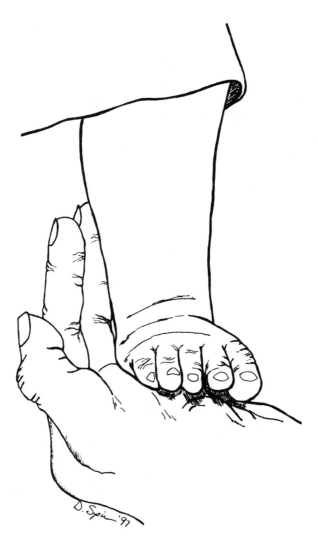

Figure 8.4
Lock heel in palm of hand before testing for tight heel cords.

studying the child's gait. Observe the anterior and posterior aspects simultaneously as the child walks toward and away from the mirror. The child should be wearing shoes or at least socks, because bare feet on a cold floor may distort the gait.

Normally a child aged 1–2 years walks with a broad-based gait, frequently with the hands out to the side—hence the name *toddler*. Gradually as the child reaches the age of 3 or 4 years, the legs are brought together and the toes are straight ahead. An older child with a broad-based gait may have abnormal mechanics of the legs or feet or may use this gait for balance if normal neural positioning and balancing mechanisms are defective. Watch for truncal ataxia as the child turns. Ask children aged more than 3 years to walk on their toes to demonstrate distal muscle weakness, a sign of peripheral neuropathy. Also ask a child this age to squat and then stand, looking for Gower sign. Ask children aged more than 4 to walk on their heels. Asymmetry suggests mild hemiparesis or hemiplegia. Ask children aged more than 5 to walk a line, heel to toe. Failure suggests a midline cerebellar lesion, a cerebellar tract defect, or gross motor incoordination.

Balance, at rest or while walking, is maintained by normal cerebellar function, normal vestibular nerve function, and good muscle, bone, and joint functions. Loss of balance may be attributed to cerebellar or vestibular disease or muscle weakness. Deviation to one side during walking may indicate cerebellar disease of that side; lack of normal swing of the arm of that side suggests cerebellar or corpus callosum involvement.

Toeing in (pigeon toe) or toeing out may be noted. Final status usually takes 3 months of independent walking. Children with pronated feet may toe in or toe out. Other orthopedic conditions causing toeing in include internal rotation of the hips, tibial torsion, and metatarsus adductus. With internal rotation at the hips, it is probably useful to have patients sit cross-legged.

A scissors gait with stiff crossing over of the legs as the child walks is evident especially in children with a spastic type of cerebral palsy or with mental delay. You can elicit this type of gait even in 7-month-old children if they are made to walk by being gripped under the shoulders and pushed along (Figure 8.5). A waddling gait may be noted in patients with bilateral dislocation of the hip or with coxa vara.

Limp

Note a limp of any type. A limp may result from local infection; muscle, nerve, bone, or joint disease; or pain, but it is most commonly caused by trauma, fatigue, or a pathologic condition of the hip. Pain in the foot, ankle, knee, hip, or spine requires careful examination of all five areas because pathologic conditions of the hip or spine may be referred to the foot or knee. A limp created by pain results in what is referred to as an antalgic gait. Children with intraabdominal inflammatory disease (e.g., appendicitis, abscess, and retroperitoneal fibrosis) may limp.

You can examine young children who limp while they sit in the parent's lap. Observe the back, hips, buttocks, and extremities. Compare the gluteal folds; look for asymmetry, swelling, and erythema of the two sides. Palpate for induration, warmth, tenderness over bones, muscle spasm, and effusion or distention of the joint capsules of the hip, knee, and ankle. Test each joint for motion, examining the suspect limb or joint last. Note restriction of flexion, extension, abduction, adduction, and rotation. Measure limb girth and length. Perform rectal and neurologic examinations.

Limp occurs with soft tissue injury anywhere in the lower extremity. Soft tissue injuries include sprains and strains. Abnormal laxity of a ligament after injury associated with local pain is characteristic of sprain; swelling occurs because of bleeding into the joint. Disruption of a muscle-tendon unit is a strain. Similar signs may be noted in cases of epiphyseal fractures and dislocation of the patella. Foreign bodies, myositis, cellulitis, hives, bruising, and other lesions in the soft tissue may cause a limp (Table 8.4).

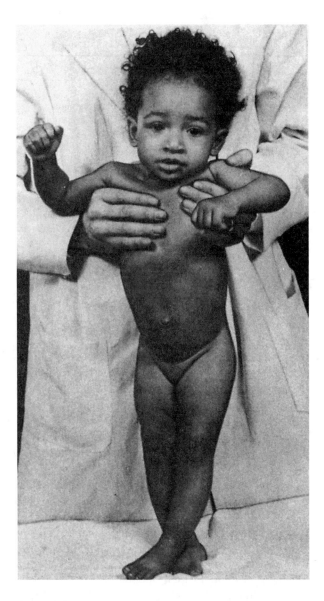

Figure 8.5
Scissors gait can be demonstrated before child can walk by
grasping under axillae and pushing patient forward.

TABLE 8.4
Common Causes of a Limp in a Child

Cause	Underlying Conditions
Generalized disorders	
Bone diseases	Rickets, infections, leukemia, primary tumors
Muscle diseases	Inflammatory, congenital, metabolic myopathies
Joint diseases	Juvenile arthritis, septic arthritis
Neurologic diseases	Cerebral palsy
Psychiatric diseases	Conversion disorder
Local causes	
Knee	Osgood-Schlatter disease, osteochondritis dissecans, tumors
Tibia	Toddler's fracture, stress fracture, fracture through a bone cyst
Foot	Tarsal coalition, Köhler disease, tight shoes, Sever disease
Hip	Congenital hip dislocation, Legg-Calvé-Perthes disease, septic arthritis, toxic synovitis, slipped capital femoral epiphysis
Back	Spondylolisthesis, osteomyelitis, Scheuermann disease
Short leg	

JOINTS

Examine the joints for heat, tenderness, swelling, effusion, redness, and limitation or pain on motion. Redness, heat, and tenderness—signs of infection—are detected by observation and palpation. Effusion in the joint, a sign of any type of joint irritation, can be best determined by ballottement of the joint or by tapping on one side of the joint and feeling protrusion on the other side as a fluid wave is elicited. In children, the most common cause of tenderness in one joint with limitation of motion but without other physical signs is synovitis of traumatic or nonspecific origin.

Swollen, hot joints are seen in children with arthritis, hemarthrosis, or osteo-chondritis. Motion is limited in these conditions, usually because of pain and spasm of the overlying muscles and tendons. Arthritis of rheumatic fever is painful without much swelling and responds to aspirin more rapidly than rheumatoid arthritis, in which the joints are stiff.

In rheumatic fever and systemic lupus erythematosus, the swelling may be reducible (Jaccoud syndrome). Pain in the joint without physical findings is arthralgia and may be caused by any condition discussed previously or by strains or overactivity.

Limitation of joint motion without pain may occur as a congenital malformation. Flexion deformities of the fingers and toes are common. Children with multiple congenital dislocations, as in arthrogryposis, may have severe flexion deformities of many joints. Limitation of joint motion is also common in children with various spastic neurologic disorders (described elsewhere in this chapter).

Trauma is the most common cause of a single swollen joint in a child. Ask about a precipitating injury.

Infections such as septic arthritis or osteomyelitis must be considered. If the child has had a fever or recent documented infection and has recently received antibiotics, you should suspect infectious arthritis, especially if marked pain, redness, and increased heat are noted in a single joint.

Consider malignancy in a child who presents with fever, weight loss, and malaise. Leukemia, lymphoma, and neuroblastoma are by far the most common possibilities.

Causes of Recurrent Joint Pain

Juvenile rheumatoid arthritis	Lupus erythematosus
Poststreptococcal arthritis	Allergic reactions
Parvovirus; other viruses	Kawasaki disease
Rubella	Hypermobility syndromes
Seronegative enthesopathy (SEA) syndrome	General debility
	Amyotonia congenita
Reflex sympathetic dystrophy	Down syndrome
Fibromyalgia	Ehlers-Danlos syndrome
Rheumatic fever	

Detect excess joint motion by hyperflexing or hyperextending the joint. Such excess motion usually results from relaxation of the structures surrounding the joint. Most children with chorea and children with rickets or malnutrition have hypermobility of the joints, especially of the wrists, because of poor muscle tone. Hyperextension of the knees (genu recurvatum) may be attributed to the intrauterine position or may be evident in children with spina bifida, arthrogryposis, agenesis of the patella, or other malformations. Marfan syndrome is also characterized by excess joint motion.

In infants, investigate the hips routinely for developmental dysplasia. With the infant on the back, flex the legs at the knees and attempt internal and external rotation by holding the knees and simultaneously rotating the thighs (Figures 8.6 and 8.7). See whether the rotation is equal on both sides. Unequal rotation is usually caused by decreased mobility of one joint. The hips can be abducted and externally rotated so that the knees touch the tabletop in most infants. With unilateral subluxation, abduction is limited on the affected side (Figure 8.7). A click heard after this maneuver may either be normal or a sign of dysplasia. Grasp the outer aspect of one thigh with the middle finger over the greater trochanter. Lift and abduct the thigh. A clunk indicates that a dislocated hip has been reduced (Ortolani click).

In a child diagnosed with congenital muscular torticollis, remember to examine the hips, because 20% of children with congenital torticollis also have developmental hip dislocation.

Determine piston mobility in children with hip joint dislocations by holding the hip region with one hand, grasping the thigh with the other hand, and pulling the hands apart gently (Figure 8.8). Motion that occurs as in a Slinky toy is piston mobility. A little motion, possibly as much as 1 cm, is normally present, but with congenital dysplasia the hip motion may have a range of 2 to more than 2 cm below the socket. As the child grows older, tightness of the adductor muscles is noted, and the gluteal folds may be uneven. Normal children may have uneven gluteal folds.

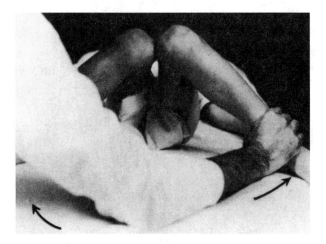

Figure 8.6
External rotation of the hips.

In addition to recognized developmental dysplasia, older children, especially those who are obese, may have progressive subluxation of the hip. The child with dislocation of the hip usually has a painless limp with apparent shortening of the leg on the involved side. When the child is asked to stand on the normal limb and raise the other leg, the pelvis on the involved side rises to maintain balance. When the patient is asked to stand on the leg with the dislocated hip and raise the normal limb, the abductor muscles cannot raise the pelvis and it drops (Trendelenburg sign) (Figure 8.9). A painless limp, worse with fatigue, occurs also with coxa plana, especially in boys.

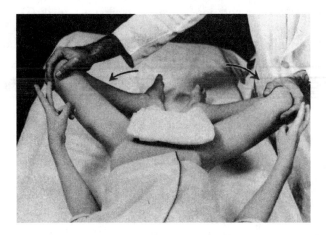

Figure 8.7
Internal rotation of the hips. Note that angles made by each leg are equal.

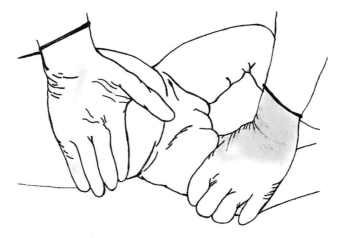

Figure 8.8
Piston mobility. Grasp thigh firmly.

A painful limp with limited motion, especially in the morning, is usually evident in children with tuberculosis of the hip. In addition, in this disease, the hip is first abducted and later adducted with flexion on the pelvis. If it appears that children are simulating limps or abnormal gaits, tell them to run, touch a spot, and return. Usually they will concentrate on your instructions and forget to simulate.

Limited motion of the elbow with weakness after injury suggests tennis elbow. Pain is felt over the lateral epicondyle because of strain. In a child aged less than 2 years, inability to supinate the hand with the arm held in flexion, along with pain in the elbow, indicates subluxation of the head of the radius. Nursemaid's elbows are created when pulling the child by the arm with the elbow fully extended.

Tenderness of the posterior aspect of the lateral malleoli suggests fracture. Tenderness over the fibular-talar ligaments, especially with internal rotation, suggests sprain.

Knee Injuries

Examine the unaffected knee first, with the patient in the supine, sitting, and standing positions. Note angular deformities, the presence of effusion, ecchymoses, abrasions, scars, and gait if weight-bearing is possible. With the knee extended, try to push fluid from the outer to the medial side of the joint with the flat part of your hand. A bulge of the synovial lining, particularly on the medial side of the knee, indicates effusion. Transillumination will help you recognize the presence of fluid. Check for muscle atrophy of the thigh or calf. Check range of motion last if effusion is present. If effusion occurs shortly after injury, suspect a serious injury with hemarthrosis. Delayed onset of effusion after injury suggests strains or an inflammatory process. Limited flexion or extension of the knee with a limp may result from dislocation or chondromalacia of the patella (peripatellar bursitis) after injury, osteochondritis, other bone disease, or all other joint diseases.

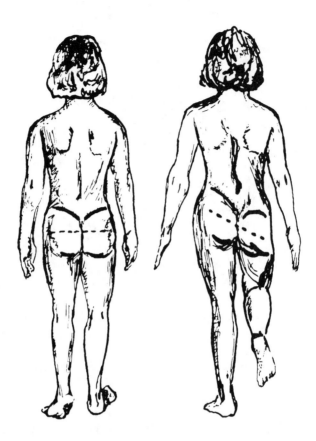

Figure 8.9
Trendelenburg sign. When the child stands on both feet,
the pelvis is level; when the child stands on the affected
side, the normal side drops.

Palpate to identify the site of maximum pain. Pain in the joint suggests a cartilage or ligament injury. Stress the joint by abducting and adducting with the patient
in the supine position and with 30° flexion. Pain elicited in a patient in the supine
position suggests medial ligament injury; at 30°, it indicates collateral ligament
injury. Test with 90° flexion, pulling on the proximal tibia. Excess displacement
indicates cruciate ligament tears.

Flex the hip and knee and rotate the foot. A click indicates a torn meniscus.
Locking of the knee suggests intraarticular loose bodies. Pain in the tibial tubercle
suggests Osgood-Schlatter disease resulting from bursitis or fracture. Pain or dislocation of the patella may indicate fracture. If the patella is not palpable, suspect peripatellar bursitis.

Shoulder Injuries

Compare both shoulders of the patient. Asymmetry may result from edema, deformity,
trauma, septic arthritis, or osteomyelitis. Squaring of the shoulder suggests dislocation.

Prominence of the distal clavicle may be attributed to acromioclavicular separation. A double bulge on the anterior surface of the upper arm when the elbow is flexed suggests rupture of the biceps tendon. Note the point of maximum tenderness and try to identify the part of the joint, tendon, muscle, or bone involved. Have the child fully abduct the arm to locate limitation. Pain and paresthesia radiating from the shoulder to fingertips relieved by shoulder elevation suggests referred pain from cervical radiculopathy. Atrophy of the deltoid muscle suggests axillary nerve injury. A prominent scapula with painful muscles suggests rotator cuff injury.

SPINE

Examine the patient's spine in routine physical examinations. Observe infants in the supine position. The infant may kick and move during the examination. Then place the infant on its abdomen. In older children, make observations with the patient in the sitting or standing position. Note the way the child stands or walks. Pain from disc disease intensifies with anterior flexion. Pain that intensifies with posterior extension suggests a bony disorder (e.g., fracture).

Causes of Scoliosis

Functional Scoliosis

Irritative or inflammatory disorders
Hysteria
Postural derangements
Herniated lumbar discs
Limb length inequality

Structural Scoliosis

Idiopathic
Congenital
Neuromuscular

Other Conditions That May Result in Scoliosis

Metabolic disorders
Osteochondrodystrophies
Neurofibromatosis
Mesenchymal disorders
Trauma, surgery, irradiation, burns
Myopathic disorders

Tufts of hair, dimples, hemangiomas, discolorations, cysts, and masses are frequently seen near the spine. A tuft of hair over a small dimple in the midline usually indicates the presence of an underlying spina bifida or may simply be an ectodermal anomaly. Spina bifida occulta can occasionally be determined by pressing carefully over the suspect area when the trunk is flexed. The spinous processes above and below the spina bifida will feel thin and well formed, whereas the spinous process of the defective vertebra may feel split.

A small dimple in the midline anywhere from the coccyx to the skull may indicate a dermoid sinus. These dimples are important to record as possible entry points of infection to the central nervous system (CNS). Any of these may be associated with tethering of the cord.

Palpate and transilluminate masses over the spine. Nontender masses of varied color and consistency with a thin covering are usually meningoceles. Meningoceles, which communicate with the CNS, can usually be distinguished from noncommunicating masses by palpation. If signs of increased intracranial pressure such as bulging of the fontanel are apparent, it is likely that the contents of the mass communicate with the spinal canal. Cystic masses that transilluminate may be teratoma, meningocele, or lipomeningocele. Nontender, noncommunicating masses near the spine are usually lipomas or fibromas. Soft masses that feel like lipomas, usually with skin dimples, may also extend into the CNS and are lipomeningoceles.

Tender masses not communicating with the spinal canal are usually infectious and include tuberculous spondylitis and tuberculous and perinephric abscesses. Deep tenderness over the spine is usually caused by trauma of the spine or surrounding structures. Localized spine tenderness is best elicited by punching with the side of your hand or by tapping with the reflex hammer. Masses covered by skin over the sacrum or coccyx may be teratomas. These are firm and can usually also be felt on rectal examination.

Causes of Localized Back Tenderness

Cord tumor	Spondylitis
Injury, bone or muscle	Spondylesthesis
Discitis	Stress fracture
Disk injury	Lumbosacral strain
Osteoarthritis	Spinal stenosis
Rheumatoid arthritis	Scoliosis
Hyperlordosis	

Examine the spine for intrinsic motion. Limitation of flexion is easily demonstrated by asking patients to sit up from a prone position. Patients with flexion limitation will turn over and maintain the position of the back with pokerlike rigidity. If patients are sitting, ask them to kiss their knees to demonstrate limitation of forward bending. If you place your fingers on several of the patient's adjoining spinous processes, the processes normally will move separately as the patient bends the trunk laterally. With stiffness of the spine, your fingers move as a unit.

The spine is stiff in children with CNS infections, especially meningitis or tetanus; in diseases or anomalies of the bones such as osteomyelitis of the spine, epiphysitis of the vertebrae, or hemivertebrae; or in patients with adjacent lesions such as peritonitis or perinephric abscesses. Occasionally, with severe trauma to the back, the spine will be rigid. Causes of limitation of motion of the spine in adults, and sometimes in adolescents, are protruding intervertebral disc and lumbosacral strain. Severe pain and tenderness over the spine, particularly at night, may result from a tuberculous abscess or cord tumor. Inflammatory disease or a tumor of or near the spine may cause referred pain to the abdomen, hips, knees, or legs.

Limitation of motion of the neck by muscle spasm is a prime neurologic sign of nervous system disease. Neurologic disorders are discussed in Chapter 18. Nonneurologic causes of limitation of motion of the neck include rheumatoid arthritis of the cervical vertebrae; adjacent infections such as cervical adenitis and retropharyngeal abscess; rotatory subluxation of the cervical vertebrae; fracture or congenital anomalies of the vertebrae, especially hemivertebrae; or shortening of the sternocleidomastoid muscle producing torticollis (wryneck).

Excess mobility of the spine is rare and is most easily demonstrated with the patient in the supine position. Place one hand beneath the patient's head and the other under the knees. As the spine is flexed, it feels unusually supple, and the knees may easily approximate the chin. Such excess mobility is evident in those states that produce generalized hypotonia and is sometimes noted in small children with acute potassium deficiency.

Winged scapulae occur when the lower borders of the scapulae extend out loosely from the back, with excess mobility. Mild degrees occur often, but marked winging may be attributed to weakness of the muscles around the scapula. This weakness may occur after injury to the long thoracic nerve, in the muscular dystrophies, or in congenital anomalies such as absence of the clavicle (cleidocranial dysostosis) and high scapula with webbed neck (Sprengel deformity).

Note posture. Lordosis and kyphosis are exaggerations of the normal anteroposterior curvatures of the spine. Lumbar lordosis is normal in children throughout childhood and mimics the appearance of children with a protuberant abdomen. Marked lordosis may be caused by rickets, muscular dystrophy, or weakness of the abdominal wall. Adolescent round back is noted in children with chronic poor posture and thoracic epiphysitis.

Kyphosis is a sharp anteroposterior angulation of the spine opposite in direction to lordosis. It is usually caused by small or collapsed vertebral bodies. It is evident in cases of tuberculosis of the spine, but it may be a diagnostic sign of mucopolysaccharidosis, Morquio disease, or aseptic necrosis of the vertebral bodies. Localized kyphosis (gibbus) is caused by disease of one or two vertebral bodies and may occur in the same disease states causing kyphosis. Lack of normal thoracic kyphosis may thrust the heart anteriorly (straight back syndrome).

Detect scoliosis, a lateral curvature of the spine. Scoliosis is detected by having the patient stand erect. Mark the tips of the spinous processes with ink. Note the deviation of these ink spots from a straight line when the patient stands upright while barebacked or in a plain tight-fitting top. Ask the child to bend forward with the knees straight and the arms hanging down. Structural scoliosis exists when (a) there is a double curvature with rotation (twisting) on the convexity, (b) the ink line does not straighten when the patient bends forward, or (c) one hip appears prominent. Note scapular asymmetry resulting from cervical or thoracic curves. Posterior ribs should be symmetric. A lump of one group of ribs indicates structural scoliosis (Figure 8.10). Two other convenient tests are checking for symmetry of shoulder height and equal distance between hands and hips while standing erect.

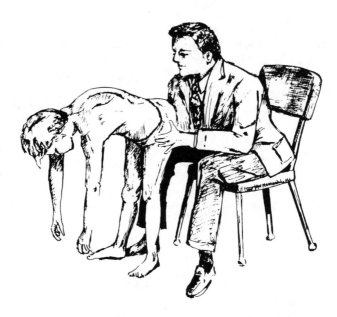

Figure 8.10
Having a patient bend forward is the fastest way to detect
scoliosis. The ribs rise. (Adapted from Netter, F., 1978, *CIBA
Clinical Symposium*, 30, 16.).

Mild scoliosis usually has no rotation, straightens in the prone position, and is
related to poor postural habits. Scoliosis in a child aged less than 5 years is usually
attributed to congenital anomalies or to lung or chest pathologic conditions. In older
children, scoliosis may be idiopathic or caused by a difference in leg length, hemivertebrae, rickets, poliomyelitis, muscular dystrophies, or neurologic disorders such as
neurofibromatosis. Some curving of the lower spine is evident in children with acute
abdominal pathologic conditions such as appendicitis or pyelonephritis. Painful scoliosis, which is relieved by aspirin, is suggestive of osteoid osteoma (Table 8.5).

Causes of Limping in Children

Skeletal System

Trauma, fracture
Foreign body
Tumor
Infections
Postinfectious condition
Hair tourniquet on toe

Joints

Synovitis
Arthralgia

Arthritis; rheumatoid, Kawasaki disease, Lyme disease, septic, parvovirus
Dislocated hip
Slipped capital femoral epiphysis
Collagen vascular disease
Henoch-Schoenlein purpura
Legg-Calvé-Perthes disease, aseptic necrosis, Osgood-Schlatter disease
Toxins
Urticaria
Foot injuries
Bursitis

Nervous System

Neuropathic conditions
Central nervous system

Spinal Conditions

Spondylitis

TABLE 8.5

Age Range and Sex Predominance for Common Musculoskeletal Disorders in Childhood

Musculoskeletal Disorders	Peak Age Range (Year)	Sex Predominance
Trauma	Any age	Male and female
Infection	Any age*	Male and female
Tumors		
Osteoma	Any age (most 10–20)	Male > female
Primary malignant bone tumor	≥10	Male and female
Secondary bone tumor	Any age	Male and female
Juvenile rheumatoid arthritis		
Polyarticular		
RF-positive	>10	Male << female
RF-negative	2–5	Male < female
Pauciarticular		
Type I	1–3	Male << female
Type II	>8	Male > female
Systemic onset	Any age	Male and female
Reflex sympathetic dystrophy	>10	Male << female
Growing pains	4–13	Male and female
Osteochondritis dissecans	>10	Male > female
Fibromyalgia	>10	Male << female
Juvenile ankylosing spondylitis	>8	Male >> female
Slipped capital femoral epiphysis	8–16	Male > female
Transient synovitis	4–8	Male > female
Legg-Calvé-Perthes disease	4–9	Male > female

*Septic arthritis is most common in children 3 years or younger.

RF, rheumatoid factor; >, greater than; >>, largely greater than.

Diskitis
Epidural abscess

Muscular System

Strain
Sprain
Myositis
Myopathic conditions

Hematologic and Oncologic Conditions

Sickle cell disease
Leukemia
Neoplasms
Hemophilia
Serum sickness
Epstein-Barr virus

Intraabdominal Conditions

Appendicitis
Infection
Inflammatory bowel disease
Ovarian tumors, torsion
Pelvic inflammatory disease
Testicular torsion
Inguinal hernia

FURTHER READING

Cassidy, J. T., & Petty, R. E. (2001). *Textbook of pediatric rheumatology* (4th ed.). Philadelphia: WB Saunders.

Engelbert, R. H., Bank, R. A., Sakkers, R. J., Helders, P. J., Beemer, F. A., & Uiterwaal, C. S. (2003). Pediatric generalized joint hypermobility with and without musculoskeletal complaints: A localized or systemic disorder? *Pediatrics 111*(3), e248–e254.

Ganel, A., Dudkiewicz, I., & Grogan, D. P. (2003). Pediatric orthopedic physical examination of the infant: A 5-minute assessment. *Journal of Pediatric Health Care, 17*(1), 39–41.

Gross, W. L., Trabandt, A., & Reinhold-Keller, E. (2000). Diagnosis and evaluation of vasculitis. *Rheumatology, 39*, 245–252.

Milojevic, D. S., & Ilowite, N. T. (2002). Treatment of rheumatic diseases in children: Special considerations. *Rheumatic Disease Clinics of North America, 28*, 461–482.

Lang, B. A., & Silverman, E. D. (1993). A clinical overview of systemic lupus erythematosus in childhood. *Pediatric Reviews 14*(5), 194–201.

Pachman, L. M. (1995). Juvenile dermatomyositis: Pathophysiology and disease expression. *Pediatric Clinics of North America, 42*, 1071–1098.

Sundel, R., & Szer, I. (2002). Vasculitis in childhood. *Rheumatic Disease Clinics of North America, 28*, 625–654.

9

HEART

Soft is the heart of a child . . . . Do not harden it.

Glenconner

BLOOD PRESSURE

The normal systolic blood pressure of an infant is between 60 and 80 mmHg in both the arm and the leg. The four methods of measuring blood pressure are (1) auscultatory, (2) palpatory, (3) visual (flush), and (4) Doppler.

Certain basic information must be part of every examination of the heart: rate, rhythm, size, shape, quality of sounds, murmurs and thrills, femoral pulses, and blood pressure (Table 9.1). In the routine examination of the heart, it is advantageous to evaluate the patient in several different positions if possible.

PULSE

Palpate the radial, femoral, and carotid pulses in young children and also the tibial pulse in older children. Absent femoral pulse indicates coarctation of the aorta; absence of the other pulses occurs with Takayusu syndrome or later stages of diabetes.

The normal pulse rate varies from 70 to 170 beats per minute (beats/min) at birth to 120–140 beats/min soon after birth (Table 9.2). Rates of 80–140 beats/min at 1 year, 80–130 beats/min at 2 years, 80–120 at 3 years and 70–115 after 3 years are within normal limits. By age 10 years, the normal rate decreases to 90 beats/min and in adolescence to 60–100 beats/min. Boys generally have slower rates than girls. After age 2 years, the pulse rate during sleep is usually 20 beats/min less than during waking. Almost always, the pulse rate during sleep as well as during waking hours is elevated in active rheumatic fever, any other active infection, or thyrotoxicosis.

Causes of Tachycardia

Excitement	Hyperthyroid
Exercise	Digitalis toxicity
Fever	Heart disease
Neuroblastoma	Pheochromocytoma
Systemic diseases	Toxins

TABLE 9.1

Normal Values of Pulse and Blood Pressure in the First Year of Life

Age Group	Pulse Rate (beats/min)		Blood pressure (mmHg)		
	Lower Limits of Normal	Average	Upper Limits of Normal	Systolic	Diastolic
Premature	80	120	170	60 (50–75)	35 (30–45)
Neonate	80	120	170	75 (60–90)	45 (40–60)
1–12 months	90	120	180	90 (75–100)	60 (50–70)

From Moller, J. H., & Neal, W. A. (1981). *Heart disease in infancy.* New York: Appleton-Century-Crofts.

In rheumatic fever, in contrast to other infections, the increased rate is usually out of proportion to the increase in temperature. The pulse rate is usually increased by 10–15 beats/min for each centigrade degree of fever. In children with upper airway obstruction, pulse rates of 140–160 beats/min are common; in those with lower airway obstruction, rates may be 180–200 beats/min or more.

Supraventricular tachycardia with rates as high as 200–300 beats/min is sometimes noted in children with congenital heart or acquired myocardial diseases or with toxic states. An idiopathic atrial tachycardia may be a cause of sudden death in infancy. Pulsus alternans, in which one beat is strong and the next weak, is a sign of severe heart strain. A slow rate (bradycardia), less than 100 beats/min in infants and less than 60 beats/min in older children, frequently means some degree of heart block. In infancy, it is usually associated with a septal defect, digitalis poisoning, severe sepsis, congenital lupus, and, occasionally, hypothyroidism. In young teenagers, sinus bradycardia, especially with sinus arrhythmia, is common. Rare causes of slow pulse include carotid sinus hypersensitivity, hypercalcemia, hyperkalemia, increased intracranial pressure, and, occasionally, acute myocarditis. The slow pulse rate sometimes noted in children with hypertension in acute nephritis may be related to an associated increased intracranial pressure. Slow rates may be noted in well-trained athletes.

TABLE 9.2

Acceptable Heart Rates in Infants and Children

Age	Resting Pulse Rates (Beats/Min)		
	Awake	Asleep	Exercise/Fever
Newborn	100–180	80–160	<220
1 week–3 months	100–220	80–200	<220
3 months–2 years	80–150	70–120	<200
2–10 years	70–110	60–90	<200
>10 years	55–90	50–90	<200

Water-hammer, or Corrigan pulse, is felt as an especially forceful beat resulting from a very wide pulse pressure. It is noted best over either the radial or femoral arteries. Capillary pulsation, or Quincke pulse, which is noted most easily after you press lightly on the tip of the nail, also results from increased pulse pressure. A method sometimes used for eliciting capillary pulsations is rubbing of the skin of the child's forehead vigorously for a minute until generalized erythema appears. Observation reveals intermittent reddening and blanching in children with increased capillary pressures. Both these pulse types are found especially in older children with patent ductus arteriosus (PDA), aortic regurgitation, or peripheral arterio-venous fistula.

Thready pulse is a rapid, weak pulse that seems to appear and disappear. It is usually a sign of circulatory failure, shock, or heart failure. A dicrotic pulse feels as though it has a notch in it. You may find it in children with sepsis. The normal pulse has this notch, but it cannot usually be palpated. Pulsus paradoxus is a marked change in pulse amplitude with respiration. Take the blood pressure several times rapidly in different parts of the respiratory cycle; alternatively, lower pressure in the cuff 1 mm/sec. Listen for the first faint sporadic sounds and the point at which all sounds are repetitive and crisp. Normally blood pressure does not increase more than 10 mmHg in expiration. Children with well-developed thoracic respiration may exhibit greater differences. An increase of more than 10 mmHg may be a sign of cardiac tamponade caused by pericardial effusion or constrictive pericarditis. A pulse pressure between two beats more than 20 mmHg is a grave sign in a child with asthma, and with cystic fibrosis such an increase reflects severity of disease. Reverse pulsus paradoxus, an increase in blood pressure with inspiration, is caused by an increase in left ventricular stroke output as in hypertrophic subaortic stenosis or during positive pressure breathing.

Almost all children, especially young adolescents, normally have sinus arrhythmia. Occasional runs of premature beats or of extrasystoles are common in childhood and may have no clinical significance. Irregular rhythm in childhood is not rare but, if present, may indicate active carditis. You will rarely see atrial fibrillation in childhood because its chief cause — rheumatic heart disease — develops in older children or adults after childhood rheumatic fever. Arrhythmias, particularly ventricular, may cause syncope and may occur in patients with long Q-T intervals. Premature contractions that disappear after exercise are benign.

Inspection

In the routine examination of the heart, inspect the chest for precordial bulging, a sign of right-sided enlargement, and the visible cardiac impulse and its localization and diffuseness. Frequently the cardiac impulse is noted in normal children or in children who are hyperactive, thin, or excited. It is not visible in many normal children. If the impulse appears diffuse, it may be normal. The position of the impulse sometimes provides a rough idea of the heart size because it may correspond to the location of the apex of the heart.

Other observations made as part of the routine examination of the heart include the appearance of respiratory distress, cyanosis, edema, clubbing of the fingers, capillary pulsations, prominence of veins, and abnormal pulsations of neck and epigastric veins. The presence or absence of femoral pulses and the blood pressure are important in determining the status of the heart.

The size of the heart is an indicator of the presence of heart disease. Heart size can be estimated by physical examination alone with careful inspection, palpation, and percussion.

Palpation

Palpation is useful in detecting the apex impulse (point of maximal impulse, PMI) of the heart. Although the PMI is an important physical sign in children and even in adolescents, it does not accurately reflect heart size. A more reliable guide is the apex beat. This is the position farthest toward the axilla and toward the lower rib margin which can be easily palpated. The apex beat is normally at the fifth interspace in the midclavicular line after age 7. Before this age, the apex beat is normally felt in the fourth interspace just to the left of the midclavicular line. The apex is usually at a lower interspace and more lateral in children with cardiac enlargement; pericardial effusion and various lung, spine, and chest wall diseases may also displace the apex.

The apex impulse may be difficult to feel in children aged less than 2 years or in children with pericardial effusion, heart failure, or emphysema. A forceful apex beat is felt in children after exercise or excitement or in those with thin chest walls, impending heart failure, fever, or hyperthyroidism.

Occasionally you can distinguish right ventricular hypertrophy from left ventricular hypertrophy by palpation. Place your palm over the child's sternum with your fingertips at the apex. Pulsation below and to the left of the apex indicates left ventricular enlargement; with right ventricular hypertrophy, you usually feel the impulse as a sharp tap or as a heave more medially. A sustained lift in the xiphoid region indicates right ventricular overwork. A slow heave suggests increased pressure work; a sharper hyperdynamic tap suggests increased volume work.

Usually the first (systolic) sound, occasionally the second (diastolic) sound, and, in a failing heart, a third sound (gallop rhythm) may be palpated. Occasionally the child will complain of tenderness when the heart area is palpated. This does not indicate that heart disease is present or absent.

Vibratory thrills and pericardial friction rubs may also be palpated. They are felt as fine or coarse vibrations, either continuously or during some part of the cardiac cycle. Record position of cardiac thrills and their timing in the cardiac cycle. Obtain timing by simultaneously feeling either the apex impulse or the carotid pulse. Thrills at the apex are more easily felt with the child lying on the left side; basal thrills are more easily felt with the child sitting up.

A high-frequency thrill along the left sternal border suggests ventricular septal defect; a low-frequency midsystolic thrill in the second left interspace indicates pulmonary stenosis; a midsystolic thrill in the second right interspace suggests aortic stenosis; and a continuous thrill indicates PDA. Feel also with one finger in the suprasternal notch. If the notch is very pulsatile, suspect PDA or aortic insufficiency. A diastolic thrill at the apex is usually caused by mitral stenosis.

Pulsus Alternans

Pulsus alternans is seen infrequently in children and when present, is invariably associated with myocardial failure. The palpating finger cannot perceive a systolic pressure difference of less than 20 mmHg, and careful observations must be made when you are recording the blood pressure in the patient with this sign. As the cuff pressure is being decreased, a systolic pressure is first encountered of only the alternate Korotkoff sounds. For example, if the blood pressure is 120 mmHg systolic with a regular rate of 50 beats/min, a regular rate of 100 beats/min is encountered as the cuff pressure is lowered further, at which time the blood pressure is 95 mmHg or possibly lower. The presence of left ventricular hypertension (aortic stenosis, systemic hypertension) increases the likelihood of eliciting this sign.

Bradycardia

If a child's pulse rate is less than 60 beats/min, complete atrioventricular (AV) block may be present. Differentiation of this condition from sinus bradycardia is usually possible at the bedside. Checking the jugular pulse is normally of little value in this age group; however, in the patient with bradycardia and possible AV block, look for cannon A waves. This procedure is performed with the child in the sitting or semi-recumbent position and the head inclined to one side. When auscultating, check for varying intensity of the first heart sound, which is caused by the varying position of the AV valves at the beginning of ventricular contraction. Also observe the effect of exercise on the child's pulse rate. In complete AV block, only a small increase occurs. An innocent murmur is frequently seen in association with bradycardia because of the increased stroke volume.

Percussion

Percussion of the heart, like percussion of the lungs, may be performed by either the direct or indirect method. Scratch percussion is an excellent way of determining cardiac borders. With the stethoscope over the heart, make longitudinal parallel scratches with a finger beginning in the axillary line and move toward the heart at about 1 cm intervals. As soon as the scratches are over the heart, you will detect a change in intensity of the scratch sound through the stethoscope (Figure 9.1).

In estimating heart size and shape, you may find a combined method of percussion and auscultation even more satisfactory. Place the stethoscope firmly on the child's chest just to the right of the sternum. Tap the chest wall lightly with your index finger, beginning in the axillary line and proceeding medially. As soon as your finger is tapping over the heart, you will note a sharp increase in sound.

The heart is usually percussed easily as a triangular area with one side of the triangle extending along the right sternal border from the second to the fifth rib, one side extending from the right sternal to the left midclavicular line along the fifth rib, and the third side extending from the right sternal border at the second rib to the left midclavicular line at the fifth rib. Usually, the heart of the infant is more horizontal, and the apex of the left border dullness is to the left of the nipple line.

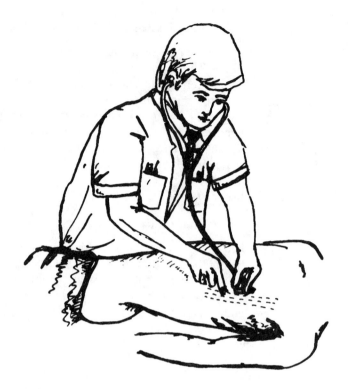

Figure 9.1
Scratch percussion. The stethoscope is near the sternum; parallel
scratches are made down the left side of the chest.

The area of heart dullness may be altered in a child with a normal or abnormal
heart size. In right or left ventricular hypertrophy, you may percuss the heart at a
lower interspace or more laterally. Percussion dullness to the right of the sternum in
the third or fourth interspace usually indicates right-sided heart enlargement or dextrocardia. Right-sided enlargement produces precordial bulging.

Causes of Heart Strain or Enlargement

Right	*Left*
Pulmonary stenosis	Coarctation of aorta
Intraatrial septal defect	Tricuspid atresia
Congenital heart lesion	Endocardial fibroelastosis
Mitral stenosis	Glycogen storage disease
	Aberrant coronary artery
	Aberrant pulmonary vein
	Hypertension
	Idiopathic hypertrophic subaortic
	stenosis (IHSS)

Dullness to the left of the midclavicular line suggests left ventricular enlargement. In children with emphysema or space-occupying lesions in the chest, the heart is pushed away from the lesion, whereas in children with atelectasis, the heart is pulled toward the side of the lesion. The heart normally moves a little as the patient is turned from side to side. If motion does not occur when the patient is turned, pulmonary masses or adhesions may be present; this physical finding is rare in childhood, however. The heart may be percussed far to the left in the second and third interspace when the child is recumbent, and it may be in the normal position when the child sits. This change in position may indicate the presence of pericardial effusion.

Small hearts, characteristic of patients with Addison disease or constrictive pericarditis, are rare in childhood. An enlarged heart is characteristic of almost all types of heart disease: congenital heart disease, anemia, myocarditis, or rheumatic heart disease. Less common causes of an enlarged heart include endocardial fibroelastosis, pericardial effusion, PDA, hypertension in nephritis, tumors, glycogen storage disease, or peripheral arteriovenous shunt. PDA may be present with a normal-sized heart.

Auscultation

Never auscultate the heart through clothing. Auscultate as you do when auscultating the lungs. Listen with the child in the sitting and supine positions. Use both the bell and the diaphragm over the entire precordium, with special reference to the valve areas as in adults: The areas shown in Figure 9.2 are the listening posts of the valve areas and not the true or anatomic valve areas. These areas regularly include the mitral valve at the apex, the pulmonary valve at the second interspace to the left of the sternum, the aortic valve at the second interspace to the right of the sternum (and at the third left interspace for diastolic murmurs), and the tricuspid valve in the fourth interspace over the sternum. In addition to auscultating in these areas, in children auscultate just to the right of the apex and several centimeters to the left of the sternum in the third interspace (frequent sites of innocent murmurs), along the sternal border (site of murmurs of septal defects), the second and third interspaces several centimeters to the left of the sternum (sites of murmurs of PDA and coarctation of the aorta), above the clavicles (sites of venous hums and transmitted murmurs), and in the axillae, along the left midaxillary line, and below the scapulae (sites of transmitted murmurs). In children, auscultation will usually yield a better measurement of the cardiac rate than will palpation at the wrist.

Evaluate the quality of the sounds. The first sound is best heard with the bell and the second is best heard with the diaphragm. In newborns, sounds should be sharp and clear. Distant sounds may indicate pericardial fluid, atelectasis, or another pulmonary disease. Sounds of poor quality, those that do not sound clear but are slurred or mushy, are almost always characteristic of severe heart disease or myocarditis, usually with heart failure. In newborns, both sounds are of approximately equal intensity. Later, the apical first sound is louder than the second, and the pulmonic second sound is louder than the first in childhood.

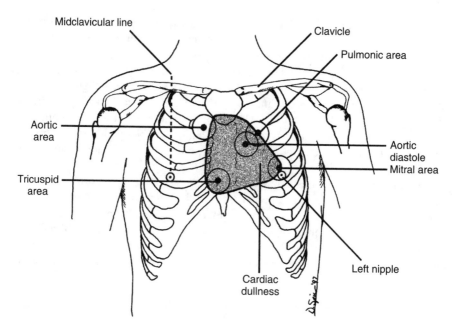

Figure 9.2
Listening areas of the heart.

A loud, snapping apical first sound is heard with mitral stenosis, left-to-right shunt, or conditions with high cardiac output; a decreased apical first sound is heard in early myocarditis.

In pulmonic stenosis, pulmonic atresia, or truncus, the pulmonic second sound usually is decreased or absent. The pulmonic second sound is normally louder than the aortic second sound during childhood and is very loud in pulmonary hypertension. You may hear the pulmonic second sound better in the third than in the second left interspace in children. The aortic second sound is usually diminished in intensity with aortic stenosis and acute myocarditis. In aortic insufficiency, the aortic second sound is often increased, but it may be decreased or absent. The aortic second sound is increased in children with hypertension of any cause. The tricuspid first sound may be obliterated with tricuspid regurgitation, a rare congenital anomaly.

The first sound, S_1, results from mitral and tricuspid (atrioventricular) valve closure. When the first sound is split, the first component is caused by mitral closure. The second sound, S_2, results from aortic and pulmonic valve closure, the aortic valve closing slightly before the pulmonic. Splitting of the second sound is heard best in the pulmonic area and is common in normal children. Deep inspiration delays pulmonic valve closure and increases the splitting of the second sound (Figure 9.3). Learn to appreciate splitting by first listening at the apex when aortic valve closure is simultaneous with mitral valve opening. Then move the stethoscope up, interspace by interspace, to the pulmonic area where the pulmonic valve closure is most distinct;

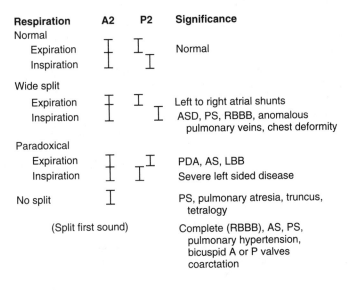

Respiration	A2	P2	Significance
Normal			
Expiration			Normal
Inspiration			
Wide split			
Expiration			Left to right atrial shunts
Inspiration			ASD, PS, RBBB, anomalous pulmonary veins, chest deformity
Paradoxical			
Expiration			PDA, AS, LBB
Inspiration			Severe left sided disease
No split			PS, pulmonary atresia, truncus, tetralogy
(Split first sound)			Complete (RBBB), AS, PS, pulmonary hypertension, bicuspid A or P valves coarctation

Figure 9.3
Second heart sounds splitting. A, aortic valve; P, pulmonic valve;
AS, aortic stenosis; ASD, atrial septal defect; LBBB, left bundle
branch block; PDA, patent ductus arteriosus; PS, pulmonic stenosis;
RBBB, right bundle branch block.

two sounds will be heard. A third heart sound, S_3, is caused by vibration of the left ventricle wall, is present in about one third of children before puberty, and occurs between the second and first heart sound early in diastole. It is best heard at the apex, with a longer interval between the second and third sounds (usually with differing intensities and qualities), and occurs in mitral insufficiency or atrial septal defect. Later in diastole, just before the first sound, a fourth sound, S_4, may be audible and indicates decreased ventricular compliance, as in fibrosis or hypertrophy.

Either the first or second sound may be split in any valvular area without being a cause of concern. Four criteria are useful in distinguishing split sounds from a third heart sound: intensity, quality, position heard, and distance between sounds. Split second sounds are of equal quality and intensity, are heard most frequently at the base of the heart, and occur with a very short interval between the sounds.

Split second sounds at the base of the heart are common in children with conditions causing left-to-right shunts such as atrial septal defect, mild pulmonic stenosis, or right bundle branch block (Figure 9.3). Splitting at the base is absent in children with pulmonic stenosis, tetralogy of Fallot, pulmonic atresia, or truncus. The wide splitting characteristically heard in children with atrial septal defects remains constant during inspiration and expiration. Paradoxical splitting, a wider split in expiration than inspiration, occurs with PDA, aortic stenosis, complete left bundle branch block, or other severe left-sided lesions.

Clicks are high-pitched sounds you may hear when valves open. They may indicate aortic, pulmonic, or mitral valve stenosis or mitral valve prolapse. Low-pitched snaps in the mitral area occur in mitral stenosis.

Occasionally it is difficult to distinguish the third heart sound from a gallop rhythm, which indicates a failing heart. You may feel the three beats of the gallop on palpation; you can never feel the third heart sound as an impulse. Differentiation between the third sound and gallop rhythm is usually based on the presence of other evidence of heart disease, when gallop rhythm would be more likely to be heard than a third heart sound. Tic-tac rhythm, or embryocardia, exists if both sounds are almost alike in quality and intensity and are equidistant from each other. Although normal in younger children, this rhythm in older children may indicate a failing heart.

Murmurs

A difficult diagnostic feature in physical examination of children is determination of the significance of murmurs. When a murmur sounds like a breath sound, it is not an innocent murmur. Many children have murmurs without heart disease, and occasionally newborns or others have severe heart disease with no murmurs. Systolic murmurs are those that occur at or after the first and before the second sound; diastolic murmurs occur at or after the second and before the first sound. Murmurs heard in systole are early systolic (regurgitant), midsystolic, or pansystolic (holosystolic). Holosystolic murmurs are caused by blood flow from a chamber with higher pressure to a chamber with lower pressure. Diastolic murmurs may be early (protodiastolic) or middiastolic or may occur late in diastole (presystolic) (Figure 9.4).

Describe quality of murmurs as soft, harsh, blowing, or whistling. Grade the intensity of murmurs. According to one system of grading, a grade 1 murmur is the softest possible murmur heard. It is not heard in all positions, especially not when the patient sits up or after exercise. A grade 2 murmur is the weakest murmur heard in all positions or after exercise. A grade 3 murmur is loud but is not accompanied by a thrill. A grade 4 murmur is loud but has a thrill. A grade 5 murmur is heard with the stethoscope barely on the chest. A grade 6 murmur can be heard with the stethoscope not touching the chest.

The intensity of murmurs alone does not indicate whether the murmur is significant of heart disease, although murmurs of grade 3 or louder usually do indicate heart disease. Following the intensity of a murmur over a period of hours, days, or weeks is helpful in determining the course of the heart disease. This is especially true in cases of rheumatic fever and bacterial endocarditis, in which the quality of the murmurs may change rapidly.

Murmurs may rumble for a short distance around the site of their maximal intensity but radiate or are transmitted if they are heard with distinct intensity some distance away from that site. Innocent murmurs usually do not radiate, and they may change in character with phase of respiration or change in position—being louder when the patient is supine than when the patient is in the sitting position. Innocent murmurs may appear or disappear during fever, exercise, excitement, or

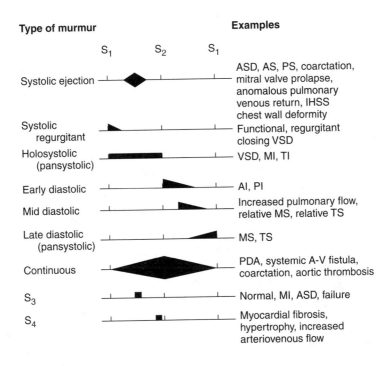

Figure 9.4
Types of murmurs and examples. AI, aortic insufficiency; AS, aortic
stenosis; ASD, atrial septal defect; A-V, arteriovenous; IHSS, idiopathic
hypertrophic subaortic stenosis; MI, mitral insufficiency; MS, mitral
stenosis; PDA, patent ductus arteriosus; PI, pulmonic insufficiency; PS,
pulmonic stenosis; TI, tricuspid insufficiency; TS, tricuspid stenosis; VSD,
ventricular septal defect.

anemia. Any diastolic murmur or a murmur that is transmitted or radiates indicates
heart disease.

Cardiopulmonary murmurs are soft, high-pitched sounds caused by the apposition of the heart and lungs, occur always in the same phase of respiration, can be
obliterated by changing position (venous shunt), and usually have no pathologic
significance but may indicate the presence of pleural adhesions. Murmurs indicating pleural adhesions are usually short, high-pitched, and squeaking, are louder
during inspiration, and project to the left sternal border. Murmurs originating from
the left side of the heart are best heard in expiration.

Short-blowing, early systolic or midsystolic murmurs of low pitch heard best in the
pulmonary area (usually in early adolescence), pulmonary flow murmurs, or vibratory murmurs that sound like musical buzzing over the precordium (in younger children) are usually innocent. If these murmurs radiate, they usually radiate downward; if murmurs of
mitral insufficiency (MI) radiate, they usually radiate laterally. In addition, the murmur
of MI is continuous during systole and is at or lateral to the apex; the innocent murmur,

which is short, is usually medial to the apex in the general area where the murmurs of septal defects are heard.

A midsystolic, crescendo-decrescendo, loud, harsh murmur ("diamond-shaped," "ejection") over the pulmonic area is characteristic of pulmonic stenosis (PS) and is also heard with atrial septal defects (ASDs) or anomalous pulmonary venous return. This murmur is usually louder, harsher, and longer than the innocent murmur resulting from pulmonary flow. Peripheral PS is accompanied by a soft systolic murmur over one or both lung fields but not over the heart. This is usually not a clinically significant condition. PS murmur may also be accompanied by a thrill and a systolic ejection click. A similar murmur in the second interspace just to the right of the sternum is characteristic of aortic stenosis (AS) or subaortic stenosis. This murmur radiates to the back. ASD is distinguished by fixed splitting of the second sound, increased intensity of the second component to the second sound at the upper left sternal edge and at the apex, and an early diastolic rumble from tricuspid flow audible at the midleft sternal border. Murmurs of aortic outflow originate in the upper right sternal border, radiate to the neck, and may cause a carotid thrill. An aortic systolic murmur, which varies in intensity, may indicate idiopathic hypertrophic subaortic cardiomyopathy, an autosomal dominant inherited trait. It increases on standing and may be associated with mitral systolic murmur. A mid- or late-blowing systolic murmur, frequently beginning with multiple systolic clicks, is characteristic of mitral valve prolapse. Murmurs of mitral valve prolapse may be honking or whooping.

The murmurs of septal defects and PS may be heard alone as isolated congenital anomalies or in combination, as in tetralogy of Fallot. The pulmonic systolic murmur with a loud tricuspid valve closure, split second sound, and prominent precordial activity may result from anterior displacement of a normal heart as in the straight back syndrome.

Holosystolic murmurs are common with mitral or tricuspid valve incompetence (MI, TI) and septal defects. In these, the first sound is not heard. Detection of this murmur very early in systole distinguishes it from innocent murmur. Marked changes in murmurs with respiration are usually caused by left heart lesions (e.g., ventricular septal defect or mitral regurgitation).

Diastolic murmurs that begin loud and then diminish in intensity are decrescendo (e.g., the murmur of aortic insufficiency, AI; or pulmonic insufficiency, PI). At the apex of the heart, murmurs starting softly and increasing in intensity are crescendo murmurs, like the murmurs of mitral stenosis (MS) or tricuspid stenosis (TS) resulting from valvular disease or increased flow secondary to a left-to-right shunt. Presystolic murmurs are usually associated with active atrial contraction and with mitral or tricuspid valve.

A continuous murmur in the second or third interspace to the left of the sternum that is widely transmitted is characteristic of PDA. A hum or high-pitched murmur anywhere along the course of the aorta may be a result of coarctation of the aorta or, rarely, a thrombosis of the aorta. A continuous murmur in the right or left parasternal areas may indicate a coronary or other arteriovenous fistula.

Rheumatic carditis is a type of acquired heart disease. A harsh, systolic, high-pitched, or soft blow, sometimes obliterating the first sound and lasting through systole up to the second sound or beginning in late systole with crescendo to the second sound at or just to the right of the apex, may be the first sign of carditis and is usually caused by MI. This murmur is usually transmitted to the axilla or back. Later, an early diastolic or middiastolic crescendo blow in the same area with a loud mitral first sound may indicate relative MS—relative because of the disproportion of the size of the valve and the ventricle. These murmurs disappear when the carditis disappears. The murmur of true MS is similar except that, in addition, early in diastole a snap is heard because of mitral valve opening. A later snap in diastole occurs with pericarditis and must be distinguished from the third heart sound.

Late signs are the blowing diastolic decrescendo murmur of AI, heard best with the diaphragm stethoscope just to the left of the sternum in the third interspace. This murmur may radiate down the left sternal border. A systolic high-pitched murmur in the third left interspace, with a decreased pulmonic second sound, is usually caused by PS.

Tricuspid murmurs are rare and are similar in character to mitral murmurs, though they may be a cause of a transient murmur in newborns; a systolic murmur indicates tricuspid insufficiency, and a diastolic murmur indicates TS.

The murmurs heard in the tricuspid area and the murmur of PS are more often congenital than acquired during childhood (Tables 9.3 and 9.4). The murmur of AS is frequently caused by congenital lesion, and the murmur of AI is rarely heard during childhood, since AI develops late in the course of rheumatic carditis.

Venous hum is a continuous, low-pitched sound originating in the internal jugular vein, heard sometimes over the clavicles. It usually radiates downward and has no pathologic significance but must be distinguished from a murmur. The hum is usually louder when the patient is sitting, disappears in recumbency, may be abolished by pressure on the internal jugular vein, and is louder on the right. Venous hums over the abdomen, especially near the umbilicus, are sometimes heard in children with cirrhosis of the liver or portal obstruction.

TABLE 9.3

Suggested Offspring Recurrence Risk for Congenital Heart Defects
Given One Affected Parent

Defect	Mother Affected	Father Affected
Aortic stenosis	18	5
Atrial septal defect	6	1.5
Coarctation of aorta	4	2.5
Endocardial cushion defect	14	1
Patent ductus arteriosus	4	2
Pulmonary stenosis	6.5	2
Tetrology of Fallot	2.5	1.5
Ventricular septal defect	9.5	2.5

TABLE 9.4
Potential Teratogens That May Result in Congenital Heart Disease

Potential Teratogens	Frequency of CV Disease (%)	Most Common Malformations
Drugs		
Alcohol	25–30	VSD, PDA, ASD
Amphetamines	75–100	VSD, PDA, ASD, D-TGA
Anticonvulsants		
Hydantoin	2–3	PS, AS, CoA, PDA
Trimethadione	15–30	D-TGA, TOF, HLHS
Lithium	10	Ebstein, ASD
Sex hormones	2–4	VSD, D-TGA, TOF
Thalidomide	5–10	TOF, VSD, ASD
Infections		
Rubella	35	PPS, PDA, VSD, ASD
Maternal Conditions		
Diabetes	3–5	D-TGA, VSD, CoA
	(30–50)	(cardiomyopathy)
Lupus	50	Heart block
Phenylketonuria	25–50	TOF, VSD, ASD

Pericardial friction rub is a grating to-and-fro sound heard through the stethoscope as though it were close to the examiner's ear. It is increased by pressure of the stethoscope on the chest or by the patient leaning forward. Intensity of the rub varies with the phase of the cardiac cycle. Rub usually indicates pericarditis (e.g., tuberculosis or acute rheumatic fever), and sometimes may be detected on palpation as a vibratory thrill. Pleuropericardial rubs are more common than pericardial rubs and are heard best in the manner described, but they vary with the phase of respiration rather than with cardiac activity. They may be confused with pericardial rubs, usually have no pathologic significance, and may be caused by the proximity of the heart and lungs but may indicate pleuropericardial adhesions. Sometimes the crunch of subcutaneous emphysema is confused with a pericardial or pleuropericardial rub.

In general, type of heart disease is not diagnosed by examination alone. First, make a tentative diagnosis by history and repeated observation and try to confirm or eliminate this diagnosis by examination and suitable laboratory studies: For example, children aged less than 5 years rarely have rheumatic fever; even if aged more than 5 years, they should have other characteristic signs of rheumatic fever such as joint pains, subcutaneous nodules, chorea, or erythema nodosum. Even in older children without fever or increased pulse rate, a diagnosis of rheumatic fever is not very likely, although it is possible. If a child has fever, increased pulse rate, and murmurs, also consider the diagnosis of fever with innocent murmurs or myocarditis secondary to infection elsewhere, as in nephritis, diphtheria, or tonsillitis.

In children aged less than 5 years, next consider whether the heart disease is cyanotic or acyanotic. Severe cyanosis at birth, which has been determined (as described in Chapter 20) in a newborn to result from heart disease, usually indicates one of the most severe congenital heart lesions such as transposition of the great vessels, truncus arteriosus, or tricuspid atresia. Cyanosis developing later in the first year of life occurs because of an increasing shunt from the right heart to the left, such as in tetralogy of Fallot, in which the increasing PS causes increasing right ventricular pressure. Cyanosis developing at age 4 or 5 years may indicate Eisenmenger complex or PS with septal defect. If cyanosis is not present unless the child exercises or cries, an atrial septal defect without PS is suggested because the right-sided pressure is not increased until the intrapulmonary pressure is increased by crying.

Differential Diagnosis of Cyanosis

- Reduced O_2 availability: high altitude (>6,000 feet), for example, air travel, ski resort, mountain travel
- Reduced O_2 transport to alveoli: respiratory failure or arrest, air flow obstruction (usually compensate for large obstruction unless complete); restrictive chest wall disease (e.g., kyphosis, weakness, or obesity)
- Abnormal ventilation
  Pneumonia, pulmonary edema, diffuse alveolar damage, alveolar proteinosis
  Asthma bronchiolitis
  Combined pathology: acute respiratory distress syndrome, bronchopulmonary dysplasia, hyaline membrane disease
- Abnormal perfusion
  Pulmonary hypertension, pulmonary embolus, abnormal anatomy (e.g., pulmonary sequestration)
- Shunt
  Intrapulmonary shunt, atrioventricular malformation
  Extrapulmonary shunt, such as time-of-flight, total anomalous pulmonary venous return (TAPVR), transposition of the great arteries
- Abnormal transport to tissue
  Abnormal hemoglobin: β-thalassemia, sickle cell disease, carbon monoxide poisoning
  Decreased blood flow: dysrhythmia, bradycardia, cardiac arrest, hypotension
- Abnormal O_2 delivery at tissue
  Mitochondrial disease, cyanide poisoning
- Chronic cyanosis starting at birth, meconium aspiration, group B streptococcus, sepsis, hyaline membrane disease
- Persistent fetal circulation

The significant noncyanotic heart diseases of infancy are toxic myocarditis from any cause, endocardial fibroelastosis, tumors of the heart, and, most commonly, PDA and coarctation of the aorta. PDA has the characteristic murmur (machinery murmur). In coarctation, pulse pressure is high in the arms and very low in the legs and femoral pulses are absent or weak. Other noncyanotic heart lesions, such as right aortic arch, dextroposition of the heart, and aortic vascular ring, are diagnosed by examination and by history suggesting obstruction of the trachea or esophagus by an extrinsic mass.

HEART FAILURE

Significance of the Age of Onset of Congestive Heart Failure

The age of onset of congestive heart failure is important in assessing the identifying cause.

- If a child becomes symptomatic because of congenital heart disease, there is a 95% probability that the symptoms will develop before the age of 3 months and usually before 2 months.
- Heart failure is rarely present at birth, because the fetal circulation allows communication between the right and left sides of the heart.
- Heart failure that develops during the first week of life, especially in the first 3 days, is usually due to an obstructive lesion or to persistent pulmonary hypertension or hypoplastic left hernia.
- Heart failure that develops 4–6 weeks after birth is invariably due to left-to-right shunting.
- If heart failure develops after 3 months it may be due to myocarditis, cardiomyopathy, and paroxysmal tachycardia.

The signs of heart failure in young children are not similar to those in adults. Early, the respiratory rate in the supine position is rapid; slight dyspnea follows. Next, the heart enlarges—best detected by scratch percussion. The liver becomes enlarged early and there may be venous engorgement and orthopnea; pulsus alternans and gallop rhythm, if present, are almost pathognomonic of heart failure. Signs of pulmonary or peripheral edema are noted late in the progression of heart failure as the failure becomes more severe. Sweating may occur.

If one's goal as a physician is limited to making a diagnosis as rapidly as possible, or patient's overall condition mandates a rapid diagnosis, then use commonly available devices. If, however, you obtain satisfaction from discovering cryptic information, develop precise examining and history-taking habits (this assumes the patient's condition allows a more deliberate approach).

Differential Diagnosis of Heart Failure

Increased Afterload

- Most common in the neonate due to left-sided obstructive lesions, which present acutely. Secondary to PDA or premature foramen ovale closure.
- Aortic coarctation is most common
  Increased pulse/blood pressure in right arm
  Decreased pulse/blood pressure in lower extremities
- Critical aortic stenosis

Poor pulses, loud murmur
- Hypoplastic left heart syndrome, aortic arch interruption

Left Heart Shunt Lesions

- Normal cardiac muscle function but overcirculation of lungs due to a congenital connection between the right and left side of the heart and low pulmonary venous return (PVR)
- Usually presents at 1–2 months of age
  PVR drops and systemic resistance becomes higher than PV pressure
  Blood shunts from left to right (systemic circulation to pulmonary circulation)
  Pulmonary overcirculation and poor systemic output (poor peripheral perfusion, low urine output)
- Ventricular septal defect (most common)
- Atrioventricular septal defect (AV canal, endocardial cushion defect), associated with Down syndrome
- PDA
- Atrial septal defect (less common)

Intrinsic Myocardial Disease

- More common cause of heart failure in older children and adolescents
- Myocarditis
  Usually postviral
  One third remain stable, one third return to normal cardiac function, and one third deteriorate
- Cardiomyopathy
  Dilated most common, but also hypertrophic and restrictive
  Multiple genetic and metabolic causes, often positive family history, some represent old, "burned-out" myocarditis
- Myocardial infarction (rare)
  Kawasaki disease
  Congenital coronary abnormalities (anomalous left coronary artery)

Chest Pain

Cardiac

Mitral valve prolapse
Pericarditis
Coronary artery insufficiency
Kawasaki disease
Aortic stenosis
Dysrhythmias
Pulmonary hypertension
Dissecting aortic aneurysm
Takayasu syndrome
Myocarditis

Embolism—thromboses
Vasculitis
Precordial catch syndrome

Noncardiac

Trauma
Muscle fatigue
Asthma
Skin infections
Collagen vascular diseases
Pneumonia—bronchitis
Pleuritis
Pneumothorax
Subcutaneous emphysema
Tietze syndrome (costochondritis)
Adolescent breast development
Cervical rib
Slipping rib
Scalenus-anticus syndrome
Tumor
Mediastinitis—pneumomediastinum
Sickle cell disease, trait
Leukemia, lymphoma
Gastrointestinal, renal conditions
Emotional/hyperventilation
Poisoning

Acyanotic Congenital Heart Defects

Patent Ductus Arteriosis

PDA is a common problem in premature infants (Figure 9.5). Clinical manifestations are asymptomatic (small shunts), congenital heart failure (large shunts), and differential cyanosis (if PVOD develops).

Atrial Septal Defect

There are three types of ASD: ostium secundum, sinus venosus defect, and ostinum primum (Figure 9.6). Physical examination reveals a slender body build, a systolic ejection murmur, and a widely split and fixed S_2.

Ventricular Septal Defect

Types of ventricular septal defect (VSD) consist of membranous (or perimembranous), muscular, and inlet (AV canal type; Figure 9.7). Clinical manifestations are, if small: asymptomatic, spontaneous closure (40–50% by 3 years of age); if large: congenital heart failure at 2–3 months. Physical examination: poor weight gain, systolic thrill with holosystolic murmur at left lateral sternal border (LLSB) with

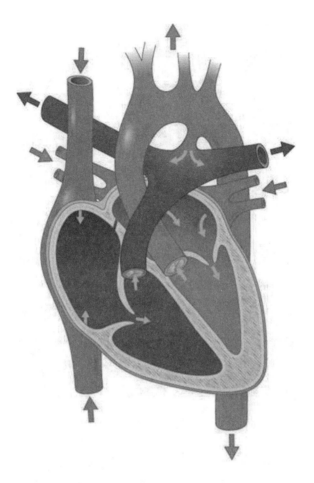

Figure 9.5
Flow of blood in a heart with patent ductus arteriosus
(PDA). (From Gilbert-Barness, E., & Debich-Spicer, D.,
2007. Congenital malformations of the heart. In
E. Gilbert-Barness, Ed., *Potter's pathology of the fetus,
infant, and child*, pp. 978–1023. New York: Elsevier.)

radiation to midclavicular line, diastolic murmur with large shunts and loud P2 with
pulmonary hypertension.

Endocardial Cushion Defect

Types consists of partial (ostium primum) and complete (atrioventricular canal).
Clinical manifestations are that 30% of the defects occur in Down syndrome, partial
(asymptomatic) and complete (congenital heart failure). Physical examination:
undernourished, hyperactive precordium with holosystolic murmur at LLSB, loud
P2, middiastolic rumble at the apex, and liver enlargement. EKG superior QRS

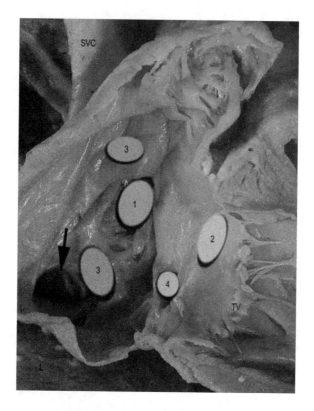

Figure 9.6
Diagram of atrial septal defect (ASD) sites: 1, ostium
secundum defect; 2, ostium primum defect; 3, sinus
venosus defect; 4, coronary sinus defects. (From Gilbert-
Barness, E., & Debich-Spicer, D., 2007. Congenital
malformations of the heart. In E. Gilbert-Barness,
Ed., *Potter's pathology of the fetus, infant, and child*,
pp. 978–1023. New York: Elsevier.)

axis; first-degree AV block, right ventricular hypertrophy (RVH) or biventricular
hypertrophy (BVH). On chest X-ray the heart size is enlarged and pulmonary vascularity is increased.

Pulmonary Stenosis

Types consists of valvular (90%), subvalvular (infundibular, rare), and supravalvular
(postpolio syndrome) (Figure 9.8). The majority are asymptomatic and usually do
not get worse. In severe cases congestive heart failure, fatigability, syncope. In newborn there is poor feeding, tachypnea, and possible cyanosis. On physical examination
acyanotic, systolic ejection click, and intensity of the murmur varies with degree of
obstruction. EKG: right axis deviation and RVH. The chest X-ray shows poststenotic
dilatation of main pulmonary artery (MPA), a normal heart size or increased (congestive heart failure, CHF), and normal pulmonary vascularity or decreased (severe PS).

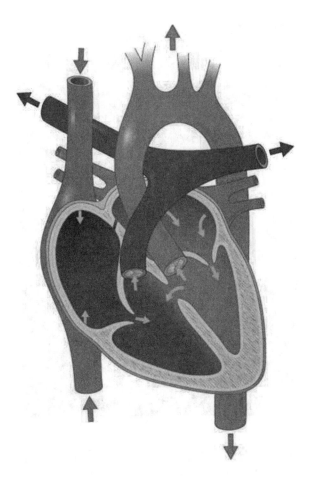

Figure 9.7
Flow of blood in a heart with VSD. (From Gilbert-Barness,
E., & Debich-Spicer, D., 2007. Congenital malformations
of the heart. In E. Gilbert-Barness, Ed., *Potter's pathology
of the fetus, infant, and child*, pp. 978–1023. New York:
Elsevier.)

Aortic Stenosis (M:F Ratio 4:1)

Types include valvular-bicuspid valve, subvalvular (membrane [discrete], long
tunnel, idiopathic hypertrophic cardiomyopathy), and supravalvular (Figure 9.9).
Clinical manifestations are mostly asymptomatic. In severe cases CHF, exertional
chest pain, syncope. Physical examination reveals acyanosis, a normal blood pressure, and a narrow pulse pressure in severe AS with a systolic thrill with murmur at
upper right sternal border, suprasternal notch, and over the carotid arteries. There is
an early ejection systolic click with valvular AS. The EKG is normal or demonstrates
LVH with strain in severe AS. On chest X-ray the heart size is normal with a dilated
ascending aorta or prominent aortic knob.

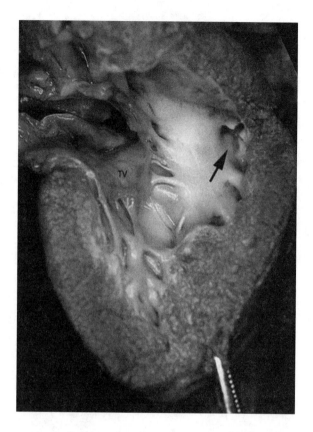

Figure 9.8
Stenosis of the pulmonic valve (arrow) with an intact ventricular septum
and decrease in size of the right ventricular cavity. The lumen of the
pulmonary artery distal to the valve is normal. Note the right ventricular
hypertrophy and endocardial fibroelastosis. TV, tricuspid valve. (From
Gilbert-Barness, E., & Debich-Spicer, D., 2007. Congenital malformations
of the heart. In E. Gilbert-Barness, Ed., *Potter's pathology of the fetus,
infant, and child*, pp. 978–1023. New York: Elsevier.)

Coarctation of Aorta (M:F Ratio 2:1)

Coarctation of the aorta (COA) is seen in 30% of Turner syndrome cases and ≥ 50%
of COA has bicuspid aortic valve (Figure 9.10). Clinical manifestations range from
asymptomatic in the majority to CHF in severe cases. On physical examination, the
pulse is absent, weak, or delayed in the legs, hypertension in the arms, and midsystolic
ejection murmur at LLSB and back.

Vascular Rings

Vascular rings are created by anomalies of the aortic arches with an anomalous vessel
coursing behind the trachea and esophagus (Figure 9.11). Symptoms are dysphagia,
hoarseness, and a shrill high-pitched cry.

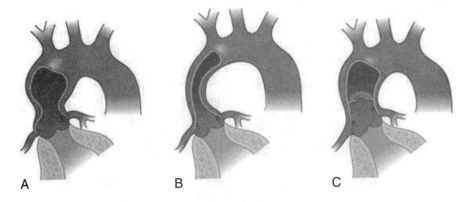

A   B   C

Figure 9.9
Diagram of three types of supravalvular aortic stenosis: A, hourglass type (most common); B, segmental type; C, fibromuscular membrane. (From Gilbert-Barness, E., & Debich-Spicer, D., 2007. Congenital malformations of the heart. In E. Gilbert-Barness, Ed., *Potter's pathology of the fetus, infant, and child*, pp. 978–1023. New York: Elsevier.)

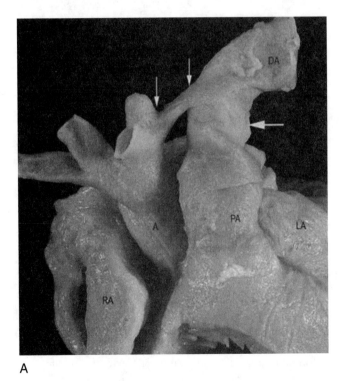

A

Figure 9.10
Preductal coarctation of the aorta (A) with tubular hypoplasia of the aortic arch (small arrows). RA, right atrial appendage; LA, left atrial appendage; PA, pulmonary artery.

Continued

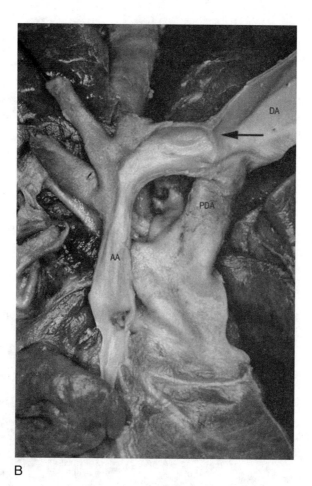

B

Figure 9.10 cont'd
Ductal coarctation. (B). There is a localized constriction of the aorta in the
region of the closure of the ductus arteriosus (arrow). AA, ascending aorta;
PDA, patent ductus arteriosus; DA, descending aorta.

Hypoplastic Left Heart Complex

There are two forms of hypoplastic left heart complex (HLHC) (Figure 9.12). In one
form with mitral atresia, a ventricular connection is absent and the LV is a trabecular
pouch. In the other form, there is mitral stenosis and the ventricular chamber is small
and shows considerable endocardial fibroelastosis. HLHC is the most common type
of cardiac malformation that is incompatible with extrauterine life.

HLHC is due to underdevelopment of the left heart and ascending aorta.
Systemic blood flow depends on a PDA. Severe CHF and death usually occur in the
first days of life. The infant is pale owing to absence of systemic blood flow, with weak
or absent pulses and blood pressure. HLHC is associated with premature closure of the
foramen ovule, which may be the cause of 10% of cases. A shunt procedure
(Norwood) has been used with limited success; cardiac transplantation offers the best
hope of survival.

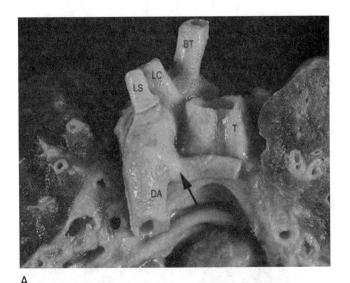

A

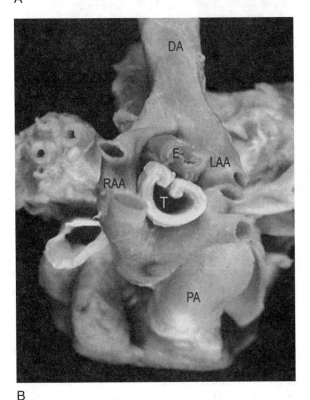

B

Figure 9.11
Vascular rings. A, Aberrant right subclavian artery coursing behind the trachea (T) and esophagus. DA, descending aorta; BT, bronchiocephalic trunk; LC, left common carotid artery; LS, left subclavian artery. B, Double aortic arch. T, trachea; E, esophagus; PA, pulmonary artery; DA, descending aorta; RAA, right aortic arch; LAA, left aortic arch. (From Gilbert-Barness, E., & Debich-Spicer, D., 2007. Congenital malformations of the heart. In E. Gilbert-Barness, Ed., *Potter's pathology of the fetus, infant, and child*, pp. 978–1023. New York: Elsevier.)

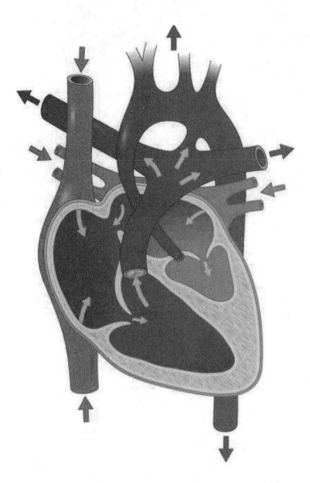

Figure 9.12
Flow of blood in hypoplastic left heart complex (HLHC). (From Gilbert-Barness, E., & Debich-Spicer, D., 2007. Congenital malformations of the heart. In E. Gilbert-Barness, Ed., *Potter's pathology of the fetus, infant, and child*, pp. 978–1023. New York: Elsevier.)

Cyanotic Congenital Heart Disease

Tetralogy of Fallot

Components of tetralogy of Fallot consist of VSD, RV outflow tract obstruction (valvular and/or infundibular), RVH, and overriding of the aorta (Figure 9.13). This malformation is due to anterior deviation with malalignment of the septum. On physical examination there is cyanosis, clubbing, and squatting. On auscultation the intensity of the systolic murmur S_2 depends on degree of obstruction. The smaller the defect, the lower the murmur as in Roger disease. The chest X-ray may show a boot-shaped heart, decreased pulmonary vascularity, or a right-sided aortic arch in 25% of the cases. Treatment for cyanotic spells includes knee-chest squatting, oxygen, IV fluids, morphine sulfate 0.1–0.2 mg/kg/SC or IM or a beta-blocker (propranolol).

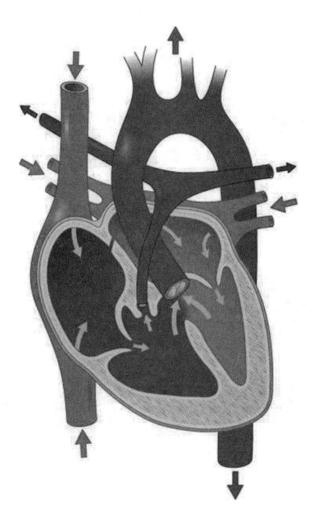

Figure 9.13
Flow of blood in tetralogy of Fallot (TOF). (From Gilbert-Barness, E., &
Debich-Spicer, D., 2007. Congenital malformations of the heart. In
E. Gilbert-Barness, Ed., *Potter's pathology of the fetus, infant, and child*,
pp. 978–1023. New York: Elsevier.)

Truncus Arteriosus

Types of truncus arteriosus include (Figure 9.14):

- MPA arises from the truncus.
- The pulmonary arteries arise from the posterior aspect of the truncus.
- The pulmonary arteries arise from the lateral aspect of the truncus.

Clinical manifestations include congestive heart failure and cyanosis. On physical
examination there is a wide pulse pressure and bounding arterial pulses and a systolic
click at the apex with harsh systolic murmur at LLSB.

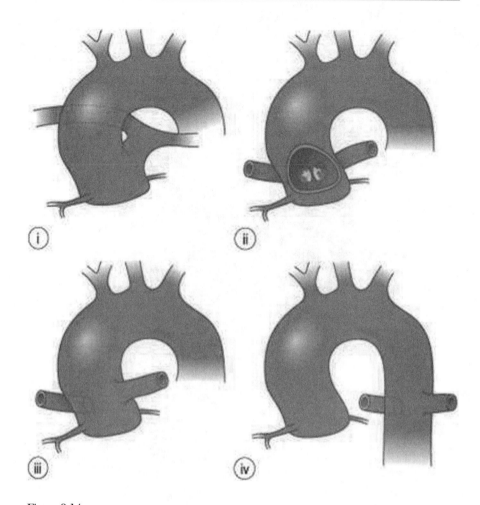

Figure 9.14
A, four types of truncus arteriosus (TA): type I, single pulmonary trunk and ascending aorta arising from a common trunk; type II, left and right pulmonary arteries (PAs) arising close together from the posterior or dorsal wall of the truncus; type III, right and left PAs arising independently from either side of the truncus; type IV, no PAs identified and there is apparent absence of the sixth arterial arch. The bronchial arteries supply the lungs.

Continued

D-Transposition of the Aorta (D-TGA)

VSD presents in 40% of cases of D-TGA (Figure 9.15). Usually a large male newborn infant (M:F ratio 3:1). There may not be a murmur. On chest X-ray there is an egg-shaped heart in 40% of cases. Intense cyanosis at birth.

Tricuspid Atresia

• Absent tricuspid valve

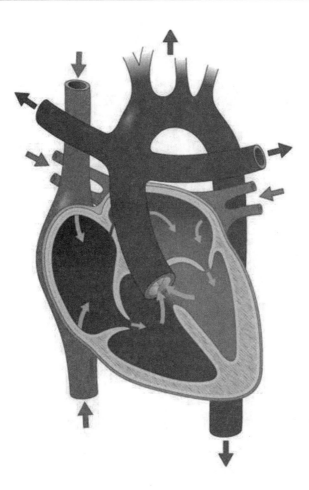

Figure 9.14 cont'd
B, flow of blood in TA. (From Gilbert-Barness, E., &
Debich-Spicer, D., 2007. Congenital malformations of the
heart. In E. Gilbert-Barness, Ed., *Potter's pathology of the
fetus, infant, and child*, pp. 978–1023. New York: Elsevier.)

- Hypoplastic RV
- Possible shunts: ASD, VSD, PDA

Most commonly tricuspid atresia with normally related great arteries, a small VSD,
and PS (Figure 9.16). Clinical manifestation is severe cyanosis. Physical examination
reveals cyanosis with or without clubbing, systolic murmur with single S_2 and hepatomegaly in case of inadequate interatrial communication.

Total Anomalous Pulmonary Venous Return

Types of TAPVR consist of supracardiac (50%), cardiac (20%), infracardiac (diaphragmatic, 20%) obstructive, and mixed type (10%). TAPVR is seen in polysplenia. With

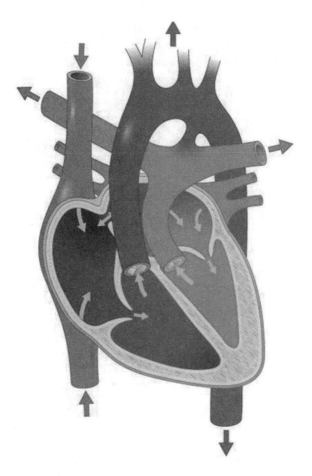

Figure 9.15
Flow of blood in the heart with transposition of the great
arteries. (From Gilbert-Barness, E., & Debich-Spicer, D.,
2007. Congenital malformations of the heart. In E.
Gilbert-Barness, Ed., *Potter's pathology of the fetus, infant,
and child*, pp. 978–1023. New York: Elsevier.)

obstruction cyanosis, heart failure and death occur in the first few months of life.
Surgical correction can be achieved.

Shock

Shock is the pathophysiologic failure of the cardiovascular system to deliver adequate blood flow to satisfy the metabolic needs of the vital organs. Shock is differentiated from CHF because the adaptive and compensatory mechanisms have become
exhausted or impaired and tissue hypoxia ensues. Septic, hypovolemic, and neurogenic are other types of shock.

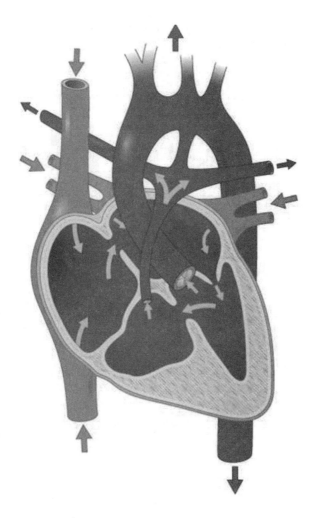

Figure 9.16
Flow of blood in tricuspid atresia. (From Gilbert-Barness, E., &
Debich-Spicer, D., 2007. Congenital malformations of the heart. In
E. Gilbert-Barness, Ed., *Potter's pathology of the fetus, infant, and child*,
pp. 978–1023. New York: Elsevier.)

Cardiogenic Shock

- Insufficient cardiac filling, impedance to venous return tachyarrhythmias
- Impaired ejection of blood from the heart, impedance to outflow, hypoplastic left heart syndrome, coarctation of the aorta
- Adequate heart rate, decreased contractility, myocardial infarction, congenital coronary anomalies
- Increased demand for blood flow, reduced arterial blood concentration of O_2, transposition of the great arteries

Endocarditis

Incidence

- Mean age in children rising
- Increase in neonates
- Adults: mean age increased from 34 to 50 years
- Children: 1930–1950 average age approximately 5 years; 1960–1980 average age approximately 8.5–13 years
- Pre- and postantibiotic era (rheumatic fever)

Risk Factors

- Patients with congenital heart disease pre- and postoperative
- Immunocompromised patients
- Neonates or others with indwelling lines
- IV drug abusers
- Rarely normal children

Microorganisms

- *Streptococcus viridans* (alpha hemolytic streptococcus) is most common
- *Staphylococcus aureus* is the second most common
- Coagulase-negative staph is uncommon, but increasing
- Other strep enterococci, pneumococci, β-hemolytic
- Gram-negative aerobes
- Fungi

The current American Heart Association risk factors requiring endocarditis prophylaxis are:

1. Cardiac transplantation
2. Artificial valves
3. History of endocarditis
4. Surgically corrected cyanotic heart disease

Laboratory diagnosis is by blood culture, which is the most valuable aid to diagnosis (Tables 9.5 and 9.6). Obtain at least three sets over 24 hours from different sites. Timing is not as important. Three cultures detect over 97% of cases. It is recommended that antibiotic prophylaxis is given for dental procedures known to produce gingival or mucosal bleeding, tonsillectomy or adenoidectomy, bronchoscopy with rigid bronchoscope, cystoscopy, urethral dilation, urethral catheterization if urinary tract infection (UTI) is present or urinary tract surgery if UTI is present, incision and drainage of infected tissue, and vaginal delivery in the presence of infection.

Myocarditis

Inflammatory process involving the myocardium. Etiology is related to group B streptococcus, coxsackievirus, echovirus, adenovirus, influenza, measles, mumps, rubella, and Rous sarcoma virus. Most patients are asymptomatic, and antecedent

TABLE 9.5
Clinical Features of Endocarditis

Finding	Frequency
Fever	++++
Nonspecific symptoms (myalgia, arthralgia, headache, malaise)	+++
Heart murmur (new or changing)	++
Heart failure	++
Petechiae	++
Embolic phenomena	++
Splenomegaly	++
Neurologic findings	++
Osler nodes (raised nodules of fingertips and toes), Janeway lesions (small nodular hemorrhagic spots on palms and soles), Roth spots (white spots in retina), splinter hemorrhages beneath the nails	+

++++, very common; +++, in a majority of cases; ++, infrequent; +, rare.

viral infection presents with flulike symptoms. Definitive diagnosis only made by endomyocardial biopsy. Other tests include mycoplasma titers, antistreptolysin, and viral cultures.

Rheumatic Fever

Sequential relationship between outbreaks of streptococcal pharyngitis (group A beta-hemolytic). Most common in young school age children and is rare in infancy. No difference in sex, race, or ethnicity. Diagnosis is established by Jones criteria. Evidence of previous streptococcal infection plus two major criteria or one major and two minor criteria.

Jones Criteria

Major criteria:

- Carditis
- Arthritis
- Syndenham chorea

TABLE 9.6
Laboratory Diagnosis

Finding	Frequency
Positive blood culture (off antibiotics)	++++
Elevated acute phase reactants	++++
Anemia	+++
Hematuria	+++
Presence of rheumatoid factor	++
Leukocytosis	++

++++, very common; +++, in a majority of cases; ++, infrequent; +, rare.

- Erythema marginatum
- Subcutaneous nodules

Minor criteria:

- Fever
- Arthralgia
- Elevated acute phase reactants
- Evidence of previous streptococcal infection
- Elevated or rising strep antibody
- Positive throat culture or rapid antigen test

Long-term treatment group beta strep prophylaxis is with benzathine penicillin IM monthly, penicillin PO daily, or erythromycin PO BID.

Kawasaki Disease (Acute Febrile Mucocutaneous Lymph Node Syndrome)

Diagnosis is by fever of at least 5 days' duration (generally high, spiking fever). Four of five major criteria (fewer if coronary aneurysms) and exclusion of other diseases.

Major criteria:

- Changes in the lips and oral cavity
- Changes in extremities
- Bilateral conjunctival injection
- Polymorphous exanthema (not vesicular)
- Cervical lymphadenopathy (usually single node >1.5 mm)
  Oropharynx (strawberry tongue)
  Extremities: erythema of palms and soles; edema of hands or feet; periungual desquamation

Laboratory findings:

- Neutrophilia and immature forms
- Elevated sedimentation rate
- Elevated α-1-antitrypsin
- Elevated serum immunoglobulin E
- Thrombocytosis
- Elevated C reactive protein (CRP)
- Elevated serum transaminases
- Hypoalbuminemia

Arrhythmias

See Figure 9.17.

Atrial Flutter

Typical saw-toothed P-waves in electrocardiogram.

A. Tachy-arrhythmias with narrow QRS:

I. Reentry tachycardias

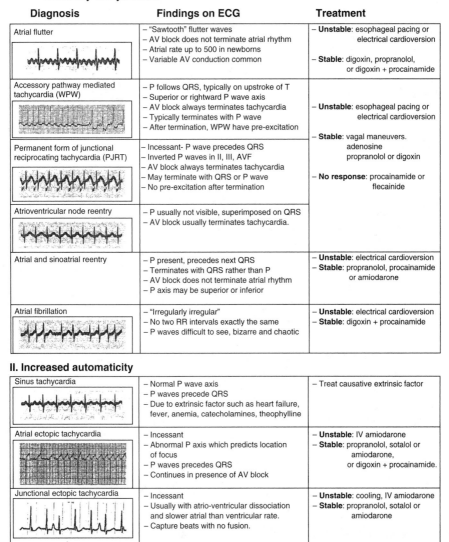

Diagnosis	Findings on ECG	Treatment
Atrial flutter	– "Sawtooth" flutter waves – AV block does not terminate atrial rhythm – Atrial rate up to 500 in newborns – Variable AV conduction common	– **Unstable**: esophageal pacing or electrical cardioversion – **Stable**: digoxin, propranolol, or digoxin + procainamide
Accessory pathway mediated tachycardia (WPW)	– P follows QRS, typically on upstroke of T – Superior or rightward P wave axis – AV block always terminates tachycardia – Typically terminates with P wave – After termination, WPW have pre-excitation	– **Unstable**: esophageal pacing or electrical cardioversion – **Stable**: vagal maneuvers. adenosine propranolol or digoxin – **No response**: procainamide or flecainide
Permanent form of junctional reciprocating tachycardia (PJRT)	– Incessant- P wave precedes QRS – Inverted P waves in II, III, AVF – AV block always terminates tachycardia – May terminate with QRS or P wave – No pre-excitation after termination	
Atrioventricular node reentry	– P usually not visible, superimposed on QRS – AV block usually terminates tachycardia.	
Atrial and sinoatrial reentry	– P present, precedes next QRS – Terminates with QRS rather than P – AV block does not terminate atrial rhythm – P axis may be superior or inferior	– **Unstable**: electrical cardioversion – **Stable**: propranolol, procainamide or amiodarone
Atrial fibrillation	– "Irregularly irregular" – No two RR intervals exactly the same – P waves difficult to see, bizarre and chaotic	– **Unstable**: electrical cardioversion – **Stable**: digoxin + procainamide

II. Increased automaticity

Sinus tachycardia	– Normal P wave axis – P waves precede QRS – Due to extrinsic factor such as heart failure, fever, anemia, catecholamines, theophylline	– Treat causative extrinsic factor
Atrial ectopic tachycardia	– Incessant – Abnormal P axis which predicts location of focus – P waves precede QRS – Continues in presence of AV block	– **Unstable**: IV amiodarone – **Stable**: propranolol, sotalol or amiodarone, or digoxin + procainamide.
Junctional ectopic tachycardia	– Incessant – Usually with atrio-ventricular dissociation and slower atrial than ventricular rate. – Capture beats with no fusion.	– **Unstable**: cooling, IV amiodarone – **Stable**: propranolol, sotalol or amiodarone

Figure 9.17
Patterns of arrhythmias. (From *Neonatal cardiac arrhythmias*, University of California, 2004.)

Continued

B. Tachy-arrhythmias with wide QRS:

Diagnosis	Findings on ECG	Treatment
Ventricular tachycardia (VT)	– Often with AV dissociation – Capture beats with narrower QRS than other beats; fusion beats	– **Unstable**: electrical cardioversion – **Stable**: lidocaine, procainamide
Ventricular fibrillation	– Complete chaotic rhythm – Rapid and irregular rhythm	(1) asynchronous cardioversion 2j/kg (2) asynchronous cardioversion 2j/kg (3) asynchronous cardioversion 4j/kg (4) lidocaine + asynch. cardioversion.
SVT with pre-existing bundle branch block	– QRS morphology similar to that in sinus rhythm – QRS morphology is that of right or left bundle branch block	– **Unstable**: esophageal pacing or electrical cardioversion – **Stable**: vagal maneuvers, adenosine, propranolol or digoxin
Antidromic SVT in WPW	– QRS morphology similar to pre-excited sinus rhythm, but wider – Never with AV dissociation	– No response: procainamide or flecainide

C. Bradyarrhythmias:

Diagnosis	Findings on ECG	Treatment
Sinus bradycardia	– Slow atrial rate with normal P waves – 1:1 conduction – Due to underlying causes such as hypoxia, acidosis, increased intracranial pressure, abdominal distension, hypoglycemia, hypothermia, digoxin, propranolol	– Vigorous resuscitation and supportive care – A B C – O_2 – Treat underlying causes
Atrioventricular block Complete atrioventricular block	– Atrioventricular dissociation – Regular R-R intervals – Regular P-P intervals – Atrial rate > ventricular rate – P which occur after T have no effect on R-R interval – Infants of maternal lupus	– **Unstable**: A B C O_2 Atropine, isoproterenol infusion Temporary trans-venous pacing – **Stable**: Treat underlying causes – Permanent pacemaker in AV bock with ventricular rate < 55 (newborn)
2nd degree atrioventricular block – Mobitz type I (Wenckebach)	– Progressive PR interval prolongation followed by a blocked beat – Usually indicates block in the AV node	
– Mobitz type II	– No characteristic PR prolongation as seen in type I. – Usually not reversible with medications. – Type II has worse prognosis than type I.	
Sinus exit block	– Sinus P waves intermittently disappear due to block of impulses leaving the node.	
Premature atrial contractions	– Premature P wave superimposed on the previous T wave, deforming it	– Usually does not need treatment.

Figure 9.17 cont'd

Continued

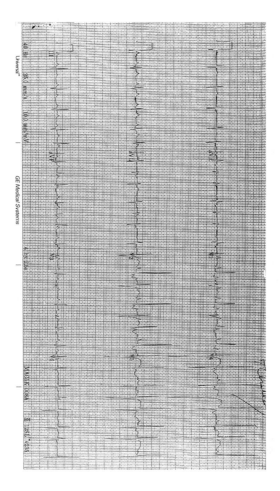

Figure 9.17 cont'd

Ventricular Tachycardia

Wide QRS tachycardia originating in the ventricle. Different morphology of QRS;
dissociation of atria from ventricle.

Long Q-T Segment

Inherited disorder of repolarization:

- Syncope
- Seizures
- Deafness
- Abnormal ECG
- Torsade de Points

Tachypnea

Tachypnea is defined as rapid breathing. The average newborn may breathe at anywhere between 30 and 80 respirations per minute, a 2-year-old at 20–40, and older children at rates close to adult averages (16–28).

CNS

- Increased "respiratory drive" usually affects rate, not just V_1
- Hypoxia, hypercapnea, acidosis: thus, hypoxia for any reason (e.g., high altitude or pneumonia) increases respiration rate

Obstruction

- Airway obstruction
- Upper airway: laryngomalacia, choanal atresia, macroglossia, micrognathia, subglottic stenosis, web, or laryngospasm
- Lower airway: tracheal stenosis, rings, slings, asthma, or foreign body

Parenchymal Disease

- Decreased lung volume (e.g., atelectasis, pulmonary edema, pneumonia, pulmonary fibrosis)

Chest Wall Disorder

- Kyphoscoliosis

Pulmonary Vascular Disease

- Hypoxia and mechanisms
- Pulmonary edema
- Pulmonary hypertension

Lymphatic System

- Lymphangiectasia
- Bronchus-associated lymphoid tissue (airway obstruction and hypoxia)

Other inflammatory mediators (e.g., cytokines or eicosanoids) may affect respiratory rate through uncertain mechanisms

FURTHER READING

Brouqui, P., & Raoult, D. (2001). Endocarditis due to rare and fastidious bacteria. *Clinical Microbiology Reviews, 14*, 177–207.

Chiappa, E. (2007). The impact of prenatal diagnosis of congenital heart disease on pediatric cardiology and cardiac surgery. *Journal of Cardiovascular Medicine, 8*(1), 12-6.

Gilbert-Barness, E., & Debich-Spicer, D. (2007). Congenital malformations of the heart. In E. Gilbert-Barness (Ed.), *Potter's pathology of the fetus, infant, and child* (pp. 978–1023). New York: Elsevier.

Guzzetta, N. A., Miller, B. E., Todd, K., Szlam, F., Moore, R. H., Brosius, K. K., et al. (2006). Clinical measures of heparin's effect and thrombin inhibitor levels in pediatric patients with congenital heart disease. *Anesthesia and Analgesia, 103*, 1131–1138.

Keane, J. F., Fyler, D. C., & Lock, J. E. (2006). *Nadas' pediatric cardiology* (2nd ed.). New York: Saunders Elsevier.

Kitterman, J. A. (1982). Cyanosis of the newborn infant. *Pediatric Review, 4*, 13–24.

Landzberg, M. J., & Underleider, R. (2006). Pediatric cardiology and adult congenital heart disease. *Journal of the American College of Cardiology, 6*(11 suppl.), 47.

Mecham, N. (2006). Early recognition and treatment of shock in the pediatric patient. *Journal of Trauma Nursing, 13*(1), 17–21.

Park, M. K. (1996). *Pediatric cardiology for practitioners* (3rd ed.). St. Louis: Mosby.

Park, M. K., & Guntheroth, W. G. (1992). *How to read pediatric ECGs* (3rd ed.). St. Louis: Mosby.

Special Writing Group of the Committee on Rheumatic Fever, Endocarditis, and Kawasaki Disease of the Council on Cardiovascular Disease in the Young of the American Heart Association. (1992). Guidelines for the diagnosis of rheumatic fever. Jones Criteria, 1992 update. *Journal of the American Medical Association, 268*, 2069–2273.

Towbin, J. A., Bricker, J. T., & Garson, A. Jr. (1992). Electrocardiographic criteria for diagnosis of acute myocardial infarction in childhood. *American Journal of Cardiology, 69*, 1545.

Wallach, J. (2000). *Interpretation of diagnostic tests* (7th ed.). Philadelphia: Lippincott Williams & Wilkins.

10

SPLEEN AND LIVER

The moving finger writes; and, having writ / Moves on; nor all
thy piety nor wit / Shall lure it back to cancel half a line / Nor all
thy tears wash out a word of it.

The Rubaiyat of Omar Khayyam

AN ENLARGED SPLEEN is usually felt as a superficial mass in the left upper quadrant. It may feel like a tongue hanging from the left costal margin, with a sharp straight border and a notch on the anterior margin. Splenic enlargement is evident in children with such diseases as septicemia, other infections, blood dyscrasias, including sickle cell or iron-deficient anemia, thalassemia major, hemolytic jaundice, infectious mononucleosis and leukemia, lysosomal storage diseases, and connective tissue diseases. A very large spleen with a less enlarged liver is evident in cases of portal vein obstruction and neonatal hepatitis. It may be normally palpable 1–2 cm below the left costal margin in newborns (because of extramedullary hematopoiesis) and in normal infants and young children. You may miss a particularly large spleen if you start palpation too high. Note the size of the spleen and whether it is tender. Floating ribs are sometimes confused with the spleen on palpation. Usually you can differentiate by palpation or percussion.

The liver is generally palpable as a superficial mass 1–2 cm below the right costal margin, with a sharp border in newborns and infants. Ask older children or adolescents to breathe in and bring the liver edge down to your finger. Note size, consistency, tenderness, and pulsation. Throughout childhood, the liver may remain palpable without having pathologic significance.

Total span by percussion is about 5 cm at 6 months of age, 7 cm at 3 years of age, 8–10 cm at 10 years of age, and 9–12 cm at adolescence. If the span is larger or more than 2 cm below the costal margin, such states as passive congestion, hepatitis, tumor or metastases, blood dyscrasias, septicemia or other infections, reticuloendothelial or metabolic disease, or pulmonary emphysema may be indicated. A rapidly enlarging liver is an early sign of right heart failure. The liver edge is usually not as sharp in heart failure as it is in pulmonary emphysema without failure. Rapidly decreasing liver size may be diagnostic of acute liver necrosis. A thrill is felt over an enlarged liver or a gurgling sound is heard with hydatid echinococcal cysts in the liver. Friction rub over the liver usually results from transmission of the impulse from the aorta, but quite rarely it may result from tricuspid regurgitation or stenosis or constrictive pericarditis.

SPLENOMEGALY

Splenomegaly is usually caused by systemic disease and not by primary splenic disease. Splenomegaly is caused by infection (excessive antigen stimulation), autoimmune disorders (disordered immunoregulation), or hemolysis (excessive destruction of abnormal blood components).

Normal Variants

15%–30% of neonates
10% of healthy children
5% of adolescents
Palpable spleen tip due to thinner abdominal musculature

Infection and Inflammation

Acute hepatitis (B or C)
Viral (Epstein-Barr virus, cytomegalovirus, HIV)
Bacterial (subacute bacterial endocarditis, cat-scratch disease, tuberculosis, histoplasmosis, toxoplasmosis, *Salmonella*)
Systemic lupus erythematosus
Rheumatoid arthritis
Inflammatory bowel disease
Celiac disease
Acidosis
Chronic granulomatous disease
Serum sickness
Protozoal infection (malaria and schistosomiasis are rare in the United States)

Hemolytic Anemias

Hereditary spherocytosis
Hemoglobinopathies
Thalassemia major
Nonspherocytic hemolytic anemias (pyruvate kinase deficiency)

Malignancy

Leukemia; 50% of children with acute lymphocytic leukemia
Hodgkin disease, non-Hodgkin lymphoma
Metastatic disease

Extramedullary Hematopoiesis

Thalassemia major
Osteoporosis (rare)
Myelofibrosis

Storage and Infiltrative Disorders

Histiocytosis

Lipidoses (e.g., Niemann-Pick, Gaucher)
Mucopolysaccharidoses (e.g., Hurler, Hunter)

Congestive

Chronic congestive heart failure
Portal hypertension; portal or splenic venous thrombosis
Hepatic fibrosis
Cirrhosis

Structural

Hematoma (trauma)
Cysts or pseudocyts

Wandering Spleen

Position on the abdomen unstable

HEPATOMEGALY

Differential Diagnosis

Inappropriate Storage

Gycogen storage diseases I–V
Lipids: Gaucher disease, Wolman disease, Niemann-Pick disease
Fat: fatty acid oxidation defects, mucopolysaccharidoses
Metals: Wilson disease (copper), hemochromatosis (iron)
Abnormal proteins: α-1 antitrypsin deficiency (store abnormal protein product)
Peroxisomal disease: Zellweger
Mucopolysaccharidoses, type I–IV

Inflammation

Most common infections: Epstein-Barr virus; hepatitis A, B, C; cytomegalovirus, TORCH syndrome
Less common infections: HIV, malaria, amebiasis, tuberculosis, toxocariasis, *Borrelia burgdorferi*
Drugs: acetaminophen (commonly used in overdoses among adolescents), NSAIDs, isoniazid, sodium valproate, propothiouracil, halothane
Toxins: tyrosinemia, galactosemia, vitamin A toxicity
Systemic lupus erythematosus
Autoimmune hepatitis

Vascular Congestion

Congestive heart failure
Budd-Chiari syndrome
Venoocclusive disease
Suprahepatic web

Biliary Obstruction

Cystic fibrosis
Primary sclerosing cholangitis
Alagille syndrome
Inspissated bile syndrome
Biliary atresia represents the most common cause of pediatric liver transplantation

Infiltration

Hepatoblastoma
Hepatocellular carcinoma
Hemangioma
Histiocytosis
Extramedullary hematopoiesis
Chronic granulomatous disease

Miscellaneous

Reye syndrome, bile acid synthetic disorder

FURTHER READING

Fishbein, M., Mogren, J., Mogren, C., Cox, S., & Jennings, R. (2005). Undetected hepatomegaly in obese children by primary care physician: A pitfall in the diagnosis of pediatric nonalcoholic fatty liver disease. *Clinical Pediatrics, 44,* 135–141.

Gartner, L. (1994). Neonatal jaundice. *Pediatric Review, 15,* 422–431.

Hilmes, M. A., & Strouse, P. J. (2007). The pediatric spleen. *Seminars in Ultrasound, CT, and MR, 28*(1), 3–11.

Provisional Committee for Quality Improvement and Subcommittee on Hyperbilirubinemia Practice Parameter: Management of hyperbilirubinemia in the healthy term newborn. (1994). *Pediatrics, 94,* 558–565.

11

CHROMOSOMAL DISORDERS AND GENETIC DISEASES

The mills of God grind slowly but they grind exceedingly small.

Charles Beard

CHROMOSOMAL ABNORMALITIES

- Extra chromosomes
- Missing chromosomes
- Deletions, duplications, translocations, unbalanced rearrangements

Down syndrome is the most common chromosome abnormality, with an incidence of 1/800 newborns. It is associated with a 1% incidence of leukemia. Risk is age-related. Mothers 20 years old have a risk of 1/2,000, 30 years 1/1,000, 35 years 1/350; 40 years 1/100; and 50 years 1/10.

Klinefelter syndrome occurs in 1/800 males, XYY in 1/1,000 males, and Turner syndrome (monosomy X) in 1/2,000 females.

Deletions, duplications, and unbalanced rearrangements are less common. Turner syndrome girls with Y material have an increased risk of gonadoblastoma.

Recurrence risk: 1% in trisomy 21; 14% if the mother carries 14/21 transloca-tion, 4% if father carries 14/21 translocation, and 100% in 21/21 translocation of either parent. The recurrence risk for a mother with trisomy 21 is 50%.

If the mother is a mosaic, the risk is 50% of the degree of mosaicism.

Down Syndrome

The most common genetic cause of mental retardation (MR) is Down syndrome. The main characteristics are hypotonia, MR, and typical craniofacial features. Well-known associated conditions include leukemia, thyroid disease (hypo- and hyperthy-roidism), altantoaxial instability/subluxation, diabetes, duodenal atresia, endocardial cushion defect, and Hirschsprung disease.

There are no phenotypic differences between Down syndrome due to regular trisomy 21 or translocations, but there are differences in their risks of recurrence.

Trisomy 18

The main characteristics of trisomy 18 include severe MR, small for gestational age (SGA), hypertonia, prominent occiput, micrognathia, low-set, malformed ears, short sternum, congenital heart disease, characteristic hand (overlapping of second finger over third finger), increased arches on fingers, and rocker-bottom feet.

Trisomy 13 (Patau Syndrome)

The main characteristics of trisomy 13 include severe MR, severe central nervous system (CNS) malformations (anencephaly, holoprosencephaly), skin defects (aplasia cutis) of posterior scalp, midline facial defects (the face predicts the brain), congenital heart disease, capillary hemangiomata, postaxial polydactyly-clenched hands, abnormal dermatoglyphics, simian crease, and rocker-bottom feet.

Deletion 4p (Wolf-Hirschhorn or 4p Syndrome)

The main characteristics of deletion 4p are growth deficiency, MR, microcephaly, peculiar face (Greek helmet appearance), hypertelorism, broad or beaked nose, cleft lip or palate, short upper lip and philtrum, fishlike mouth, simple ears, preauricular tag or pit, and hypoplastic dermal ridges.

Deletion 5p (Cri-du-Chat or 5p Syndrome)

Main characteristics of deletion 5p include slow growth, MR, microcephaly, catlike cry, round face, hypertelorism, epicanthal folds, antimongoloid slant of palpebral fissures, strabismus, low-set ears, and micrognathia.

Turner (45,X, Monosomy X) Syndrome

The main characteristics of Turner syndrome include short stature (short stature homeobox containing genes located in Xpter involved in Turner, Leri-Weill syndrome, Langer syndrome, idiopathic proportional short stature, idiopathic mesomelic short stature); gonadal dysgenesis and infertility, broad webbed neck, broad chest with widely separated nipples, minor skeletal anomalies (cubitus valgus, short fourth metacarpal), benign renal malformations, cardiac malformations (coarctation of aorta/bicuspid aortic valve), and lymphedema of hands and feet at birth (Table 11.1). Treatment involves hormonal therapy at puberty for development of secondary sexual characteristics. There is a risk of minor cognitive defects, with 10%–15% or more learning disorders. Patients with paternal X (=20%) have higher verbal IQ scores and better social cognition than do those who receive the X from the mother (=80%) (imprinting).

Karyotype	Phenotype
45,X	Turner (40–60%)
45,X/46,XX	proximal portions of Xp are missing (2%–25%)

TABLE 11.1
Differential Diagnosis of Turner and Noonan Syndromes

	Main Common Findings	
	Turner	Noonan
Webbed neck	+	+
Cubitus valgus	+	+
Short stature	+	+
Lymphedema	+	+
Pectus excavatum	+	+

	Main Differential Findings	
	Turner	Noonan
Coarctation aorta	+	−
Pulmonic stenosis	−	+
Mental retardation	−	+
Etiology	45,X	A.D.

46,X,del (X)(p)	Turner (especially if the most distal or proximal portions of Xp are missing (2%–25%)
46, X,del(X)(q)	Amenorrhea, greater stature
46,X,iso(X)(q)	Turner (15%–20%)
46,X,r(X)	Turner (7%)
45,X,/46,XY	Female, ambiguous, or male

47,XYY

- Incidence 1/1,000 but normal phenotype
- Height above average
- Increased risk of educational difficulties
- Risk of possible psychosocial adjustment problems

47,XXX

- Incidence 1/1,000 but normal phenotype
- Educational difficulties
- Deficits in verbal abilities
- Normal or borderline low range IQ

For patients with 48, 49, or more chromosomes involving sex chromosomes, the greater the number of Xs, the more severe the manifestations simulating an autosomal aberration (MR, growth retardation, dysmorphic features, and malformations).

Fragile X Syndrome (Martin-Bell Syndrome)

Fragile X affects 1 in 1,250–1,500 males and 1 in 2,500 females, making it the single most common form of inherited MR. About 30% of female heterozygotes (carriers) and 80% of male hemizygotes are mentally impaired. Also, 20% of males carrying the mutation may be phenotypically and cytogenetically normal (transmitting males).

Main characteristics include MR, craniofacial dysmorphism (large ears, prominent chin, relative macrocephaly), macroorchidism (sometimes prepubertal) (total volume >25 ml in almost 90% of postpubertal affected males). Abnormal speech (perseverative, jocular, retarded, high pitched); the diagnosis is suspected clinically and confirmed by the DNA-based test.

Russell-Silver Syndrome

Main characteristics include short for gestational age and intrauterine growth retardation, short stature (pre- and postnatal), skeletal asymmetry, triangular facies, clinodactyly (Figure 11.1) and late closure of anterior fontanel.

Heterogeneous conditions may be due to: UPD 7 (~10%), chromosomal translocation (17q25), deletion 15q26.1→qter, ring chromosomes, chromosomal mosaicism of the placenta, placental insufficiency, autosomal dominant inheritance, and X-L inheritance.

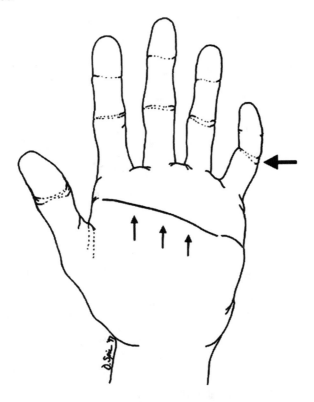

Figure 11.1
Clinodactyly (large arrow), or incurving of the fifth finger, results from hypoplasia of the middle phalanx. Note that this child with Down syndrome has only a single flexion crease of the fifth finger and single transverse palmar crease (small arrows).

INBORN ERRORS OF METABOLISM
PRESENTING IN THE NEWBORN

For practical purposes, inborn errors of metabolism (IEM) seen in the newborn period can be divided into seven groups (Tables 11.2, 11.3):

1. Aminoacidurias and organic acidemias (AA/OA)
2. Primary lactic acidosis (PLA)
3. Fatty acid oxidation defects (FAO)
4. Galactosemia (GAL)

TABLE 11.2
Newborn Screening

Disease	Level	Diagnostic Tests	Immediate Clinical Response
Phenylketonuria	Phe 4–6 mg/dl Phe 6–12 mg/dl Phe >12 mg/dl	Plasma amino acids (Phe, Tyr); phenyl acids; genotyping	For mild elevation: Evaluate nutritional, developmental, neurologic status, hepatic and renal function. Repeat screening test.
Maple syrup urine disease	Leu 4 mg/dl Leu 4–8 mg/dl Leu >8 mg/dl	Plasma amino acids (valine, leucine, isoleucine)	For moderate elevation: Consult referral center and send frozen urine and plasma.
Homocystinuria	Meth 2–6 mg/dl Meth >6 mg/dl	Plasma amino acids (Tyr, Phe); blood spot for succinylacetone	For high levels: Arrange for hospitalization and diagnostic evaluation.
Tyrosinemia	Tyr 6–12 mg/dl Tyr 12–20 mg/dl Tyr >20 mg/dl		Repeat testings and treat.
Galactosemia	Beutler test, positive; *Escherichia coli* phage test, negative; Beutler test, positive; *E. coli* phage test, positive	Galactose-1-phosphate uridyltransferase; galactokinase; uridine diphosphate galactose 4-epimerase; galactose-1-phosphate	Evaluate for jaundice, sepsis, cataracts, urine-reducing substances. Send blood for enzyme analysis. Remove lactose from diet.
Hypothyroidism	RIA: T_4 = 5.0–7.6 µg/dl; TSH <25 µIU/ml RIA: T_4 <5 µg/dl; TSH >25 µIU/ml	T_2, T_3, TSH, TBG, thyroid antibodies, bone age	Evaluate for hypothermia, hypoactivity, poor feeding, jaundice, constipation.

Ileu, isoleucine; Leu, leucine; Meth, methionine; Phe, phenylalanine; RIA, radioimmunoassay; T_2, diiodothyronine; T_3, triiodothyronine; T_4, thyroxine; TBG, thyroid-binding globulin; TSH, thyroid-stimulating hormone; Tyr, tyrosine; Val, valine.

TABLE 11.3
Inborn Errors of Metabolism

Disorder	AA/OA	PLA	FAO	GAL	NKHG	PER	UCD
pH	Metabolic acidosis	Metabolic acidosis	Metabolic acidosis	Normal	Normal	Normal	Respiratory alkalosis
Ammonium	<500 mmol/dl	Normal	Normal	Normal	Normal	Normal	>500 mmol/dl
Lactic acid	+	+++	+	+/−	−	−	−
Anion gap	Elevated	Elevated	Elevated	Normal	Normal	Normal	Normal
Hypoglycemia	+	+	+	+	−	−	−
Ketone bodies	+	+	−	+/−	−	−	−
Urine		−	−	Reducing substances	−	−	−
Hyperbilirubinemia	+	−	−	+	−	+	−
LFTs	+	−	−	+	−	+	−
Neutropenia	+	−	−	−	−	−	−
Thrombocytopenia	+						
Anemia	+						
Amino acids	Plasma	−	−	−	CSF	−	Plasma
Organic acids	+	+	−	−	−	−	−
Carnitine profile	+	−	+	−	−	−	−
VCLFA	−	−	−	−	−	+	−
CNS affected	+	+	+	+	+	+	+
Tachypnea	+	+	+	−	−	−	+
Cataracts	−	−	−	+	−	−	−
Odor	+	−	−	−	−	−	+
Dysmorphic	−	−	−	−	−	+	+
Cardiac failure	−	−	+	−	−	−	−
S&S in the first day	−	+	−	−	−	−	−

LFT, liver function test; VLCFA, very long chain fatty acids; CNS, central nervous system; CSF, cerebrospinal fluid; S&S, signs and symptoms; +, present; −, absent.
From Soliz, A., Chandler, B. D., & Vasconcellos, E. (2007). The enigmatic baby: A practical approach to the diagnosis of inborn errors of metabolism. *International Pediatrics*, 22(4), 193.

5. Nonketotic hyperglycinemia (NKHG)
6. Perixosomal diseases (PER)
7. Urea cycle defects (UCD)

AMINO ACID DISORDERS

Alkaptonuria

Deficiency of Homogentisic Oxidase

Melanin-like pigment deposited in

- Heart valves → calcification
- Mycardium, endocardium, and pericardium
- Aorta → potentiates atherosclerosis in coronary elastic and muscular arteries
- Veins and capillaries

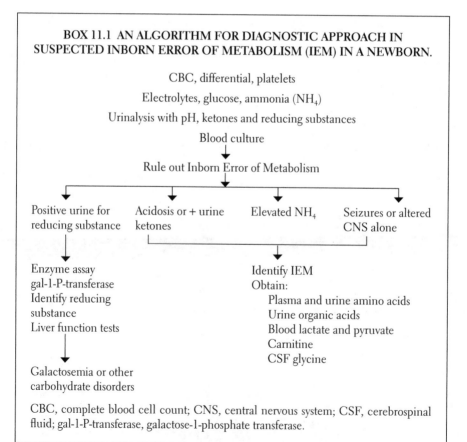

BOX 11.1 AN ALGORITHM FOR DIAGNOSTIC APPROACH IN SUSPECTED INBORN ERROR OF METABOLISM (IEM) IN A NEWBORN.

CBC, differential, platelets

Electrolytes, glucose, ammonia (NH_4)

Urinalysis with pH, ketones and reducing substances

Blood culture

Rule out Inborn Error of Metabolism

| Positive urine for reducing substance | Acidosis or + urine ketones | Elevated NH_4 | Seizures or altered CNS alone |

Enzyme assay
gal-1-P-transferase
Identify reducing
substance
Liver function tests

Identify IEM
Obtain:
  Plasma and urine amino acids
  Urine organic acids
  Blood lactate and pyruvate
  Carnitine
  CSF glycine

Galactosemia or other
carbohydrate disorders

CBC, complete blood cell count; CNS, central nervous system; CSF, cerebrospinal fluid; gal-1-P-transferase, galactose-1-phosphate transferase.

Phenylketonuria, Due to Phenylalanine Hydroxylase Deficiency

Clinical symptoms are characterized by neurologic symptoms, neurodegenerative symptoms, developmental delay, failure to thrive, dermatologic abnormalities (newborn screening). Incidence is 1/14,000. Serum phenylalanine level ≥ 20 mg/dl. Urine ferric chloride test results are positive, and chromatography confirms presence of orthohydroxyphenylacetic acid. Definitive diagnosis is by DNA tests and liver phenylalanine hydroxylase levels.

Tyrosinemia Type I (Fumarylacetoacetate Hydrolase Deficiency; Hepatorenal Tyrosinemia)

Clinical symptoms include acute neonatal crisis, neurologic symptoms, hepatocellular disease, visceromegaly, renal dysfunction, renal Fanconi syndrome, gastrointestinal disease, failure to thrive, hypoglycemia, metabolic acidosis or hyperammonemia, coagulation disorders, and psychiatric disorders.

Diagnostic studies include amino acid quantitation in blood and urine: increased blood and urine tyrosine and methionine levels. Prenatal diagnosis is by measurement of succinylacetone in amniotic fluid.

Tyrosinemia Type II (Oculocutaneous)

Clinical symptoms include developmental delay, palmar and plantar hyperkeratosis, corneal ulcers, and photophobia, which may occur within the first months.

Tyrosinemia Type III (4-Hydroxyphenylpyruvate Dioxygenase Deficiency)

This form is very rare and may be accompanied by developmental delay, seizures, ataxia, or self-mutilation, tyrosinemia, and tyrosyluria. Urine contains 4-hydroxyphenyl pyruvic, 4-hydroxyphenyl lactic, and 4-hydroxyphenylacetic acids. Enzyme activity is decreased in liver biopsy specimen.

Transient Tyrosinemia

This is due to incomplete development of tyrosine-oxidizing system, especially in premature or low-birth-weight infants. Usually asymptomatic but suggested by positive newborn phenylalanine screening test results. Tyrosine metabolites in urine are ≤ 1 mg/ml (parahydroxyphenyl lactic and parahydroxyphenyl acetic acids); reversed within 24 hours by administration of ascorbic acid.

Homocystinuria (Cystathionine Synthase Deficiency)

Clinical symptoms consists of failure to thrive, developmental subluxed lenses and other eye defects, marfanoid stature, malar flush, osteoporosis, and thromboembolism, increased methionine and homocystine levels in blood and urine (homocystine should be measured in fresh urine), and enzyme assay in liver biopsy specimen.

Urea Cycle Disorders

Persons with urea cycle disorders are typically normal at birth with no prenatal warning signs. Onset is after 24 hours with irritability, feeding intolerance, and labored breathing. If diagnosis is delayed, permanent brain damage or death occurs. Presentation is hyperammonemia and respiratory alkalosis with absence of acidosis and ketones. Hyperammonemia causes brain damage (Table 11.4). The urea cycle consists of five enzymes responsible for the elimination of ammonia as urea. Ornithine transcarbamylase (OTC) deficiency—X-linked, citrullinemia (AR); arginosuccinic aciduria (AR); carbamoyl phosphate synthase deficiency (AR); arginase deficiency (AR); and N-acetyglutamate synthase deficiency (AR).

BRANCHED-CHAIN AMINO ACID DISORDERS

The three branched-chain amino acids, leucine, isoleucine, and valine, are essential amino acids and have similar metabolic pathways (Table 11.5). In one group, deficiency of the branched-chain α-keto acid dehydrogenase complex results in the metabolic block of the three amino acids. This results in maple syrup urine disease. A group involving leucine transamination and decarboxylation results in the formation of a number of organic acids.

Isovaleric Acidemia

Clinical symptoms include episodic vomiting, natural aversion to protein foods, lethargy, coma, odor of sweaty feet, psychomotor retardation, and seizures.

Laboratory findings include acidosis, ketosis, anion gap increased, ammonia (blood) increased, neutropenia, thrombocytopenia, pancytopenia; organic acids: isovalerylglycine and its metabolites in urine; volatile short-chain organic acids: isovaleric acid in plasma; abnormal levels of total and free carnitine (plasma), and increased level of esterified carnitine (plasma).

TABLE 11.4
Hyperammonemia

Respiratory distress prior to 24 hours of age		
Present		Absent
Transient hyperammonemia of the newborn		Inborn error of metabolism Acidosis and/or ketosis
Present		Absent
Organic acidemias		Inborn error of ureagenesis Plasma citrulline level
Absent, trace Urinary orotate	100–300 μmol/L Argininosuccinate and anhydrides in plasma	>1,000 μmol/L
Low High CPS OTC	AL	AS

AL, argininosuccinase deficiency; AS, argininosuccinic acid synthetase deficiency; CPS, carbamoyl phosphate synthetase deficiency; OTC, ornithine transcarbamylase deficiency.

TABLE 11.5
Tissue Required for Prenatal Diagnosis of Branched-Chain Amino Acid Disorders

Disorder	Tissue	Trimester of Pregnancy
Maple syrup urine disease	CV sampling, cultured AFC	I, II
Isovaleric acidemia	AF, cultured AFC	II
Isolated 3-methylcrotonyl-CoA carboxylase deficiency	AF, cultured AFC, CV tissues	I, II
3-Methylglutaconic aciduria type I (3-methylglutaconyl-CoA hydratase deficiency)	AF, cultured AFC	II
3-Methylglutaconic aciduria, other types (3-methylglutaconyl-CoA hydratase, normal activity)	AF[a]	II
3-Hydroxy-3-methylglutaric aciduria (3-hydroxy-3-methyglutaryl-CoA lyase deficiency)	AF, cultured AF, CV tissue	I, II
Mevalonic aciduria (mevalonate kinase deficiency)	AF, cultured AFC, CV tissue	I, II

AF, amniotic fluid; AFC, amniotic fluid cells; CV, chorionic villus.
[a]Thus far, studies have been limited to patients categorized as having 3-methylglutaconic aciduria, unclassified form.

Maple Syrup Urine (Branched-Chain α-Ketodehydrogenase Deficiency)

Maple syrup urine disease is an autosomal-recessive disorder of the mitochondrial multienzyme complex branched-chain α-keto acid dehydrogenase that results in increased concentrations of branched-chain amino acids and α-keto acids. Estimated incidence is 1/120,000 to 1/400,000 live births, and the disease is most common among the Mennonites of North America, in whom the incidence is 1/176. Untreated, the patient with classic maple syrup urine disease usually dies with apnea or coma.

OTHER AMINO ACID DISORDERS

Nonketotic Hyperglycinemia

Main characteristics include an autosomal recessive defect in glycine cleavage; increased CSF glycine-to-plasma glycine ratio, onset before 24 hours; it presents clinically with hypotonia, seizures, encephalopathy, and burst suppression EEG. Treatment is by sodium benzoate or dextramethorphan.

Organic Acidemias

Organic acidemias constitute a large group of inborn errors of metabolism that are caused by various enzyme defects in the catabolic pathways of amino acids, fatty acids, vitamins, and other compounds. They can present as a metabolic crisis in the neonatal period or later.

Glutaric Academia Type I (Glutaryl CoA Dehydrogenase Deficiency)

Main characteristics include neurological deterioration, dystonia, choreoathetosis, and ketoacidosis. Diagnosis is by abnormal MRI (striatal necrosis). Treatment is diet, riboflavin, and carnitine.

Hereditary Fructose Intolerance (Fructoaldolase Deficiency; Autosomal Recessive)

Symptoms can occur after fructose ingestion including vomiting, lethargy, sweating, and coma with hypoglycemia. Patients tend to avoid sucrose (fructose-glucose) and have no dental caries. Diagnosis is by fructoaldolase assay. Treatment is to avoid fructose.

Glutaric Acidemia Type II (Multiple Acyl CoA Dehydrogenase Deficiency)

Main characteristics include hypoketotic hypoglycemia, hyperammonemia, cystic kidneys, dysmorphic features; death in early infancy is common; sweaty feet odor. Treatment is with diet, carnitine, and riboflavin but is not usually successful, and the chance of survival is poor.

FATTY ACID OXIDATION DEFECTS

Carnitine Metabolism Disorders

- Carnitine/acylcarnitine translocase deficiency
- Carnitine palmitoyltransferase deficiency (CPT I and II)
- Carnitine transport defect

Children with organic acidemias excrete excess carnitine as esters and may present with signs of carnitine deficiency.

Clinical symptoms include acute neonatal crisis, neurologic symptoms, developmental delay, hepatocellular disease, visceromegaly, gastrointestinal disease, skeletal myopathy, cardiomyopathy, failure to thrive, hypoglycemia, metabolic acidosis, Reye syndrome, and hyperammonemia.

Diagnostic studies include carnitine species identification and quantitation in blood, urine, or tissue, and amino and organic acid quantitation in blood or urine (Table 11.6).

INBORN ERRORS OF METABOLISM AND METABOLIC DISEASES

IEMs are single gene defects with enzyme deficiency, usually autosomal recessive, some X-linked. Investigations for metabolic diseases in the neonate and newborn screening are shown in Table 11.7.

DISORDERS OF CARBOHYDRATE METABOLISM

Galactose Metabolism Disorders

There are defects in liver and red blood cells (RBCs) of galactose-1-phosphate uridyltransferase, which converts galactose to glucose, resulting in accumulation of

TABLE 11.6

Characteristic Features of Fatty Acid Oxidation Defects

MIM No.	Disorder	Tissue Distribution	Chromosome Location	Symptoms and Signs	Laboratory Findings
212140	Carnitine deficiency	Kidney, heart, muscle, FB, liver		Cardiomyopathy, coma muscle weakness, Reye-like syndrome, sudden infant death	Glucose (P) ⌐, ammonia (B) ↑, acidosis +, carnitine (P) ↑, long-chain acylcarnitine (P) N, cellular carnitine uptake ⌐
255120	Carnitine palmitoyl	Liver, FB	11q22–q23	Coma, liver insufficiency, hepatomegaly	Glucose (P) ⌐, ammonia (B) N or ↑, acidosis +, carnitine (P) N or ↑, long-chain acylcarnitine (P) N
212138	Acylcarnitine translocase	FB, liver, heart, muscle		Coma, cardiac abnormalities, liver insufficiency, vomiting	Glucose (P) ⌐, ammonia (B) ↑, acidosis ±, free carnitine (P) ⌐, acylcarnitine (P) ↑, long-chain acylcarnitine (P) ↑, seizures ±
255110	Carnitine palmitoyl	Muscle, heart, liver, FB	1p32	Coma, Reye-like syndrome, hepatomegaly, exercise intolerance, myalgia, cardiomyopathy, developmental delay ±, sudden death	Glucose (B) ⌐, ketosis ↑, liver enzymes (P) ↑, CK (P) ↑, myoglobin (P, U) ↑, dicarboxylic acids (U) ±, carnitine (P) ⌐, long-chain acylcarnitine (P) ↑
	Very-long-chain acyl-CoA dehydrogenase			Cardiomyopathy, coma, respiratory arrest, Reye-like syndrome, muscle weakness, muscle pain	Glucose (B) ⌐, acidosis +, CK (P) ↑, dicarboxylic acids (U) ↑, C₁₄:₁ acylcarnitine (P) ↑, carnitine (P) ⌐, long-chain acylcarnitine (P) ↑
201450	Medium-chain acyl-CoA dehydrogenase	Muscle, liver, FB, WBC	1p31	Coma/lethargy, hepatopathy, hypotonia, apnea/respiratory arrest, sudden death, seizures ±, mental retardation, attention deficit disorder	Glucose (B) ⌐, ketosis ±, acidosis +, transamines (P) ↑, ammonia (B) ↑, uric acid (P) ↑, dicarboxylic acids (U) N or ↑, glycine conjugates (U, P) ↑, decanoate (P) ↑, acylcarnitines (U) ↑, carnitine (P) N or ⌐, long-chain acylcarnitine (P) N

Continued

TABLE 11.6

Characteristic Features of Fatty Acid Oxidation Defects (*Continued*)

MIM No.	Disorder	Tissue Distribution	Chromosome Location	Symptoms and Signs	Laboratory Findings
201470	Short-chain acyl-CoA dehydrogenase	Muscle, liver, FB, WBC	12q22-qtr	Muscle weakness, lethargy, failure to thrive, mental retardation	Ketosis +, acidosis +, ethylmalonic acid (U) N or ↑, carnitine (P) ¬ or N
143450	Long-chain 3-hydroxyacyl-CoA	Liver, muscle, heart, FB, WBC	7	Coma/lethargy, hepatopathy, cardiomyopathy, neuropathy, retinopathy, muscle weakness, sudden death	Glucose (B) ¬, acidosis ±, lactate (P) ↑, myoglobin (P, U) ↑, CK (P) ↑, dicarboxylic acids (U) ↑, hydroxy-dicarboxylic acids (U) ↑, long-chain 3-hydroxy fatty acids (P) ↑, carnitine (P) ¬, long-chain acylcarnitine (P)
600890	Short-chain 3-hydroxyacyl-CoA dehydrogenase deficiency	Muscle, FB		Cardiomyopathy, muscle weakness, lethargy	Glucose (B) ¬, myoglobinuria +, CK (P) ↑, AST/ALT (P) ↑, ketosis +, ketones (U) ↑, dicarboxylic acids (U) N or ↑

↑, increased; ¬, decreased; +, present; ±, sometimes present; AST, aspartate transferase; ALT, alanine transferase; B, blood; CK, creatine kinase; CoA, coenzyme A; FB, fibroblasts; MIM, Mendelian Inheritance in Man system; N, normal; P, plasma; U, urine; WBC, white blood cells.

TABLE 11.7
Investigations for Metabolic Disease in the Neonate

Presentation	Possible Metabolic Disorders	Suggested Investigations
Unexplained hypoglycemia	Organic acid disorders Amino acid disorders Glycogen storage disorder (type 1) Disorders of glycogenesis Congenital adrenal hyperplasia Congenital lactic acidosis Galactosemia	Organic acids (U) Amino acids (U, P) 3-Hydroxybutyrate (P) Free fatty acids (P) Lactate (P) Insulin (P) Cortisol (P) 17-Hydroxyprogesterone (P) Galactose-1-phosphate uridyltransferase (B)
Acid-base imbalance Metabolic acidosis (exclude primary cardiac and respiratory disorders)	Organic acid disorders Congenital lactic acidosis	Organic acids (U) Lactate (P) Amino acids (U, P)
Respiratory alkalosis	Urea cycle disorders	Ammonia (P) Orotic acid (U) Amino acids (U, P)
Liver dysfunction (often associated with hypoglycemia and galactosuria)	Galactosemia Fructose 1,6-diphosphatase deficiency Hereditary fructose intolerance Tyrosinemia (type I) Glycogen storage disorder (type I) Disorders of gluconeogenesis α_1-Antitrypsin deficiency	Galactose-1-phosphate-uridyltransferase (B) Sugars (U) Amino acids (U, P) Succinyl acetone (U) α-Fetoprotein (P) Lactate (P) Oligosaccharides (U) Organic acids (U) α_1-Antitrypsin (P)
Neurologic dysfunction Seizures Depressed consciousness Hypotonia with Zellweger syndrome Organic acid disorders Cardiomyopathy	Nonketotic hyperglycinemia Urea cycle disorders Xanthine/sulfite oxidase deficiency Homocystinuria (remethylation defect) Congenital lactic acidosis Glycogen storage type 2 (Pompe disease) Fatty acid oxidation disorders Tyrosinemia (type I)	Amino acids (U, P, C) Orotic acid (U) Ammonia (P) Urate (P, U) Sulfite (U) Lactate (P) Organic acids (U) Very-long-chain fatty acids (P) Lactate (P) 3-Hydroxybutyrate (P) Free fatty acids (P) Oligosaccharides (U) Organic acids (U) Carnitine (P) Amino acids (U, P)

B, whole blood; C, cerebrospinal fluid; P, plasma; U, urine.

galactose-1-phosphate; seen less frequently are galactokinase and galactose epime-rase deficiency.

Clinical symptoms include acute neonatal crisis, neurologic symptoms, developmental delay, hepatocellular disease, visceromegaly, renal dysfunction, renal Fanconi syndrome, gastrointestinal disease, failure to thrive, ophthalmologic disorders, hypoglycemia, metabolic acidosis, coagulation disorders, cataracts, and gonadal dysfunction.

Diagnostic studies include increased urine galactose of 500–2,000 mg/dl (normal is <5 mg/dl), positive urine reaction with clinitest but negative with clinistix; and tes-tape; this may be useful for pediatric screening up to 1 year of age.

Reduced RBC galactose-1-phosphate uridyltransferase establishes the diagnosis.

Galactose tolerance test is positive but not necessary for diagnosis and may be hazardous because of induced hypoglycemia and hypokalemia.

Laboratory findings include albuminuria, jaundice (onset at age 4240–10 days), severe hemolysis, coagulation abnormalities, vomiting, diarrhea, failure to thrive, hyperchloremic metabolic acidosis, cataracts, and mental and physical retardation.

Screening incidence is 1 in 62,000 live births. Prenatal diagnosis is made by measurement of galactose-1-phosphate uridyltransferase in cell culture from amniotic fluid. Parents show <50% enzyme activity in RBCs.

Glycogen Storage Diseases

See Table 11.8 for a review of the most common glycogen storage diseases.

Type IA (Von Gierke Disease): Glucose-6-Phosphatase Deficiency

Main characteristics include: hepatomegaly, hypoglycemia, lactic acidosis presenting in early infancy, and growth delay. Diagnosis is by liver biopsy and assay of enzyme. Treatment is by frequent carbohydrate feedings, nasogastric night feeds, and cornstarch feedings.

Note: Glucose oxidase filter strip detects only glucose; Benedict solution detects all sugars.

Type IB

Type IB is similar to type IA but also has neutropenia; type IB is due to defective compartmentalization of glucose-6-phosphatase.

Type II (Pompe Disease)

Classic infantile form. Main characteristics include deficiency of alpha glucosidase, infantile form presenting with hypotonia, weakness, cardiac hypertrophy, short P-R, large QRS, death usually in the first year; milder forms exist, usually normal glucose and lactate. Diagnosis is based on glycogen in muscle and assay of enzyme. Treatment is with enzyme replacement therapy in some cases.

Type III (Debrancher Deficiency)

Autosomal recessive disease. Main characteristics include: similar to type I but milder; hepatomegaly is prominent; cardiac and skeletal muscle may be involved. Diagnosis is confirmed by liver and muscle biopsy specimens that show biochemical findings of increased glycogen and absence of specific enzyme activity. Treatment is mainly avoidance of fasting and feedings of uncooked cornstarch.

TABLE 11.8

Glycogen Storage Diseases: Most Frequent Types

MIM No.	Type	Inheri-tance	Enzyme Defect	Clinical/Pathologic Features	Pathology	Tissue for Diagnosis[a]
240600	0	AR	Glycogen synthetase	Hypoglycemia, failure to thrive, liver fibrosis	Glycogen is present (0.5% after meal)	Liver, muscle, RBC
232200	1a (von Gierke disease)	AR	Glucose-6-phosphatase	Hepatosplenomegaly, hypoglycemia, hyperlipidemia, acidosis, eruptive xanthomas, hepatic adenomas, hepatocellular carcinoma, no response to glucagon or epinephrine, kidney and GI mucosa involved	Uniform distribution of glycogen with distention of liver cells, mosaic pattern, small and large fat vacuoles, nuclear glycogenation; electron microscopy—uniform increase in normal-appearing glycogen, lipid droplets with glycogen particles within them, normal muscle	Liver
232210	1s (1asp)	AR	Stabilizing protein for glucose-6-phosphatase	Very early clinical onset		Liver
232220	1b	AR	Glucose-6-phosphate transporter protein	Like 1a plus neutropenia, recurrent infections, Crohn disease	Similar to type 1a	Liver
232240	1c		Microsomal phosphate transporter	Hepatomegaly	Uniform distribution of glycogen, mosaic pattern	Liver
232500	1d		Microsomal glucose transporter	Hepatomegaly	Uniform distribution of glycogen, mosaic pattern	Liver

Continued

TABLE 11.8

Glycogen Storage Diseases: Most Frequent Types (*Continued*)

MIM No.	Type	Inheri-tance	Enzyme Defect	Clinical/Pathologic Features	Pathology	Tissue for Diagnosis[a]
232300	2 (Pompe disease)	AR	α-1,4-glycosidase (acid maltase)	Cardiomegaly, hepatomegaly, hypotonia, no hypoglycemia, macroglossia, generalized glycogenosis, CNS involvement, death usually by 1–2 yr	Uniform slight distention of liver cells, microvacuolation due to accumulation, nonmosaic pattern, fat absent; electron microscopy—glycogen vesicles surrounded by membranes (so-called lysosomes), muscle—marked glycogen deposition; muscle electron microscopy—excessive glycogen (free and in vesicles), loss of myofibrils	Liver, muscle, WBC, amniocytes, fibroblasts
232330	2b	?AR *vs.* XLR	Not established	Cardiac glycogenesis with survival to 2nd decade	Similar to type 2	Liver, muscle, WBC, amniocytes, fibroblasts
	2 (Antopol disease)	AD	Not established	Survival to 2nd to 4th decade	Similar to but milder changes than in type 2	Liver, muscle, WBC, amniocytes, fibroblasts
	2 (Skeletal muscle type)	AR	Acid maltase	Childhood/adult onset, muscle weakness, cerebral aneurysms in adults	Changes in muscle similar to those in type 2	Muscle, WBC, amniocytes, fibroblasts

232400	3 (Forbes disease/ Cori disease/ limit dextrinosis)	AR	Amylo-1,6-glucosidase	Liver, skeletal muscle, heart involvement, hypoglycemia Response to glucagon	Uniform distension of liver cells due to glycogen, mosaic pattern, nuclear glycogenation, fibrous septa formation, small droplets of fat; electron microscopy— same as type 1 (lipid vacuoles less frequent); muscle electron microscopy—glycogen subsarcolemmal and between myofibrils	Liver, muscle, WBC
232500	4 (Andersen disease/ amylopectinosis)	AR	Amylo-1,4-1, 6-transglucosidase (brancher enzyme)	Cirrhosis, jaundice hepatosplenomegaly, CNS involvement, portal hypertension, sudden death in infancy; adult females with cardiomyopathy are heterozygotes; allelic form with clinical picture like muscular dystrophy in adults	Liver—pale, amphophilic, hyaline or vacuolated, PAS-positive, diastase-resistant material (amylopectin), particularly in periportal hepatocytes; variable, large lipid vacuoles, prominent septa formation progressing to cirrhosis; electron microscopy— fibrillar appearance of amylopectin; muscle— amylopectin deposits	Muscle, WBC, amniocytes, fibroblasts
232600	5 (McArdle disease)	AR	Myophosphorylase (1,4-α-D-glucan, orthophosphate α-glucosyl transferase, D-glycanorthophosphatase-α-D-glucosyl transferase)	Muscle pain, weakness after exercise, myoglobinuria, good prognosis	Muscle—subsarcolemmal glycogen; electron microscopy—same as in light microscopy; liver—normal	Muscle enzyme

Continued

TABLE 11.8
Glycogen Storage Diseases: Most Frequent Types *(Continued)*

MIM No.	Type	Inheri-tance	Enzyme Defect	Clinical/Pathologic Features	Pathology	Tissue for Diagnosis[a]
232700	6 (Hers disease)	AR	Hepatophosphorylase	Hepatomegaly, mild to moderate hypoglycemia, good prognosis	Liver—nonuniform distention of hepatocytes due to glycogen, mosaic pattern, septa formation, small fat droplets; electron microscopy—burst appearance of glycogen, rosettes, lipid vacuoles with glycogen; muscle—normal	Liver, WBC, RBC
232800	7 (Tarui disease)	AR	Muscle phosphofructokinase	Muscle cramps, myoglobinuria, good prognosis	Muscle—subsarcolemmal glycogen; electron microscopy—same as in light microscopy	Muscle enzyme
261750	8	AR	Hepatic phosphorylase	Hepatomegaly, growth retardation, lipidemia, progressive neurologic deterioration	Nonuniform distention of hepatocytes due to glycogen, mosaic pattern; electron microscopy—same as in type 6, less frequent lipid vacuoles with glycogen in them; muscle—subsarcolemmal glycogen; electron microscopy—same as in light microscopy	Liver, CNS (glycogen in axons)

AD, autosomal dominant; AMP, adenosine monophosphate; AR, autosomal recessive; CNS, central nervous system; MIM, Mendelian Inheritance in Man system; PAS, periodic acid–Schiff; RBC, red blood cells; WBC, white blood cells; XLR, X-linked recessive; S, serum.

[a] Tissues should be fixed in alcohol for preservation of glycogen. Lipid stains should be done on frozen sections. Tests for absence of myophosphorylase in type 5 and phosphofructokinase in type 7 done on snap-frozen (−70°C) muscle biopsy specimen by enzyme histochemistry. Biochemical studies done on tissue wrapped in aluminum foil and fresh-frozen (−70°C) (liver or muscle). Transport on dry ice by overnight mail to reference laboratory. WBC skin fibroblasts and amniocytes should be shipped at room temperature; avoid freezing or overheating.

Type IV (Anderson Disease, Brancher Disease, Amylopectinosis)

Due to the absence of amylo $(1,4 \rightarrow 1,6)$-transglucosidase. Hypoglycemia is not present. Main characteristics are failure to thrive, hepatomegaly, splenomegaly, cirrhosis, and death usually by 2 years of age. Biopsy specimen from liver may show a cirrhotic reaction to glycogen of abnormal structure. Definitive diagnosis is by enzyme assay. Treatment is by liver transplantation.

Type V (McArdle Disease, Muscle Phosphorylase Deficiency)

Autosomal recessive disease. Main characteristics include cramping, exercise intolerance, weakness, and possibly myoglobinuria due to rhabdomyolysis with no hepatomegaly or hypoglycemia. Treatment is by avoiding strenuous exercise.

Type VII (Phosphofructokinase Deficiency)

Similar clinical picture to Type V. Autosomal recessive disease with deficiency of muscle phosphofructokinase.

STORAGE DISEASES

See Table 11.9 for a review of mucopolysaccharidoses (MPS).

Mucolipidoses

I-cell (inclusion-cell) disease is differentiated from Hurler syndrome by the absence of mucopolysacchariduria. I-cell disease is so named because of numerous phase-dense inclusions in the cytoplasm of cultured fibroblasts from affected individuals. Similar inclusions have since been seen in cells from patients with mucolipidosis I and pseudo-Hurler polydystrophy (mucolipidosis III).

Mucolipidosis II is characterized by a deficiency of multiple lysosomal enzymes in cultured fibroblasts and an increased concentration in culture medium, serum, and other body fluids.

The diagnosis of both mucolipidosis II and mucolipidosis III can be confirmed by measuring the activities of lysosomal enzymes in serum or in cultured fibroblasts. Tenfold to 20-fold increases in β-hexosaminidase, iduronate sulfatase, and arylsulfatase A are characteristic of both mucolipidosis II and mucolipidosis III. Lysosomal enzyme activities in white blood cells (WBCs) are not reliable for diagnosis. The level of N-acetylglucosamine phosphotransferase activity in WBCs or cultured fibroblasts can be measured directly with commercially available substrates.

Activity of plasma hyaluronidase, an endoglycosidase of presumably lysosomal origin, is not increased in the plasma from individuals with mucolipidosis II and III, unlike most lysosomal enzymes.

Hurler Syndrome

Main characteristics include regression of development, large head, coarse facial features, corneal clouding, hepatosplenomegaly, radiologic picture of dysostosis multiplex, and dermatan and heparin sulfate in urine. It is autosomal recessive. Treatment is by bone marrow transplantation or enzyme replacement.

TABLE 11.9

Mucopolysaccharidoses (MPS)

MIM	Chromosome		Inheritance	Defective Enzyme	Clinical Pathologic Features
252800	4p16.3	MPS IH (Hurler)	AR	ʟ-Iduronidase	Abnormal facies, visceromegaly, skeletal changes, cardiovascular disease, mental retardation, corneal clouding
		MPS IS (Scheie)	AR	ʟ-Iduronidase	Cardiac valve disease, corneal clouding, joint stiffness, (defect allelic with above) normal intelligence
		MPS IH/Is genetic compound	AR	ʟ-Iduronidase	Intermediate between above
309900	X.q28	MPS IIA (Hunter, clinically severe subset)	XLR	Sulfoiduronate sulfatase	Abnormal facies, growth retardation, hepatosplenomegaly, cardiovascular disease, death by second decade
		MPS IIB (Hunter, clinically milder subset)	AR	Sulfoiduronate sulfatase (? defect allelic with IIA)	Features less severe than above with longer survival
252900		MPS IIIA (Sanfilippo A)	AR	Heparan sulfate sulfatase	Visceral/skeletal features slight, defect severe
252920		MPS IIIB (Sanfilippo B)	AR	N-acetyl-ᴅ-glucosaminidase	Similar to above
252930		MPS IIIC (Sanfilippo C)	AR	Acetyl CoA: glucosaminide N-acetyltransferase	Similar to above
252940	12q14	MPS IIID (Sanfilippo D)	AR	N-acetylglucosamine 6- sulfate sulfatase	Similar to above
253000	16q24	MPS IVa (Morquio A)	AR	Galactosamine-6-sulfate sulfatase	Thoracic skeletal deformity, aortic valve disease, corneal clouding

253010	MPS IVB (Morquio B)	AR	Galactosidase (presumably allelic with forms of generalized GM_1 gangliosidosis)	Skeletal disease, clouding mild, intellect normal
	MPS V–now MPS IS	AR	Arylsulfatase B	Skeletal, corneal clouding severe, intellect Normal until late in course
253200	MPS VI (Maroteaux-Lamy)			Short stature, major feature
253229	MPS VII (Sly)	AR	Glucuronidase	Short stature, hepatomegaly, mental retardation, normal corneas
253230	MPS VIII		Glucosamine-6-sulfate sulfatase	

AR, Autosomal recessive; XLR, X-linked recessive.

Hunter Syndrome (Iduronate Sulfatase Deficiency; MPS II)

This is similar to Hurler but there is no corneal clouding. Dermatan and heparin sulfate are in the urine, and it is X-linked inheritance as opposed to Hurler syndrome. Treatment is by enzyme replacement.

San Filippo Syndrome (MPS III)

This syndrome has less severe somatic features, developmental delay, behavioral problems, and neurologic regression.

Morquio Syndrome (MPS IV)

Type A: galactose-6-sulfatase deficiency
Type B: β-galactosidase deficiency

Main characteristics are short stature, joint laxity, multiple skeletal deformity, and odontoid hypoplasia.

Marotaux-Lamy Syndrome (MPS VI)

Main characteristics are Hurler-like skeletal features, dystosis multiplex, and relative sparing of CNS.

Sly Disease (MPS VII)

Main characteristics include variable features, including hydrops, hepatosplenomegaly, and corneal clouding.

LYSOSOMAL LIPID STORAGE DISEASES

For a review of lysosomal lipid storage diseases, see Table 11.10.

Gaucher Disease Type I

Type I (nonneuronopathic) is the chronic form of Gaucher disease. Clinical manifestations are highly variable. The disease has been diagnosed from infancy to adulthood. The incidence in the Ashkenazi Jewish population is between 1 in 600 and 1 in 2,500. The disease is inherited as an autosomal recessive trait.

Painless splenomegaly, thrombocytopenia, anemia, and leukopenia are the usual initial presenting symptoms. Platelet counts may be $<50 \infty 10^9$/L without an accompanying bleeding diathesis. The liver frequently does not become significantly enlarged until later in the course of the disease. Erlenmeyer flask deformity of the distal ends of the femur is considered diagnostic of Gaucher disease. Diffuse yellow-brown skin pigmentation may involve the face and legs. Renal involvement, pulmonary hypertension, and cardiac abnormalities are less frequent.

Gaucher Disease Type II

Type II Gaucher disease (acute neuronopathic, infantile), an autosomal recessive disorder, has no ethnic predilection. It is rapidly progressive, with severe neurologic complications and signs of cranial nerve nuclei and extrapyramidal tract involvement beginning by 3–6 months after birth.

TABLE 11.10

Lysosomal Lipid Storage Diseases

MIM	Disease	Inheritance	Deficient Enzyme	Clinicopathologic Features
Cholesteryl Ester Storage Diseases				
278000	Wolman, infantile	AR	Acid lipase (cholesterol ester hydrolase)	Failure to thrive, hepatomegaly, malabsorption, adrenal insufficiency, rapid course; storage of triglyceride, cholesterol ester in liver, spleen, lymphoid tissues, adrenal, marrow, lungs, intestinal lamina propria, renal epithelium, enteric and central neurons, placental trophoblast; adrenal necrosis with calcification
278000	Wolman, late infantile juvenile	AR	Acid lipase	Later onset, slower course (presumably allelic)
215000	Cholesteryl ester storage disease	AR	Acid lipase	Splenomegaly, atheromas, esophageal varices, pulmonary hypertension, hepatic failure (allelic)
Sphingomyelin Storage Diseases				
257200	Niemann-Pick A (infantile cerebral type)	AR	Sphingomyelinase	Visceromegaly, cerebral deterioration, rapid course; lysosomal storage in reticuloendothelial cells (foam cells), hepatocytes, bone marrow, lungs, peripheral and central neurons, epicenter in Eastern Europe, with disease most frequent in Ashkenazi Jews; ? congenital Niemann-Pick disease is variant
607616	Niemann-Pick B (juvenile noncerebral type)	AR	Sphingomyelinase	Visceromegaly, lung infiltration; storage cells and sea-blue histiocytes, but neurons not involved; survival to at least late first decade
	Niemann-Pick B (neonatal malignant cholestatic jaundice)	AR	Presumably sphingomyelinase subset of NP-A	Cholestatic jaundice with giant cell transformation of liver (neonatal hepatitis) early; findings as in NP-A and NP-C or NP-D if survival adequate; possible epicenter in Hispanics in western United States

Continued

TABLE 11.10
Lysosomal Lipid Storage Diseases (Continued)

MIM	Disease	Inheritance	Deficient Enzyme	Clinicopathologic Features
257220	Niemann-Pick C (subacute juvenile neuronopathic type)	AR	Deficient esterification of exogenous cholesterol	Visceromegaly, cerebellar ataxia, seizures, psychotic features; Western European epicenter; positive OTAN stain of storage cells useful
257220	Niemann-Pick D (subacute juvenile/adult neurono pathic type	AR	Deficient esterification of exogenous cholesterol	Visceromegaly, cerebellar ataxia, seizures, psychotic features; Eastern European epicenter; positive OTAN stain of storage cells useful
607616	Niemann-Pick E (adult noncerebral type)	AR	Same as above	Survival into second decade; epicenter in Nova Scotia region epicenter. Storage cells as in NP-B; possible Mediterranean
Other Neural Lipidoses				
213700	Cerebral dystonic lipidosis	AR	CYP27A1	Onset 4–9 yr, dementia, seizures, dystonic movements, normal fundi; foam cells in marrow
213700	Cerebrotendinous xanthomatosis (cerebral cholesterolosis, normolipemic xanthomatosis)	AR	Mitochondrial sterol 27-hydroxylase	Onset in second decade; cerebral deterioration, cerebellar ataxia, cataract, atherosclerosis; cholesterol, cholestanol deposits in tendons (especially Achilles tendon), lungs, cerebellar white matter, cerebral peduncles
269600	Neurovisceral disease with supranuclear opthalmoplegia, xanthomatosis	AR	Sphingomyelinase	Supranuclear ophthalmoplegia, hepatic cirrhosis; foam cells, sea-blue histiocytes, in marrow*; neuronal lipid storage
Cerebroside Storage Diseases				
230800	Gaucher 1 (adult Gaucher disease)	AR	Glucocerebrosidase β-D-glucosyl-N-acyl sphingosine hydrolase	Hepatosplenomegaly, osteoporosis with liability to fracture; onset in first decade with survival to sixth decade or later; Gaucher cells are macrophages of spleen, liver, nodes, thymus, marrow; storage lysosomes have elongated tubular shape; Eastern European epicenter, with greater frequency in Ashkenazi Jews (possible West African epicenter)

Note similar disease can be due to saposin C (sphingolipid activator protein 2) deficiency

230900	Gaucher 2A (infantile cerebral type)	AR	Glucocerebrosidase	Visceral disease similar to type I, rapidly progressive cerebral damage without neuronal cerebroside storage; short survival; no apparent epicenter
	Gaucher 2B (rapidly progressive with ichthyosis)	AR	Glucocerebrosidase	Neonatal rapidly progressive ichthyosis, nonimmune hydrops, death by 5 mo; Gaucher cells in reticuloendothelial system and central nervous system
231000	Gaucher 3 (chronic neuropathic or Norrbottnian type)	AR	Glucocerebrosidase	Both visceral and progressive neurologic dysfunction; survival into second or third decades; storage cells as in Gaucher 1 and adventitia of vessels of cortex and cerebral white matter
230800	Pseudo-Gaucher disease	AR	Glucocerebrosidase	Corneal opacities, hydrocephalus, valvular heart disease, deafness, supranuclear ophthalmoplegia, visceral infiltration mild; specific mutation not known, ? allelic with Gaucher 1
245200	Krabbe, infantile type	AR	Galactocerebroside β-galactosidase	Onset 4–6 mo with rapid, severe neurologic damage; storage "globoid body" cells in central white matter
245200	Krabbe, late infantile/juvenile type	AR	Galactocerebroside β-galactosidase	Onset by 5 yr, course more rapid if onset by 3 yr; visual failure, cerebellar ataxia, spastic hemi/paraparesis, peripheral neuropathy with reduced nerve conduction velocity; storage cells in central and peripheral neural tissue; epicenter in Sicily reported
301500	Farber lipogranulomatosis			
	a. Early onset	AR	Ceramidase	Subcutaneous nodules, arthritis, laryngeal
	b. Infantile type	AR	Ceramidase	Periarticular, no lung involvement, normal intelligence
	c. Late onset	AR	Ceramidase	Survival into second decade, macroglossia, laryngeal, joint but not lung involvement and less cerebral dysfunction
	d. Neonatal type	AR	Ceramidase	Psychomotor retardation, hepatomegaly, debility

Continued

TABLE 11.10
Lysosomal Lipid Storage Diseases (*Continued*)

MIM	Disease	Inheritance	Deficient Enzyme	Clinicopathologic Features
	e. Malignant histiocytosis type	AR	Ceramidase	Death before 6 months; psychomotor retardation at 1–2 yr; hoarseness, arthritis, macular cherry-red spot
301500	Fabry (angiokeratoma corporis diffusum)†	XLR	α-Galactosidase A (ceramide trihexosidase)	Onset in males in first decade, later with slower course in female heterozygotes; nephrotic syndrome, progressive to renal failure, cardiomegaly with cardiomyopathy (especially in young adult females), episodic abdominal pain, angiokeratomas of skin; storage in renal glomerular and tubular epithelium, cardiac myocytes, enteric and brain stem/spinal cord neurons, blood vessel walls
Gangliosidoses				
230500	GM₁ type 1 gangliosidosis, infantile	AR	β-Galactosidas	Onset birth/early infancy; survival ±1–2 yr; abnormal facies, skeletal changes (especially vertebrae), visceromegaly, cerebral deterioration; storage of ganglioside and/or mucopolysaccharide in reticuloendothelial cells, liver cells, renal glomerular and tubular epithelium, pancreatic and mucoserous gland epithelium, central and peripheral neurons
230600	GM₁ gangliosidosis, type 2 infantile (Derry)	AR	As above, presumably allelic	Onset later, course slower than above; visceromegaly, skeletal changes less marked; neuronal storage as above
230650	GM₁ gangliosidosis type 3, adult	AR	As above, presumably allelic	Mental deterioration, visual loss, myoclonic seizures; angiokeratomas may be early feature

Note above three conditions presumably allelic with mucopolysaccharidosis IVB (Morquio B, q.v.)

272800	GM₂ type I gangliosidosis, infantile (Tay-Sachs disease, B form)	AR	Hexosamidase A (α-unit mutation)	Rapidly progressive dementia, blindness, macular cherry-red spot; epicenter in Eastern Europe with high frequency in Ashkenazi Jews; most frequent gene abnormality is 4 basepair in section in *Hex A* gene, second is G-C substitution
272750	Tay-Sachs disease, AB form	AR	Hexosaminidase activator protein (Saposin)	Later onset than Tay-Sachs (B form); epicenter in Portugal; Affected persons from other for a TS mutation and B1 mutation
272800	Tay-Sachs disease, B1 form, GM₂ type 3 (juvenile type)	AR	Hexosaminidase A, α-unit (mutation gives gly 269 ser change in Hex A gene) (allelic with Tay-Sachs α-unit mutations)	Neuronal storage like that of Tay-Sachs disease with modest degree of visceral storage
268800	GM₂ type 2 gangliosidosis, infantile generalized 0 form (Sandhoff)	AR	Hexosaminidases A and B (β-unit mutation)	Progressive dementia, ataxia; picture can resemble X-linked bulbospinal muscular atrophy
230700	GM₂ gangliosidosis, juvenile, β-unit mutation	AR	Same as above	Similar to above
230710	GM₂ gangliosidosis, juvenile, α-unit mutation	AR	Hexosaminidase A α-unit	
	GM₂ gangliosidosis, chronic	AR	As above	Can be spinocerebellar degeneration resembling Friedreich ataxia, juvenile spinal muscular atrophy resembling Kugelberg-Welander disease, or like amyotrophic lateral sclerosis
	GM₂ gangliosidosis, chronic, α-unit mutation	AR	Hexosaminidases A and B	Dementia, ataxia, pyramidal tract signs, amyotrophy; psychotic features regular; rectal biopsy for neurons useful
256540	Galactosialidosis (Goldberg)	AR	β-Galactosidase, neuraminidase early and late infantile forms deafness; due to deficiency of "protector protein" for above lysosomal hydrolases, adult type due to abnormality of processor protein)	Abnormal facies, mental retardation, seizures, corneal clouding lysosomal storage, especially in macrophages

Continued

TABLE 11.10

Lysosomal Lipid Storage Diseases (*Continued*)

MIM	Disease	Inheritance	Deficient Enzyme	Clinicopathologic Features
Sulfatide Storage Diseases				
250100	Metachromatic leukodystrophy, infantile	AR	Arylsulfase A (cerebroside sulphate sulfate) (allele 1 mutation)	Onset at ±2 yr, survival to ±5 yr; hypotonia, muscle weakness, mental deterioration, peripheral nerve involvement (prolonged nerve conduction time); storage cells in liver, kidney, epithelium, rectal lamina propia, central white matter, nerves; sulfatide shows brown metachromasia with cresyl violet, toluidine blue stains
250100	Metachromatic leukodystrophy, juvenile	AR	As above; presumably allelic with above (allele A mutation); genetic compound of allele 1 and allele A mutations presumably occurs	As above, clinical onset 4–10 yr, with slower course; reduced nerve conduction velocity
250100	Metachromatic leukodystrophy, adult onset	AR	Same as above (? in spectrum of severity with other forms); pseudodeficiency gene occurs; some patients presumably genetic compound of MLD mutation and pseudodeficiency gene	Onset in second decade with schizophrenia-like behavior; visceral and central nervous system involvement

| 249900 | Metachromatic leukodystrophy | AR | Saposin B (sulfatase activator protein I) | Variably as other forms |
| 272200 | Multiple sulfatase deficiency (Austin mucosulfatidosis) | AR | Arylsulfatases A, B, and C; clinical type 1: onset in first yr, survival to 6–10 yr; 2: onset in later infancy, survival into second decade; 3: onset in second decade, survival to third-fourth decades; probably due to continuous spectrum of severity rather than allelic differences | Like those of metachromatic leukodystrophy with ichthyosis and somatic features suggesting mucopolysaccharidosis |

From Gilbert-Barness, E. (2007). *Potter's pathology of fetus, infant and child* (2nd ed., pp. 479–483). New York: Elsevier.

*Sea-blue histiocytes also occur in Hermansky-Pudlak albinism, hemorrhagic tendency, pigmented lipid histiocyte syndrome (q.v.), and Norum lecithin: cholesterol acyltransferase (LCAT) deficiency.

†Cutaneous angiokeratomas also occur in fucosidosis, adult gangliosidosis, GM$_1$ aspartylglycosaminuria, galactosialidosis (Goldberg syndrome), later onset multiple sulfate deficiency, α-galactosidase β deficiency (Schindler syndrome and Kanzaki glycoaminoacid storage disease), and β-mannosidosis, fucosidosis.

AR, autosomal recessive; XLR, X-linked recessive.

Niemann-Pick Disease, Types A and B

The most common and severe variant of Niemann-Pick disease is type A, the acute neuropathic form. These patients, often of Eastern European Jewish ancestry, present early in life. Often the skin has a yellow-brown pigmentation, lymph nodes are enlarged, and ocular manifestations (cherry-red macula and corneal opacifications) are evident. Few survive beyond 4 years of age.

The type B variant (an allele variant of type A) features a pattern of visceral involvement similar to that in type A yet spares the CNS.

The diagnosis of types A and B Niemann-Pick disease can be made by foam cells in the marrow and enzymatic determination of sphingomyelinase activity in cell or tissue extracts.

Niemann-Pick Disease Types C and D

Patients with Niemann-Pick disease types C and D may present with neonatal jaundice, appear to recover, then suffer progressive neurodegeneration.

Krabbe Disease

Krabbe disease is an autosomal recessive disorder caused by deficiency of galactocerebrosidase, the lysosomal enzyme responsible for the degradation of galactocerebroside. Galactocerebroside (galactosylceramide) is a sphingoglycolipid consisting of sphingosine, fatty acid, and galactose, and is normally present almost exclusively in the myelin sheath.

This disorder usually presents between 3 and 6 months of life after a normal neonatal period and has a rapidly progressive course with irritability, hypersensitivity to external stimuli, and severe mental and motor deterioration. Patients rarely survive beyond 2 years.

Wolman Disease

Deficiency of acid lipase results in storage of cholesterol esters and triglycerides in lysosomes. Clinically, infants fail to thrive and show pernicious vomiting, hepatosplenomegaly, and steatorrhea. Adrenal glands are calcified. Death occurs early in the severe form of the disease.

Gangliosidoses

Tay-Sachs Disease (G_{M2} Gangliosidosis)

Classical picture is infant with hypotonia, exaggerated startle to sound. By one year of age, rapid neurological decline with blindness and deafness and eventually decerebrate rigidity. Due to hexosaminidase A deficiency. Prenatal screening in communities with high Jewish population.

Sulfatidoses

Metachromatic Leukodystrophy

Metachromatic leukodystrophy is an autosomal recessive lysosomal storage disease caused by deficiency of the enzyme arylsulfatase A. Frequency is estimated to be

1 in 40,000. There are several forms, the most common being the late infantile form. There is gradual loss of speech at about 2 years of age, delayed walking and mental regression, eventual spastic quadriplegia, and lack of awareness of surroundings. Death usually occurs by about 7 years of age. Treatment is by bone marrow transplantation in some patients.

MITOCHONDRIAL DISORDERS

Acute neonatal crisis, neurologic symptoms, neurodegenerative symptoms, developmental delay, hepatocellular disease, visceromegaly, renal Fanconi syndrome, gastrointestinal disease, skeletal myopathy, cardiomyopathy, cardiac symptoms, failure to thrive, ophthalmologic disorders, deafness, hypoglycemia, metabolic acidosis or hyperammonemia (or both), diabetes, psychiatric disorders at any age (Table 11.11). Healthy relatives who are silent carriers may have no symptoms.

TABLE 11.11
Examples of Mitochondrial Disorders

Disorder	Systemic Lesions	CNS Lesions
Leigh disease	None reported	Deep and periventricular gray matter spongy change; vascular proliferation; cystic lesions
Pyruvate dehydrogenase complex		
Pyruvate decarboxylase deficiency	None reported	Cerebrum; deep and periventricular gray matter cystic lesions in white more than in gray matter
Pyruvate carboxylase deficiency	Hepatic steatosis	Cerebral white matter; neocortex; paucity of myelin; neuronal loss
Glioneuronal dystrophy (some cases of Alpers disease)	Hepatic fibrosis	Neocortex spongy change and neuronal loss
Respiratory chain enzymes deficiency	Cardiomyopathy	
Biotin-dependent enzymes; biotinidase deficiency	Skin rash; alopecia	Insufficient data
Carnitine deficiency	Lipid myopathy	None reported
Carnitine palmitoyl transferase deficiency	Rhabdomyolysis	None reported
Ragged red fiber–related diseases		
Kearns-Sayre disease	Ragged red fibers	Brain stem, cerebellar white matter; spongy change
Luft disease	Ragged red fibers	None reported
MERRF	Ragged red fibers	Dentate nucleus; brain stem neuronal loss; tract degeneration
MELAS	Ragged red fibers	Neocortex microinfarcts

MELAS, mitochondrial encephalopathy, lactic acidosis, and stroke; MERRF, myoclonic epilepsy with ragged red fibers.
From Powers, J. M., & Haroupian, D. S. (1996). Central nervous system. In I. Damijnov & J. Linder (Eds.), *Anderson's pathology.* St. Louis: Mosby.

PURINE AND PYRIMIDINE DEFECTS

Hypoxanthine-Guanine Phosphoribosyltransferase Deficiency

Lesch-Nyhan syndrome is the severest form. It is distinguished by self-mutilating activity, spasticity, choreoathetosis, MR, and gout.

Hereditary Orotic Aciduria

Main characteristics include hypochromatic, megaloblastic anemia, leucopenia, and developmental delay and crystalluria.

PERIOXISOMAL DISORDERS

General Features of Peroxisomal Defects

Dysmorphic features, acute neonatal presentation, neurologic symptoms, neurodegenerative symptoms, hypotonia, developmental delay, hepatocellular disease, visceromegaly, renal dysfunction, gastrointestinal disease, skeletal myopathy, skeletal abnormalities, failure to thrive, ophthalmologic disorders, deafness, coagulation disorders, endocrine disorders.

Diagnostic Studies

Diagnostic tests for peroxisomal disorders include the following:

1. Increased levels of long-chain fatty acids in plasma, RBCs, or cultured skin fibroblasts, except in rhizomelic chondrodysplasia punctata.
2. Diminished levels of plasmalogen in RBCs and defective plasmalogen synthesis.
3. Elevated pipecolic acid levels in plasma.
4. Elevated levels of plasma phytanic acid in Refsum disease.
5. Absent or abnormal peroxisomes in liver biopsy specimens by electron microscopy.

Prenatal Diagnosis

Except for type I hyperoxaluria, all peroxisomal disorders can be identified prenatally in the first or second trimester of pregnancy by measurement of very-long-chain fatty acids and bile acid intermediates, and by assays of plasmalogen synthesis in cultured amniocytes or cultured chorionic villus cells.

The prenatal diagnosis of type I hyperoxaluria requires measurement of alanine-glyoxylate aminotransferase activity in biopsy specimens of fetal liver due to absent or minimal activity of the enzyme in fibroblasts and in cell cultures from chorionic villus biopsy specimens or amniotic fluid.

Peroxisomal Diseases

Neonatal and infantile main characteristics include hypotonia, seizures, dysmorphism, skeletal changes, and hyperbilirubinemia, for example, Zellweger syndrome, neonatal adrenoleukodystrophy, and rhizomelic chrondrodysplasia punctata.

Later-onset peroxisomal diseases include adrenoleukodystrophy (X-linked), which presents in later childhood with behavioral changes, cognitive regression, and demyelination. Refsum disease presents in later childhood with visual decline, hearing loss, and peripheral neuropathy.

Oxalosis, Primary Oxalosis

Autosomal recessive due to deficiency of glyoxalate enzyme in liver resulting in deposition of calcium oxalate crystals in kidney, bones, and conduction system of heart. Renal transplantation only temporarily effective. Death from renal failure usually by age 7 years.

Zellweger Syndrome

Severe peroxisomal phenotype with characteristic facial dysmorphism, disturbances of neuronal migration (polymicrogyria, neuronal heterotopias), corneal clouding, nystagmus, cataracts, congenital heart disease, poor feeding, failure to thrive, and death within a few months.

Neonatal Adrenoleukodystrophy

Severe peroxisomal phenotype with more subtle facial dysmorphism, disturbances of neuronal migration (polymicrogyria, neuronal heterotopias), chemical evidence of adrenal insufficiency, poor feeding, failure to thrive; survival for up to a few years.

Infantile Refsum Disease

Severe peroxisomal phenotype with facial dysmorphism, subtle disturbances of neuronal migration (polymicrogyria, neuronal heterotopias), decreased plasma cholesterol, prominent retinal degeneration and sensorineural hearing impairment; survival for up to many years.

Hyperpipecolic Acidemia

Severe peroxisomal phenotype with prominent retinal degeneration, cirrhosis; survival for up to many years.

Single Enzyme Defects

Rhizomelic Chondrodysplasia Punctata

Severe peroxisomal phenotype with facial dysmorphism, severe shortening of proximal limbs, chondrodysplasia punctata (stippled epiphyses), skin lesions, cataracts; survival highly variable.

METAL DISORDERS

Wilson Disease

Main characteristics include excessive accumulation of copper in the body; autosomal recessive. Organs that are affected by copper toxicity include the liver (mild hepatitis to fulminant liver), neurologic (ataxia, dysarthria, flapping failure), kidney (renal failure, renal tubular acidosis), eyes (Kayser-Fleischer rings), and hematologic, skeletal, and endocrine problems. Diagnosis is by Kayser-Fleischer rings; low copper and low ceruloplasmin in plasma, increased copper in urine, liver biopsy shows increased copper deposition. Treatment is by chelation with D-penicilla-mine.

Menke Disease

Main characteristics include: X-linked, abnormal tissue distribution of copper, decreased copper in liver and brain; increased copper in some other organs, severe developmental delay, dysmorphic facial features; distinguished clinically by brittle, twisted hair known as pili torti, low copper, and low ceruloplasmin in plasma and low hepatic copper.

Acrodermatitis Enteropathica

Main characteristics include autosomal recessive zinc deficiency, characteristic der-matitis, failure to thrive, and neurological problems. Treatment is with zinc.

GENETIC MENDELIAN DISORDERS: AUTOSOMAL DOMINANT DISORDERS

Neurofibromatosis (NF)

Heterogeneous group (Table 11.12):

1. NF-1, peripheral or von Recklinghausen NF
2. NF-2, central NF or bilateral acoustic NF (BANF)
3. Schwannomatosis

Other forms:

1. NF-3, mixed central and peripheral NF
2. NF-4, variants or atypical forms

TABLE 11.12
Differential Diagnosis Between NF-1 and NF-2

	NF-1	NF-2
Incidence	1/3–4,000	1/40,000
CAL spots	Frequent	Few, large pale
Cutaneous lesions	Frequent	Few
Lisch nodules	Present	—
Optic neuroma	19% (CT)	—
Bilateral vestibular schwannomas	Exceptional	Characteristic
Malignancies	2%–10%	30%–50%
Age of onset	Early	Late
Gene location	Chromosome 17	Chromosome 22
Gene product	Neurofibromin	Merlin or schwannomin

Neural crest-derived tissues affect cell growth, resulting in neurofibromas and neurofibroscarcoma.

Diagnostic Criteria for NF-1

At least two of the following findings are present:

1. Six or more café-au-lait macules (over 5 mm on prepubertals and 15 mm in postpubertals
2. Multiple freckles (axillary or inguinal regions, Crowe sign)
3. Two or more neurofibromas or one plexiform NF
4. Optic glioma
5. Two or more Lisch nodules (iris hamartomas)
6. Distinctive osseous lesion (sphenoid dysplasia or thinning of long bone cortex)

NF-2

Autosomal dominant pattern of inheritance with over 95% penetrance; 25–50% of all cases represent new mutations. Main clinical features include progressive hearing loss (usually unilateral, in the teens or early 20s), ringing in the ears, neurological problems such as unsteadiness in walking, facial weakness, sensory change, ache, change in vision. Few café-au-lait spots (CALS) and neurofibroma, cataracts (may precede the onset of symptoms of the vestibular schwannoma), tumors of the CNS. Basic problem is the CNS tumor. Gadolinium-enhanced MRI is the most important diagnostic test. The NF-2 gene constitutes a novel class of tumor suppressor genes. It encodes a novel protein related to the moesin (membrane-organizing extension spike protein)-ezrib (cytovillin)-radixin family of cytoskeleton-associated proteins. The protein was named "merlin" (moesin-ezrin-radixin-like protein) or Schwannomin.

Diagnostic Criteria for NF-2

1. Bilateral vestibular schwannomas (= 85%)
2. Meningioma, glioma, schwannoma, juvenile posterior subcapsular lenticular opacities/juvenile cortical cataract (1) or (2, and 3, or 4).

Tuberous Sclerosis

Two-thirds of cases are new mutations. Mutations in TSC1 are on 9q34 and TSC2 on 16p13-encoding proteins hamartin and tuberin respectively. May affect 1/6,000 newborns instead of 1/150–300,000. Many carriers may be totally asymptomatic. The classic triad (MR, seizure, adenoma, sebaceum) may not be present.

Main characteristics include: hamartomatous involving brain, eyes, skin, bone, and kidneys. Intracranial calcifications (basal ganglia or periventricular), retinal phakomas (astrocytic tumors) (mulberry-like appearance), bone lesions, depigmented nevi, café-au-lait spots, shagreen patches, and gray or white patches of scalp. The hypomelanotic macules (achromic patches or ash-leaf spots) are the most common and earliest cutaneous sign of tuberous sclerosis. Periungual and digital fibromas (characteristic lesion seen in 20% of the postpubertal patients). Cardiac rhabdomyomas suggest this diagnosis. Patients and parents should be examined with Wood's lamp, also CT/MRI, skeletal survey, ophthalmologic and dental evaluations, renal ultrasound and echocardiogram.

Marfan Syndrome

Autosomal dominant. Mutation in the fibrillin gene (FBN1), located in chromosome 15q21.1. Mutation in the transforming growth factor-beta receptor 2 (TGFBR2).
   Revised diagnostic criteria for Marfan syndrome:

- More stringent requirements for diagnosis of Marfan syndrome in relatives of an unequivocally affected individual to avoid overdiagnosis
- Skeletal involvement as a major criterion if at least four of eight typical skeletal manifestations are present
- Potential contribution of molecular analysis to the diagnosis of Marfan syndrome
- Delineation of initial criteria for diagnosis of other heritable conditions with partially overlapping phenotypes

Infantile form:

- Sporadic
- More severe
- Dolichocephaly (43%)
- Peculiar facies (38%)
- Ectopia lentis (63%)
- Megalocornea (30%)
- Myopia (42%)
- Aortic dilatation at birth (82%–92%)
- Mitral valve prolapse (82%)
- Arachnodactyly (87%)
- Joint laxity (59%)
- Joint dislocation (36%)

Differential diagnosis (Table 11.13):

- Marfan II: TGFBR2 (3p25-p24.2)

Ehlers-Danlos Syndrome

Main characteristics include skin hyperextensibility, articular hypermobility, and tissue fragility (Table 11.14). The most common types are I, II, and III. All three are autosomal dominant.

Achondroplasia

Main characteristics include dwarfism (4f)-short limbs-rhizomelia, normal intelligence, megalocephaly and hydrocephaly, characteristic face/frontal bossing/mid-facial hypoplasia (MFH), lumbar lordosis, T-L-kyphosis, caudal narrowing of spinal canal,

TABLE 11.13
Differential Diagnosis of Marfan Syndrome and Homocystinuria

	Marfan Syndrome	Homocystinuria
Skeletal anomalies	+	+
Lax joints	+	−
Tight joints	−	+
Ectopia lentis	+ (up)	+ (down)
Aorta dilation	+	−
Thromboembolism	−	+
Mental retardation	−	+
Psychiatric disturbance	−	+
Cyanide nitroprusside	−	+
Inheritance	AD	AR

and short trident hand (Table 11.15). Mutation on the *FGFR3* (fibroblast growth factor receptor 3) gene located on 4p16.3. New mutation in 80%–90% of cases.

Cleidocranial Dysplasia/Dysostosis

About two thirds are inherited. Wide clinical variability. Main characteristics include aplasia or hypoplasia of clavicles, late closure of fontanelles and ossification of cranial sutures, and multiple dental anomalies with late eruption.

Treacher Collins Syndrome

Autosomal dominant. Incidence 1/50,000 live births. Main characteristics include malar hypoplasia, with cleft in zygomatic bone, down-slanting palpebral fissures, lower lid coloboma, mandibular hypoplasia, and malformation of external ear.

Waardenburg Syndrome Types I, II, III, and IV

Autosomal dominant. Variable penetrance and expressivity. Main characteristics in type I include hearing impairment in about 25% in type I and 50% of type II and white forelock. Types I and II are caused by mutations in the *PAX3* gene at 2q35. Type II is caused by mutations in the human microphthalmia (*MITF*) gene at 3p12.3–p14.1. Type IV is either autosomal recessive or autosomal dominant.

Van Der Woude Syndrome (Lip Pit-Cleft Lip Syndrome)

Autosomal dominant form of cleft lip or cleft palate. Gene interferon regulatory factor-6 (*IRF6*) on chromosome 1q.32. About 80% penetrance, 30%–50% de novo mutations. Main characteristics include lower lip pits (fistulas of small accessory salivary glands), cleft lip with or without cleft palate, and hypodontia.

Osteogenesis Imperfecta (OI)

Seven types of osteogenesis imperfecta have been described (Table 11.16).

Be careful when diagnosing osteogenesis imperfecta. Consider it as a differential in cases of fractures and suspected child abuse. To confirm the diagnosis, perform collagen synthesis studies in skin fibroblasts.

TABLE 11.14
Ehlers-Danlos Syndromes

New Type	Clinical Abnormality	Abnormal Gene	Inheritance
I. Classical	Skin hyperextensibility Wide atrophic scars Joint hypermobility	COL5A1, COL5A2, Other	Autosomal dominant
II. Hypermobility	Spectrum of skin involvement General joint hypermobility	No collagen abnormality detected; Mutations of TNX (tenascin-X)	Autosomal dominant
III. Vascular	Thin translucent skin Organ fragility Sudden death	COL3A1	Autosomal dominant
IV. Kyphoscoliosis	Generalized joint laxity Severe hypnotic from birth Congenital progressive scoliosis	PLOD gene (collagen- modifying enzyme)	Autosomal recessive
V. Arthrochalasia	Severe generalized hypermobility with recurrent subluxations ? Congenital hip dislocation	COL1A1, COL1A2 (both skip exon 6)	Autosomal dominant
VI. Dermatospraxis	Sagging, redundant skin Severe skin fragility with substantial bruising	Procollagen 1, N-terminal peptidase	Autosomal recessive
Stickler Syndrome*			
Type I	COL2A1 μ	12q13.11–q13.2	Congenital ocular abnormalities (high risk retinal detach- ment); normal hearing or mild sensorineural hearing loss; preco- cious osteoarthritis; from mild nasal anteversion to PRS
Type II	COL11A1 μ	1p21	Typical phenotype; severe hearing loss; vitreous anomaly
Type III	COL11A2 μ	6p21.3	No ocular involvement

*This is an autosomal dominant connective tissue disorder. It is heterogeneous (several genes or different allelic mutations) with wide interfamilial variation.

TABLE 11.15
Craniosynostosis Syndromes

Disorder	Gene	Chromosome	Major Manifestations Craniosynotosis PLUS:
Apert Acrocephalo- syndactyly type I, most new mutations	FGFR2	10q25.3–26	Coronal, hypertelorism, maxillary hypoplasia, supraoribital protrusion, symmetric syndactyly hands and feet, abnormal shoulder girdle, other malformations (CHD, GU, CP)
Crouzon 75% inherited	FGFR2	10q25.3–26	Hypertelorism, exophthalmos and external strabismus, beaked nose, short upper lip, hypoplastic maxilla, relative prognathism, usually no hands/feet malformations
Jackson-Weiss	FGFR2	10q25.3–26	Foot abnormalities, type of Crouzon/ Pfeiffer allelic with Crouzon
Pfeiffer	FGFR2 FGFR1 (5%)	10q25.3–26 8p11.2–12	Several sutures (turricephaly, cloverleaf skull), hyper/hypotelorism, beaked nose, MFH, broad great toes, broad thumbs, or symphalangism, syndactyly, short fingers
Saethre-Chotzen	TWIST FGFR2 FGFR3	7p21–25 7p21–22 10q25.3–26 4p16.3	Coronal synostosis, facial asymmetry, 1% ptosis, deviated nasal septum, low frontal hairline, small ears with prominent crura, brachydactyly, partial cutaneous syndactyly
Adelaide type	FGFR3? MSX1?	4p16.3	Similar to Jackson-Weiss, but Coned epiphysis, distal and mbd, carpal bone malsegmentation, hallux valgus, absence of metatarsal fusions
Greig	GL13 (Zn)	7p13	Pre- and postaxial polysyndactyly of hands, preaxial polysyndactyly of feet, macrocephaly, prominent forehead, broad base of the nose, mild hypertelorism, 5% craniosynostosis
Boston type	MSX2	5qter	Various synostosis (brachycephaly- turribrachycephaly-cloverleaf skull deformity)
Muenke	FGFR3	4p16.3	May have unilateral coronal synostosis or megalencephaly without craniosynostosis, ± carpal and/or tarsal fusion and broad great toes
Baere-Stevenson	FGFR2	10q25.3–26	Normal hands and feet, MR, anogenital, cutis gyrate and acanthosis nigricans

TABLE 11.16
Characteristics of Different Types of Osteogenesis Imperfecta

Type	Inheritance	Characteristics
Type I	Dominant	Mild, typically no bone deformities, bone fragility may have vertebral compression fractures, blue sclerae, easy bruising
Type II	Dominant New mutation	Lethal in perinatal period, usually caused by respiratory compromise/rib fracture, beaded ribs and crumpled bones, blue sclerae
Type III	Recessive	Extreme short stature, limb and spine deformities caused by multiple fractures usually in utero, bluish gray sclerae
Type IV	Dominant	Moderate bone deformities and variable short stature
Type V	Dominant	Moderate-to-severe bone fragility, calcification of interosseous membrane at the forearm, and a predisposition to develop hyperplastic calluses
Type VI		Moderate-to-severe, unknown, inheritance pattern; bone histology shows increased amount of osteoid and an abnormal pattern of lamellation
Type VII		Has only been observed in a community of Native Americans in northern Quebec; bone fragility, rhizomelia, coax vera, autosomal recessive

AUTOSOMAL RECESSIVE DISORDERS

Meckel-Gruber Syndrome

Main characteristics include encephalocele, microcephaly, polydactyly, abnormal genitalia, and large cystic dysplasic kidneys. Autosomal recessive.

Smith-Lemli-Opitz Syndrome

The incidence is limited at 1 in 20,000, making it the third most common lethal genetic disorder behind cystic fibrosis and phenylketonuria. Main characteristics include MR, microcephaly, ptosis of eyelids, anteverted nostrils, micrognathia, hypospadias and cryptorchidism, cystic kidneys, syndactyly in the second and third toes, high frequency of whorls on finger patterns, and occasional stippled epiphyses. Fifty percent have congenital cardiac defects, principally endocardial cushion defect, hypoplastic left heart, axial and ventricular septal defects, and patent ductus arteriosus.

There is a defect in last step of cholesterol metabolism (low cholesterol and high 7-dehydrocholesterol levels) and results from a deficiency of 7-dehydrocholesterol reductase (DHCR7), the gene localized to chromosome 11q12–13. Prenatal diagnosis by 16 weeks gestation is possible by reduced amniotic fluid, cholesterol, elevated 7-dehydrocholesterol with undetectable amniotic fluid unconjugated estriol.

CHROMOSOMAL FRAGILITY SYNDROMES

- Xeroderma pigmentosum
- Bloom syndrome

- Fanconi pancytopenia
- Ataxia telangiectasia

Major common characteristics are growth failure, congenital anomalies, immunologic deficiencies, and high rates of cancer. Most are autosomal recessive. Main characteristics of Fanconi pancytopenia are radial hypoplasia with hypoplasia to aplasia of thumb, pancytopenia, hyperpigmentation, urinary tract anomalies, malignancies, and chromosomal breakage. The skeletal anomalies are similar to those of thrombocytopenia absent radius (TAR) syndrome. However, in TAR the thumbs are always present.

X-LINKED SYNDROMES

Lesch-Nyhan Syndrome

This X-linked recessive syndrome is characterized by MR, progressive spasticity, choreoathetosis, self-mutilation, elevated serum uric acid levels, and deficiency of hypoxanthine guanine phosphoribosyl transferase (HGPRT). Heterozygous women are mosaic.

X-Linked Hypophosphatemic Rickets

X-L dominant hypophosphatemia; females are less severely affected. Main characteristics include mild to moderate growth deficiency, bowing of lower extremities, rickets, and hypophosphatemia. There is unresponsiveness to physiologic dosage of vitamin D.

Incontinentia Pigmenti Syndrome

X-L dominant, lethal in the hemizygous affected male. Main characteristics include irregular pigmented skin lesions (bullous lesions in early infancy, achromic stains in adulthood), patchy alopecia, dental anomalies (anodontia, delayed eruption), and CNS abnormalities.

SOME SPORADIC DISORDERS

Rubinstein-Taybi Syndrome

Main characteristics include short stature and MR, broad thumbs and halluces, sometimes other fingers and toes, microcephaly, antimongoloid slanting of palpebral fissures, mild ptosis, hypertelorism, long eyelashes, hypoplastic maxilla with narrow palate, beaked nose, patella dislocation, congenital heart disease, respiratory infections, and feeding difficulties in infancy; neural and developmental tumors are common.

Cornelia De Lange Syndrome

Main characteristics include intrauterine growth retardation, MR, microbrachycephaly, synophrys, long curly eyelashes, thin down-turned upper lip, micromelia, and hypertrichosis. Mutation on *NIPBL* gene is seen in 40% (sister chromatid cohesion protein on 5p13.1).

Proteus Syndrome

May be mistaken for neurofibromatosis as in the "elephant man," who had proteus syndrome.

Main characteristics include asymmetric partial gigantism of hands and feet, macrodactyly-cerebriform thickening of palms and soles, bony prominences of skull, macrocephaly, hemihypertrophy, pigmented epidermal nevi, subcutaneous hamartomatous tumors, mostly lipomas, and accelerated growth and muscular atrophy.

Sturge-Weber Sequence

Main characteristics include flat facial hemangiomata (capillary hemangiomas) involving the ophthalmic division of the trigeminal nerve, and angiomas of the meninges (arachnoid and pia mater). Complications include seizures, MR, intracranial calcifications, and ocular anomalies (glaucoma).

Klippel-Feil Sequence

Main characteristics include anomalies of cervical vertebrae (fusion, hemivertebrae), short neck, low posterior hair line, thoracic defects with scoliosis, webbed neck, torticollis, facial asymmetry, deafness, cleft palate, heart defects, renal anomalies, and MR. Most cases are sporadic; some are autosomal dominant. May be part of specific syndromes.

ASSOCIATIONS

These are disorders due to anomalies of blastogenesis, which can be diagnosed and counseled with low recurrence risk because of their overwhelmingly sporadic nature.

VATER Association (or VATERS, VACTERLS)

V	Vertebral defects, ventricular septal defect
A	Anal atresia
T	Tracheo-
E	Esophageal fistula
R	Radial and renal dysplasia
S	Single umbilical artery

CHARGE Association

C	Coloboma
H	Heart anomalies
A	Atresia of the choanae

R   Retarded growth and development
G   Genital anomalies
E   Ear anomalies

Most cases are sporadic, but similar cases are due to chromosomal abnormalities, AR inheritance mutations, X-L inheritance, and new AD mutations involving the chromodomain chromosome 8q12.1.

ONLINE INFORMATION ON GENETIC DISORDERS

An extremely useful and convenient resource for information on genetic disorders is Online Mendelian Inheritance in Man (OMIM; www.ncbi.nlm.nih.gov/sites/entrez?db=OMIM), an online database derived from the pioneering catalogue of Mendelian diseases compiled by Dr. Victor McKusick. Entering OMIM in your browser takes you to the search page, where entry of disease names or symptoms will yield the appropriate entries. McKusick assigned a unique number to each Mendelian or single gene disorder and started with 1 for autosomal dominant, 2 for autosomal recessive, 3 for X-linked, 4 for Y-linked, and 5 for mitochondrial diseases. Newer entries all start with a 6 that does not reflect the mechanism of inheritance. Another caveat about the OMIM catalogue is that some multifactorial or chromosomal disorders are listed, in part to record progress in finding single gene markers that are predictive of disease susceptibility (e.g., diabetes mellitus or schizophrenia) or are located within key chromosome regions (e.g., the RB retinoblastoma gene that was found through study of a chromosome 13 deletion).

Entering "Wilson disease" on the OMIM search page yields entry #277900, which summarizes the history, clinical findings, and relevant biochemical and molecular data when available. Key references are provided, as well as links to PubMed for relevant abstracts, to www.genetests.org to see which laboratories offer DNA testing for the condition, and even to chromosome location or DNA sequence data available in the human genome database at the time of collating, December 2007.

FURTHER READING

American Academy of Pediatrics, Committee on Genetics. (1996). Health supervision of children with Marfan syndrome. *Pediatrics, 98,* 978–982.

American Academy of Pediatrics, Committee on Genetics. (2001). Health supervision for children with Down syndrome. *Pediatrics, 107,* 442–449.

American Academy of Pediatrics, Committee on Genetics. (2003). Health supervision for children with Turner syndrome. *Pediatrics, 111,* 692–702.

Epstein, C. (2003). Genetic disorders and birth defects. In A. M. Rudolph, C. D. Rudolph, et al. (Eds.), *Rudolph's pediatrics* (21st ed.). Norwalk, CT: Appleton and Lange.

Gilbert-Barness, E., & Barness, L. A. (2000). *Metabolic diseases: Foundations of clinical management, genetics and pathology* (Vols. 1 and 2). South Natick, MA: Eaton.

Gilbert-Barness, E., & Barness, L. A. (2007). Metabolic disorders. In E. Gilbert-Barness (Ed.), *Potter's pathology of the fetus, infant, and child* (pp. 463–572). New York: Elsevier.

Gilbert-Barness, E., & Oligny, L. (2007). Chromosomal abnormalities. In E. Gilbert-Barness (Ed.), *Potter's pathology of the fetus, infant, and child.* New York: Elsevier.

Gorlin, R., Cohen, M., & Hennekan, R. (2001). *Syndromes of the head and neck* (4th ed.). New York: Oxford University Press.

Seidel, H. M., Rosenstein, B. J., & Pathak, A. (2001). *Primary care of the newborn* (3rd ed.). St. Louis: Mosby.

12

HEMATOLOGIC DISORDERS

If a man will begin with certainties he shall end in doubt, but if he will be content to begin with doubt he shall end in certainties.

NORMAL VALUES OF HEMOGLOBIN (Hb)

Age	Hb
32 weeks gestation	16.0 (18.5 ± 2.0)
Newborn	16.8 (13.7271–20.1)
3 months	12.0 (9.5–14.5)
6 months–6 years	12.0 (10.5–14.0)
7–12 years	13.0 (11.0–16.0)
Adult (female)	14.0 (12.0–16.0)
Adult (male)	16.0 (14.0–18.0)

Site of Sampling

Capillary samples give higher Hb/hematocrit (Hct) values than venous samples (see Figure 12.1). Differences average 3.5 gm/dl (5–25%) during first year of life. Age, hypotension, ambient temperatures, infants younger than 30 weeks of gestational age, small sick infants, acidosis, and red cell mass less than 35 ml/kg are factors that may influence these differences.

Capillary/venous Hct differences gradually decrease with gestational age. In healthy infants, the variations are only about 2.5% by one week of life.

Correct interpretation of Hb/Hct in the newborn is important in polycythemia. Hct higher than 65% (venous) can precipitate hyperviscosity syndrome, leading to hypoglycemia, central nervous system injury, and hyperbilirubinemia.

Pallor in the newborn may be due to asphyxia, acute severe blood loss, or hemolytic disease (Table 12.1).

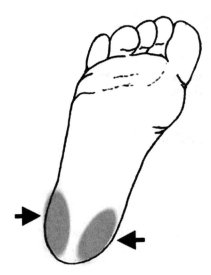

• Use for infants up to 12 months

• Performed only on the medial or lateral (inner or outer) plantar surface of either heel.

• Always perform puncture perpendicular to lines of footprint.

• *Precautionary Note:* If collecting from an infant's heel, do not force the blood to the puncture site by sliding the finger or thumb along the infant's sole. To do so is to risk damage to the undeveloped tendons of the foot. Instead, force the blood to the puncture site by gently rolling the thumb along the infants's sole from the middle of the foot to the heel.

• Neonates and infants should not be bandaged after the puncture - skin is much more sensitive to the effects of the adhesive and because of the risk of ingestion and/or airway obstruction should bandage become dislodged.

Figure 12.1
Procedure for doing a heelstick.

BLOOD LOSS IN THE NEWBORN

Fetomaternal hemorrhage diagnosed by Kliehauer-Betke test (presence of fetal red blood cells in maternal blood). If greater than 1% of fetal hemoglobin = approximately 50 ml fetal blood. Detectable in 50% of pregnancies but only causes anemia in 1% (Table 12.2).

• Fetofetal transfusion in twins—monoclonal pregnancies have 15% chance.
• Obstetric accident
• Neonatal blood loss

Isoimmune—Rh or ABO incompatibility and minor blood group incompatibilities, infection, disseminated intravascular coagulation, microangiopathy, galactosemia, red cell membrane defect (spherocytosis), enzyme deficiencies, glucose-6-phosphate dehydrogenase (G6PD), phosphate kinase (PK). Hemoglobinopathies—alpha thalassemia syndromes, Hb Barts.

ANEMIA OF INFANCY

Hb decreases in all newborns over the first few weeks of life with nadir at 10 weeks.

Premature infants may have exaggerated and more dramatic decrease in Hb called anemia of prematurity. Complex changes occur in Hb in response to availability of oxygen. Better oxygen availability after birth is due to various factors, including decrease in fetal hemoglobin (Hb F) and higher Hb A. There is increased

TABLE 12.1

Causes of Anemia

Classification of Anemia			
Reticulocyte Count	Microcytic Anemia	Normocytic Anemia	Macrocytic Anemia

Low	Iron deficiency
	Lead poisoning
	Chronic disease
	Aluminum toxicity
	Copper deficiency
	Protein malnutrition
	
	Pyridoxine deficiency
		Chronic deficiency
		RBC aplasia (TEC,
		  infection, drug induced)
		Malignancy
		Juvenile rheumatoid
		Arthritis
		Endocrinopathies
		Renal failure
			Folate deficiency
			Vitamin B_{12} deficiency
			Aplastic anemia
			Congenital bone marrow
			  dysfunction (Diamond-
			  Blackfan or Fanconi
			  syndrome)
			Drug induced
			Trisomy 21
			Hypothyroidism

Normal	Thalassemia trait Sideroblastic anemia	Acute bleeding Hypersplenism Dyserythropoietic anemia II	—

High	Thalassemia
	  syndromes
	Hemoglobin C
	  disorders
		Antibody-mediated
		  hemolysis
		Hypersplenism
		Microangiopathy (HUS,
		  TTP, DIC, Kasabach-
		  Merritt syndrome)
		Membranopathies
		  (spherocytosis,
		  elliptocytosis)
		Enzyme disorders (G-6-PD,
		  pyruvate kinase
		  deficiencies)
		Hemoglobinopathies
			Dyserythropoietic
			  anemia I, III
			Active hemolysis

DIC, disseminated intravascular coagulation; G-6-PD, glucose-6-phosphate dehydrogenase; TEC, transient erythroblastopenia of childhood; HUS, hemolytic-uremic syndrome; RBC, red blood cell; TTP, thrombotic thrombocytopenic purpura.
From Gilbert-Barness, E., & Barness, L. A. (2003). *Clinical use of pediatric diagnostic tests.* Baltimore: Lippincott Williams & Wilkins.

cardiac output, redistribution of flow, increased oxygen extraction, and left shift of oxygen dissociation curve.

Iron deficiency is the most prevalent hematological disease and occurs in 5%–10% of infants. Decreased mean corpuscular volume (MCV), decreased serum Fe, and decreased ferritin and increased fetal iron-binding capacity are usual.

In lead poisoning there is basophilic stippling of the erythrocytes with denatured RNA and interferences with heme synthesis through δ-ALA and ferrochelatase. Lead and FEP levels are increased with IQ/neurologic sequelae. Current accepted toxic range of lead is ≥0.5 μg/ml.

Diagnosis of thalassemia minor (β or α) is the presence of basophilic stippling, target cells, and by Hb electrophoresis that shows increased hemoglobin A2 in β thalassemia minor (Table 12.3).

TABLE 12.2

Hematologic Parameters of Frequent Causes of Anemia

	Iron Deficiency	β Thalassemia Trait	Chronic Inflammation	Lead Poisoning	Sickle Disease
Reticulocyte count	Low	Low	Normal	Low	High
RDW	↑	↓	Normal	↓	↑
Ferritin	↓	Normal to ↑	Normal	↓ to normal	↑ or normal
FEP	↑	Normal	↑	↑	Normal
Iron	↓	Normal	↓	↓ to normal	↑
TIBC	↑	Normal	↓		Normal or ↓
Electrophoresis	Normal	↑ HbA$_2$ or F	Normal	Normal	HbSS
ESR	Normal	Normal	↑	Normal	Low
Smear	Hypochromic, target cells	Normochromic, microcytic	Varies	Basophilic stippling	Sickle

↑, increased; ↓, decreased; ESR, erythrocyte sedimentation rate; F, fetal hemoglobin; FEP, free erythrocyte protoporphyrin; HbA$_2$, hemoglobin A$_2$; HbSS, hemoglobin SS; RDW, red cell distribution width; TIBC, total iron-binding capacity.
From Gilbert-Barness, E., & Barness, L. A. (2003). *Clinical use of pediatric diagnostic tests*. Baltimore: Lippincott Williams & Wilkins.

Congenital (Erythrocyte Underproduction)

- Diamond-Blackfan anemia
  Macrocytic anemia in first year
  Associated with other anomalies: short stature, musculoskeletal, heart defects
  Absent erythroid precursors on bone marrow aspirate
  Chronic transfusion therapy, steroids, bone marrow transplant
- Fanconi aplastic anemia
  Autosomal recessive
  Musculoskeletal abnormalities
  Chromosomal instability
  Progressive pancytopenia
  Predisposition to leukemia or lymphoma
  Treatment: bone marrow transplant

TABLE 12.3

D/D Microcytic Anemia

	MCV	RBC	MCV/RBC	FEB	Hb Electrophoresis
Iron deficiency	↓	↓	>13.0	30–150 mg	—
Lead poisoning	↓	↓	—	↑ 150	—
Thal trait	↓	↑ or N	<13.0	Normal	↑ A2

MCV, mean corpuscular volume; RBC, red blood cell; FEB, free erythrocytic protoporphyrin.

TABLE 12.4
Hemolytic Anemias

Hereditary Disorders	
Membrane defects	Hereditary spherocytosis, hereditary elliptocytosis, stomatocytosis, hereditary xerocytosis, pyropoikilocytosis, Macleod syndrome, Rh deficiency syndrome, other rare membrane disorders
Enzyme defects	G-6-PD deficiency, pyruvate kinase deficiency, glutathione pathway deficiency, deficiencies of the pentose pathway
Hemoglobin defects	Amino acid substitutions: hemoglobin S, hemoglobin C, etc.; decreased production; thalassemia
Acquired or extrinsic	
Infection, trauma	Bacterial: *Clostridium perfringens* infection
	Protozoal: malaria
	Viral: *Mycoplasma*, infectious mononucleosis
	Physiochemical damage: burns, oxidative and nonoxidative
	Mechanical damage: heart valve prosthesis (aortic), ulcerative colitis, hemolytic-uremic syndrome, TTP, DIC, hypersplenism
Antibody	Alloantibody: incompatible transfusion, fetal-maternal blood group incompatibility
	Autoantibody: idiopathic, secondary to malignant lymphomas, collagen vascular diseases, viral infections, secondary to drugs
Other	Paroxysmal nocturnal hemoglobinuria

DIC, disseminated intravascular coagulation; G-6-PD, glucose-6-phosphate dehydrogenase; TTP, thrombotic thrombocytopenic purpura.
From Gilbert-Barness, E., & Barness, L. A. (2003). *Clinical use of pediatric diagnostic tests.* Baltimore: Lippincott Williams & Wilkins.

Acquired

- Erythroid aplasia
  Aplastic crisis of hemolytic disease
  Parvovirus B-19 (erythema infectiosum, fifth disease)
- Aplastic anemia
  Maternal drug ingestion (azathioprine)
  Chloramphenicol
  Infectious (hepatitis)
  Trimethaprim-sulfate
- Folic acid and vitamin B_{12} deficiency
  Macrocytosis with or without anemia
  Hypothyroidism, trisomy 21, asplenia
  Differential diagnosis in neonate: goat milk anemia, methylmalonic aciduria, orotic aciduria, congenital folate malabsorption, transcobalamin II deficiency, short gut

Isoimmunization

- ABO incompatibility (Table 12.5)
  May occur in first pregnancy, without progression in subsequent pregnancies

TABLE 12.5

Differential Diagnosis of ABO and RL Isoimmunization

Findings	ABO	Rh_0
Clinical		
Pregnancy associated with disease	Any, including the first	After the first pregnancy
Clinical severity	Unpredictable, generally worse with B	Most severe with each antigen-positive pregnancy
Prenatal evaluation	None needed	Sequential anti-Rh_0 titers, amniocentesis
Onset of jaundice	3–4 days after delivery	Intrauterine or immediately after delivery
Treatment (options listed by increasing severity of hemolysis)	None; phototherapy or rarely exchange therapy	None; early delivery, phototherapy, exchange transfusion, or intrauterine transfusion
Laboratory		
Direct Coombs test	± to 1+	2+ to 4+
Fetal blood group	A, B, or AB	Rh_0 positive
Antibody causing hemolysis	Anti-A or anti-B	Anti-Rh_0 (anti-D)
Maternal blood group	O, A, B	Rh_0 or D^u negative
Maternal antibody screening	Negative	Positive
Peripheral blood (newborn)	Microspherocytes	Not diagnostic

From Gilbert-Barness, E., & Barness, L. A. (2003). *Clinical use of pediatric diagnostic tests.* Baltimore: Lippincott Williams & Wilkins.

Mild hemolysis; direct Coombs test may be positive
Microspherocytes in the peripheral smear
Late anemia (after first month)
• Rh incompatibility
Three linked genes with allele expression: C, c, D, E, e
ABO incompatibility may be protective
Clinical severity increases with each pregnancy; maternal antibody not predictive of severity; prior sensitization may have occurred from silent miscarriage
Prophylactic RhIG (Rhogam) at 28 weeks and delivery

Sickle Cell Anemia

Sickle cell anemia is a chronic hemoglobinopathy transmitted genetically, marked by moderately severe chronic hemolytic anemia, periodic acute painful episodes, and increased susceptibility to intercurrent infections, especially with encapsulated bacteria such as *Streptococcus pneumoniae*. The heterozygous condition (HbA/HbS) is called *sickle cell trait* and is usually asymptomatic, with no anemia.

Sickle cell anemia is autosomal recessive; therefore a homozygous presence is necessary for disease expression. The variant hemoglobin is HbS, sickle hemoglobin. Approximately 1 in 500 African Americans and 1 in 1,000 Hispanics have sickle cell anemia; 9% of African Americans have sickle cell trait.

Signs and Symptoms

Sickle cell anemia is often asymptomatic in the early months of life; after 6 months of age, the earliest symptoms are pallor and symmetric, painful swelling of the hands and feet (hand-foot syndrome). Chronic hemolytic anemia develops. Symptoms include painful crises involving bones, joints, abdomen, back, and viscera. These crises account for 90% of all hospital admissions of patients with sickle cell anemia. Mild scleral icterus; increased susceptibility to infections, especially pneumococcal sepsis and staphylococcal or *Salmonella* infections; osteomyelitis; functional asplenia; and delayed physical and sexual maturation, especially in boys, are common. Many multisystem complications may occur, particularly in later childhood and adolescence, especially episodes of acute chest syndrome (which presents a clinical picture consistent with pneumonia or infection).

A variety of crises and infections occur. The bases may be as follows:

1. Vasoocclusive ("painful crisis"): most common; pain results from tissue necrosis secondary to vascular occlusion and tissue hypoxia. Progressive organ failure and acute tissue damage result from repeated vasoocclusive episodes.
2. Aplastic crisis: temporary suppression of RBC production of bone marrow by severe infection such as parvovirus B19 infection.
3. Hyperthermolytic crisis: accelerated hemolysis; increased RBC fragility and shortened RBC life span.
4. Sequestration crisis: splenic sequestration of blood (only in infants and young children).

Patients with sickle cell anemia have susceptibility to infection with impaired or absent splenic function and a defect in the alternate pathway of complement activation.

Risk factors in sickle cell anemia include:

1. Vasoocclusive crisis: hypoxia, dehydration, infection, fever, acidosis, cold, anesthesia, strenuous physical exercise, smoking
2. Aplastic crisis: severe infections, human parvovirus B19 infection, folic acid deficiency (therefore, routine folic acid supplementation is recommended).
3. Hyperhemolytic crisis: acute bacterial infections and exposure to oxidant drugs

DIAGNOSIS OF HEMOGLOBINOPATHIES

Hemoglobinopathies are diagnosed by electrophoretic analysis of hemoglobin: isoelectric focusing, electrophoresis in cellulose acetate at alkaline pH and agar gel at acid pH, and electrophoresis of separated globin chains. Prenatal diagnosis by means of molecular tests with probes for the common mutations is possible.

In addition to the well-recognized HbA of normal adult erythrocytes, HbF of the normal fetus, and HbS of sickle cell anemia, many other abnormal hemoglobins have been discovered by electrophoresis. Hemoglobulins recognized in addition to these are designated C, D, E, G, H, I, J, and K. Disorders in which combinations of abnormalities have been seen include sickle cell anemia with HbC, HbD, HbE, and HbG; thalassemia with HbS, HbC, HbE, and HbG; spherocytosis with HbS; and elliptocytosis with hemoglobinopathy.

Hb Electrophoresis

HbS predominates, variable amount of HbF, no HbA. (In sickle cell trait, both HbS and HbA are present.)

Screening Tests

Sodium metabisulfite reduction test; Sickledex test.

Anemia

Hemoglobin level of approximately 8 g/dl (1.24 mmol/L); RBC indices usually normal but MCV > 75 μm^3 (75 fL). Reticulocytosis of 10%–20%, leukocytosis, bands normal in absence of infection, and thrombocytosis are typical. Peripheral smear shows few sickled RBCs, polychromasia, and nucleated RBCs. The peripheral smear in HbC disease shows numerous target cells and occasional microspherocytes and HbC crystals after splenectomy. The smear in HbC trait contains 65% HbA and 35% HbC, whereas in HbSC disease it contains approximately 52% HbS and 48% HbC. Target cells are seen in thalassemia, HbC disease, and HbS disease. Serum bilirubin level is mildly elevated (2–4 mg/dl [34–68 $\mu mol/L$]); fecal and urinary urobilinogen levels are high. Erythrocyte sedimentation rate is low; serum lactate dehydrogenase level is elevated; and haptoglobin is absent or present at very low levels.

If HbF, HbS, and HbA are present in a newborn, the differential diagnosis includes sickle cell trait or HbS/β^+ thalassemia. Repeat studies at 1 year of age may clarify the diagnosis.

Prenatal diagnosis can be accomplished using recombinant DNA techniques. Cells from the amniotic fluid can be tested for the aberrant gene at 16–20 weeks' gestation or chorionic villi can be sampled as early as 8–12 weeks.

THALASSEMIA SYNDROMES: HEMOGLOBINOPATHIES

- Alpha thalassemia
  Severity based upon number of genes expressed
  Alpha globin chains predominate from midgestation; therefore defects may be detected at birth
- Beta thalassemia
  Not usually diagnosed before 6 months unless blood loss or red cell destruction creates an unusually high demand for replacement of red cells

The thalassemias are a heterogenous group of inherited disorders, all characterized by a failure to synthesize one of the two globin chains (α or β) of HbA. The α globin chain gene resides on chromosome 16, and the β gene chain resides on chromosome 11.

The thalassemias can be classified clinically according to the degree of clinical severity, genetically according to their abnormal globin synthesis, or at the molecular level according to their particular gene mutation. Classification of the thalassemias is also complicated by the high frequency with which other structural hemoglobin abnormalities are associated with thalassemia, such as the presence of HbS, HbC, and HbE.

Two main clinical forms of alpha thalassemia are due to α globin chain deficiency. The first is one for which there is no production of α chain owing to the deletion of both chain genes in both alleles of chromosome 16. This form of alpha thalassemia is incompatible with life and produces fetal death associated with hydrops fetalis syndrome (Bart disease). The second is characterized by a reduced production of α globin due to deletion of three of four α chain genes. In this form (HbH disease), the anemia is moderate to severe. Examination of the peripheral blood smear shows, in addition to target cells, the inclusion of rod-shaped bodies in the RBCs. These bodies represent precipitates of HbH. Individuals who lack two α globin genes have thalassemia trait, and those who lack one α globin gene are silent carriers.

Thalassemia major (Cooley anemia), thalassemia intermedia, and thalassemia minor are due to a deficiency of the β chain of hemoglobin. The characteristic laboratory finding is mild hypochromic microcytic anemia. The beta thalassemia trait is clinically silent and is diagnosed when a peripheral blood smear is examined for other causes. Laboratory findings in thalassemia minor include hypochromic microcytic anemia (hemoglobin levels of 9–10 g/dl and MCV <75 fL) and elevated red cell diameter or distribution width. The peripheral blood smear shows anisopoikilocytosis. Target cells, in which the cell surface is increased in disproportion to its volume, are the characteristic RBC form. Resistance to falciparum malarial infections in carriers of thalassemia genes may have been a selective force for their survival.

RED CELL MEMBRANE DISORDERS

- Hereditary spherocytosis
  Autosomal dominant
  Neonatal jaundice with splenomegaly; spherocytes not always present
  Incubated osmotic fragility test positive
- Hereditary elliptocytosis
  Autosomal dominant
  Oval-shaped red blood cells
  Normal osmotic fragility
- Vitamin E deficiency
  Fat-soluble vitamin, antioxidant
  Reticulocytosis, thrombocytosis, acanthocytosis

BLEEDING DISORDERS

Differential diagnosis of bleeding includes the following (Table 12.6):

- Leukemia, malignancies
- Disseminated intravascular coagulation—sepsis

TABLE 12.6
Common Bleeding Disorders

	B.T.	P.T.	P.T.T.	Platelet Count	Diagnosis
Henoch-Schönlein purpura	N	N	N	N	History, physical, skin biopsy
Factor VIII deficiency	N	N	↑	N	Factor assay
Factor IX deficiency	N	N	↑	N	Factor assay
Von Willebrand	↑	N	↑ (mild)	N	Factor assay, VW platelet aggregation
Vitamin K deficiency	N	↑	↑	N	↓ factors VII, IX
DIC	↑	↑	↑	↓	Smear abnormal ↓ Factors V, VIII ↓ Fibrinogen ↑ FSP
Liver disease	↑	↑	↑	↓	↓ Liver-dependent factors
Platelet function defect	↑	N	N	Often N	Function studies

From Nathan, D. G., Orkin, S. H., Look, A. T., & Ginsburg, D. (2003). *Nathan and Oski's hematology of infancy and childhood* (6th ed.). Philadelphia: WB Saunders.

- Storage disorders
- Henoch-Schönlein purpura (HSP)
- Cavernous hemangioma (Kasabach-Merritt syndrome)
- Epstein-Barr virus infection with thrombocytopenia
- Vasculitis—systemic lupus erythematosus
- Drugs, particularly anticonvulsants
- Aplastic or hypoplastic anemia
- Thrombotic thrombocytopenic purpura
- Hemolytic uremic syndrome
- Child abuse

Causes of Neonatal Thrombocytopenia

- Maternal idiopathic thrombocytopenic purpura, autoimmune disorders
- Blood group incompatibility (isoimmune)
- Sepsis, disseminated intravascular coagulation
- Intrauterine viral infections, HIV
- Drugs
- Thrombocytopenia, absent radius (TAR) syndrome
- Congenital leukemia
- Histiocytosis X

Platelet Disorders

- Neonatal isoimmune thrombocytopenia purpura
  Prevalence of 1:2,000
  Mother, with normal platelet count, is platelet antigen PLA 1-negative in 2%

Infant possesses platelet antigen of paternal origin
Transplacental passage of IgG antibodies leads to sensitization of fetal platelets
Antenatal intracranial hemorrhage is possible
Treat with washed maternal platelets

- Autoimmune thrombocytopenia purpura
Passively acquired maternal antibodies
Mother may be thrombocytopenic, or have a normal platelet count if she has had splenectomy
Infant may require corticosteroids and IgG; but usually a self-limiting disorder in the neonate

Disseminated Intravascular Coagulation

- Paradoxical association of hemorrhage and thrombosis; normal delicate balance altered
- Activation of clotting system (bacterial endotoxins, hemolysis, AgAB complexes, neoplastic cells)

Etiology is related to infection (bacterial, viral), malignancy, Kasabach-Merritt syndrome, shock, burns, snakebite, or trauma.

Diagnosis is by clinical picture, anemia, schistocytes in the peripheral blood smear, increased prothrombin time, partial thromboplastin time (TT). Increased fibrin split products (FSP), decreased platelets, decreased factors V and VIII.

von Willebrand Disease

von Willebrand disease may present initially as recurrent epistaxis or hypermenorrhagia. Patients manifest increased bleeding time, increased partial thromboplastin time (mild), decreased factor VIII activity, and abnormal platelet aggregation. von Willebrand factor (vWF), an autosomally inherited factor, is a large multimeric glycoprotein that is essential in platelet adhesion to damaged vessel walls. There are types I, IIa, IIb, and III.

Hypercoagulable States

Manifestations are sick neonate, central line, homocystinuria, dehydration, protein C, protein S, antithrombin III deficiency, and immobilization. Causes are umbilical catheters and birth control pills.

WHITE BLOOD CELL DISORDERS

Most Common Cause of Acquired Neutropenia: Viral Infection

Patients with congenital neutropenia have severe, recurrent, and often fatal infections. Neonates may develop neutropenia from maternal factors such as hypertension, drug treatments given to the mother during late gestation, and maternal antibodies that cross the placenta and attack fetal granulocytes. A variety of distinct constitutional neutropenic disorders may manifest during the neonatal period and include rare hereditary disorders (Table 12.7). Severe sustained neutropenia characterizes

TABLE 12.7

Constitutional Disorders Associated With Neutropenia

Disorder	Age of Onset	Type of Defect
Cyclic neutropenia	Early infancy	Proliferation
Kostmann syndrome	Birth/early infancy	Proliferation
Shwachman-Diamond syndrome	Birth/early infancy	Proliferation
Immunodeficiency disorders, reticular dysgenesis	Early infancy	Proliferation
Chédiak-Higashi syndrome	Early infancy	Maturation
Myelokathexis	Early infancy	Maturation
Fanconi anemia	Infancy/childhood/ adulthood (rare)	Proliferation
Dyskeratosis congenita	Infancy	Proliferation

From Gilbert-Barness, E., & Barness, L. (2003). *Clinical use of pediatric diagnostic tests.*
Baltimore: Lippincott Williams & Wilkins, pp. 411–412.

Kostmann syndrome and Chédiak-Higashi syndrome, whereas patients with cyclic neutropenia exhibit episodic loss of neutrophils followed by a rebound recovery. As with neonates, infection is a common cause of neutropenia in older children. Because of the variety of underlying causes, patients with neutropenia have diverse clinical manifestations.

Neutropenia Causes

Neonatal Infections

Maternal hypertension or drug treatment
Maternal antibody production (e.g., in systemic lupus erythematosus)
Constitutional disorders such as cyclic neutropenia
Infantile genetic agranulocytosis
Kostmann syndrome
Chédiak-Higashi syndrome
Phenotypic abnormalities

Infant/Child Infections

Autoimmune neutropenia
Neoplasms replacing bone marrow
Idiosyncratic drug reactions
Myeloablative therapies
Constitutional neutropenic disorders
Megaloblastic anemias, adult-type pernicious anemia
Copper deficiency (rare)
Hypersplenism
Metabolic disease (e.g., aminoacidemia, organic acidemia)
Aleukemic leukemia
Aplastic anemia
Idiopathic

TABLE 12.8
Serologic Profile in Infectious Mononucleosis
(Epstein-Barr Virus Infection)

Antibody	Acute (0–3 mo)	Recent (3–12 mo)	Past (>12 mo)
Heterophil	+	–	–
EBV specific			
VCA IgM	+	–	–
VCA IgG	+	+	+
EA	+ or –	+ or –	–
EBNA	–	+	+

EA, early antigen; EBNA, Epstein-Barr nuclear antigen; EBV, Epstein-Barr virus; Ig, immunoglobulin; Negative, no detectable antibody; Positive, detectable antibody; VCA, viral capsid antigen.
From Gilbert-Barness, E., & Barness, L. A. (2003). *Clinical use of pediatric diagnostic tests.* Baltimore: Lippincott Williams & Wilkins.

Infectious Mononucleosis

For a serologic profile of mononucleosis, see Table 12.8.

LEUKEMIA

Types of Leukemia Seen in Children

- Acute lymphoblastic leukemia (ALL)—70% (Table 12.9)
- Acute nonlymphoblastic leukemia (ANLL)—27%
- Chronic myelogenous leukemia (CML)—3%
- All subtypes:
  Early Pre-B ALL (65%–70%): common phenotype, null, negative SIg, negative Cig, CALLA positive/negative
  Pre-B ALL (15%–20%): negative SIg, positive Cig, negative T
  T-cell ALL: positive T-cell antigens
  B-cell ALL: positive SIg, B-cell antigens

Common Presenting Symptoms

Fever
Pallor
Bleeding
General malaise
Bone pain
Abdominal pain
Joint pain
Lymphadenopathy
Hepatosplenomegaly

TABLE 12.9

French-American-British (FAB) Classification and Histochemical Features of the Acute Nonlymphoblastic Leukemias

Designation	Predominant Cell Type (S)	Histochemistry
M1 (undifferentiated myelocytic)	Myeloblasts	MP+, SB+
M2 (myelocytic)	Myeloblasts, promyelocytes, myelocytes	MP+, SB+
M3 (promyelocytes)	Hypergranular promyelocytes	MP+, SB+
M4 (myelomonocytic)	Promyelocytes, myelocytes, promonocytes, monocytes	MP+, NSE+, SB+
M5a (monoblastic)	Monoblasts	NSE+
M5b (differentiated monocytic)	Monoblasts, promonocytes, monocytes	NSE+
M6 (erythroleukemia)	Erythroblasts	MP+, PAS+, SB+
M7 (megakaryocytic)	Megakaryocytes	NSE+, PAS+

PAS, periodic Acid-Schiff; MP, myeloperoxidase; SB, Sudan black; NSE, nonspecific esterase.

Abnormal Physical Findings

Pallor
Purpura
Fever
Lymphadenopathy
Hepatosplenomegaly

POLYCYTHEMIA

- Venous hematocrit >65%, hemoglobin >22 grams percent
- Affects 1.5%–4% of all newborns in first week of life
- Possible causes:
  Twin-twin transfusion
  Maternofetal transfusion
  Delayed cord clamping
- Associations include
  Placental insufficiency: small for gestational age, postmaturity, toxemia of pregnancy
  Placenta previa
  Maternal diabetes

HEMOSTASIS: HEMORRHAGIC DISEASES

Hemorrhagic Disease of the Newborn

- Vitamin K deficiency
- Secondary to liver disease, malabsorption, antibiotics, coumadin
- Breast-fed infants at higher risk
- Occurs at 1–7 days, rarely with intracranial hemorrhage

- Late disease occurs at 1–3 months presenting with intracranial bleed
- Prevention: prophylaxis with vitamin K

Hemophilia A and B

- X-linked disorder, incidence 1:10,000 males
- Hemophilia A (VIII) 70%, hemophilia B (IX) 30%
- Factors do not cross placenta
- Bleeding from venipuncture sites, umbilical stump, circumcision; intracranial hemorrhage
- Milder forms (B) may be missed in infancy

Differential Diagnosis of Petechiae

Antibody Mediated

- Thrombotic thrombocytopenic purpura
- Immunologic disorders
- Infection

Coagulopathy

- Disseminated intravascular coagulation
- Sepsis
- Necrotizing enterocolitis
- Cavernous hemangioma (Kasabach-Merritt syndrome)

Congenital

- Fanconi anemia: pancytopenia usually does not occur until after the age of 5; associated with short stature, hyperpigmentation, thumb anomalies, renal problems, and microcephaly; autosomal recessive
- Wiskott-Aldrich syndrome: immune defects with increased IgE and IgA and decreased IgM; associated with eczema and thrombocytopenia; X-linked
- Thrombocytopenia absent radii (TAR): autosomal recessive
- May-Heglin anomaly: giant platelets and leukocyte inclusions
- Bernard-Soulier disease: giant platelets
- Glanzmann thrombocytopenia
- Metabolic disorders
- Osteopetrosis

Acquired Decreased Production

- Leukemia or other malignancy
- Aplastic anemia
- Folate or vitamin B_{12} deficiency

Other Causes

- Hemolytic uremic syndrome
- Thrombotic thrombocytopenic purpura

- Drug-induced
- Hypersplenism
- Respiratory distress syndrome
- Uremia
- Progressive pigmentary dermatosis (Schamberg disease): Petechiae typically over the lower extremities

LYMPHOMAS

Lymphomas are generally classified into two main histologic types: Hodgkin lymphoma and non-Hodgkin lymphoma (NHL). Hodgkin lymphoma is extremely rare in children less than 3 years of age. NHL is frequently associated with leukemia or immunodeficiency disease (Tables 12.10, 12.11). Blast cells in peripheral blood and bone marrow make the differentiation of lymphoma from ALL difficult. Lymph node biopsy is required for the diagnosis of lymphomas.

TABLE 12.10
Clinical Features of Common Pediatric Lymphomas

Clinical Features	Diagnosis	Comment
Mediastinum		
Child or teenager, male, rapid growth	Lymphoblastic (convoluted) T lymphoma	May have respiratory failure, pleural or pericardial effusion, superior vena caval syndrome, rapid response to steroids
Teenager or young adult, female, rapid growth	Large B-cell lymphoma	May have compression symptoms
Teenager or young adult, female, slow growth	Hodgkin disease, nodular sclerosing type	May have superior vena caval obstruction, tracheal compression, parasternal mass
Abdomen, Gastrointestinal Tract, Ovary		
Child or young adult, rapid growth	Small transformed (noncleaved) lymphoma, Burkitt type	Nonendemic form
Nodes, Cervical or Axillary		
Child or teenager, slow growth	Hodgkin disease, lymphocyte-predominant type	
Child or teenager, rapid growth	Anaplastic large-cell lymphoma, CD30+	May present with small-cell variant with clinical features suggesting infection
Bone		
Child, rapid growth	Small transformed (noncleaved) lymphoma, Burkitt type	Endemic form

Modified from Collins, R. D., & Swerdlow, S. A. (2001). *Pediatric hematopathology.* New York: Churchill Livingstone.

TABLE 12.11

Cell of Origin, Major Genotypic and Karyotypic Abnormalities, and Epstein-Barr Virus
Association in Major Types of Pediatric Lymphomas

Diagnosis	Cell Type and Other Important Cellular Constituents	Major Genotypic or Karyotypic Abnormalities	EBV Association
Burkitt lymphoma	B cell similar to those in follicular center or transformed memory-type B cell	*MYC* rearrangement from 8q24 immunoglobulin heavy chain (14q32) or, less often, to κ (2p11) or λ (22q11); *MYC* mutations	Endemic: almost all EBV positive Sporadic: 10%–40% EBV positive
T-lymphoblastic lymphoma	Thymic type I lymphoblast	Translocations involving T-cell receptor (α, β, γ, or δ chains on 14q11, 7q32, 14q11, or 7p15, respectively) and protooncogenes (mostly transcription factors)	None
Anaplastic large-cell (Ki-1 antigen positive) lymphoma	Cytotoxic T cell; less often, "null" (indeterminate) cell	t(2;5)(P23;P35) involving *nucleophosmin* gene (5) and anaplastic lymphoma kinase gene (2) with *NPM/ALK* fusion product ("p80")	Usually none
HD, nodular lymphocyte predominance	Follicular center B cell ("L and H" Reed-Sternberg variants)	No consistent abnormality in these clonal B cells	None
HD, nodular sclerosis and mixed cellularity types	Reed-Sternberg cells in some cases resemble follicular center cells but do not show immunoglobulin gene expression; some cases of T-cell origin; others undefined Reactive cellular elements that, like Reed-Sternberg cells, are important in cytokine secretion	No consistent abnormality but typically aneuploid	>50% EBV positive, with highest proportion in children <10 years old

HD, Hodgkin disease.
From Collins, R. D., & Swerdlow, S. H. (2001). *Pediatric hematopathology.* New York: Churchill Livingstone.

NHL in childhood is virtually limited to three histologic types:

1. Lymphoblastic lymphoma: 30%–35% small noncleaved cell (undifferentiated)
2. Burkitt and non-Burkitt types: 40%–50%
3. Large-cell lymphoma: 15%–20%

FURTHER READING

Bellinger, D. C. (2004). Lead. *Pediatrics 113*(4 suppl.), 1016–1022.

d'Amore, E. S., Menin, A., Bonoldi, E., Bevilacqua, P., Cazzavillan, S., Donofrio, V., et al. (2007). Anaplastic large cell lymphomas: A study of 75 pediatric patients. *Pediatric and Developmental Pathology, 10*(3), 181–191.

Felix, C. A., & Lange, B. J. (1999). Leukemia in infants. *Oncologist, 4*, 225–240.

Hoffbrand, A. V., & Herbert, V. (1999). Nutritional anemias. *Seminars in Hematology, 36* (4 suppl. 7), 13–23.

Isaac, H. Jr. (2003). Fetal and neonatal leukemia. *Journal of Pediatric Hematology and Oncology, 25*, 348–361.

Italiano, J. E. Jr., & Shivdasani, T. A. (2003). Megakaryocytes and beyond: The birth of platelets. *Journal of Thrombosis and Haemostasis, 1*, 1174–1182.

Mannucci, P. M. (2004). Treatment of von Willebrandt's disease. *New England Journal of Medicine, 351*, 683.

Motta, M., Tincani, A., Lojacono, A., Faden, D., Gorla, R., Airò, P., et al. (2004). Neonatal outcome in patients with rheumatic disease. *Lupus, 13*, 718–723.

Panagiotou, J. P., & Douros, K. (2004). Clinicolaboratory findings and treatment of iron-deficiency anemia in childhood. *Pediatric Hematology and Oncology, 21*, 521–534.

Paraskevas, F. (2004). Clusters of differentiation. In J. P. Greer, J. Foerster, I. N. Lukens, et al. (Eds.), *Wintrobe's clinical hematology* (11th ed., pp. 27–98). Philadelphia: Lippincott Williams & Wilkins.

Perkins, S. L. (2000). Diagnosis of anemia. In C. Kjeldsberg (Ed.), *Practical diagnosis of hematologic disorders* (3rd ed., pp. 3–22). Chicago: ASCP Press.

Perkins, S. L. (2004). Pediatric red cell disorders and pure red cell aplasia. *American Journal of Clinical Pathology, 122*(suppl.), S70–S86.

Reddy, K. S., & Perkins, S. L. (2004). Advances in the diagnostic approach to childhood lymphoblastic malignant neoplasms. *American Journal of Clinical Pathology, 122*(suppl.), S3–S18.

Russell, J. B. (2003). Fetal and neonatal cytopenias: What have we learned? *American Journal of Perinatology, 20*, 425–431.

Saxena, R., Kannan, M., & Choudhry, V. P. (2003). Neonatal thrombosis. *Indian Journal of Pediatrics, 70*, 903.

Sosothikul, D., Seksarn, P., & Lusher, J. M. (2007). Pediatric reference values for molecular markers in hemostasis. *Journal of Pediatric Hematology and Oncology, 29*(1), 19–22.

Tefferi, A. (2005). Blood eosinophilia: A new paradigm in disease classification, diagnosis and treatment. *Mayo Clinic Proceedings, 80*, 75–83.

van den Akker, E. S., & Oepkes, D. (2008). Fetal and neonatal alloimmune thrombocytopenia. *Best Practice and Research, Clinical Obstetrics and Gynaecology, 22*, 3–14.

Zeidler, C., Schwinzer, B., & Welte, K. (2003). Congenital neutropenias. *Reviews in Clinical and Experimental Hematology, 7*, 72–83.

13

INFECTIONS

How much better it is to get wisdom than gold; to get understanding rather than silver.

Proverbs 15:16

BACTERIAL PATHOGENS

Gram-Positive Rods
   Clostridium botulinum
   Clostridium tetani
   Corynebacterium diphtheriae
   Listeria monocytogenes
Gram-Positive Cocci
   Staphlococcus aureus
   Streptococcus pneumoniae
   Streptococcus pyogenes (GAS)
   Streptococcus agalactiae (GBS)
   Enterococcus

Gram-Negative Cocci
   Neisseria meningitidis
   Neisseria gonorrhoeae

Gram-Negative Rods
   Bastonella henselae
   Bordetella pertusis
   Haemophilus influenzae
   Yersinia pestis
   Pasteurella multicida
   Escherichia coli
   Pseudomonas spp.
   Salmonella spp.
   Shigella spp.
   Campylobacter jejuni
Viruses
Herpes simplex virus
Influenza
Mumps
Rotavirus
Rous sarcoma virus
Roseola
Rabies

Botulism

Clostridium botulinum causes neurotoxin production (A, B, E, and F). Its spores are ingested from contaminated food products. Infection is acquired from honey (if < 1 year old), canned foods, and corn syrup. Clinical manifestations include weak cry, respiratory failure, constipation, hypotonia, poor feeding, and decreased gag reflex. Laboratory diagnosis is based on stool culture and on toxin detection in stool. Treatment includes botulism immune globulin intravenous and avoidance of antibiotics.

Tetanus—*Clostridium tetani*

Tetanus is acquired by wound contamination with *Clostridium tetani*, which then produces tetanospasmin. Clinical manifestations include trismus from muscular spasms (lockjaw). There is generalized, localized, cephalic, and neonatal boardlike abdominal wall. Treatment is administration of metronidazole, tetanus antitoxin, or penicillin and wound debridement. Penicillin is an alternative antibiotic.

Diphtheria—*Corynebacterium diphtheriae* (Gram-Positive Pleomorphic Bacilli)

Diphtheria is transmitted by droplets or fomites with an incubation period of 2–4 days. The toxin inhibits protein synthesis with subsequent tissue necrosis. The toxin can spread hematogenously and produce injury in distant sites. Clinical manifestations include nasal diphtheria, pharyngeal or tonsillar diphtheria with severe lymphadenopathy (bull neck), distinctive mousy odor, and laryngeal diphtheria (pseudomembrane). Other sites include skin, conjuctiva, and genitals. Myocarditis occurs at 2 weeks of illness and central nervous system (CNS) manifestations occur later. Laboratory diagnosis requires culture on Loeffler media, Tellurite, or blood agar. Treatment requires intravenous equine antitoxin and penicillin or erythromycin for 7 days and immunization with diphtheria toxoid after recovery.

Listeriosis—*Listeria monocytogenes*

Listeriosis is more frequently observed at the extremes of life. Clinical manifestations in neonates may be in utero infections (spontaneous abortion), granulomatosis infanti septica, and premature onset of labor associated with prematurity. Later onset is associated with meningitis and other manifestations including purulent conjunctivitis, papular rash, and jaundice. Older children may have bacteremia and meningitis, especially in immunosuppressed individuals, thomboencephalitis, brain abscesses, and endocarditis are linked to underlying gastrointestinal disease. The organism is susceptible to ampicillin and TMP-SMX.

Streptococcus pneumoniae—Gram-Positive Diplococci (Alpha-Hemolytic Colonies)

There are over 90 serotypes of *Streptococcus pneumoniae*. Most common in the United States are 19, 6A, 23, 14, 3, 9N, 11, and 18. Spread is by nasopharyngeal route. Clinical manifestations include otitis media, occult bacteremia, sinusitis, pharyngitis, meningitis, and pneumonia. Laboratory diagnosis is by Gram stain and culture from clean sites (blood, cerebrospinal fluid [CSF], middle ear), repeat lumbar puncture after 48 hours of treatment in case of meningitis, leukocytosis with white blood cell count >15,000. Susceptibility tests to penicillin and ceftriaxone or cefotaxime should be performed on all isolates. Recent addition of conjugate vaccine has reduced invasive disease. S. pneumoniae has had a sharp increase in penicillin resistance.

Group A Streptococcus—*Streptococcus pyogenes*

M-proteins are major antigenic determinants. Clinical manifestations include rhinitis, pharyngotonsillitis, scarlet fever, pyoderma (cellulitis), toxic shock syndrome, necrotizing fasciitis, suppurative cervical adenitis, peritonsillar abscess, retropharyngeal abscess, pneumonia with empyema and nonsuppurative complications, and perianal cellulitis. Rheumatic fever has (associated with tonsillopharyngitis) as major manifestations carditis, arthritis (migratory), nodules (subcutaneous), chorea (Sydenham), and erythema marginatum; acute glomerulonephritis is associated with pyoderma and tonsillopharyngitis and pediatric autoimmune neuropsychiatric disorders associated with streptococcal infection. Minor manifestations for rheumatic fever include previous rheumatic fever or rheumatic heart disease, arthralgia, and fever. Laboratory diagnosis includes throat culture, rapid tests (nitrous acid extraction of group A carbohydrate), antistreptolysins O, anti-DNAse B, and streptozyme. Rapid antigen detection tests provide results at the time of the office visit, though backup throat culture of negative rapid streptococcal tests (RST) is still recommended.

Group B Streptococcus—Classified Into Serotypes (1a, 1b, II, III, IV, V, and VI)

Serotype III is associated with neonatal meningitis. Early onset is infection 0–7 days of life. Late-onset infection is 8 days–3 months of life. Clinical manifestations with early onset include lethargy, apnea or bradycardia, poor feeding, hypothermia, hyperthermia, septicemia, pneumonia, meningitis; late onset includes meningitis, osteomyelitis, cellulitis, adenitis, and arthritis. Laboratory diagnosis includes leukocytosis or leucopenia, left shift, GBS in maternal amniotic fluid, blood, or CSF cultures, latex agglutination tests, and minimum inhibitory concentration (MIC) to penicillin to rule out tolerant strains. All pregnant women should be screened at 35–37 weeks gestation. If the mother is GBS positive, she needs to receive antibiotics more than four hours prior to delivery.

Staphylococcus Spp.—*Staphylococcus aureus*

Clinical manifestations of staph include localized infections: cellulitis, furuncles, impetigo, lymphadenitis, and wound infections. Invasive infections include bacteremia, septicemia, endocarditis, pericarditis, pneumonia, pleural empyema, pyomyositis, osteomyelitis, and arthritis. Toxin-mediated syndromes include toxic shock syndrome, staphylococcal scalded skin syndrome, and food poisoning. Treatment for methicillin-sensitive *Staphylococcus aureus*) includes β-lactamase-resistant antimicrobials (nafcillin, oxacillin) and first- or second-generation cephalosporins (cefazolin or cefuroxime); MRSA (methicillin-resistant *Staphylococcus aureus*) treatment includes vancomycin, clindamycin, TMP-SMX, and linezolid. MRSA is the most prevalent form of *Staphylococcus aureus* in many parts of the country.

Coagulase Negative—Staphylococcus *Spp.*

A major cause of nosocomial infections, especially in the presence of indwelling devices, and are the most common organisms in vascular catheter and ventriculo-peritoneal (VP) shunt infections, sensitive to vancomycin, linezolid, vancomycin and rifampin, or vancomycin and gentamicin.

Enterococcus—*Enterococcus faecalis, Enterococcus faecium*

Infection may occur in hospitalizations, prior use of antibiotics, or in immunocompromised patients. During the neonatal period, septicemia, meningitis, early-onset infection (0–7 days), and late-onset infection (>7 days) may occur. In older children, cytomegalovirus (CMV) infections, endocarditis, urinary tract infection, peritonitis, and intraabdominal abscesses can occur. It may be sensitive to ampicillin, ampicillin and aminoglycoside (if high-level aminoglycoside resistance is excluded), or vancomycin (if β-lactamase resistance is documented). Linezolid (if vancomycin and β-lactamase resistance are documented).

Note that cephalosporins are not effective against enterococcal infections.

Neisseria meningitidis

Fifty percent of cases occur in children younger than 16 years of age. Transmission may occur up to 24 hours after initiation of treatment. The major risk factors are complement deficiencies (C5–C9, properdin) and asplenia, and for military recruits and college freshmen in dorms. Most severe are meningococcemia (disseminated intravascular coagulation [DIC], Waterhouse-Friderichsen syndrome), meningitis, pneumonia, febrile occult bacteremia, endophthalmitis, septic arthritis, myocarditis, and pericarditis. Diagnosis requires cultures of blood, CSF, body fluid (pleural, synovial), petechial lesions, and CSF antigen detection by latex agglutination. Treatment requires high doses (IV) of penicillin G, cefotaxime, or ceftriaxone. Chemoprophylaxis includes rifampin, ceftriaxone, azithromycin, or ciprofloxacin. Immunoprophylaxis is obtained with polysaccharide meningococcal vaccine, which includes serogroups A, C, Y, and W-135, licensed for use in children older than 2 years, and meningococcal C conjugate vaccine.

Neisseria gonorrhoeae—Gram-Negative Oxidase-Positive Diplococci

Transmission by genital contact. Clinical manifestations in the newborn are ophthalmia neonatorum, bacteremia, and meningitis. In prepubertal children, if due to genital tract colonization or infection, strongly consider sexual abuse. In adolescents it is usually an asymptomatic infection (more common in females), though urethritis, cervicitis, salpingitis, pharyngitis, pelvic inflammatory disease, perihepatitis (FitzHugh-Curtis syndrome), and disseminated infection (arthritis-dermatitis syndrome) can occur. Diagnosis is by Gram-stained smear of exudates or lesions, culture (inoculate on culture media immediately after collection, using chocolate agar, Thayer-Martin media, or NYC media), polymerase chain reaction (PCR), and ligase chain reaction. Newborns are treated with extended spectrum cephalosporin (ceftriaxone sodium), ophthalmia neonatorum 125 mg ceftriaxone, and hospitalization.

Disseminated infection requires ceftriaxone/cefotaxime for 7 days. Cefotaxime should be used in case of hyperbilirubinemia and meningitis with ceftriaxone/cefotaxime for 14 days. In older children, ceftriaxone and azithromycin and in complicated infection with ceftriaxone for 7 days, doxycycline for 14 days, and endocarditis with ceftriaxone for 28 days. Prophylaxis for ophthalmia neonatorum is 1% silver nitrate, 1% tetracycline, or 0.5% erythromycin ophthalmic ointment.

Pertussis—*Bordetella pertussis*

Infants younger than 6 months of age are most frequently affected; adults with waning immunity are a significant reservoir and vaccine-induced immunity is not likely after 12 years. For this reason, pertussis vaccine is now reported in adolescents. Clinical manifestations include three stages: catarrhal, paroxysmal, and convalescent. Laboratory diagnosis: blood white cell count includes leukocytosis with lymphocytosis; culture is the gold standard (Regan-Lowe, Stainer-Scholte); direct fluorescent antibody and PCR. Treatment is with erythromycin esolate 40 mg/kg/day every 6 hours for 14 days. Treatment with erythromycin is associated with hypertrophic pyloric stenosis. Clarithromycin and azithromycin are effective. Prophylaxis and erythromycin is required for all close contacts.

Haemophilus influenzae Type B

Clinical manifestations include cellulitis, meningitis, pneumonia, epiglottitis, septic arthritis, and occult febrile bacteremia. Laboratory diagnosis is by blood culture, CSF culture, synovial fluid cultures, chocolate agar enriched with factors X and V, and latex particle agglutination for detection of type capsular antigen in CSF. All isolates from sterile sites should be serotyped. Treatment is cefotaxime or ceftriaxone, and dexamethasone for children with meningitis. In children suspected to have epiglottitis, be prepared to establish an airway. Invasive *Haemophilus influenzae* has become quite infrequent since conjugate vaccinations.

Yersinia pestis—Plague

More common in New Mexico, Arizona, California, and Colorado. Enzootic infection is in squirrels, prairie dogs, and wild rodents. The vector is fleas. Clinical manifestations include bubonic plague, septicemic plague, and pneumonic (primary vs. secondary) plague. Laboratory diagnosis includes "safety pin" appearance on Gram stain, fluorescent antibody test, cultures from blood or tissue, and PCR. Treatment is with streptomycin sulfate the treatment of choice, with gentamicin sulfate, doxycycline or tetracycline (>8 years old), or chloramphenicol preferred for meningitis.

Pasteurella multicida—Gram-Negative Rod/Coccobacilli

Pasteurella multicida is transmitted by animal bites. Clinical manifestations include cellulitis, lymphadenopathy, osteomyelitis, septic arthritis, and tenosynovitis. Treatment is with penicillin, amoxicillin-clavulanate, TMP-SMX, or doxycycline.
Note: Do not use clindamycin, erythromycin, or first-generation cephalosporins.

Pseudomonas aeruginosa

Major associations are with cystic fibrosis, chronic granulomatous disease, burns, and immunocompromised (ecthyma gangrenosum) children. Treatment is with ceftazidime (or cefepime) and aminoglycoside, or anti-*Pseudomonas* penicillin and aminoglycoside.

Escherichia coli — *E. coli* 0157:H7

Shiga toxin-producing *E. coli* (STEC) is associated with bloody diarrhea and with hemolytic uremic syndrome (see Chapter 7). MacConkey agar with sorbitol is used for screening. Antibiotic therapy is contraindicated. Enteric gram negative infections are listed in Table 13.1.

OTHER INFECTIOUS AGENTS

Treponema pallidum — Syphilis

Manifestations include hepatosplenomegaly, snuffles, lymphadenopathy, mucocutaneous lesions, and osteochondritis. Late congenital manifestations include Hutchinson triad (keratitis, deafness, Hutchinson teeth), Clutton joints, Mulberry molar, and rhagades. Acquired syphilis manifestations: in primary stage, painless chancre; secondary stage, rash on palms and soles involvement and condyloma lata; tertiary stage, gumma, cardiovascular involvement; neurosyphilis can occur at any stage.

Laboratory diagnosis consists of using dark field microscopy, nontreponemal tests, which includes VDRL, RPR, and ART; treponemal tests include FTA-ABS and TP-PA. Treatment in congenital infected patients is with penicillin G for 10 days; early syphilis with penicillin G benzathine × 1; more than 1 year with penicillin G benzathine weekly × 3 weeks and neurosyphilis with penicillin G IV for 10–14 days (±) or with benzathine penicillin weekly × 3.

Ticks — *Borrelia burgdorferi* (Lyme Disease)

Tick vectors: *Ixodes scapularis* and *Ixodes pacificus*, located in the Northeast, Midwest, and West Coast of the United States.

Clinical manifestations include:

- Early localized: erythema migrans (single lesion), headache, malaise, fever, and arthralgias
- Early disseminated: erythema migrans (multiple lesions), cranial nerve palsies (facial), carditis with heart block, and conjunctivitis.
- Late manifestations: recurrent arthritis (pauciarticular), CNS manifestations

Diagnosis includes:

- Early: mainly clinical
- Late and disseminated disease: clinical and serology
- Serology: high probability of false positive results in low-risk patients

TABLE 13.1
Enteric Gram Negative Infections

	Campylobacter jejuni	Salmonella Spp.	Shigella Spp.	Yersinia enterocolitica
Reservoir	Poultry, dogs, cats, hamsters, birds	Poultry, reptiles, livestock	Humans	Swine
Special populations		Hemoglobinopathies		Hemoglobinopathies desferrioxamine use
Transmission	Food, water, unpasteurized milk, fecal-oral	Food, pet contact, water	Fecal-oral, food, flies	Water, food, (chitterlings), RBC transfusions
Treatment	Erythromycin Azithromycin Doxycycline	Uncomplicated: Do not treat Complicated: TMP-SMX Cefotaxime Ceftriaxone	TMP-SMX Ampicillin Ceftriaxone	TMP-SMX Aminoglycosides Cefotaxime Doxycycline
Bloody diarrhea	++	+	+++	++
Laboratory tests	Dark field, Gram stain, stool, blood culture	Blood, stool, tissue cultures	Shiga toxin, stool culture	Blood, stool, body fluid culture, antibody titers
Bacteremia	+ infants	+	+	≤1 year
Methylene-blue in stool WBC	++	++	+++	++
Focal infections	Uncommon	Meningitis, reactive arthritis		Abscesses, meningitis
Other clinical manifestations	E. nodosum, Reiter syndrome, Guillain-Barré		HUS, Reiter syndrome	E. nodosum, reactive arthritis, HLA-B27
Toxic megacolon	–	–	+	–
Mesenteric adenitis	–	–	–	+
Encephalopathy	–	–	+ (Ekiri syndrome)	–

Treatment with early localization is with doxycycline if >8 years or amoxicillin <8 years.

Rocky Mountain Spotted Fever—*Rickettsia rickettsii*

Manifestations include systemic small-vessel vasculitis, centrifungal rash before the sixth day of illness, and may have systemic complaints. Symptoms last up to 3 weeks with severe neurologic sequelae. Disease is transmitted by tick bite (dog or wood tick) and usually affects children <15 years of age. Peak season is summer months in Southeast and central United States.

Diagnosis is by serology. Treatment with decision based on clinical grounds and if suspicious, treat with doxycycline regardless of age of patient.

Mycobacterium tuberculosis

High-risk groups include those who are foreign born or homeless. Transmission is by inhalation. A pediatric case equals an adult or adolescent index case. Incubation period is between 2 and 12 weeks. Clinical manifestations include, for TB infection (LTBI), a positive tuberculin skin test but otherwise asymptomatic. Active TB manifestations include fever, failure to thrive, cough, chills, night sweats, or extrapulmonary manifestations such as meningitis.

Diagnosis is by purefied protein derivative (PPD) (interpretation in patients with previous bacille Calmette-Guérin [BCG] administration is the same), culture of early morning gastric aspirate, sputum culture, or chest x-ray (A/P and lateral).

Tuberculin Skin Test

Reaction	Applies to the following groups
≥5 mm	TB contact, TB suspect (X-ray, clinical), immunosuppressed (HIV, steroid, medications)
≥10 mm	Age <4 years, medical risk factors (DM, RF, malnutrition), high prevalence area
≥15 mm	All

Treatment for latent TB (i.e., positive PPD and no disease) is with isoniazid for 9 months or with rifampin if contact with patients harboring INH-resistant M tuberculosis. There is an increasing incidence worldwide of multidrug-resistant TB.

ATYPICAL MYCOBACTERIA

Mycobacterium marinum

Mycobacterium marinum is associated with injury during water-related activities with development of purpuric/bluish lesions. Diagnosis is based on clinical suspicion subsequently proved by biopsy and culture. Treatment is by excision, rifampin, and clarithromycin.

Mycobacterium avium Complex

Associated with cellular immunosuppression.

Mycobacterium scrofulaceum and *Mycobacterium kansaii*

Associated with suppurative cervical lymphadenitis.

Mycobacterium fortuitum, Mycobacterium kansasii, and *Mycobacterium cheloneae*

Associated with central catheter bacteremia.

Helicobacter pylori

General characteristic consists of gram-negative spiral bacillus with rates of infection higher in underdeveloped countries. It is associated with the development of gastric and duodenal ulcers. There is an increased risk of gastric cancer. Diagnosis is made by urease testing of gastric specimens, culture of gastric tissue, Warthin Starry stain of gastric tissue, specific IgG titer, and urea breath test. It is sensitive to amoxicillin, clarithromycin, or metronidazole, and omeprazole protein pump inhibitor or bismuth subsalicylate.

Infectious Mononucleosis

Symptoms, signs, and lab of infectious mononucleosis include fever, exudative pharyngitis, lymphadenopathy, hepatosplenomegaly, and atypical lymphocyotsis (>10%). Complications include splenic rupture, thrombocytopenia, airway obstruction, agranulocytosis, hemolytic anemia, pancreatitis emophagocytic syndrome, orchitis, myocarditis, lymphoma (Burkitt), nasopharyngeal carcinoma, lymphoproliferative disorder (posttransplant, X-linked), chronic infectious mononucleosis, encephalitis, aseptic meningitis, and Guillain-Barré syndrome. Diagnosis consists of heterophile antibody test (usually negative <4 years or if infective <6 days), Epstein-Barr virus serologies and PCR. Treatment is supportive. Patients should avoid contact sports for 1 month because of risk of splenic rupture. Steroids are given for airway obstruction, massive splenomegaly, myocarditis, hemolytic anemia, and hemophagocytic syndrome. Antiviral treatment has no proven value.

Measles (Rubeola)

Measles is normally a severe disease and occurs predominantly in infants and young children. It is transmitted by direct contact with respiratory secretions and is highly contagious 1–2 days before symptoms to 4 days postrash. Incubation period is 8–12 days. Clinical manifestations of measles are fever, Koplik cough, and Koplik coryza. The rash is maculopapular and nonvesicular on the face, trunk, and extremities. Also present is mucositis: Koplik conjuctiva, oral (Koplik spots). Complications include otitis media, bronchopneumonia, laryngotracheobronchitis, and diarrhea. Mortality is 1–3:1,000 due to respiratory or neurologic complications. The diagnosis is by serology (IgM, IgG), antigen detection, and virus isolation and histology. Isolation is standard plus airborne care until 4 days after the rash resolves. Prevention includes routine vaccination (two doses), or vaccination up to 72 hours postexposure and IG (up to 6 days postexposure), IM. Almost eliminated with childhood immunization.

Rubella

Rubella is mostly benign except when the fetus is affected. Transmission is from contact with infected droplets. It is infectious beginning a few days before to 7 days after the rash. Incubation period is 16–18 days (14–23 days).

Of acquired rubella cases, 25% are asymptomatic. Those that are symptomatic are characterized by generalized, fine maculopapular rash, fever, lymphadenopathy (suboccipital, postauricular, cervical), polyarthralgia/polyarthritis (adolescents and adults). Complications can consist of encephalitis and thrombocytopenia.

Congenital rubella syndrome (CRS) may present with miscarriage, fetal death, hepatosplenomegaly, thrombocytopenia, purpura, blueberry muffin rash, cataracts, retinopathy, glaucoma, patent ductus arteriosus, peripheral pulmonary artery stenosis, behavioral disorders, meningoencephalitis, and mental challenge.

Risk of Congenital Rubella Syndrome

Gestational age	Risk of CRS
<4 weeks	85%
1–2 months	20%–30%
2–4 months	5%

Diagnosis is made by serology (IgM, IgG), viral culture, and PCR. Care includes isolation and droplet precautions for 7 days after rash. To prevent CRS, contact precautions are required for 1 year. Vaccination (MMR) is practiced for prevention, with near total elimination of congenital rubella syndrome in the United States.

FUNGAL

Candida

Mild infections consist of thrush and diaper rash.

The risk group for invasive *Candida* infection is immunosuppressed patients with indwelling catheters, with a high mortality of 40%–60%. Treatment is amphotericin B with follow-up conazole and removal of indwelling catheters.

Blastomycosis

Geographic distribution of blastomycosis is in the eastern half of North America. It resides in the soil. It rarely occurs in children. The major organs involved are pulmonary 66%, skin 27%, bone 16%, kidney 7%, and liver 3%. Treatment is with amphotericin B or intraconazole.

Coccidioidomycosis

Coccidioidomycosis is found in the desert soil in the southwestern United States. The infection may be asymptomatic or self-limited in 60%–70% of cases. The primary disease is a respiratory infection, with 20%–25% having pneumonia, pleural effusion, or pulmonary nodule or cavity. Also, primary cutaneous infection or lymphadenopathy

<1%, disseminated infection involving skin and soft tissue infection, bone and synovial infection, meningitis, genital or pelvic infection, and infection of other organs are seen.

Diagnosis is by culture and serology. If diffuse pneumonia occurs, treat with amphotericin B followed by fluconazole, intraconazole, or ketoconazole.

Histoplasmosis

Histoplasmosis is endemic in the Mississippi, Ohio, and Missouri river valleys (soil, bird feces, bat guano).

Clinical presentation may be asymptomatic with mediastinal granuloma and fibrosis. Cavitary pulmonary disease, acute pericarditis, and acute or progressive disseminated disease might develop. Diagnosis includes positive skin test, urinary histoantigen, serum buffy coat for histoantigen, and tissue biopsy. Treatment, if necessary, may use amphotericin B or intraconazole.

Aspergillosis

Invasive disease occurs almost exclusively in immunocompromised patients. The clinical presentation consists of aspergilloma, invasive disease, and malignant otitis externa. Treatment is with amphotericin B or intraconazole.

Sporotrichosis *Sporothrix schenckii*

Sporotrichosis is usually cutaneous although it can be pulmonary. It is also known as Rose-grower's disease. Tracks along lymphatic channels develop. Diagnosis is by culture. Treatment is with intraconazole or saturated solution of potassium iodide.

Pneumocystis jiroveci (carinii)

P. jiroveci occurs in immunocompromised patients, especially HIV-positive children between 3 and 6 months of age. It presents as diffuse pneumonitis with desaturation with minimal exertion.

Diagnosis is with methamine silver stain or blue toluidine blue O stain on bronchoscopic or induced sputum specimen. Treatment is with trimethoprim/sulfamethoxazole 15–20 mg/kg divided every 6–8 hours.

PARASITES

Giardia lamblia

Manifestations include occasional days of acute watery diarrhea or foul-smelling stools with flatulence and abdominal distention with an incubation period of 1–4 weeks. It is a common cause of diarrhea in day care. Most community-wide epidemics are the result of contaminated water supply.

Diagnosis is by identification of cysts or trophozites in stool examination, immunofluorescence of stool or duodenal aspirates, or string test, or it may require duodenal biopsy (Figure 13.1). Treatment is with metronidazole for 5–7 days.

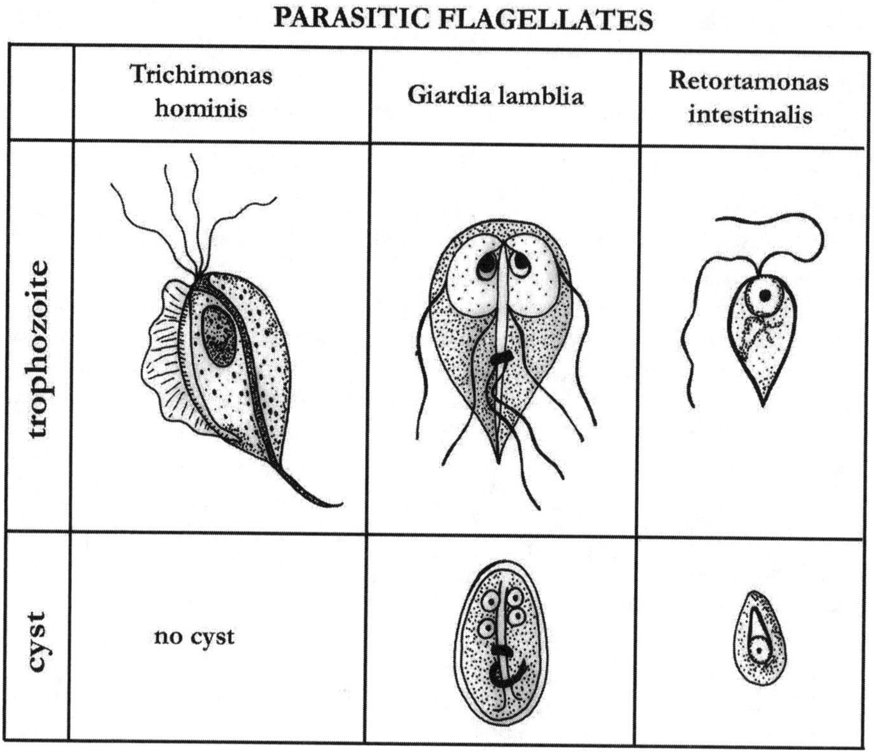

PARASITIC FLAGELLATES

	Trichimonas hominis	Giardia lamblia	Retortamonas intestinalis
trophozoite			
cyst	no cyst		

Figure 13.1

Toxoplasma gondii

Infants with congenital infection are 70%–90% asymptomatic at birth, although large portion of patients develop learning disabilities, visual problems, or mental retardation over time. Signs at birth include maculopapular rash, generalized lymphadenopathy, hepatomegaly, splenomegaly, jaundice, and thrombocytopenia. One may see cerebral calcifications radiographically. Congenital infection occurs as a result of primary maternal infection during pregnancy.

Acquired infections are usually asymptomatic, but nonspecific symptoms similar to mononucleosis may occur. Humans become infected by ingestion of undercooked meat or accidental ingestion of sporulated oocysts from soil. Immunocomprised reactivation disease with encephalitis or pneumonitis or systemic infection.

Diagnosis: IgG appears 1–2 months after infection; though can test IgM for acute infection with enzyme immunoassays most sensitive for IgM. For prenatal detection, test for the parasite in fetal blood or amniotic fluid or for a positive IgM or IgA in fetal blood. Postnatal evaluation should include ophthalmologic, auditory, and neurologic exams; lumbar puncture; CT of the head. Also attempt to isolate the organism from placenta, umbilical cord, or blood. Treatment for those with acute or reactivation is pyrimethamine, sulfadiazine, and folinic acid.

Trichomoniasis

Manifestations include infection that is usually asymptomatic in 90% of men and 50% of women. In females there might be a frothy vaginal discharge with a musty odor and a "strawberry cervix"; in males there is urethritis, prostatitis, and epididymitis. It is sexually transmitted.

Diagnosis is by wet-mount preparation and rarely culture. Treatment is with metronidazole. It is most important to also treat sexual partner.

Toxocara—Visceral Larva Migrans

Most who are infected lightly are asymptomatic. It typically occurs in children 1–4 years of age, usually with history of pica (ingestion from soil). Clinical manifestations include fever, leukocytosis, eosinophilia, hypergammaglobulinemia, and hepatomegaly. It can also cause ocular disease (endophthalmitis or retinal granulomas).

Treatment is albendazole or mebendazole.

Enterobius vermicularis—Pinworm

Pinworm usually presents as pruritus ani, though some are asymptomatic.

Diagnosis is by visualization of the adult worms in the perinatal region 2–3 hours after the child goes to sleep (Figure 13.2). Alternatively one can do the "tape test" to look for eggs three times early in the morning before washing. Treatment is with mebendazole or pyrantel pamoate or albendazole given as a single dose and then repeated in 2 weeks. All household members should be treated if patient has had repeated infections.

Plasmodium Spp.—Malaria

Malaria is endemic throughout the tropical world, with the highest risk in sub-Saharan Africa, Papua New Guinea, the Solomon Islands, and Vanuatu. It is acquired from the bite of the anopheles mosquito (nocturnal-feeding female). Chloroquine-resistant strains of *P. falciparum* are found throughout the world and chloroquine-resistant strains of *P. vivax* are found in Indonesia, Papua New Guinea, India, Guyana, and the Solomon Islands. It should be suspected in any traveler returning from endemic area with fever. The Centers for Disease Control Website (cdc.gov) gives up-to-date information on resistance patterns and malaria endemic areas.

Manifestations are high fever with rigors, sweats, and headache, possibly in a cyclic pattern. Below is a brief summary of symptoms for each species.

- *Plasmodium falciparum*: cerebral malaria, hypoglycemia, renal failure
- *P. vivax* and *P. ovale*: hypersplenism, relapse 3–5 years later
- *P. malariae*: nephritic syndrome, chronic asymptomatic infection

Diagnosis is by thick and thin peripheral blood smears. Treatment is based on infecting species, severity of disease, and likelihood of resistance.

MOST COMMON WORM INFESTATIONS

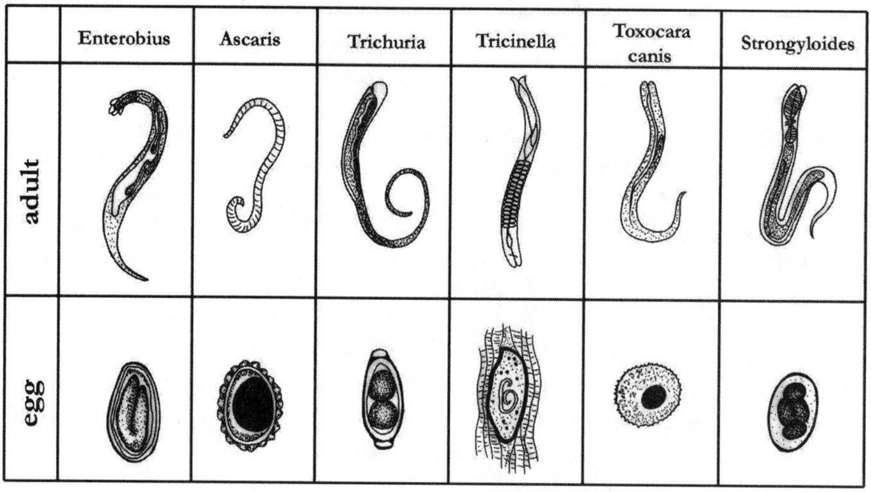

	Enterobius	Ascaris	Trichuria	Tricinella	Toxocara canis	Strongyloides
adult						
egg						

Figure 13.2

Prophylaxis: begin 1 week prior to arrival in endemic area (except doxycycline and atovaquone-proguanil). Choices include chloroquine, mefloquine, doxycycline, and atovaquone-proguanil. Prophylaxis generally once weekly until 4 weeks after leaving endemic area.

Entamoeba histolytica

Clinical symptoms include a noninvasive intestinal infection, intestinal amebiasis, ameboma, and liver abscess. It is more severe in the very young or old or pregnant patients with 1–3 weeks of increasing watery diarrhea progressing to bloody dysentery. It is transmitted via fecal-oral route and the incubation period is variable.

Diagnosis is by examination of stool specimens for trophozoites or cysts (Figure 13.3). Consider serum antibody assay for amebic colitis or liver involvement. If a liver abscess is present, one needs to look at tissue at rim of the abscess. Treatment for asymptomatic shedders is iodoquinol, paromomycin, or diloxanide furoate. In symptomatic infection, metronidazole is followed by one of the above luminal amebicides.

Bartonella heneselae—Gram-Negative Bacillus

Infection is more common during the fall and winter. Cat fleas transmit the infection among cats. It may be manifested as cat-scratch disease, bacillary angiomatosis, or peliosis hepatic disease. Diagnosis is made by serology (IFA, EIA), PCR, Warthin-Starry silver stain, and granulomas in tissue biopsy. It is sensitive to azithromycin, TMP-SMX, rifampin, and gentamicin.

AMEBAE

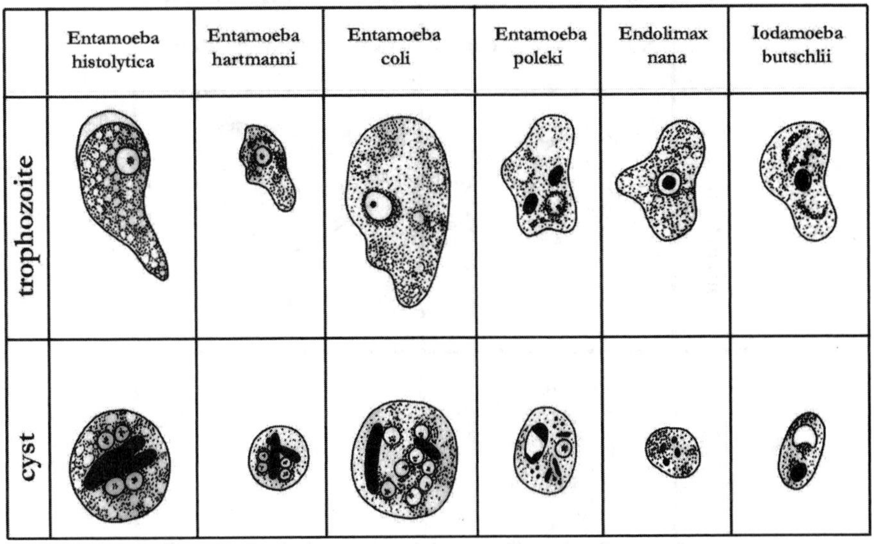

	Entamoeba histolytica	Entamoeba hartmanni	Entamoeba coli	Entamoeba poleki	Endolimax nana	Iodamoeba butschlii
trophozoite						
cyst						

Figure 13.3

TAPEWORMS

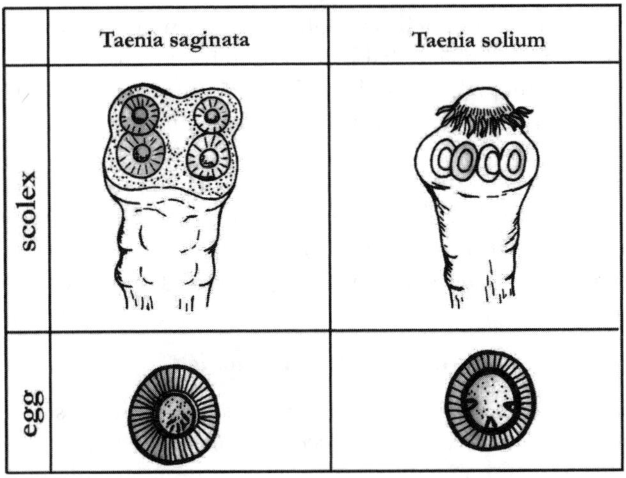

	Taenia saginata	Taenia solium
scolex		
egg		

Figure 13.4

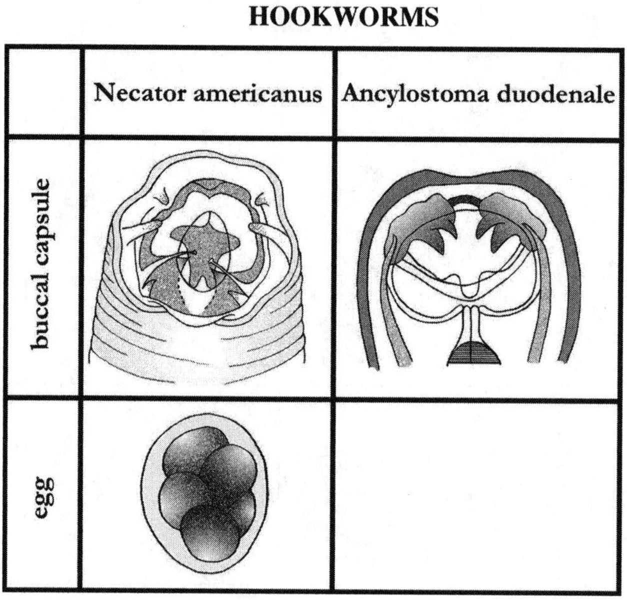

HOOKWORMS

	Necator americanus	Ancylostoma duodenale
buccal capsule		
egg		

Figure 13.5

Chlamydia trachomatis Obligate Intracellular Bacteria

Chlamydia is the most common reportable sexually transmitted infection in the United States. It may be manifested by oculogenital disease (serovars A–K), lymphogranuloma venereum (serovars L1–L3), trachoma (serovars A–C), perinatal infections (serovars B, D–K), conjunctivitis, and pneumonia.

Diagnosis is made by culture or PCR, ligase chain reaction, DNA probe, DFA, EIA, Giemsa stain of conjunctival scrapings, or peripheral eosinophilia. Treatment of neonates is by oral erythromycin base or ethylsuccinate 50 mg/kg/day for 14 days (potential association between erythromycin treatment and pylori stenosis). Genital tract infection is treated by doxycycline 100 mg bid for 7 days or azithromycin 1 g oral as a single dose.

Mycoplasma pneumoniae

M. pneumoniae is manifested as pneumonia, otitis media, sinusitis, maculopapular rash, transverse myelitis, encephalitis, Stevens-Johnson syndrome, and arthritis. Diagnosis is by enzyme immunoassay, complement fixation, culture, and fourfold increase in serum cold hemagglutinin. Treatment is by macrolides or doxycycline. Tetracycline may be used in children older than 8 years.

STREPTOCOCCAL PHARYNGITIS

Newer technologies, specifically rapid antigen detection tests (RADTs), provide results at the time of the office visit. Although the specificity of RADTs is very high, their lower sensitivity compared with throat culture makes them unreliable for ruling out disease.

GAS pharyngitis typically has an abrupt onset. Presenting symptoms may include sore throat, fever, headache, fatigue, abdominal pain, nausea, vomiting, and rash. In general, cough and rhinorrhea suggest an alternate diagnosis. The most common findings on physical examination are fever, pharyngeal injection, palatal petechiae, and cervical lymphadenopathy. Occasionally tonsillar exudates, perioral pallor, or scarlatiniform rash may be present.

Rarely GAS may lead to suppurative complications, including peritonsillar and retropharyngeal abscesses, cervical lymphadenitis, otitis, sinusitis, and bacteremia. Nonsuppurative complications such as acute rheumatic fever and acute glomerulonephritis may occur.

Approximately 10%–20% of school-aged children are carriers. It is clinically difficult to distinguish between carriers and disease. Treatment of carrier state is controversial.

Causes of Pharyngitis in Children

Viruses

Herpes simplex virus in adolescents
Respiratory viruses including influenza virus, parainfluenza virus, and rhinovirus
Epstein-Barr virus
Adenovirus

Bacteria

Mycoplasma pneumoniae
Corynebacterium diphtheriae (rare in the United States)
Neisseria gonorrhoeae in sexually active persons
Group A streptococcus (Streptococcus pyogenes)
Group C streptococcus (Streptococcus equisimilis) in college students
Arcanobacterium hemolyticum in adolescents (rarely)

Ticks

Remove the tick as soon as possible to minimize or interrupt the transfer of infectious material. Prevent the tick from regurgitating infectious material into the patient. Minimize damage or pain to the patient undergoing the procedure.

Many infectious diseases are transmitted by ticks. Lyme disease is the best known, but others that may not sound so familiar include Rocky Mountain spotted fever, ehrlichiosis, tularemia, and tick paralysis. Not all ticks carry disease, and not all that can make you or your child sick, will.

SCABIES AND LICE

This is caused by the eight-legged human mite *Sarcoptes scabiei*, whose length is up to 4 mm. The adult lives 30–40 days. The eggs reach maturity in 10–14 days. Those infested develop prurilic papules on the abdomen, dorsa of the hands, flexural surface of the wrist, elbows, periaxillary skin, genitalia, and interdigital webs.

Treatment

First choice: Permethrin; toxicity; pruritus and rash.

Alternatives: Lindane; system absorption can lead to aplastic anemia, seizures, or cardiac arrhythmias.

Pediculosis capitis—Head Lice

This louse only infests the human head, sucking blood and selecting saliva. The eggs are laid and attached to the hair shaft at the scalp. The eggs hatch within 1 week. The empty egg shells are called nits and move with the hair as it grows 1 cm per month.

Treatment

Various combing techniques and the use of topicals such as permethrin, pyrethrin, and malathion.

Pediculosis Pubis—Crab Lice

Crabs are caused by the louse *Pthirus pubis*. The nymphs and adult lice feed on human blood. The infestation may present as anogenital pruritis. The louse can reside on many hair areas such as eyelashes, eyebrows, beard, axilla, perianal, and rarely scalp as characteristic sign is the presence of a blush or slate-colored maculae (known as maculae cerulae).

Treatment

Use of pediculicides such as permethrin 1% or 5% (not FDA approved) with retreatment 7–10 days later.

VIRAL PATHOGENS

Herpes Simplex Virus (HSV)

- HSV-1: Mucocutaneous, 80%–100%
- HSV-2: Genital, 20%–30%

HSV-1 primary infection causes herpetic gingivostomatitis, herpetic whitlow, herpes gladiatorum, conjunctivitis, and keratitis. Recurrent infection causes mucocutaneous vesicles. It may be severe (disseminated) in immunodeficient host.

HSV-2 infection causes genital herpes: primary and recurrent and Mollaret meningitis; congenital from another with genital herpes: 1% shed at time of delivery.

Early diagnosis and treatment are essential. Laboratory diagnosis includes antigen detection (FAb, EIA; especially vesicles), HSV-PCR (especially CNS disease), viral culture (especially neonates; takes 2–3 days); of limited value are serologic test, CSF culture, and Tzanck prep. Treatment is acyclovir (IV, PO), and ophthalmic drugs (trifluridine, iododeoxyuridine, vidarabine).

Management of Child Born to Mother With HSV

Mother history HSV but no lesions	No treatment
Mother HSV lesions cesarean <4–6 hours ROM	Observation, Cx 24–48 hours
Mother HSV lesions cesarean >4–6 hours ROM	Cx 24–48 hours, observation (vs. Tx)
Mother HSV lesions, primary, vaginal	Cx 24–48 hours, Tx (vs. observation)
Mother HSV lesions, recurrent, vaginal	Cx 24–48 hours, observation No treatment if membranes ruptured less than 4 hours

ROM = rupture of membranes, Cx = culture, Tx = treatment.

Vaccination for Human Papillomavirus

Infection with 1 of approximately 15 oncogenic human papillomavirus (HPV) types is required for the development of cervical cancer. This has permitted primary prevention efforts via vaccination. Two vaccines based on HPV L1 protein viruslike particles (VLPs) are available. One vaccine (Gardasil) is a quadrivalent HPV-16/18 cervical cancer candidate vaccine that contains VLPs from two oncogenic HPV types, HPV-16 and HPV-18, and also contains VLPs from HPV types 6 and 11, which are not involved in cervical cancer pathogenesis but are linked to benign genital warts. This vaccine has been approved for use in women aged 9–26 years in the United States and several other countries. The second vaccine (Cervarix) is a bivalent HPV-16/18 cervical cancer candidate vaccine that contains VLPs only from the two oncogenic HPV types, HPV-16 and HPV-18. High levels of antibodies are observed systemically and in the genital tract after vaccination in humans.

Most HPV infections, regardless of type, clear spontaneously, typically within 6 months to 2 years. Risk of progression to in situ disease and invasive cancer is highest among the small subset of women with persistent infections beyond this period.

In women positive for HPV DNA, HPV-16/18 vaccination does not accelerate clearance of the virus and should not be used to treat prevalent infections.

Varicella Zoster Virus

Varicella zoster primarily causes varicella (chicken-pox). Recurrent infection causes herpes zoster, a reactivation of the latent virus. Varicella is transmitted by contact with infected skin with droplets. It is contagious 1–2 days before rash appears and until lesions become crusted. Incubation period is 14–16 days (10–21 days). The lesions are usually benign. They are macular or vesicular in different stages with centripetal spread. They heal in 7 days. Most common complication is superimposed skin bacterial infection with GAS, Reye syndrome, and encephalitis (cerebellar ataxia). It is most severe in adults, especially in pregnancy and the neonatal period, when it may become disseminated. Congenital risk is 2% with maternal infection in the first 20 weeks, with limb atrophy, scarring of the skin extremities, CNS, and eye symptoms as manifestations.

Herpes Zoster

Grouped vesicular lesions, involving 1–3 dermatomes. Herpes zoster is more frequent in immunocompromised hosts but also can be seen in normal hosts and in infants, usually secondary to in utero exposure. Postherpetic neuralgia occurs. Diagnosis includes fluorescent antibody (especially skin lesions), Tzanck prep, serology (best to determine natural immunity), and viral culture. Treatment is acyclovir if treatment started within 24 hours. Varicella vaccine for prevention at 12–18 months of age using a live vaccine up to 72 hours postexposure or varicella zoster immunoglobulin (VZIG) up to 96 hours postexposure, IM. This blood product is expensive, is restricted, and is not for treatment, only for prevention. Indications for VZIG include neonates born to mothers with varicella −5, +2 days peripartum, preterm ≤28 weeks or with no maternal history of VZG, nonimmune pregnant women exposed to VZG, and ID patients exposed to VZG. Isolation includes standard, contact, airborne precautions, with a minimum of 5 days after onset of rash, exposed individuals 8–21 days postexposure (28 days if VZIG). In zoster use contact precautions for duration of eruption.

Cytomegalovirus

CMV is very common and usually asymptomatic. Intermittent shedding for life is normal. Natural secretions are oral, vaginal, urine, semen, and human milk. It can be present in blood transfusion and organ donation. Incubation is unknown for horizontal transmission; in blood (3–12 weeks) and in transplant (1–4 months).

Congenital CMV

The most common congenital infection occurs in 1%–2% of newborns and is 90% asymptomatic (shedding in urine, saliva, and other secretions). It may result in growth retardation, microcephaly, cerebral calcifications (periventricular), deafness, retinitis, hepatosplenomegaly, jaundice, thrombocytopenia, petechia, and rash (blueberry muffin baby). It is largely asymptomatic, though an infectious mononucleosis-like syndrome (heterophile antibody negative) with lymphadenopathy occurs. Diagnosis may be made by fluorescent antibody, viral culture (tissue, secretions), serology (limited, insensitive, IgM unreliable), or urine (sediment in epithelial cells). Treatment for symptomatic patients is ganciclovir (Valganciclovir) or foscarnet CMV-IVIG.

Epstein-Barr Virus

Epstein-Barr is very common. Most symptomatic cases occur in adolescents. It is transmitted by oral secretions. Incubation period is 30–50 days.

Influenza Virus

Epidemic influenza is caused by type A or B.

- Hemagglutinin (HA) and neuraminidase (NA) are the surface antigens by which influenza A is subclassified.
- Antigenic drift (minor) occurs continuously and results in new strains of A or B. Major changes in HA or NA occur only in influenza A and can lead to a pandemic.

Transmission is contact with infected droplets and surfaces. The infectious period is 24 hours before symptoms to 7 days. Incubation period is 1–3 days. Clinical manifestations of influenza include fever (sudden); malaise, myalgias, headache, dry cough, sore throat, rhinitis, conjunctival injection, abdominal pain, nausea and vomiting, pneumonia, croup, wheezing, bronchiolitis, sepsis-like picture, Reye syndrome, encephalitis, and myositis. Diagnosis is by blood culture, CSF (especially first 72 hours), antigen detection (rapid, modest sensitivity/specificity), and serology (limited value). Treatment is by antivirals. Antibiotics are reserved for secondary bacterial infections. Prevention is by administration of annual vaccine. A cold-adaptive live vaccine administered nasally has recently been approved down to 2 years of age, though not for patients with asthma.

Respiratory Syncytial Virus

Onset under age 2 years may result in a more serious illness. The peak season is winter and early spring, though less seasonal in warmer latitudes.

Transmission is by contact with infected secretions or fomites. The incubation period is 4–6 days (2–8 days). Communicability is 3–8 days (3–4 weeks in neonates). Clinical manifestations are upper respiratory infection, bronchiolitis, pneumonia, and apnea (neonates). Excessive mortality occurs in patients with underlying conditions such as congenital heart disease (especially pulmonary hypertension), bronchopulmonary dysplasia, prematurity or low birth weight, and immunodeficient host. Diagnosis is by culture and antigen detection. Management is supportive and antivirals: ribavirin aerosol (very selective use). Prevention is by palivizumab.

Hepatitis Virus

Hepatitis A is transmitted by fecal-oral; B route by bloody fluids, percutaneous (40%), perinatal (5%–20% to 70%–90%) and as a sexually transmitted disease; C is transmitted by parenteral exposure to blood (3%–5%). Perinatal is 5% higher for HIV+. Infectious period for hepatitis A is 1–2 weeks before onset of illness to 1 week after. Hepatitis B is infectious as long as HBsAg (variable); hepatitis C, as long as viremic ("always").

Incubation of Hepatitis

A: 25–30 days (15–50 days)
B: 90 days (45–160 days)
C: 40–50 days (14–160 days)

Risk factors for hepatitis A include exposure to infected household member and travel to endemic areas; hepatitis B is exposure perinatally, household contacts, multiple sexual partners, and immigrants from endemic areas; hepatitis C includes repeat blood transfusions, IV drug abuse, multiple sexual partners, and perinatal, with no risk for breast-feeding. In most cases there is no known source. Hepatitis A is asymptomatic in 30% of exposed children versus symptomatic in 70% of adults; acute, self-limited, and never chronic. It is rarely fulminant. Hepatitis B is acute and chronic. The younger the child, the more likely the child will be asymptomatic but develop to a chronic infection. Extrahepatic manifestations include arthralgias, arthritis, macular rash, thrombocytopenia, and papular acrodermatis (Gianotti-Crosti syndrome). Hepatitis C is an acute infection, usually mild or asymptomatic, with a persistent infection in 60% and chronic infection (10%–70%) leading to cirrhosis or hepatocellular carcinoma.

Age at Infection	Risk of Chronicity
Perinatal	>90%
1–5 years	25%–50%
Children/adults	6%–10%

Diagnosis of hepatitis A is made by serology of IgM and IgG. Hepatitis B is made by serology of HBsAg, HBeAg, Anti-HBs, anti-HBe, or anti-HBc (total and IgM). Hepatitis C serology is determined by ELISA and RIBA. PCR may be used early as well as perinatal test by PCR. Maternal antibodies can last 18 months.

Treatment for hepatitis A is supportive. Hepatitis B is treated with interferon alpha, antivirals (lamivudine, adefovir), no corticosteroids, and immunize against HAV. Hepatitis C is treated with interferon alpha (pegylated), plus ribavirin, no corticosteroids, immunize against HAV and HBV.

Prevention for hepatitis A is vaccine (2 years and older), IG (within 2 weeks); hepatitis B with vaccine, HBIG; for hepatitis C there is no vaccine.

Rotavirus

Rotavirus infection is the most common cause of diarrhea in infants. Age of onset is under 2 years. Peak of the season is the wintertime. Mode of transmission is by fecal-oral route. Incubation period is between 2 and 5 days. There are four serotypes.

Clinical manifestations include acute gastroenteritis (fever and vomiting followed by diarrhea, 3–8 days). Stools rarely contain blood. Rotavirus infection with fever may trigger seizures in children who have a propensity for febrile seizures. Dehydration and electrolyte disturbances are the major sequelae of rotavirus infection and occur most often in the youngest children. Cleaning hands with soap and water and then an alcohol-containing hand rub should be used. Diagnosis is by antigen testing (stool)—Rotazyme. Treatment is supportive and rehydration. Vaccination is the only control measure likely to have a significant impact on the incidence of severe, dehydrating rotavirus disease. The current approved vaccine is an oral attenuated vaccine initiated at 2 months of age.

Enterovirus

Enteroviruses include coxsackieviruses, echoviruses, and polioviruses. Transmission is by fecal-oral, respiratory, and peripartum routes. Incubation period is 3–6 days. Clinical manifestations include protean manifestations, nonspecific fever, rhinitis, pharyngitis, herpangina, stomatitis, pneumonia, and pleurodynia. Skin reaction consists of exanthema (nonvesicular). Neurologic symptoms such as aseptic meningitis, encephalitis, and paralysis occur. Gastrointestinal symptoms consist of vomiting, diarrhea, abdominal pain, and hepatitis. The eye symptoms consist of acute hemorrhagic conjunctivitis and heart symptoms of myocarditis.

Diagnosis is via culture (throat, stool, rectal, or other) and PCR (especially CSF and tissues). Serology is of limited value. Treatment is supportive and antiviral (pleconaril).

Polio consists of serotypes 1, 2, and 3. It is asymptomatic in 95%, though a nonspecific febrile illness (5%–10%), aseptic meningitis, paresthesias (1%–5%), and acute flaccid paralysis (0.1%–1%) occur. Postpolio syndrome is 30–40 years later (muscle pain and weakness). Prevention is through vaccination.

Mumps

The mumps are a relatively benign disease with different manifestations depending on age and sex. It is transmitted by contact with infected respiratory secretions, 1–2 days before to 5 days after parotid swelling. Incubation period is 16–18 days (12–25 days). Clinical manifestations consist of parotitis, which is most common, orchitis (after puberty), pancreatitis, and meningoencephalitis (50% pleocytosis and 10% symptoms). Complications are more common in older children and adults, including neurosensory hearing loss.

Diagnosis is by serology (IgM, IgG) and virus isolation (throat wash). Treatment is supportive and prevention is by vaccination.

Parvovirus B19

Clinical manifestations of parvovirus are fever in 15%–30% and rash (slapped cheek, circumoral pallor, symmetric, maculopapular, lacelike, pruritic rash on the 3 trunk and moves peripherally). Arthralgia and arthritis occur in adults especially. This is the immune phase; actual infection is 7–10 days prior. Once rash is present, the patient is no longer contagious. Congenital infection may cause fetal death or fetal hydrops in 2%–6%.

Diagnosis is through serology (IgM, IgG) and PCR. Treatment is supportive. Blood transfusion and IVIG have proven effective.

Roseola (HHV-6)

Clinical manifestations of roseola consist of fever (high) for 3–7 days followed by erythematous maculopapular rash that may be fleeting. Seizures may occur in 10%–15% during febrile stage. Immunocompromised host develops fever, hepatitis, bone marrow suppression, pneumonia, and encephalitis. Treatment is supportive.

Rabies

Epidemiology consists of exposure to secretions (saliva) from infected animals, including bats, raccoons, skunks, foxes, or coyotes, but not from small rodents or lagomorphs and no person-to-person transmission. Clinical manifestations are acute, progressive CNS involvement, anxiety, dysphagia, seizures, paralysis, or death.

Diagnosis is through antigen detection (immunofluorescence), postmortem or skin biopsy from nape (Negri bodies), or culture from saliva, brain, or other tissues. Serology by serum, CSF, or PCR. Treatment is supportive. Prevention is through wound care (cleanse, Td, with no suture), vaccine (depending on circumstances, species, with tests), and rabies immunoglobulin.

Arboviruses

Arthropod-borne viruses (ticks, mosquitoes, sandflies) are causes of California encephalitis (LaCrosse), eastern and western equine encephalitis, Powassan encephalitis, St. Louis encephalitis, Venezuelan equine encephalitis, West Nile encephalitis, Colorado tick fever, dengue, Japanese encephalitis, and yellow fever. The geographic variation is seasonal.

Diagnosis is by serology (serum, CSF), culture, or PCR. Treatment is supportive. Prevention is vaccination (yellow fever, Japanese encephalitis) and avoidance of contact with vectors and repellants.

Parainfluenza (Types 1, 2, and 3)

Clinical manifestations consist of laryngotracheobronchitis (croup), pneumonia, and bronchiolitis. Rarely aseptic meningitis, encephalitis, and parotitis.

Diagnosis is by antigen detection, culture, and serology (limited value). Treatment is supportive.

Adenovirus

Mode of transmission: close contact with infected secretions and fomites. Incubation period is 3–10 days. The peak season and epidemics are late winter, spring, and summer.

Clinical manifestations consist of common cold, pharyngitis, tonsillitis, otitis media, pharyngoconjunctival fever, acute hemorrhagic conjunctivitis, hemorrhagic cystitis, pertussis-like syndrome, croup, bronchiolitis, and gastroenteritis. Rarely pneumonia, meningitis, and encephalitis develop.

Diagnosis is by antigen detection, culture, and serology (for epidemiology studies). Treatment is supportive.

Caliciviruses—Novoviruses (Formerly Norwalk and Safoviruses)

Most common cause of diarrhea outbreaks in children and adults, notably on cruise ships.

Novovirus infection symptoms include diarrhea, vomiting (commonly with fever), headache, malaise, myalgia, and abdominal cramps. The symptoms last 1 day to 2 weeks. Incubation period is 12–72 hours.

Research and reference labs employ enzyme immunoassay for detection of viral antigens in stool or antigens in semen (Centers for Disease Control and Prevention). Treatment is supportive.

Ehrlichiosis

There are three pathogens: *Ehrlichia chaffeensis* (human monocytic), *Anaplasma phagocytophilia* (human granulocytic), and *Ehrlichia ewingii.*

Manifestations are similar to Rocky Mountain Spotted Fever (RMSF) but with increased incidence of anemia, thrombocytopenia, and elevation in transaminases; less commonly there is a rash. Epidemiology: lone star tick in the southeastern and south central states; deer tick in north central and northeastern states.

Diagnosis is by serology, isolation in the blood, positive PCR, and presence of a morulae (intraleukocytoplasmic microcolonies of bacteria) with serology of at least a single IFA (immunofluorescent antibody titer) of 1:64. Treatment is with doxycycline.

FURTHER READING

Bratton, R. L. (2005). Tick-borne disease. *American Family Physician, 71,* 2323.

Daugherty, R. J., Posner, J., Henretig, F. M., McHugh, L. A., & Tan, C. G. (2005). Tick paralysis: Atypical presentation, unusual location. *Pediatric Emergency Care, 21,* 677–680.

des Vigns, F., Piesman, J., Heffernan, R., Schulze, T. L., Stafford, K. C. 3rd, & Fish, D. (2001). Effect of tick removal on transmission of *Borrelia burgdorferi* and *Ehrlichia phagocyophilia* by *Ixodes scapularis* nymphs. *Journal of Infectious Diseases, 183,* 773.

Feigin, R. D., Cherry, J., Demmler, G., & Kaplan, S. (2003). *Textbook of pediatric infectious diseases* (5th ed.). Philadelphia: Saunders.

Gilbert-Barness, E., & Barness, L. A. (2003). *Clinical use of pediatric diagnostic tests.* Baltimore: Lippincott Williams & Wilkins.

Long, S. S., Pickering, L. K., & Prober, C. G. (Eds.). (2007). *Principles and practice of pediatric infectious disease* (3rd ed.). Philadelphia: Saunders, Elsevier.

Pickering, L. K. (Ed.). (2003). *Report of the committee on infectious diseases* (26th ed.). Elk Grove Village, IL: American Academy of Pediatrics.

Shapiro, E. D., Gerber, M. A., Holabird, M. B., Berg, A. T., Feder, H. M. Jr., Bell, G. L., et al. (1992). A controlled trial of antimicrobial prophylaxis for Lyme disease after deer-tick bites. *New England Journal of Medicine, 17,* 1769.

Steele, R. W. (2007). *Clinical handbook of pediatric infectious disease* (3rd ed.). New York: Informa Healthcare USA.

14

URINARY TRACT

Sunlight unto moonlight is as water unto wine.

Alfred, Lord Tennyson

EXAMINATION OF THE URINE

Clarity

Turbidity usually is normal due to crystal formation at room temperature. Uric acid crystals form in acidic urine, phosphate crystals in alkaline urine. Cellular material and bacteria can also cause turbidity.

Dipsticks and Test Tapes

IRIS Chemstrips (Roche; Basel, Switzerland) and Multistix (Bayer; Tarrytown, NY)

For the determination of specific gravity, pH, leukocytes, nitrite, protein, glucose, ketones, urobilinogen, bilirubin, and blood in urine.

Storage and Stability

Store IRIStrips at temperatures below 30°C. Do not freeze. Opened IRIStrips are stable until the expiration date when stored in the original capped vial. The vial must be closed immediately after removal of each strip.

Procedure

Dip test areas in urine completely but briefly to avoid dissolving out the reagents. If using strips visually, read test results carefully at the times specified, in a good light (such as fluorescent) and with the test area held near the appropriate color chart on the bottle label.

After dipping the strip, check the pH area. If the color on the pad is not uniform, read the reagent area immediately, comparing the darkest color to the appropriate color chart. All reagent areas except leukocyte areas may be read between 1 and 2 minutes after dipping to identify negative specimens and to determine the pH and specific gravity. A positive reaction (a reading of "small" or greater) at <2 minutes on the leukocyte test may be regarded as a positive indication of leukocytes in urine. Color changes that occur after 2 minutes are of no diagnostic value. If the strips are analyzed instrumentally, the instrument will automatically read each reagent area at the specified time.

The following lists the generally detectable levels of analytes in urine; however, because of the inherent variability of clinical urines, lesser concentrations may be detected.

Reagent area	Sensitivity
Glucose	75–125 mg/dl glucose
Bilirubin	0.4–0.8 mg/dl bilirubin
Ketone	5–10 mg/dl acetoacetic acid
Blood	0.015–0.062 mg/dl hemoglobin
Protein	15–30 mg/dl albumin
Nitrite	0.06–0.1 mg/dl nitrite ion
Leukocytes	5–15 cells/high-power field (hpf) in clinical urine

Visual Appearance of Urine

Color	Cause
Dark yellow	Concentrated urine, bile pigments, riboflavin
Red	Doxorubicin hydrochloride (Adriamycin), methyldopa, beets in anemic individuals, blackberries, deferoxamine mesylate (with elevated serum iron), phenytoin, red food coloring, hemoglobulin, phenazopyridine hydrochloride (acid urine), phenolphthalein (alkaline urine), phenothiazines, porphyrins, chloroquine, rifampin, phenazopyridine hydrochloride (Pyridium), pyrvinium pamoate (Povan), red blood cells, red diaper syndrome (nonpathogenic *Serratia marcescens*), urates
Yellow-brown	Antimalarials (pamaquine, primaquine, quinacrine), sulfasalazine (Azulfidine) (alkaline urine), B-complex vitamins, bilirubin, carotene, cascara, metronidazole, nitrofurantoin, sulfonamides
Brown-black	Hemosiderin, homogentisic acid (alkaptonuria), melanin (especially in alkaline urine), myoglobin, old blood, quinine sulfate
Purple-brown	Porphyrins (old urine)
Orange	Phenazopyridine, rifampin, urates, warfarin sodium
Blue-green	Doxorubicin hydrochloride, amitriptyline hydrochloride, blue diaper syndrome (familial metabolic disease, nephrocalcinosis), biliverdin

(seen in chronic obstructive jaundice), indomethacin, methylene blue, *Pseudomonas* urinary tract infection (rare), riboflavin

CAUSES OF ASYMPTOMATIC PROTEINURIA

Benign Proteinuria (Most Common)

- Often orthostatic
- Transient with fever, acute illness

Silent Renal Disease

- Glomerular diseases
- Tubulointerstitial diseases
  Reflux nephropathy
  Chronic pyelonephritis
  Interstitial nephritis
  Nephrotoxicity
  Fanconi syndrome

NEPHROTIC SYNDROME

- Proteinuria is in excess of 3.5 g/1.73 m^2/day.
- Hypoalbuminemia (loss, enhanced renal catabolism, decreased hepatic synthesis).
- Hyperlipidemia (stimulated by decreased plasma oncotic pressure).
- Insidious onset of edema (loss of intravascular volume).
- Homeostatic adjustments to correct the resulting deficit in effective plasma volume lead to an increase in sodium or water retention.
  - Activation of renin-angiotensin-aldosterone system
  - Enhanced vasopressin secretion
  - Sympathetic nervous system stimulation
  - Alteration in secretion or in the renal response to atrial natriuretic peptide
  - Loss of important proteins in addition to albumin
- Thyroid-binding globulin abnormality (abnormal thyroid function test results or clinical hypothyroidism)
- Cholecalciferol-binding protein abnormality (vitamin D deficiency and secondary hyperparathyroidism leading to hypocalcemia, hypocalciuria)
- Transferrin abnormality (iron-resistant microcytic, hypochromic anemia)
- Metal-binding protein abnormalities (deficiency of zinc and copper)
- Multifactorial hypercoagulable state: loss of antithrombin III, protein C, protein S, fibrinogen; enhanced platelet aggregation; increased α- and β-globulins

Minimal-Change Disease

Ninety percent of children respond to prednisone treatment. Nonresponse suggests focal glomerulosclerosis. Cyclophosphamide may produce remission in cases with frequent relapses. Male preponderance is seen. If diagnosis is in doubt, renal biopsy should be performed.

Causes of Nephrotic Syndrome

Primary Glomerular Diseases

- Minimal-change disease (70%–80% of affected children, 15%–20% of adults) caused by foot process defects (formerly called lipid nephrosis or nil disease)
- Mesangial proliferative glomerulonephritis (GN)
- Focal and segmental glomerulosclerosis
- Membranous GN
- Membranoproliferative GN
- Other proliferative GNs (e.g., focal, IgA nephropathy, mesangial)
- Rapidly progressive GN

Infection

- Poststreptococcal GN, malaria, hepatitis B, infectious mononucleosis, secondary syphilis, acquired immunodeficiency syndrome

Drugs

- Organic gold, penicillamine, NSAIDs, contrast media
- Probenecid, captopril
- Contrast media
- Mercury (organic, inorganic, and elemental)
- Street heroin (including impurities)
- Antivenoms and antitoxins

Neoplasia

- Hodgkin disease, non-Hodgkin lymphoma, melanoma, leukemias
- Wilms tumor

Multisystem Diseases

- Systemic lupus erythematosis, Henoch-Schönlein purpura, vasculitides, dermatomyositis, rheumatoid arthritis, Goodpasture syndrome, Alport syndrome, inflammatory bowel disease
- Diabetic glomerulosclerosis
- Amyloidosis
- Kwashiorkor

Hereditofamilial or Congenital Diseases

- Malignant obesity
- Renovascular hypertension
- Thyroiditis
- Chronic allograft rejection
- Myxedema

- Bee sting allergies
- Chronic interstitial nephritis with vesicoureteric reflux
- Sickle cell disease
- Preeclamptic toxemia
- Berger disease
- Polyarteritis (rare)
- Takayasu disease
- Sarcoidosis
- Sjögren syndrome
- Wegener granulomatosis
- Cryoglobulinemia
- Obstruction of inferior vena cava (thrombosis, tumor)
- Constrictive pericarditis
- Tricuspid stenosis
- Congestive heart failure

Causes of Glomerulonephritis

Poststreptococcal GN	1%–2% of cases progress to chronic GN
Rapidly progressive GN	90% of cases progress to chronic GN
Membranous GN	50% of cases progress to chronic GN
Focal glomerulosclerosis	50%–80% of cases progress to chronic GN
Membranoproliferative	50% of cases progress to chronic GN
IgA nephropathy	30%–50% of cases progress to chronic GN

Laboratory Findings

The presence of red cell casts with or without proteinuria is usual. Measurement of the third component of the complement system, C3, used in conjunction with measurements of C4 and total hemolytic complement (C5H50), helps distinguish the type of GN (Table 14.1). Activation of the classical pathway results in low concentrations of C3 and C4, whereas activation of the alternate pathway leads only to low C3 values. Deficiencies of other complement components result in normal C3 and C4 levels, but a low C5H50 level. The GNs commonly associated with low C3 concentrations include systemic lupus erythematosis, membranoproliferative GN, GN caused by chronic infections such as bacterial endocarditis or infected ventriculoperitoneal shunts, postinfectious nephritis, and inherited abnormalities of the complement system. Diseases usually associated with normal C3 concentrations include Henoch-Schönlein purpura, Berger disease (Ig A nephropathy), epidemic hemolytic-uremic syndrome, Goodpasture syndrome, and hereditary nephritis.

POLYCYSTIC KIDNEY DISEASE

Polycystic kidney disease occurs in two forms, autosomal dominant and autosomal recessive.

The autosomal dominant form is usually slowly progressive and asymptomatic until patient is >50 years old; accounts for approximately 10% of transplant or

TABLE 14.1

Differentiation of Types of Glomerulonephritis

Clinical Manifestations	Poststreptococcal GN	IgA Nephropathy	Membranoproliferative GN	RPGN
Age and sex	All ages, mean 7 yr, 2:1 male	15–35 yr, 2:1 male	15–30 yr, 6:1 male	Mean 58 yr, 2:1 male
Acute nephritic syndrome	90%	50%	90%	90%
Asymptomatic hematuria	Occasionally	50%	Rare	Rare
Nephrotic syndrome	10%–20%	Rare	Rare	10%–20%
Hypertension	70%	30%–50%	Rare	25%
Acute renal failure	50% (transient)	Very rare	50%	60%
Other	Latent period of 1–3 wk	Follows viral syndromes	Pulmonary hemorrhage; iron deficiency anemia	None
Laboratory findings	↑ASO titers (70%); Positive streptozyme (95%); ↑C3–C9, normal C1, C4	↑Serum IgA (50%); IgA in dermal capillaries	Positive anti-GBM antibody	Positive ANCA
Immunogenetics	HLA-B12, D "EN"	HLA-Bw 35, DR4	HLA-DR2	None established
Renal pathology	Diffuse proliferation	Focal proliferation	Focal proliferation with crescents	Crescentic GN
Immunofluorescence	Granular IgG, C3	Diffuse mesangial IgA	Linear IgG, C3	No immune deposits
Electron microscopy	Subepithelial humps	Mesangial deposits	No deposits	No deposits
Prognosis	95% resolve spontaneously; 5% RPGN or slowly progressive	Slow progression in 25%–50%	75% stabilize or improve if treated early	75% stabilize or improve if treated early
Treatment	Supportive	None established	Plasma exchange, steroids, cyclophosphamide	Steroid pulse therapy

↑, increased; ANCA, antineutrophil cytoplasm antibody; ASO, antistreptolysin-O; GBM, glomerular basement membrane; GN, glomerulonephritis; IgA, immunoglobulin A; IgG, immunoglobulin G; RPGN, rapidly progressive glomerulonephritis.

[a]Relative risk.

Modified from Couser, W. G. (1992). Glomerular disorders. In J. B. Wyngaarden, L. H. Smith, & J. C. Bennett (Eds.), Cecil textbook of medicine (19th ed., Vol 1). Philadelphia: WB Saunders.

dialysis cases. Usually does not manifest until adult life. Some cases have been diagnosed in the neonatal period and in childhood. It may present as polyuria.

- Polyuria is present.
- Hematuria may be gross and episodic or an incidental microscopic finding (50%).
- Proteinuria occurs in approximately one third of patients and is mild (<1 mg/24 hrs).
- Renal calculi may be associated (≤30% of patients).
- Hypertension may be present (affects 30% of children, ≤60% of adults before onset of renal insufficiency, and >80% with end-stage renal failure).
- Anemia of renal failure is less severe than that in other forms of kidney disease.
- Prenatal diagnosis is possible using DNA obtained by amniocentesis or chorionic villus sampling.

The autosomal recessive form is usually more severe and becomes manifest earlier with fewer patients surviving as adults. It is characterized by very large cystic kidneys that can be diagnosed prenatally. It is associated with oligohydramnios. The Potter sequence and pulmonary hypoplasia are incompatible with life. Some patients have undergone successful kidney transplantation at birth.

HEMATURIA

Hematuria is defined as at least 5 red blood cells (RBCs) per milliliter in the urine. It can be determined by a urinary dipstick that is capable of detecting 3–10 RBC/ml urine.

Prevalence of Microscopic Hematuria

- 0.1%–0.5% in schoolchildren
- Slightly higher in girls than in boys
- Not age dependent

Definition

- ≥3 RBC/hpf in uncentrifuged urine
- ≥10 RBC/0.9 mm^3 in centrifuged urine

Dipstick

- Very sensitive, may detect as few as 2 RBC/hpf
- More sensitive for free Hgb than RBCs

Localization of Hematuria

Renal

- Brown or cola-colored urine
- Cellular casts

Lower Urinary Tract

- Terminal gross hematuria
- Passage of blood clots

Causes of Asymptomatic Hematuria

Renal

- Glomerular
  Benign familial hematuria
  Acute poststreptococcal GN
  IgA nephropathy
  Chronic GN
  Alport syndrome
  Exercise induced
- Nonglomerular
  Hypercalciuria
  Neprholithiasis/nephrocalcinosis
  Interstitial nephritis
  Renal malformations, cystic diseases
  Sickle-cell disease or trait
  Trauma (rare with normal anatomy)
  Tumors (Wilms, leukemia)

Lower Urinary Tract

- Bacterial/viral urinary tract infection (UTI)
- Structural (obstruction, ureterocele)
- Trauma

Other Rare Causes of Hematuria

- Coagulopathy
- Vascular accidents (mainly newborns)

URINARY TRACT INFECTION

The incidence of UTI is lower in the first 72 hours than after 72 hours of life. In the first 72 hours of life, 90% of the UTIs are accompanied by bacteremia, suggesting the presence of disseminated sepsis. In the newborn, UTI is found in about 0.7% of normal term infants and 2.2%–3.4% of premature, postmature, and high-risk infants. The symptoms and signs of UTI are nonspecific and may be similar to those of septicemia or meningitis.

Newborns with UTI may present with diarrhea, vomiting, abdominal disten-tion, and refusal of feeding with or without lethargy, hypothermia, fever, metabolic acidosis, dehydration, and jaundice. Jaundice is only present in <20% of infants with UTI.

Maternal factors may be important in the development of pyelonephritis as a part of sepsis in the newborn infant. These conditions include prolonged rupture of the amniotic membranes over 18 hours, uterine tenderness, premature labor, UTI of the mother at the time of labor, or near term, fever, and positive vaginal culture for group B hemolytic streptococci.

Definite diagnosis of early neonatal UTI is made by culture of properly collected urine sample. Cultures of urine samples collected by bag are inappropriate. Properly catheterized urine samples are considered suitable for culture by some, while others consider reliability of catheterized urine no better than bag urine, with possibility of iatrogenic infection with catheterization. Appropriate method of obtaining urine for culture in a neonate is suprapubic bladder aspiration (SPA) under sterile technique. For bladder aspiration, determine that the bladder contains urine by palpation and percussion.

Any growth from a bladder aspirate, even a single colony, is considered positive, while a count of 10 or higher from a catheterized urine sample is indicative of UTI.

Urine sample obtained needs to be sent for immediate culture, or refrigerated overnight, but must not be frozen.

Escherichia coli is responsible for the majority (67%) of UTIs in newborns, followed by *Klebsiella pneumoniae* (21%) and *Proteus mirabilis* (2%).

Predisposing factors for UTI in the newborn include vesicoureteric reflux (VUR), ureterocele, and obstructive uropathies such as ureteropelvic junction obstruction, ureterovesicular obstruction, phimosis, and posterior urethral valve. The tip of the penis should be slitlike. Ask the parent about the distance the boy can shoot his stream.

Among females, 60%–80% will have recurrent UTI; 75% of males have an anatomic abnormality.

Pyuria

Pyuria may occur in children with renal tubular acidosis, dehydration, GN, renal stones, or following any form of instrumentation, appendicitis, or other extrinsic ureteral irritation in the absence of demonstrable microbial infection.

Recurrent UTI

Consider functional disorder, such as unstable bladder, especially in a child with enuresis.

Vesicoureteral Reflux

Etiology is related to 1°, deficiency of ureterovesical junction, 2°, reflux with increased intravesical pressure, neurogenic bladder, dysfunctional elimination or detrusor instability or posterior urethral valves. Incidence of 1° reflux is about 30%–50% of children with UTI. Diagnosis can only be made by voiding cystogram. Resolution: I, 87%; II, 63%; III, 25%; IV, 33%.

VUR affects up to 0.5% of all normal newborns. Most of these refluxes are of low grade I or II and will disappear spontaneously by the end of the first year of life.

The International Reflux Study Committee grades the VUR into five grades:

Grade I: Urine refluxes to the ureter only (Figure 14.1).
Grade II: Urine refluxes into the ureter, renal pelvis, and calyceal fornices.
Grade III: Urine refluxes into the ureter, renal pelvis, and calyces with mild to moderate dilatation or tortuosity of the ureter and mild to moderate dilatation of the renal pelvis, with only slight or no blunting of the fornices.

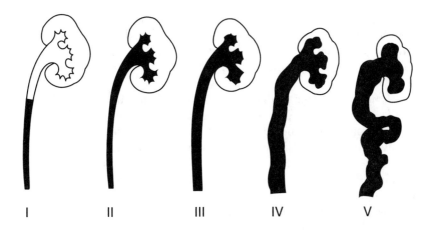

Figure 14.1
Grading of vesicoureteral reflux. Stages I through V. From the International
Reflux Study.

Grade IV: Urine refluxes into the ureter, renal pelvis, and calyces with moderate
  dilatation or tortuosity of the ureter, and moderate dilatation of the pelvis and
  calyces. There is complete obliteration of the sharp angles of the fornices but
  the papillary impression in the majority of the calyces is maintained.
Grade V: Urine refluxes into the ureter, renal pelvis, and calyces with gross dilatation and tortuosity of the ureter, pelvis, and calyces. The papillary impressions
  are no longer visible in the majority of the calyces.

Imaging Investigation

Renal ultrasound is performed after diagnosis of a first UTI. This noninvasive procedure can demonstrate most of the anatomical abnormalities of the urinary tract. The
ultrasonogram is normally obtained within the first 48 hours of the diagnosis of UTI
if the condition of the infant allows this. However, ultrasonography is believed not
to be sensitive enough to detect the presence of hydronephrosis, hydroureter, VUR,
and renal scarring.

Newborns with established UTI will need to have a micturation cystourethro-
gram.

Consider isotope renal scanning using 99m technetium-dimercaptosuccinic
acid (DMSA) early to identify any residual parenchymal damage. Such an early
study may also be used to identify the presence of pyelonephritis if there was any
difficulty in establishing the diagnosis.

Laboratory Investigation

Laboratory investigation includes complete blood count (CBC), C-reactive protein
(CRP), electrolytes, blood urea nitrogen (BUN), serum creatinine, urine culture,
blood culture, and possibly cerebrospinal fluid culture as part of the sepsis workup.

From 2 months to 2 years UTI is characterized by unexplained fever. Diagnosis is best by obtaining a urine sample by SPA or by transurethral bladder catheterization, which has a sensitivity of 95% and specificity of 99% when compared to SPA sample. Urine samples collected by urine bag for culture have a very high false-positive rate, around 85%.

Escherichia coli is the predominant microorganism causing UTI (80%–85%). *Klebsiella, enterococcus,* and *Proteus mirabilis* account for the other 15%.

In addition to the urine culture, laboratory investigations will include CBC, ESR, CRP, electrolytes, BUN, serum creatinine, and blood culture.

In 2–5-year-old children, unexplained fever may suggest UTI especially if the focus of infection is not evident on physical examination. With cystitis the common manifestation includes symptoms such as dysuria, urgency and frequency, localized suprapubic pain, and hematuria. Dysuria alone can also be due to pinworm infestation, bubble bath, vaginitis, and urethritis.

Diagnosis is established by finding positive microorganisms in the urine culture. A urine sample obtained by clean catch midstream method may be used for culture. Colony count (pure culture) of $> 10^4$/ml of urine obtained by clean catch for culture in boys, and $\geq 10^5$/ml in girls is highly suggestive of infection.

Escherichia coli comprises about 90% of infections in girls, and 45% in boys, while *Proteus mirabilis* infection in girls is only 5% and up to 45% in boys.

In children age 5 years and above, the overall incidence of UTI is 1.7 per 1,000 in boys and 3.1 per 1,000 in girls.

There may be repeated UTI in sexually active female teenagers due to *Chlamydia trachomatis.* Chlamydia and gonococcus may be diagnosed by urine tests.

URETEROCELE

Ureteral duplication with upper-pole ureterocele and reflux into lower-pole ureter is called a ureterocele.

- This anomaly is a deformity of terminal ureter, usually associated with duplication/upper pole.
- The incidence is 1 in 5,000–12,000 pediatric admissions.
- The patient usually presents with a UTI and urethral obstruction (more common cause in females). It may be diagnosed by prenatal ultrasound.
- It may be associated with lower-pole VUR in 50%, contralateral obstruction in 10% of cases.

POSTERIOR URETHRAL VALVES

Posterior urethral valves are caused by paired leaflets in the prostatic urethra that cause obstruction of the bladder as well as both kidneys. They may be diagnosed prenatally in 1 in 8,000 pregnancies with bilateral hydroureteronephrosis and oligohydramnios or in infants <6 months old in 50% of cases. They rapidly lead to renal failure with bladder distention and urinary retention, UTI, and sepsis.

ENURESIS/NEUROGENIC BLADDER

Normal Bladder Function

- Storage:
- Low-pressure filling with adequate sphincter tone
- Emptying: volitional bladder contraction with sphincter relaxation

Neurophysiology of Lower Urinary Tract

- Parasympathetic: bladder contraction
- Sympathetic:
  Bladder relaxation
  Increased tone in proximal urethra
- Somatic (pudendal nerves): voluntary control of external urinary sphincter

INCONTINENCE

Etiology of Incontinence

- Diurnal and nocturnal incontinence
  Urologic anomaly: urine bypasses bladder, or bladder neck or urethra deformed
- Ectopic ureter or ureterocele
- Epispadias or bladder exstrophy
- Urogenital sinus anomaly
  Posttraumatic or postsurgical damage to lower urinary tract
  Neurogenic
- Overt (e.g., myelodysplasia, cerebral palsy)
- Occult (e.g., tethered cord)
  Nonneurogenic
- Detrusor instability: bladder contraction or increased tone during filling (symptoms include squat, squirm, dance, stare—may occur with reflux)
- Decreased bladder capacity for age
- Detrusor-sphincter discoordination
- Fecal retention → detrusor instability
- Psychogenic

Nocturnal Enuresis

- Maturational delay is very common—15% at 5 years, will resolve spontaneously in 15%–20% per year.
- Major causes of nocturnal enuresis:
  Decreased nocturnal awareness of bladder fullness
  Polyuria, most commonly 2° nocturnal alcohol dehydrogenase dysfunction
  Decreased bladder capacity or instability
  Constipation

Diurnal Enuresis

- Unstable bladder: uninhibited bladder contractions in a child who should have voluntary control of urination

Diurnal enuresis occurs in 15%–20% of 5-year-olds, 10% of 10-year-olds, and 1% of 15-year-olds. Of these children, 60% have a family history of delayed nighttime dryness; the problem is more common among lower socioeconomic groups. More common in larger families of 5 or more children. Etiologies include maturational variation, UTI, emotional disturbances, and anatomic or functional variations. It is a heterogeneous disorder. Autosomal dominant inheritance with 90% penetrance; one third of cases are sporadic. Four gene loci have been identified. There will be 10%–20% spontaneous remission per year. Self or parent awakening program results in 92% remission.

HEMOLYTIC UREMIC SYNDROME

HUS (hemolytic uremic syndrome) is the most common cause of acute renal failure in young children and is characterized by microangiopathic hemolytic anemia, thrombocytopenia, and uremia. It has features common to thrombotic thrombocytopenic purpura, except the latter usually occurs in adults. The more frequent etiologic organism associated with HUS is *E. coli* 0157:H7 (Figure 14.2).

EDEMA

Causes of Edema

- Kidney disease (nephrotic syndrome)
  Insidious onset, periorbital and lower extremity edema, abdominal distention
  Various types include minimal change nephritic syndrome, local segmental glomerulosclerosis, acute and chronic GN
- Chronic renal failure
- Liver disease—impaired production of albumin
- Congestive heart failure
- Protein-losing enteropathy
  Ménétrier disease (typically cytomegalovirus), inflammatory bowel disease, neuroblastoma, intestinal lymphangiectasia, trypsinogen deficiency
- Celiac disease
- Sepsis
- Hereditary angioneurotic edema
  Intermittent swelling of extremities
  Often preceded by trauma
  Decreased C4 and C1 esterase inhibitor
- Rocky Mountain spotted fever
- Stevens-Johnson syndrome
- Vitamin E deficiency
- Hypothyroidism
- Severe malnutrition

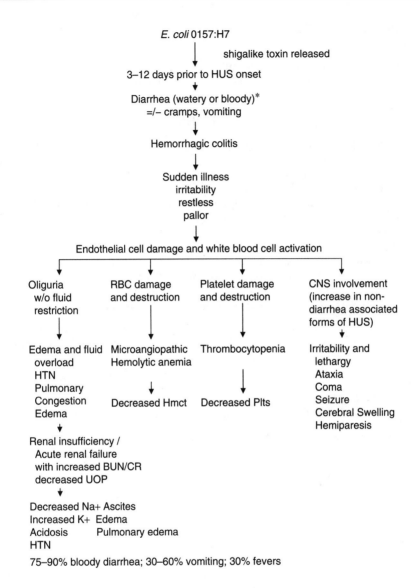

Figure 14.2
Hemolytic Uremic Syndrome.

Marasmus (calorie deficiency)
Kwashiorkor (protein deficiency)
- Zinc deficiency
- Hydrops fetalis
- Impaired lymphatic drainage
  Milroy disease
  Meigs syndrome

Yellow nail syndrome

Lymphedema praecox

- Filariasis (nematode infection resulting in elephantiasis)
- Immobility including placement of casts and paralysis

FURTHER READING

American Academy of Pediatrics, Committee on Quality Improvement, Subcommittee on Urinary Tract Infection. (1999). Practice parameter: The diagnosis, treatment, and evaluation of the initial urinary tract infection in febrile infants and young children. *Pediatrics, 104*(4 Pt. I), 843–852.

Amirlak, I., & Amirlak, B. (2007). Urinary tract infection in different pediatric age groups: An overview of diagnosis, investigation, management and outcome. *International Pediatrics, 22*(3).

Hoberman, A., & Wald, E. R. (1997). UTI in young children: New light on old questions. *Contemporary Pediatrics, 14,* 140–156.

Robson, W. L. M. (1997). Nocturnal enuresis. *Pediatric Review, 18,* 407–412.

Scarpero, H., & Ortenberg, J. (2007). Urinary tract infections. In R. Steel (Ed.), *Clinical handbook of pediatric infectious disease* (3rd ed.). New York: Informa Healthcare USA.

15

GENITALIA

*The miracle of life transcends our scientific understanding. We can only
marvel at the awesome possibilities that are created in each new life.*

Elizabeth Gilbert-Bono

FEMALE GENITALIA

Inspect the genitalia. The mother of the patient or another woman should be in the
room when you perform a vaginal examination. Ask the mother to pull the pants or
undergarments below the knee while a blanket covers the patient. Always wear
gloves. Answer succinctly any questions the patient raises. Inspect pubic hair, mons
pubis, labia majora, labia minora, clitoris, urethral meatus, and vaginal introitus for
presence, location, infestations, appearance, and discharge. A large clitoris (a glans
wider than 10 mm) may be normal or an isolated physical finding; however, it may
indicate adrenal hyperplasia or any of the conditions associated with precocious puberty
defined as occurring before age 8 years (7 years in African Americans) in girls. The
clitoris may not develop in adolescent girls with hypopituitarism or gonadal dysgenesis. The external genitalia grow very little until adolescence starts. In early puberty,
a rectal examination and an examination with the girl on the examining table with
the knees bent and the soles of the feet flat allows the patient to hold the labia apart
when this exam is indicated. Show the equipment to be used and explain any expected
pain or pressure. Pubic hair stages (Figure 15.1) are useful in quantifying development. Urethral discharges are always pathologic in childhood and may indicate
infection anywhere in the urinary tract. A flaming red area around the end of the
urethra may be caused by prolapse of the urethral mucosa. An eccentric mass near
the urethra may be a cyst, urethral polyp, papilloma, caruncle, condyloma, sarcoma
botryoides, prolapsed ureterocele, or periurethral abscess.

Inspect the vaginal orifice (Figures 15.2, 15.3) with the girl in the knee-chest
position. In preschool and primary school girls the opening is about $1-4 \times 3-8$ mm;
in preadolescent girls, it is about $1-2$ mm larger. Rough vaginal borders or an orifice
larger than 1 cm in diameter may indicate manipulation or abuse. Small tender
ulcers may be indicative of herpes simplex or other infections, including other sexually transmitted diseases.

Adhesions of the labia majora in a newborn may be a congenital malformation
or may occur in children with congenital adrenal hyperplasia (CAH). Imperforate

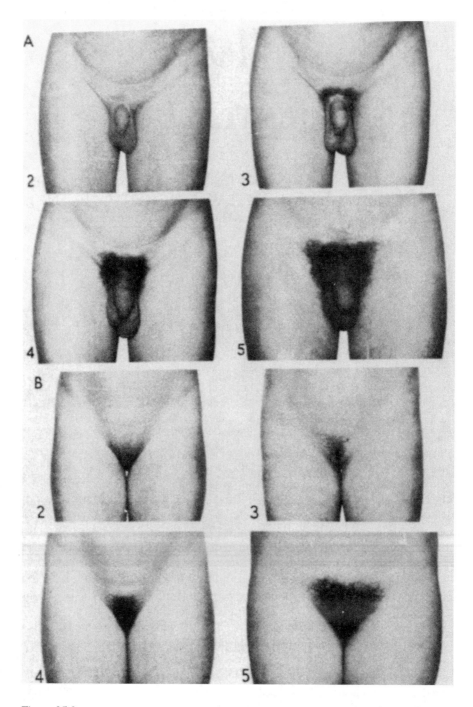

Figure 15.1
Pubic hair stages in males (A) and females (B). Stage 1 (not shown): preadolescent (no pubic hair). Stage 2: sparse, long, slightly pigmented. Stage 3: darker, coarser, more curled. Stage 4: adult type but smaller area. Stage 5: adult. (From Tanner, J. M., 1962. *Growth at adolescence*. Philadelphia: F. A. Davis.)

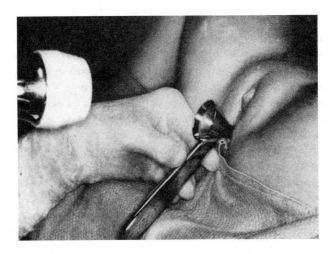

Figure 15.2
Inspection of the vagina with a vaginascope for children and
simple illumination with a flashlight.

hymen may be noted; this may cause hydrocolpos in young girls or hematocolpos in
pubertal girls. Have the patient cough. With imperforate hymen, the hymen bulges.
With absent vagina, the vaginal area is retracted upward and the hymen does not
move. Vaginal septa may cause similar signs. The labia minora are prominent in
newborns, then atrophy, and are virtually absent until estrogens are produced at
adolescence. Adhesions of the labia in older girls are common and may be caused
by infections, irritation, or local trauma, including abuse, and may cause dysuria.

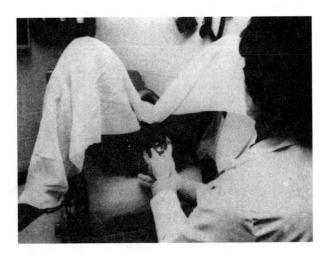

Figure 15.3
Proper draping for a pelvic examination.

A bloody vaginal discharge is normal (most often dime-sized on the 5th day) but not common up to the 4th week of life and at menarche. Vaginal bleeding in children aged less than 8 years is usually attributable to foreign bodies, injury, or constitutional isosexual precocity; ovarian tumors, botryoid sarcoma, and carcinoma of the cervix may present similarly. A mucoid vaginal discharge is frequently noted. In children still in diapers, this usually results from irritation caused by the diaper or the powder used in the diaper region. In older girls a foul discharge may be due to tight panties or pants, intertrigo, masturbation, pinworms, infection secondary to a foreign body, or allergy. A thin watery discharge is common in girls for 2–3 years before onset of menstruation. Redness of the perineum may be caused by irritation of physical or chemical agents such as bubble baths but may also signal a urinary tract infection.

Discharge accompanied by red inflammation in the surrounding vaginal and urethral structures usually indicates disease (Table 15.1). A white, practically odorless discharge has no significance.

A purulent discharge may be attributable to gonorrhea. Profuse, frothy, foul-smelling pruritic discharges may be due to *Trichomonas* organisms. White adherent discharge suggests *Candida* infection (Table 15.2).

Foreign bodies are usually toilet paper. Solids may be palpated by rectal examination. Urethral caruncle or prolapse of the urethra may be noted.

Vaginal palpation is usually omitted until near puberty. Note vaginal discharge or foreign body, size of uterus, and presence of ovaries. The normal uterus measures 1–2 cm, and the ovaries measure 0.5–1.0 cm until puberty. In older girls, use the lithotomy position with stirrups. Palpate the vaginal orifice before inserting the warmed speculum. Feel for enlarged glands, a sign of sexually transmitted infectious

TABLE 15.1

Categories of Prepubertal Vulvovaginitis

	Infections	
Noninfectious	**Nonvenereal Pathogens**	**Venereal Pathogens**
Poor hygiene	Bacterial respiratory and/or skin pathogens	Bacterial pathogens
Physiologic leukorrhea*	Gastrointestinal pathogens	*Chlamydia trachomatis**
	Candida species	*Gardnerella vaginalis**
	Shigella species*	*Neisseria gonorrhoeae**
	Enterobius vermicularis	?Genital mycoplasmas
Frictional trauma	Viral pathogens	Viral pathogens
Contact dermatitis	Varicella-Zoster virus	Herpes simplex
(allergic vulvitis)	Adenovirus*	Papilloma virus
Chemical irritant	Echovirus*	Protozoans
Sympathetic inflammation	Bacterial pathogens Group A	
and fistulas*	beta-hemolytic streptococcus*	
Vaginal foreign body*	*Streptococcus pneumoniae**	
	*Hemophilus influenzae**	

*Conditions in which vaginal discharge is prominent.

TABLE 15.2

Clinical and Laboratory Features of Vaginal Discharge in Adolescents

	Physiologic	Candida	Trichomonas	*Gardnerella vaginalis*
Appearance	White, gray or clear; flocculent	White; curdlike with adherent plaques	Gray, yellow or creamy; ± frothy or homogeneous	Gray, white; homogeneous
Amount pH of discharge	Variable ≤4.5	Scant ≤4.5	Large >5.0	Large >4.5
Vulvar and vaginal irritation	None	Common	Occasional	Rare
Amine odor with 10% KOH (Whiff test)	Absent	Absent	Present	Present
Microscopy	Epithelial cells, few WBCs, lactobacilli	↑ WBCs, +KOH: pseudohyphae and budding yeast	↑ WBCs, motile trichomonads (in saline prep) in 80%–90% of symptomatic patients	Few WBCs, +clue cells on saline prep

diseases. Do not lubricate the speculum before insertion, since this precludes obtaining cultures. Use a vaginoscope with a 1 × 11 cm blade. Press down on the introitus with one finger, insert the blade vertically, and then turn it horizontally; open it slowly with most pressure posteriorly. Maneuver the speculum until the cervix is seen. Do not stretch the hymen. Regardless of findings, do not use terms to describe the uterus such as *small*, *infantile*, or *underdeveloped*, since these terms may frighten the patient. The normal ratio of fundus to cervix is 1:3 in infants, 1:1 in pubertal girls, and 3:1 in mature women.

Organisms Thought to Constitute Normal or Nonpathogenic Vaginal Flora

Anaerobes and Facultative Anaerobes

Diphtheroids
Lactobacilli (newborn and postmenarchial)
Klebsiella species
Staphylococcus epidermidis
Beta-hemolytic streptococcus group B
Proteus species
Staphylococcus aureus
Pseudomonas species

Anaerobes

Peptococcus species
Bacteroides species
Peptostreptococcus species

It is currently unclear whether or not *Mycoplasma hominis, Ureaplasma,* and *Gardnerella vaginalis* can constitute normal flora or if they should be regarded as primarily pathogenic.

Examination

The cervix is normally pink and smooth, but columnar epithelium may extend over the junction, resembling erosion. There is an age-dependent migration of this border. The color becomes blue during pregnancy. Tenderness on moving the cervix or in the area of the fallopian tubes suggests pelvic inflammatory disease. An adnexal mass may be abscess, ectopic pregnancy, endometriosis, or ovarian cyst. An enlarged uterus occurs with intrauterine or ectopic pregnancy. Observe the vaginal wall for discharge or ulcers. Take cultures of any discharge, and endocervical swab for Papanicolaou (PAP) smear. Remove the speculum slowly. Proceed with bimanual examination; rectal examination is discussed below. Use a clean glove after rectal examination. Cover the gloved index and middle fingers with sterile lubricant and press posteriorly. Note any firmness or masses in the vagina. Note whether the cervix is firm or soft and whether the os is open or closed. Palpate the uterus between the abdomen and vagina: note its size, shape, and position and whether it is soft, firm, smooth, or tender. Palpate the adnexa on either side for enlargement, tenderness, or masses. The size of the ovaries normally is less than 1 cm before puberty and as much as 3 cm at puberty, and they may not be palpable unless they are enlarged.

Average adolescent development in girls proceeds as follows: breast development after age 8 years, pubic hair development at about age 12 years, increase in height velocity at age 12 years, menarche and axillary hair before age 13 years, and pubarche starts 6 months after thelarche.

MALE GENITALIA

In males, make a note if the position of the urethral orifice is not at the tip of the glans. *Hypospadias* exists if the opening is on the ventral (inferior) surface, and *epispadias* exists if the opening is on the dorsal surface of the penis. Examine the prepuce for infection, posthitis, and *phimosis* (adhesions preventing full retraction of foreskin). Some adhesions of the prepuce to the glans are normal until about age 4 years. Foreign body may be felt as a hard mass in the urethra. The prepuce may be inflamed, swollen, and tender. Inflammation of the glans (balanitis) may cause urinary obstruction. Pink pearly papules (1–3 mm elongated papillae on the corona of the penis) are normal in adolescents. Venereal warts are less uniform in size. Herpes simplex may resemble a small tender pimple, whereas a syphilitic chancre is a larger, less tender ulcer.

An enlarged penis may be noted in children with precocious puberty, CNS lesions, some testicular tumors, and adrenal hyperplasia. In CAH, the penis is large but the testes are of normal size. The penis may appear small if it is obscured by fat in corpulent boys. The penis is small in adolescent boys with hypopituitarism.

Observe the meatal opening. Stenosis may cause the opening to appear round instead of slitlike. Ulcers may cause obstruction to urinary flow. Note strength of stream. Slow stream indicates obstruction.

Next look at the scrotum. Normally the scrotum of a child who is not cold or frightened is loose and the testes and cords can be felt in it. Anything else in the scrotum is abnormal. If the scrotum appears large, suspect hernia or hydrocele or both. Often, especially in premature infants, the scrotal sac appears small, empty, and underdeveloped. Make an inverted V with your index finger and thumb together, place them about half an inch above the center of the inguinal ligament, and gently push toward the scrotum. Somewhere along the inguinal canal, a soft mass will be felt. Then try to push this mass into the scrotum. Once the mass is in the scrotum, grasp the mass with the thumb and forefinger of the opposite hand. If it can be brought to this position even though it may immediately retract, the mass is normally undescended testis. Repeat the procedure on the opposite side. If the mass is palpable in the inguinal canal but cannot be pushed down or if the testis is not felt, suspect an undescended or abdominal testis. In an older boy, one maneuver to bring the testis down is as follows: Have the boy sit in a chair with his heels on the seat, grabbing his knees. The extra abdominal pressure may push the testis into the scrotum. A small, flat, underdeveloped scrotum is probably the most accurate indication of true maldescent (cryptorchidism), usually resulting from defects in the inguinal canal but possibly signaling hypogonadism.

The testes are smooth; their size is usually about 1 cm until puberty. At stage II of puberty, testes length is 2–3.2 cm; at stage III, it is 3.3–4.0 cm; at stage IV, it is 4.1–4.9 cm; and at stage V, it is 5 cm. They remain small in children with hypopituitarism. They are large in boys with fragile X syndrome and are uneven and enlarged with infection or tumor of the testis. They are large with precocious puberty, defined as occurring before age 9 years in boys, but not with precocious puberty secondary to adrenal hyperplasia. A hard, enlarged testis without pain suggests tumor.

Average penile length as measured with a ruler at the base of the gently pulled penis is 4 cm at birth, 5 cm at age 4 years, 6 cm at age 11 years, and 12 cm at the end of adolescence. Micropenis is found in children with chromosome abnormalities, Prader-Willi syndrome, and other dysmorphic syndromes. If the penis is normal or small and the testes are firm and small in the adolescent, gonadal dysgenesis (Klinefelter syndrome) may be present. The left testis is usually lower than the right; the opposite may indicate complete situs inversus. It is believed they are not at the same level to avoid knocking against each other, especially when running.

If the scrotum appears large, changes size, or enlarges with coughing or crying, place one finger on the external inguinal ring and palpate the scrotum. If the mass in the scrotum feels firm, it is probably normal testis. If something is palpated in addition to the testis and cord, try to determine whether the sensation obtained is that of fluid, gas, or solid structure. Try to reduce the mass in the scrotum by pushing the contents back through the external ring. Masses that cannot be reduced include incarcerated hernia, hydrocele, varicocele, and spermatocele, in addition to normal structures.

Next, shine a light through the mass. An otoscope works well. Also darken the room. If the mass (except the testis) transilluminates and is irreducible, fluid is probably present. If the mass does not transilluminate and is irreducible, hernia is probably present. The use of transillumination in young children may be misleading because bowel in a hernial sac may transilluminate.

If a bulge occurs in the inguinal canal, and if a mass that is neither testis nor fluid is found in the scrotum, or you have the sensation of gas (crepitus) on palpation, the patient has a visible hernia. If you feel crepitus when you try to push the mass through the external ring, hernia is likely. Tenderness may be noted. In contrast to hydroceles, hernias are usually tender. Next, auscultate over the scrotal sac. Peristaltic sounds help indicate the presence of a hernia.

Hernias that cannot be reduced despite careful manipulation are said to be incarcerated. Hernias that feel swollen or have become gangrenous are strangulated from the tight constriction of the neck of the sac.

Finally, if a hernia or hydrocele is suspected, feel over the internal ring with the flat part of the index finger and roll the spermatic cord beneath the fingers as it lies in the inguinal canal. Although the ring is normally open, only a thin 1–2 mm solid structure should be felt extending through the ring. If the cord feels thickened or like silk being rubbed on silk, peritoneum is going through the ring, denoting a hernia that may be invisible. The size of the structures in the canal can be determined, and thickened structures may indicate polyarteritis, hernia, or other abnormality. Occasionally a hydrocele of the spermatic cord can be felt and may be mistaken for an incarcerated hernia. Careful palpation of the mass helps separate the upper end of the hydrocele from the internal ring, which is not possible with a hernia.

If an observer reports the presence of a hernia but none is found, the following maneuvers may make the hernia obvious: Have the patient stand on the examining table, and place the flat of your hand on the patient's abdomen. Pump the abdomen in and out with several short frequent strokes, and the hernial sac will become apparent. An older child may sit on a stool and hold the knees while you try to straighten the legs. The hernial sac will then fill.

Fluid in the scrotum usually indicates the presence of a hydrocele. Hydroceles are found frequently in children aged less than 2 years, are usually not tender, and with closed tunica vaginalis testis usually do not change size when reduction is attempted. Fluid fluctuating in volume denotes the presence of a patent tunica vaginalis testis or indirect inguinal hernia. *Varicocele* feels like a "bag of worms" because of the dilation of the pampiniform veins and usually occurs on the left. *Spermatocele* is a benign cyst on the head of the epididymis.

Acute swelling of the scrotum with discoloration may occur in those with Mediterranean fever or may result from torsion of the spermatic cord, a surgical emergency. Acute painful swelling also occurs in boys with orchitis, epididymitis, Henoch-Schönlein purpura, or rarely, torsion of the testis appendages. With torsion, the testicle is higher in the scrotum than it should be and may appear to lie transversely. With epididymitis, the testicle is in the normal position, and the long axis usually is in the axis of the body. The spermatic cord is tender and swollen with epididymitis and tender but not swollen with torsion. Elevation of the swollen tender mass decreases the pain in epididymitis and increases the pain with torsion. Epididymitis is usually caused by infection and accompanied by signs of urethral infection, but it may be a presenting sign of sarcoid. The testis may be dislocated into the inguinal canal after trauma.

Differential diagnosis of testicular torsion, incarcerated inguinal hernia, epididymitis, and orchitis—all of which cause scrotal swelling—may be difficult. With testicular torsion, the spermatic artery on the involved side does not pulsate. Pulsation is increased with orchitis, epididymitis, and torsion of the testicular appendix. Orchitis is usually accompanied by mumps or other viral infection.

The cremasteric reflex is tested by stroking the inner aspect of the thigh. The testis will rise in the scrotum, sometimes rising into the canal. This reflex is normal at any age. Absence may indicate a low spinal cord lesion, as in poliomyelitis, or testicular torsion, but it is also frequently absent in normal boys, especially at age less than 6 months and more than 12 years.

Examine the lymph nodes in the inguinal region for size and tenderness. Ordinarily three or four 0.5–1.0 cm glands are not abnormal. Tenderness or enlargement always indicates infection or any of the systemic diseases associated with generalized enlarged nodes.

The average adolescent development in boys proceeds as follows: testicular enlargement at age 11.5 years; pubic hair development at age 12.5 years; increase in height velocity at age 14 years; and development of facial and axillary hair at age 14.5 years.

Micropenis

Appearance of genitalia at birth: micropenis
Karyotype: XY
Levels of androgens: insufficient
Clinical evolution: delayed puberty

Micropenis at birth may imply a sufficient amount of testosterone to cause normal differentiation but an insufficient amount from the third month of gestation to birth.

Cryptorchidism

The etiology of cryptorchidism is related to hormonal-fetal hypothalamic-pituitary dysfunction during the third trimester or mechanical maldescent to an ectopic location. Location of cryptorchidism in 80% of cases is palpable in mid-upper scrotum or inguinal/ectopic and 20% impalpable intraabdominal or agenesis/torsion during descent. If bilaterally the testes are impalpable, rule out anorchia. Majority show spontaneous descent usually at 3–6 months, not after 1 year and not after previous inguinal surgery.

Retractile testis is descended testis but active cremasteric reflex. It needs to be distinguished from cryptorchidism. It is present in 75% percent of older males with empty scrotum. Testis descends to lower scrotum in cross-legged or squatting position. No treatment is necessary. A gliding testis can be pulled into the scrotum but retracts when released. It is a marginal undescended testis. The absence of demonstrable testes may be the result of "vanishing testes."

Malignancy is 40 times increased if the testis remains undescended; it is not reported if descended by 2 years. The peak incidence of malignancy is 20–40 years; in intersex cases it may occur in childhood. Tumors are usually painless.

Acute Scrotal Pain

Scrotal pain is caused by testicular torsion until proven otherwise. Differential diagnosis for the child or adolescent: torsion—testis (some present with recurrent pain), torsion of appendix testis/epididymus.

Epididymitis/orchitis—bacterial/viral/ureaplasma; trauma may cause hematocele/testicular rupture (severe injury).

Differential diagnosis for neonate: torsion—perinatal, hernia with incarceration, or birth trauma.

Varicocele

Etiology is related to defect in valves of left internal spermatic vein that causes blood pooling with increased temperature. Incidence is 5–15% in adolescents. An upright position examination will detect a varicocele usually on left; 10% are bilateral.

Newborn Circumcision

Benefits

- Decreased urinary tract infection—decreased 10–20×, in infancy
- Decreased penile carcinoma
- Decreased balanitis 3% (versus 6%)
- Decreased incidence of venereal disease and HIV
- Decreased risk of cervical cancer in spouse

Risks

- Meatal stenosis—8%–31%
- Penile adhesions
- Surgical complications—buried penis
- Defer circumcision if penile anomaly, such as concealed penis or hypospadias/chordee

Hypospadias

Hypospadias occurs in about 1 in 50 male newborns. In the mildest cases the urethra opens on the ventral surface of the glans with the presence of a dorsal hood. With increasing severity the penis is curved ventrally to form chordee and the penile urethra is short. Etiology is related to the endocrine-endogenous defect, environmental antiandrogen, or dysmorphic process.

Epispadias

Epispadias is present when the urethral opening is on the dorsal surface of the glans. It is frequently associated with cloacal extrophy.

AMBIGUOUS GENITALIA

Most newborns presenting with ambiguous genitalia are genetic females with CAH due to 21-hydroxylase deficiency (Figure 15.4).

- Apparent male:
  Bilateral nonpalpable testes in a full-term infant
  Severe hypospadias associated with bifid scrotum
  Undescended testis with hypospadias

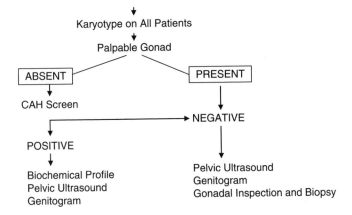

Figure 15.4
Intersex disorder.

- Indeterminate ambiguous genitalia
- Apparent female:
  Clitoral hypertrophy of any degree
  Foreshortened vulva with a single opening
  Inguinal hernia containing a gonad

Principal causes of ambiguous genitalia are:

- Ovary:
  CAH
  Placental aromatase deficiency
  Maternal source of virilization
- Testes:
  Leydig cell hypoplasia
  Testosterone biosynthesis defect
  5-α-reductase deficiency
  Androgen insensitivity
- Ovary and testes:
  True hermaphroditism
- Dysgenetic gonads
  Gonadal dysgenesis
  Denys-Drash and Frasier syndromes
  Smith-Lemli-Opitz syndrome
  Campomelic dwarfism

CAUSES OF DELAYED PUBERTY

I. Transient (Table 15.3)
   Constitutional Delay

TABLE 15.3

Relative Frequencies of the Causes of Delayed Puberty
in Males and Females

	Males (%)	Females (%)
Constitutional delay	50	20
Hypothalamic-pituitary	30	30
Gonadal puberty	10	40
Systemic pathology	10	10

II. Reversible
   A. Chronic systemic diseases
      1. Endocrine
      2. Nonendocrine
   B. Malnutrition
III. Permanent
   A. Hypothalamic disease
      1. Congenital deficiency of gonadotropin-releasing hormone (GnRH)
         a. Kallmann syndrome
         b. Prader-Willi syndrome
         c. Laurence-Moon-Biedl syndrome
         d. CNS anomalies (holoprosencephaly)
      2. Acquired deficiency of GnRH; infection, neoplasia, and so on
   B. Pituitary disorders
      1. Congenital deficiency of gonadotropin
      2. Acquired deficiency of gonadotropin; trauma, infection, neoplasia, and so on
   C. Gonadal disorders
      1. Congenital
         a. Turner syndrome
         b. Pure gonadal dysgenesis
         c. Resistant ovary syndrome
         d. Testicular feminization
      2. Acquired
         a. Ovarian insufficiency—autoimmune
         b. Trauma, infections, postsurgical, radiation

FURTHER READING

Busiah, K., Belien, V., Dallot, N., Fila, M., Guilbert, J., Harroche, A., et al. (2007). Diagnosis of delayed puberty. *Archives de Pédiatrie, 14,* 1101–1110.

Gilbert-Barness, E., & Gunasekaran, S. (2007). Male reproductive system. In E. Gilbert-Barness (Ed.), *Potter's pathology of the fetus, infant, and child* (pp. 1414–1426). New York: Elsevier.

Ibáñez, L., Jaramillo, A., Enriquez, G., Miró, E., López-Bermejo, A., Dunger, D., et al. (2007). Polycystic ovaries after precocious pubarche: Relation to prenatal growth. *Human Reproduction, 22,* 395–400.

McCann, J., Miyamoto, S., Boyle, C., & Rogers, K. (2007). Healing of nonhymenal genital injuries in prepubertal and adolescent girls: A descriptive study. *Pediatrics, 120*(5), 1000–1011.

Van Howe, R. S., & Robson, W. L. (2007). The possible role of circumcision in newborn outbreaks of community-associated methicillin-resistant *Staphylococcus aureus. Clinical Pediatrics (Philadelphia), 46,* 356–358.

16

ENDOCRINE

If contentment is the theme, Life's melody is sweet.

PITUITARY

The pituitary is the master hormone responsible for the activity of many of the other hormones, including human growth hormone, which is responsible for growth. Pituitary agenesis may be familial in rare instances and may be associated with one variety of congenital hypopituitarism or with major craniofacial anomalies (e.g., alobar holoprosencephaly or facial clefts) and in anencephalics. Infants with isolated pituitary aplasia may have normal intrauterine growth but present with neonatal hypoglycemia.

Anencephaly

The sella turcica is shallow or may be obliterated by vascular tissue that covers the base of the skull. Fetal growth in anencephalics is not significantly reduced.

Severe Perinatal Anoxia

In severe perinatal anoxia, ischemic damage to the pituitary may occur and also may elevate intracranial pressure. Some newborn infants with intracranial hemorrhage develop a syndrome of inappropriate secretion of antidiuretic hormone associated with fluid retention and hyponatremia.

Cysts and Tumors

Cysts are caused by the remnants of Rathke pouch and parapituitary craniopharyngiomas as well as teratomas replacing the pituitary gland.

Growth Hormone Deficiency

Children with growth hormone (GH) deficiency have retarded bone age and decreased growth rate (below 4.5 cm/year before puberty), documented during at least 1 year follow-up.

Growth Retardation: Causes by Age

Infancy

- Intrauterine growth retardation

- Calorie deficiency (malnutrition, malabsorption)
- Essential nutrient deficiency or excess (unbalanced diet)
- Metabolic diseases, renal failure
- Hypothyroidism
- Hypopituitarism

Childhood

- Genetic short stature
- Calorie deficiency (psychosocial dwarfism, malabsorption)
- Chronic diseases
- GH deficiency
- Inflammatory bowel disease
- Hypothyroidism
- Essential nutrient deficiency or excess
- Genetic bone disease
- Syndromes (girls):
  Turner syndrome
  Hypercorticism, hyperandrogenism
  Cushing syndrome

Puberty

- Constitutional delay
- Turner syndrome
- Essential nutrient deficiency or excess
- Hypopituitarism
- Anorexia nervosa
- Chronic diseases

THYROID DISORDERS

Hypothyroidism in Infancy

Normal Values of Thyroid Function Tests

- T_4 6.0–16.0 µg/dl > after 1 week
- TSH 0.5–5 µU/ml > in term infants
- 25% premature infants have T_4 values less than 6.5 µg/dl
- 50% premature <30 weeks gestation have values <6.5 µg/dl

Transient Hypothroxinemia

- Hypothalamic immaturity of prematurity
- Low T_4, normal TSH
- Prevalence: 25% of all prematures >50% <30 weeks gestation
- Free T_4 levels, relatively low, similar to adult normals 50% of term normals
- Treatment not indicated

Transient Hypothyroidism

- Temporary acute iodine deficiency
- Use of iodide, radiocontrast materials containing iodine, antithyroid drugs, and maternal TSH receptor-blocking antibodies
- May last for 2–3 months
- Usually seen in premature infants
- More common in Europe (20% premature > infants in Belgium)
- Low iodine availability relative to the needs
- Low free T_4 levels
- Therapy indicated

Euthyroid Sick Syndrome

- Low T_4, low T_3, high gamma-T_3, normal TSH
- Normal free T_4 in mild to moderate illnesses
- Birth trauma, acidosis, hypoxia, hypoglycemia, infection, malnutrition
- No therapy indicated

Secondary/Tertiary Hypothroidism

- Low T_4, low or low normal TSH
- Low free T_4
- Other hormone deficiencies: GH, adrenocorticotropic hormone (ACTH), luteinizing hormone, follicle-stimulating hormone
- Other coexisting findings
  Hypoglycemia
  Microphallus

Thyroxine-Binding Globulin Deficiency

- Common 1:10,000
- When thyroxine-binding globulin levels change, there is a parallel change in total T_4 levels
- Misinterpretation—hypo- or hyperthyroidism
- Free T_4 level to clarify

PARATHYROID GLANDS

Abnormalities of the parathyroid glands are common in DiGeorge syndrome (or the III–IV pharyngeal pouch syndrome). The parathyroid abnormalities range from functional deficits to complete absence of parathyroid tissue. This results in neonatal tetany. In addition to the parathyroid abnormalities, thymic abnormalities (absence or extreme hypoplasia), aortic arch abnormalities, and abnormal facies may be present.

Hypoparathyroidism

Hypoparathyroidism may occur in the newborn as a reactive phenomenon in response to maternal hypercalcemia. The elevated maternal calcium levels depress fetal parathyroid function. Infants may present with tetany and seizures toward the end of the first week of postnatal life, but some may present later with convulsions, precipitated by feeding of formula. Prolonged therapy with vitamin D and calcium may be needed before recovery occurs. Parathyroid function may be suppressed for as long as 3 months.

Hyperparathyroidism

Hypercalcemia becomes evident only after about 1 week. Skeletal radiographs show some demineralization and osteopenia; fractures and renal calcinosis may also be present.

Primary hyperparathyroidism in infancy may have an autosomal dominant or recessive pattern of inheritance. Secondary hyperparathyroidism occurs with vitamin D deficiency rickets, vitamin D-dependent rickets due to 1-α-hydroxylase deficiency, hepatic disease, renal disease, maternal hypoparathyroidism, furosemide therapy, and infants fed humanized cow's milk (with a high phosphorus load).

Hypocalcemia in the Newborn

Hypocalcemia in the neonate is not always associated with parathyroid disease, but may be associated with delayed development of a renal parathyroid receptor in preterm infants or with elevated calcitonin levels. However, most cases of neonatal hypocalcemia, including those with tetany, are related to infants fed formulas that do not meet their calcium and phosphorus requirements.

Hypercalcemia

Hypercalcemia is defined as total serum calcium concentration of >2.7 mmol/L (10.8 mg/dl) or serum ionized calcium concentration of >1.4 mmol/L (5.6 mg/dl). In pathologic hypercalcemia, elevation of serum Ca^{2+} usually occurs simultaneously with elevation of total calcium; however, elevated total calcium may occur without elevation of Ca^{2+}.

Hyperphosphatemia

Hyperphosphatemia in infants up to 18 months of age is defined as serum phosphorus concentrations of >2.7 mmol/L (8.4 mg/dl). In older children and adolescents, serum phosphorus concentration >2 mmol/L (6 mg/dl) are considered to be in the hyperphosphatemic range. Hyperphosphatemia may be caused by a decreased urinary phosphorate excretion or by sudden release of intracellular phosphorus into the extracellular space or an increase in dietary phosphate.

Calcium and Phosphorus Levels in Newborn

The third trimester is the time of maximal intrauterine calcium and phosphorus accretion. Daily accretion rates of 117–150 mg calcium/kg and 74 mg P/kg have been estimated for near-term fetuses. Interruption of the placental supply of these minerals at the time of delivery therefore predisposes the neonate to hypocalcemia at a time when oral feeding is limited. Parathyroid hormone level increases markedly at birth.

Serum 1,25-dihydroxyvitamin D [1,25(OH)$_2$D] concentrations rise steadily during the first day of life.

ADRENAL GLANDS

Adrenal Cortex

Zona glomerulosa → aldosterone
Zona fasciculata → cortisol
Zona reticularis → androgen

Aldosteronism

Aldosteronism is characterized by hypertension, hypokalemia, and decreased rennin. It may be due to an aldosterone-secreting adenoma or adrenal hyperplasia.

Cushing Syndrome

Cushing syndrome is due to chronic exposure to excessive amounts of cortisol or overproduction of ACTH as a consequence of hypothalamic-pituitary disease or ectopic ACTH secretion from nonadrenal tumors. Due to increased circulating levels of ACTH, the patients have bilateral adrenal hyperplasia. Cushing syndrome may be caused by adrenal adenomas or adrenal carcinomas.

Clinical features include moon face, increased adipose tissue in the neck and trunk, central weight gain, emotional lability, hypertension, osteoporosis, purple striae on the skin, and diabetes or glucose intolerance with fasting hyperglycemia or glycosuria or increased catabolism, and skeletal growth retardation; easy bruising and hirsutism also occur.

Function of Fetal Adrenal Cortex

The major factor that regulates steroidogenesis in the fetal adrenal gland is fetal pituitary ACTH stimulation, and the feedback mechanisms that exist in normal adults operate in the fetus. The relatively low unit output of cortisol induces an ACTH-triggered hypertrophy of the gland, especially the cells of the fetal zone.

Absence of Adrenal Glands

Absence of adrenal glands is extremely rare. Obviously, without treatment, the condition is not compatible with life.

Hemorrhage and Necrosis

Hemorrhagic necrosis of the adrenal gland frequently is due to birth trauma with breech deliveries and other varieties of severe birth trauma. However, the most important factors in its development, even in the presence of massive birth trauma, are severe intrauterine and intrapartum asphyxia and hypotension.

Other Features

Some examples of adrenal hemorrhage have been detected antenatally: renal vein thrombosis and coexistent adrenal hemorrhage.

Wiedemann-Beckwith Syndrome

In Wiedemann-Beckwith syndrome there is a triad of lesions characterized by exomphalos, visceromegaly, and macroglossia. There is massive enlargement of the fetal zone, with numerous diffusely scattered cells with enlarged nuclei.

Hyperplasia of the Adrenal Gland

True hyperplasia of the gland occurs in congenital adrenal hyperplasia associated with abnormal steroid synthesis.

Hypoplasia of the Adrenal Gland

Three histologic variants are described: anencephalic, cytomegalic, and miniature types. The genetics of the lesions may be X-linked, autosomal recessive, variable, or sporadic. Symptoms present shortly after birth, with early death if untreated, and hypogonadism at puberty if the child survives.

ADRENOMEDULLARY DISORDERS

Adrenal Medulla

Disorders of the adrenal medulla include neuroblastoma and pheochromocytoma. The diagnosis of these conditions depends principally on the measurement of their metabolites.

Evaluation of Adrenal Medullary Function

Total catecholamines, free catecholamines (norepinephrine, epinephrine, and dopamine), metadrenalines, homovanillic acid, and 4-hydroxy-3-methoxygenamphetamine excretion in urine are used to diagnose neuroblastoma and pheochromocytoma (Table 16.1).

Neuroblastoma

Neuroblastoma accounts for 7%–10% of all pediatric malignancies and is predominantly a disease of infancy. It is the most common nonhematopoietic tumor in the first 2 years of life.

Neuroblastomas are tumors derived from cells of neuroectodermal origin. They are classified clinically into types I to IV, depending on the primary site and degree of spread. This classification has prognostic significance. Stage IV-S is a congenital form involving bone marrow, skin, and liver and usually has a good prognosis.

Pheochromocytoma

Pheochromocytomas are catecholamine-secreting tumors. Patients present with intermittent headache, hypertension, profuse sweating, and diarrhea.

Tumors are found more frequently in boys (male-female ratio 1.8:1.0), and 35%–40% are single tumors of the adrenal medulla. Also, 10% of children have bilateral adrenal tumors; 10% of the tumors are malignant.

TABLE 16.1

Reference Ranges for Catecholamines and Their Metabolites

Age (Years)	Upper Limit* of Normal Excretion (mmol/mol Creatinine [µg/mg Creatinine])			
	Norepinephrine	Dopamine	HMMA (VMA)	HVA
<1	0.25 (0.37)	1.8 (2.4)	15.0 (26.3)	22.0 (35.5)
1–2	0.2 (0.3)	1.5 (2.0)	12.0 (21.1)	17.0 (27.4)
3–4	0.15 (0.22)	0.90 (1.22)	8 (14)	15.0 (24.2)
5–9	0.14 (0.21)	0.80 (1.08)	7.0 (12.3)	10.0 (16.1)
10–15	0.11 (0.16)	0.70 (0.95)	7.0 (12.3)	7.0 (11.3)

Note: These reference ranges were derived from urine collected over 18–24 hours into sufficient acid to reduce pH to <3.0. The reference population consisted of patients in whom an adrenal medullary tumor was suspected but whose final diagnosis excluded neuroblastoma or pheochromocytoma. Analysis was by high-pressure liquid chromatography with electrochemical detection.
HMMA, 4-hydroxy-3-methoxymandelic acid; HVA, homovanillic acid; VMA, vanillymandelic acid.
*The upper limit of normal is defined as the 0.95 fractile, determined using nonparametric methods.

Familial pheochromocytomas are recognized either as separate entity or in association with disorders such as multiple endocrine neoplasia, neurofibromatosis, and von Hippel-Lindau syndrome.

Elevated levels of total metadrenalines and free catecholamine in 24-hour urine tests are diagnostic.

FURTHER READING

Brewer, D. B. (1957). Congenital absence of the pituitary gland and its consequences. *Journal of Pathology and Bacteriology, 73*, 59.

Burke, B. (1992). The pituitary, pineal, adrenal, thyroid and parathyroid glands. In J. Stocker & L. P. Dehner (Eds.), *Pediatric pathology* (p. 980). Philadelphia: JB Lippincott.

Isaacs, H. Jr. (2007). Tumors of endocrine glands. In E. Gilbert-Barness (Ed.), *Potter's pathology of the fetus, infant, and child* (pp. 1657–1676). New York: Elsevier.

Lacson, A., & deSa, D. (2007). Endocrine glands. In E. Gilbert-Barness (Ed.), *Potter's pathology of the fetus, infant, and child* (pp. 1595–1656). New York: Elsevier.

Lucas, A., Bloom, S. R., & Aynsley-Freen, A. (1983). Metabolic and endocrine consequences of depriving preterm infants of enteral nutrition. *Acta Paediatrica Scandinavica, 72*, 245.

Mallett, E., Basutau, J. P., Brunelle, P., et al. (1978). Neonatal parathyroid secretion and renal receptor maturation in premature infants. *Biology of the Neonate, 33*, 304.

Paes, B. A., deSa, D. J., Hunter, D. J. S., & Pirani, M. (1982). Benign intracranial teratoma: Prenatal diagnosis influencing delivery. *American Journal of Obstetrics and Gynecology, 143*, 600.

Robinson, H. B., Jr. (1975). DiGeorge's or the III–IV pharyngeal pouch syndrome: Pathology and a theory of pathogenesis. *Perspectives in Pediatric Pathology, 3*, 173.

17

THE EYE

Mary Milne Gilbert-Lawrence

*A blind man's world is bounded by the limits
of his touch; an ignorant man's world by the limits of his
knowledge; a great man's world by the limits of his vision.*

E. Paul Hovey

A PRACTICAL APPROACH TO OFFICE VISION SCREENING

The American Academy of Pediatrics (AAP) and American Academy of Ophthalmology both recommend that infants and young children have periodic vision screening to detect amblyopia, glaucoma, astigmatism, and other conditions that can lead to vision loss if not treated. Newborns should have an eye examination performed by a pediatrician or other primary care provider and all children should be evaluated by 6 months of age for visual behavior and ocular alignment. Specific screening for visual acuity should be performed by 3½ years and repeated annually until age 10 years. Accurate, thorough screening for amblyopia and visual acuity can be difficult and time consuming, especially in preschool children. Several new technologies and a new nationwide screening program may help improve the vision screening rate among young children.

An illustration of the eye and its components are shown in Figures 17.1 and 17.2. Figures 17.3A and B show the structure of the eye.

The AAP has endorsed the use of photoscreening technology, which can help detect vision problems early in infants and children, as one option for increasing the vision screening rate among young children. Pediavision distributes one such device that rapidly screens infants and children for vision problems as they peer into a handheld binocular infrared camera system with a light target on which patients involuntarily fix their gaze. The Pediavision S04 Vision Screener is the only available photoscreener that performs binocular testing and combines autorefraction with video retinoscopy. A Website, www.infantsee.org, is available for information about a new program, InfantSEE, that provides free vision screening for infants 6–12 months of age.

This chapter written by Mary Lawrence, MD, MPH, Associate Professor of Ophthalmology, University of Minnesota Medical School, Associate Chief of Opthalmology, Minneapolis Veterans Affairs Medical Center, Glaucoma, Cataract, and Visual Rehabilitation, Minneapolis, Minnesota.

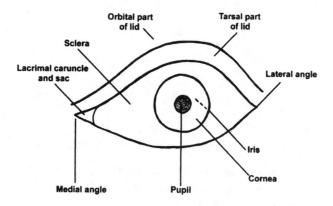

Figure 17.1
The eye.

Development of Visual Acuity

Age of Infant	Behavior
Term	Focuses on face, briefly tracks vertically and horizontally, turns toward diffuse light source, widens eyes to object or face at 8–12 inches
1 month	Blinks at approaching object "looming," tracks 60° horizontally, 30° vertically
2 months	Tracks across midline, follows movement 6 feet away, smiles to a smiling face, raises head 30° if prone

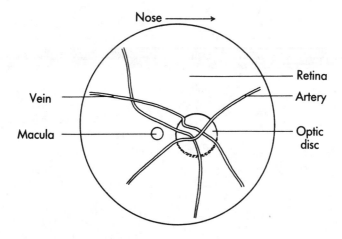

Figure 17.2
Diagram of the retina.

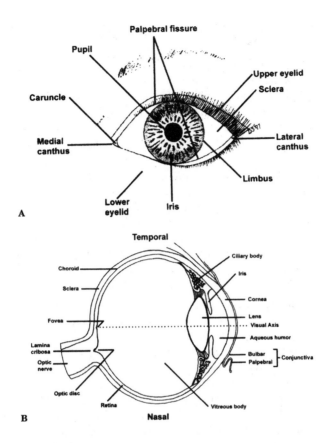

Figure 17.3
Normal structure of the eye. **A,** Frontal view of eye. **B,** Section through the orbit.

3 months	Eyes and head track 180°, looks at hands, looks at objects placed in hands
4–5 months	Reaches for object (12-inch cube) 12 inches away, notices raisins 1 foot away, smiles at familiar adult
5–6 months	Smiles in mirror
7–8 months	Rakes at raisin
8–9 months	Notes visual details, pokes holes in pegboard and at elevator buttons
9 months	Neat pincer grasp
12–14 months	Stacks blocks, places peg in round hole

The eye is not only the most important sensory organ, but is also a window to the brain. A careful examination of the eyes of a small child is basically made without the cooperation of the child and is difficult. Infants less than 1 year may be kept quiet with a bottle, but for children 1–4 years of age, you must use other devices.

Even in a small child, the examination is best performed if you use your left hand carefully. Hold the ophthalmoscope in your right hand and keep your left hand far from the patient's eye to attract attention. The natural tendency is to try to hold the eye open forcibly. This results only in a wet eye that is impossible to hold open, a distraught child, and an overheated examiner. If the child starts to cry when the light approaches the eye, put the light away or let the child play with it and perform this part of the examination later.

The *sclera* is the white of the eye; the *cornea* is the pigmented area. The clear area of the cornea is round. A small pigmented curtain (the iris) normally is also round and, by constricting and relaxing, it controls the amount of light that penetrates to the retina and through the pupil. The space inside the iris is designated the pupil.

Vision may be assessed in very young children by noting the child's interest in a light or bright object and noting the pupillary response to light. A newborn sees only light; by 1 month of age, an infant can see smaller objects and by 2 months of age can see rough outlines and follow moving fingers. By 6 months of age, the infant should focus for short periods but is farsighted. In older children, vision can be estimated by the child's interest in brightly colored objects in the room. The eye may be examined by having the child fix, if even for a moment, on some familiar object such as the parent's nose or face. Apparent blindness in a child less than 4 months may be due to developmental delay.

If more detailed tests of vision are desired in young children, they should be made before one proceeds further with the examination of the eye. Infants can respond to light and darkness. Observe children 1–2 years while they pick up different-sized colored objects from the floor. You can test a child older than 2 years with a letter E chart by asking the child which way the bars point. At age 3–5 years, both the child's eyes should see at least 20/40 and, after 5 years, 20/30 in both eyes, with no more than a two-line difference between eyes. The infant may also be tested by rotating a cylinder on which black and white lines are painted. An infant who sees will develop nystagmus as the cylinder is rotated; the blind infant's eyes will remain stationary. This cylinder test is also useful in distinguishing hysterical from organic blindness in older children. Blindness or varying degrees of decreased visual acuity may be due to optic nerve lesions, lesions anywhere in the eye including refractive errors, cortical atrophy, or CNS defects. Occasionally, temporary blindness may occur after head trauma, with no sequelae. Unilateral visual defect should direct your attention to lesions that are peripheral to the optic chiasm and in the eye.

If there is any question of a brain lesion, test visual fields by confrontation. Hold a piece of cotton in your hand, sit opposite the child, and have the child cover one eye while you close your eye. The child then looks at your open eye. Hold the cotton at arm's length and slowly bring it in, moving it through various planes midway between the child and you toward your eyes. As soon as the cotton is seen, the child will make a sudden movement toward it. This should occur at about the same time you see the cotton. Younger children may be asked to pick up small bright objects.

Vertical defects are termed *vertical hemianopia*. Heteronymous defects are almost always bitemporal, due to pressure on optic fibers at the chiasm. Homonymous defects usually indicate lesions posterior to the chiasm or in the visual cortex; temporal defects usually indicate lesions near the chiasm. Sudden onset of blind spots (scotoma) that enlarge and then resolve may be an early sign of migraine. Central scotoma may be due to pressure on the chiasm or to poisons. Constricted visual fields that are fixed in size, regardless of the distance from the patient, may be caused by hysteria.

The next part of the routine eye examination consists of observation of the eye. Blinking normally occurs bilaterally when a quick movement is made toward the eyes or when one cornea is touched. This is the basis of the corneal reflex. Spasmodic blinking is usually due to habit spasm.

The sclerae should be completely white, but they are blue in many normal children because of the normal thinness of the sclera. Children with osteogenesis imperfecta, iron deficiency, and Ehlers-Danlos syndrome have blue sclerae. Yellow or mud-colored sclerae may be the first sign of clinical jaundice. Red sclerae occur with conjunctivitis or glaucoma or may be due to drug or alcohol abuse. In carotenemia, the skin is yellow but the sclerae are clear. The top of the sclera is visible below the upper eyelid in children with the setting sun sign, which may be noted in normal premature infants, at times in normal full-term infants, and in some with abuse of phencyclidine. If marked, it is suggestive of hydrocephalus, increased intracranial pressure, or kernicterus. The bulbar conjunctiva covers the sclera.

Note exophthalmos or enophthalmos. Suspect exophthalmos if the eye appears large or protruding. Exophthalmos due to lid retraction occurs with hyperthyroidism, which is rare in childhood. In children with exophthalmos, the distance from the angle of the eye to the front of the cornea is more than 15 mm. Exophthalmos may be unilateral. The eyes may appear to bulge.

Apparent Bulging: Proptosis

Congenital glaucoma
Glaucoma
Orbital cellulitis, abscess
Retroorbital tumors, hemorrhage, metastases
Orbital tumors, optic glioma
Hand-Schüller-Christian disease
Neurofibromatosis
Lymphangioma, hemangioma
Cerebral sinus thrombosis
Hyperthyroidism

Suspect enophthalmos if the eye appears sunken or small. Enophthalmos is usually due to cervical sympathetic nerve damage, as in Horner syndrome or microphthalmos, but apparent retraction of the eyeballs is observed in children with chronic malnutrition or acute dehydration.

Note the position of the eyes at rest. When the child looks straight ahead, the irises should be between the lids. The iris may appear to be beneath the lower lid in children with the setting sun sign.

Note strabismus. The eyes should be parallel when the child glances in any direction. If there is less parallelism when the eyes move in one direction, suspect muscle paralysis. If the deviation from parallelism is equal when the eyes move in all directions, the squint is nonparalytic or concomitant. An easy method of observing squint is to look at the eyes when the child is looking toward a light about 3 feet away. The reflection of the light should come from approximately the same part of each pupil.

Degree of strabismus can be estimated by degree of deviation of light reflection from the center of the pupil. Deviation is approximately 15° if the reflection appears at the edge of the pupil, 30° if the reflection is halfway between the edge of the pupil and the limbus (outer edge of the cornea), and 45° if the reflection is at the edge of the limbus.

Another simple test for squint is the cover test. Hold a light about 2–3 feet from the child's eyes and sit directly in front of the child. Ask the child to focus on the light. Then cover one eye; the opposite eye is noted for motion. That eye is then covered, and the first eye is noted for motion. Motion indicates the presence of strabismus or tropia. Eye dominance can be determined by noting which eye moves a little during the cover test. Resistance to movement on covering of one eye more than the other may be an indication of defective central vision in one eye.

In strabismus, one eye (monocular) or both eyes (alternating) may be involved. Involvement can be determined by the constancy of the deviation in the cover test. Strabismus may be present only when the patient is tired (intermittent). Test for strabismus with distant and near objects. Squint may be present for only one of these planes of focus and still be concomitant.

In children with paralytic strabismus, the involved eye does not complete the full range of motion. In nonparalytic strabismus, each eye can move to all quadrants, but the eyes do not move simultaneously. Paralytic strabismus also occurs with retrobulbar pain and otitis in children with petrositis. Always check the child's vision carefully when strabismus is present, especially for equality of vision in both eyes.

Causes of Strabismus

Paralytic	Nonparalytic
Lesion of third, fourth, or sixth cranial nerve	Unilateral refractive error Nonfusion
Meningitis	Focusing difficulties
Botulism	Anatomic differences in eyes
Increased intracranial pressure	
Muscle weakness	

Strabismus is frequently present in newborns but should be minimal after 6 months of age. Even in very young children, however, fixed strabismus needs a careful ophthalmologic examination to exclude lesions that cause limitation of vision, such as optic atrophy, tumor, and chorioretinitis. Large epicanthal folds partly cover the globe of the eye and may be confused with squint. A unilateral epicanthal fold may be associated with torticollis.

Loss of upward gaze may be a sign of generalized increased intracranial pressure, pineal tumor, or lesions in the superior colliculi (Parinaud syndrome). It may be a late sign of kernicterus. Slow movements of the eyes may be observed in any condition causing paresis or paralysis of the eye muscles or with hyperthyroidism. In comatose patients, deviation of the eye downward and laterally with the pupil dilated suggests cranial nerve dysfunction with tentorial herniation. In such patients, rotate the head quickly. Eyes normally show conjugate movements to the side opposite to the direction of rotation. Absence of this response (doll's eye sign) indicates brain stem or oculomotor nerve dysfunction.

Nystagmus

Absence of a normal red reflex in the deviating eye may be a sign of a retinoblastoma or a cataract.

Note nystagmus by observing the constant motion of the eyes. Rarely, attempt to induce horizontal nystagmus by having the patient focus on an object from the outer angle of the eye. Record the direction of the fast and slow components of the nystagmus, as well as whether the nystagmus is spontaneous or induced. Circular, elliptical, and latent nystagmus are congenital. Rotatory nystagmus suggests a lesion in the medulla.

In infancy, spontaneous nystagmus may occur in hypothyroidism or may be congenital or of unknown etiology. The infant may be blind and have a peculiar searching type of nystagmus. Nystagmus is characteristic of cerebellar lesions and brain tumors and also occurs in the degenerative neurologic diseases and vestibular diseases. Vestibular nystagmus is always jerky, not pendular. The fast jerks are directed away from the involved ear. It may be evident in children with severe refractive errors. Bilateral, asymmetric nystagmus, pronounced in one eye and hardly discernible in the other, may be a sign of spasmus nutans. It is found in those who consume such drugs as marijuana, alcohol, benzodiazepines, or phencyclidine. Nystagmus present in a child with the eyes shut is congenital or should be considered vestibular in origin. Seesaw nystagmus, in which one eye moves rhythmically up while the other goes down, suggests a lesion near the third ventricle.

Ptosis of the lid may be congenital. It may represent birth injury to the brain or peripheral oculomotor nerve. If it is associated with a sunken eyeball, constricted pupil, anhidrosis, and facial pallor, it is due to cervical sympathetic paralysis (Horner syndrome). Ptosis may be an early sign of myasthenia gravis, botulism, amyotonia congenita, and myotonic dystrophy and occurs in children with heroin use, encephalitis, or tendon injury to the levator palpebra superior. It may occasionally be noted in children recovering from tetany.

Only slight ptosis results from sympathetic paralysis. Third-nerve paralysis results in severe ptosis. Ptosis associated with automatic elevation of the lid during chewing (the jaw-winking or Gunn phenomenon) is a congenital anomaly. Because of weakness of the orbicularis oculi, the palpebral fissures are more widely spaced on the involved side in children with facial palsy.

Other abnormalities of the eyelids should be noted. Hemorrhagic discoloration of the lids may be due to injury, neuroblastoma, or any bleeding dyscrasia such as scurvy and leukemia. Distortion of the lid may be due to edema, retrobulbar tumor, or metastases such as neuroblastoma. Extensive infection of the lids may be due to deep abscess formation or osteomyelitis around the sinuses. Fistulas near the lids may be congenital or may be due to chronic infection. Hemangiomas of the lids are common. Violaceous eyelids may be noted in children with dermatomyositis and scleroderma. Crepitation of the lids (emphysema) is due to air trapping and may follow fracture of the nose or sinuses. Look for distichiasis, a congenital anomaly of the eyelids with double rows of eyelashes or occasional aberrant hairs.

Dark circles under the eyes may be noted. Their significance is uncertain, but they may indicate tiredness, insufficient sleep, or allergy, or they may be a residual of edema in the face. Infraorbital eyelid creases (Morgan lines) are found in allergic children.

Examine the conjunctivae for inflammation, conjunctivitis, hemorrhages, and foreign body. Conjunctivitis alone does not usually produce severe pain—only burning, soreness, or itching. If a foreign body is suspected, use a magnifying lens with good lighting. Photophobia may be present with conjunctivitis. The usual causes of redness of the conjunctivae in childhood are:

Bacterial or viral infection (pink eye)	Vitamin D poisoning
	Measles
Allergy	Kawasaki disease (bulbar)
Foreign body	Eye strain
Crying	Acrodynia
Marijuana smoke	Erythema multiforme

An early sign of measles, seen occasionally even before Koplik spots appear in the mouth, is the appearance of small red transverse lines in the conjunctivae (Stimson lines).

Conjunctivitis is common in newborns and may be due to gonorrhea, chemical irritation, or inclusion blennorrhea, which is probably caused by *Chlamydia oculogenitale*. Noting the extent of the conjunctivitis is important. In gonorrheal conjunctivitis or with any acute iritis, the bulbar and palpebral conjunctivae are inflamed; in conjunctivitis due to chemical irritation, the bulbar conjunctivae are usually spared and only the palpebral conjunctivae are inflamed. Children with vitamin A deficiency manifest dry wrinkled conjunctivae with foamy, yellow patches (Bitot spots). Small comma-shaped vessels in the lower bulbar conjunctivae are characteristic of vascular stasis and sickle cell disease.

Small hemorrhages in the conjunctivae may be significant signs of bacterial endocarditis, scurvy, and meningococcemia. They are also seen in the bleeding diseases. They are commonly seen in the normal newborn and in children following cough or trauma.

Pingueculae are small, yellowish, wedge-shaped areas near the cornea. They occasionally occur with the xanthomatoses or Gaucher disease. *Pterygium*, a wing-shaped white area that may cover the cornea, is an abnormal extension of the conjunctiva.

Sties (hordeolum) usually occur on the lower lid as tender, reddish-yellow pustules at the root of the hair follicle. Recurrent sties may be a sign of eyestrain, exposure to dust or dirt, general debility, or hay fever. A sty may be an early sign of diabetes. A nonpainful, yellow swelling of the eyelid edge (chalazion) is due to inclusion cyst. Scaling of the lid margins (blepharitis) may be due to seborrhea, allergy, or infection.

The cornea should be crystal clear and is best examined with good room illumination or with an open bulb placed about 2 feet in front of the patient. The cornea is about 10 mm in diameter at birth and about 12 mm at adulthood. Any inflammation, ulceration, or opacity is abnormal. The cornea is clear in a child with conjunctivitis.

Note redness of the cornea due to vessel engorgement. If the redness is less near the cornea and increases toward the conjunctiva, superficial inflammation (keratitis) is probably present. If redness is greater near the cornea and fades toward the periphery, deep (ciliary) inflammation (iritis) is present, and the eye is painful.

Opacities in the cornea are usually due to ulcerations. White, Swiss cheese–like superficial membranes at the periphery of the cornea are band keratopathy due to deposition of calcium and are observed in children with hypercalcemia, chronic uveitis, or juvenile rheumatoid arthritis.

Yellow opacities usually indicate active ulcerations; bluish-white opacities are healed ulcerations. Note depth of ulceration. Active ulcerations are usually associated with pain, photophobia, redness of the eye, and a small pupil. If inflammation or opacity is present, suspect foreign body, trauma, or infection. Corneal ulceration may occur with riboflavin deficiency or may be due to herpes.

Pinhead grayish ulcerations with conjunctivitis (phlyctenular conjunctivitis) is a rare painful form of tuberculosis or tuberculin sensitivity. It begins at the corneal-scleral junction and then invades the cornea. Deep ciliary inflammation is especially common in children with interstitial keratitis due to late congenital syphilis. The entire cornea may appear steamy white. Keratoconjunctivitis also occurs with measles and other viral diseases and with rheumatoid arthritis. A gray-green-orange ring around the cornea—the Kayser-Fleischer ring—is seen in hepatolenticular degeneration (Wilson disease).

The cornea is hazy in children with glaucoma, drug abuse, or avitaminosis A, and in children with metabolic diseases such as mucopolysaccharidoses and cystinosis, although slit lamp examination is usually necessary to demonstrate crystal formation in the cornea. A large cornea may also be a sign of glaucoma.

Foreign bodies on the cornea or conjunctiva may be detected easily unless they lie over the pupil. If you suspect a foreign body, evert the lids and swing the light in different directions while carefully examining the eye. You will observe either the foreign body or its shadow. The eyelids can be everted by asking the patient to look down. Place an applicator stick just over the edge of the upper eyelid and pull the eyelid forward and upward. If the suspected foreign body or abrasion cannot be located, fluorescein sticks may be placed in the eye. On oblique illumination, the injured area of the cornea will stand out with a greenish fluorescence.

With the light in the same position, evaluate the anterior chamber. Blood or small white spots may be observed. Blood is usually due to injury. White spots may be an early sign of uveitis. Light sensitivity suggests iritis or keratitis.

Note discharges from the eye. An infant ordinarily does not have tears before 1 month of age, and the lacrimal duct opens several weeks later. A watery discharge in infancy, usually from one eye, may signify a blocked tear duct. Press on the tear sac, which is just below the inner canthus of the eye. At the same time, slightly evert the lower lid so that you can observe the small opening (punctum). If fluid escapes when you apply pressure, there may be obstruction below the lacrimal sac. Fixed, red, painful swelling and induration in the area of the lacrimal sac indicate abscess formation with blockage (dacryocystitis). Obstruction without infection is usually a congenital anomaly; with infections, it is an acquired disease. A bluish swelling over the lacrimal sac may be a dacryocystocele and should be differentiated from a hemangioma. Tearing with a wet nose, however, may be a sign of infantile glaucoma; when a tear duct is blocked the nose is usually dry.

Watery discharges (epiphora) are also seen with allergy, sinusitis, sties, and drug abuse. Purulent discharges are due to infections. In newborns, the pus due to the chemical irritants placed in the eye may easily be confused with gonorrheal ophthalmia. Absence of tears has been noted as a characteristic of children with familial dysautonomia or Sjögren syndrome.

The iris contains two muscles that control the size of the pupils and is usually blue at birth and becomes pigmented within 6 months. Inequality of pigmentation may be a congenital anomaly or may be due to metallic foreign bodies. In Horner syndrome, the involved side remains blue and the opposite side acquires pigment. Different-colored irises (heterochromia) may indicate Waardenburg syndrome. Observe the iris to determine any fluttering, which may occur with subluxation or detachment of the lens. Absence of a part of the iris (coloboma) may be associated with other anomalies or with Wilms tumor. Adhesions may be seen from the iris toward the lens. These may be congenital, due to persistence of the pupillary membranes, or may occur with chronic iritis, as in rheumatoid arthritis. Black and white spots (Brushfield spots) in the iris are usually evident in children with Down syndrome. Pigmented nodules (Lisch nodules) are characteristic of children with neurofibromatosis. In the iris, nodules may be due to tuberculosis, and hypopigmented spots are evident in tuberous sclerosis. When a light shines on the iris of patients with albinism, the eye lights up as if a switch had been thrown.

Compare the pupils for size and shape. They should be round, regular, clear, and equal. The pupil controls the quantity of light reaching the retina, minimizes aberrations of the peripheral cornea and lens, and increases depth of field. Irregularities in the pupil are usually due to congenital malformations. The sudden appearance of an irregular pupil should make you immediately suspect a penetrating foreign body through the cornea. White bands over the pupil may be due to congenitally persistent pupillary membranes. Unequal pupils (anisocoria) are usually congenital, but if they appear suddenly in the presence of equal illumination, they usually indicate acute intracranial disease.

Note reaction to light of the pupils. Size and light reaction are controlled by the sympathetic nervous system and the parasympathetics carried by the third cranial nerve. Children's pupils should react to light quickly. Reaction of the pupil in which the light shines is the direct reaction. The reaction of the opposite pupil is the consensual reaction. Absence of consensual reaction on one side occurs with optic nerve or retinal lesion and on both sides with a midbrain lesion. The pupils of newborn infants are constricted until about 3 weeks of age, so light reaction, while always sluggish in an infant with congenital glaucoma, is not a good test of glaucoma in newborns. Acute pain or excitement may cause dilation of pupils.

A fixed, dilated pupil indicates sympathetic stimulation, blindness, or poisoning. It may be caused by pressure on the midbrain due to acute increase in intracranial pressure. It may indicate a homolateral extradural or subdural hematoma, or meningitis. Injury to the ciliary ganglion can result in a dilated pupil that reacts poorly to light but constricts to near accommodation (Adie pupil). This does not indicate intracranial injury and usually follows injury to the eye. Dilated, unreactive pupils are seen with atropine or deep barbiturate poisoning, cocaine or amphetamine use, or anoxia. Dilatation of the contralateral pupil on light stimulation of one eye suggests injury to the eye and poor vision of the opposite eye, even in a comatose or uncooperative patient (Marcus Gunn sign). Pupils that react to accommodation but not to light (Argyll Robertson pupils) indicate a midbrain lesion, as occurs in Lyme disease, viral encephalopathies, syphilis, and granulomatous diseases.

Dilated pupils do not react in children whose coma is due to compressing lesions of the brain, but they are usually reactive in comatose children with metabolic disease. The pupils remain dilated in children with partial blindness, but the pupils respond to light in children with cortical blindness. Pupils may react slowly or not at all in those consuming illicit drugs. The pupils do not react during a petit mal episode, in contrast to those in children who are staring or daydreaming.

Constricted, unreactive pupils are noted in children with cervical sympathetic palsy (Horner syndrome) or acute iritis, or in opiate, light barbiturate, or cholinesterase enzyme poisoning. In neurosyphilis of childhood, the pupils remain fixed and small because of parasympathetic injury. Constricted pupils generally indicate that the third-nerve impulses are intact.

Hippus is exaggerated rhythmic contraction and dilatation of the pupils. It may be a normal variant but also occurs with CNS disease.

Accommodation can be tested even in young children by having them look first at a shiny colored object at a distance and quickly bringing the object toward the eye. The pupil contracts as the object is brought near the eye. This reaction is known as the *convergence reaction*. Various neurologic disorders including diphtheria, as well as alcohol and other drugs, cause loss of the accommodation reflex. Most infants are hyperopic, but occasionally very young infants will play with objects within 2–3 inches of their eyes. Such infants will probably be myopic when their vision develops fully.

Examine the lens with direct light from the unshaded bulb. White or gray spots usually indicate opacities (cataracts) in the lens. In persons with cataracts, almost nothing can be seen beyond the white membrane of the lens when a light shines into the eye.

Successful internal examination of the eye depends on your having gained the confidence of the child and having learned to develop a picture image of what you see in a flash. (This same technique is useful in examination of the pharynx in children.) Tell the patient that the room will be darkened, that a light will shine in the eyes, but that nothing painful will be done. Eye drops should be avoided but may be necessary. If the child is old enough, ask the child to look at a brightly colored picture across the room. Children who are somewhat younger can be given a flashlight and asked to turn it on and shine it on the picture across the room.

First, use a $+8$ to $+2$ lens to examine the cornea, iris, and lens and then a 0 to -2 lens for examination of the disc and retina. Use your right eye to examine the patient's right eye and your left eye for the patient's left eye. Start about a foot away from the patient's eye and, as you approach the eye, change the ophthalmoscope lenses so that they become less positive. The retina is usually best visible with a 0 to -2 lens in infants and children and is usually seen first as a red area (the red reflex). The details become obvious as you move closer. With this type of illumination, opacities in the cornea, anterior chamber, or lens will usually be seen as black spots against the red reflex of the retina. The anterior chamber is hazy with iritis, shallow with glaucoma, and dark with blood (hyphema).

With direct light, pearly gray, opaque, round areas in the center of the lens are typical of cataracts (Table 17.1). Lenticular cataracts are usually lamellar (zonular) in children.

The lens may appear clear but misshapen. The posterior eye structures will be seen with difficulty. The lens may be dislocated upward, as in patients with Marfan syndrome, or downward, as in patients with homocystinuria. Other syndromes with

TABLE 17.1
Causes of Cataracts in Infants and Children

Metabolic Disorders	**Skin Disorders**
Galactosemia	Cockayne syndrome
Galactokinase deficiency	Incontinentia pigmenti
Diabetes mellitus	Ichthyosis
Mannosidosis	**Craniofacial Disorders**
Hypoparathyroidism	Hallermann-Streiff syndrome
Homocystinuria	Smith-Lemli-Opitz syndrome
Fabry disease	Rubinstein-Taybi syndrome
Refsum disease	Marshall syndrome
Cerebrotendinous xanthomatosis	Cerebro-oculo-facial syndromes
Wilson disease	Chromosome abnormalities,
Glucose 6-phosphatase deficiency	including trisomy 21
Renal Disorders	**Central Nervous System**
Lowe syndrome	Marinesco-Sjögren syndrome
Alport syndrome	Rubella syndrome
Musculoskeletal Disorders	**Ocular Disorders**
Chrondrodysplasia punctata	Retinoblastoma
Myotonic dystrophy	Glaucoma
Stickler syndrome	Trauma
Robert syndrome	
Congenital	
Retinopathy of prematurity	
Maternal diabetes	
Maternal thyroid disease	
Maternal parathyroid disease	

dislocated lenses include Sturge-Weber, Ehlers-Danlos, Crouzon, Weill-Marchesani, sulfite oxidase deficiency, and mandibulofacial dysostasis.

The appearance of the red reflex from the retina provides important information. Ordinarily, the fundus will be pink and shiny, but it may be gray in deeply pigmented or anemic children. The retina becomes gray and loses its shine whenever it becomes avascular. Absence of the red reflex or the appearance of a white-opaque reflex (leukocoria) is noted in children with opacities of the cornea or lens, cataracts, persistent posterior fibrovascular sheath of the lens, retrolental fibroplasia, retinal detachment, or retinoblastoma. Darkly pigmented freckles in the retina occur in children with familial polyposis; a lighter pigment may indicate retinitis pigmentosa, which is accompanied by the complaint of night blindness.

Veins and arteries are of almost equal size, or the veins are slightly larger than the arteries. In the hypertensive diseases, especially nephritis, the arteries are narrow. The vessels are dilated and cyanotic in children with cyanotic heart disease. Venous distention is an early sign of increased intracranial pressure. The veins pulsate normally. Exaggerated pulsations of the arteries, however, may indicate arteriovenous fistula, aortic regurgitation, or other causes of increased pulse pressure. All vessels of the disc are engorged with inflammation of the optic nerve (optic neuritis) and may appear small and thickened with arteritis, as in the collagen diseases.

Fresh hemorrhages on the retina in newborns may indicate trauma or anoxia or may be a cardinal sign of subdural hematoma. In older infants and children, fresh hemorrhages almost always indicate child abuse (shaken baby syndrome) but they are also seen in those with rare metabolic diseases, such as glutaric acidemia. They appear as red spots alone or with a surrounding white haze. These spots are also seen with sinus thrombosis, leukemia, scurvy, bacterial endocarditis, and other bleeding diseases. Multiple, gray, mulberrylike tubercles in the retina are seen in children with tuberous sclerosis, tuberculosis, and neurofibromatosis.

Patchy areas of white and red indicate chorioretinitis. They may appear in various infections but are characteristic of infection with toxoplasmosis, cytomegalic inclusion disease, syphilis, tuberculosis, and chronic brucellosis. Grayish-brown streaks radiating out from the disc are angioid streaks, seen in pseudoxanthoma elasticum.

The disc is most easily found if you relax and gaze from the temporal side of the patient's eye toward the posterior aspects of the eye. The edges of the disc usually have a sharp border around half the circumference and then fade. Blurring indicates increased intracranial pressure. The entire disc may be surrounded by a melanin ring, and this is usually normal. Gray stippling around the optic disc is a sign of lead poisoning. The disc is usually in the same plane as the retina in children. It is usually a little less pink than the surrounding retina. It is very pale in patients with anemia.

The disc may appear large and swollen; the edges may appear blurred; and the retinal vessels may appear to bend down from the disc to the retina in children with papilledema. Use the green filter to detect minimal blurring. Such "choked" or bulging discs indicate increased intracranial pressure or optic neuritis. Brain tumors or abscesses, except those originating in the anterior fossa, usually cause papilledema. Pulmonary insufficiency, especially that associated with obesity, may be associated with papilledema (a form of pseudotumor cerebri).

The disc appears white in children with optic neuritis or optic atrophy.

Glaucoma (Infantile or Congenital)

A rare but important ocular disease often manifesting as tearing and photophobia (an inability to tolerate normal daylight) can be mistaken for lacrimal duct obstruction, but the photophobia and increased corneal size help make the correct diagnosis. Treatment is urgent and often surgical. Amblyopia is also associated.

Causes of White Optic Disc (Leukocoria)

Optic neuritis

Optic nerve atrophy

Meningitis

Encephalitis

Generalized infections

Neurofibroma

Osteopetrosis

Localized lesion of the
    posterior pole, retinoblastoma

Toxocara canis (visceral larva
    migrans), retinal toxoplasmosis

Cataract, big posterior coloboma

Retinoblastoma

Cataract, retinal detachment

Sarcoid or *Candida vitritis*

Uveitis with cataract and glaucoma

Cataract

Retinopathy of prematurity

Cystic fibrosis

Thiamine deficiency

Brain tumors

Optic nerve tumors

Fibrous dysplasia

Poisons

Septooptic dysplasia

Leukocoria may precede other signs of multiple sclerosis, or it may be an isolated finding. Unilateral papilledema with contralateral optic atrophy may be due to a frontal lobe tumor (Foster-Kennedy syndrome). If the retina appears opalescent, retinal detachment may be present. Cupping of the disc in which the vessels appear to dip down from the retina toward the disc may be physiologic or may be exaggerated with glaucoma or in children with any of the conditions causing white disc.

Just to the temporal side of the disc is a small yellow-red area devoid of vessels — the macula. Because the macula is the most light-sensitive area of the eye, the pupil constricts as the macula is approached. In an older child, the macula can be visualized if the child is told to look at the ophthalmoscope light. This area appears to be cherry-red in reticuloendothelial diseases such as Tay-Sachs and Niemann-Pick disease and in other lysosomal storage diseases. The macula may be brown and appear fragmented in children with the juvenile form of macular degeneration. Bruit over the eyeball may occur with congenital arteriovenous fistulas in the brain.

Later in the examination, obtain the corneal reflex by touching the cornea with a piece of cotton or suddenly bring an object toward the child's eyes. Both eyes normally shut. Failure to obtain the corneal reflex indicates trigeminal (sensory component) or facial (motor component) nerve injury. Pontine injuries and anesthesia and many drugs depress this reflex.

In general, complete cooperation is impossible with young children. As the child grows older, devices for obtaining attention should be used. However, with or without the child's cooperation, you should explore these areas of the eye (Table 17.2). If you note a defect in any area, refer the patient to an ophthalmologist, who can use other instruments and anesthetics (Table 17.3).

Periorbital Edema: Differential Diagnosis

- Periorbital cellulitis
  Usually pathogens are streptococcal species, *Staphylococcus aureus*, and *Haemophilus influenzae*
- Orbital cellulitis
  Bacterial pathogens are the same as periorbital cellulitis
  May be accompanied by orbital abscess and may spread via the sinuses to the brain
- Other infections
  Conjunctivitis
  Sinusitis

TABLE 17.2
Ocular Findings in Dysmorphology

Feature	Conditions to Watch For	
Orbits (the set of the eyes)	Hypoterlorism/hypertelorism	Prominent/deeply set eyes
	Palpebral fissures: size and slant (up, down)	Prominent /flat supraorbital ridges
Eyebrows	High arched	Thick
	Synophrys (eyebrows that meet in the middle)	Thin
	Medial flare	Absent
Eyelids	Long	Absent
	Epicanthal folds	Ptosis
	Telecanthus	Coloboma or dermoid
Globe	Anophthalmia	Microphthalmos
Cornea	Corneal clouding	Microcornea
Lens	Cataract	Dislocated lens
	Stellate pattern	
Iris	Aniridia	Brushfield spots
	Coloboma	Lisch nodules
	Heterochromia	
Sclerae	Blue sclerae	Telangiectasis
Retina	Albinism	Optic atrophy
	Pigmentary changes	Coloboma
	Cherry-red spot	Detachment
Motility	Nystagmus	Strabismus

TABLE 17.3
Main Examination Techniques by Age Group

Technique	Newborn/Infant (0–1 year)	Toddler (Up to 3 Years)	Preschool and Older
Pupillary red reflex	Yes	Yes	Yes
Corneal light reflex	Yes	Yes	Yes
Vision	Face follow, OKN*	Cover test HOTV†	HOTV
Ocular movement	Spin baby	Head twist	Frame
Visual fields		Wiggly fingers	Count fingers
Funduscopy	4 quadrants red reflex	4 quadrants red reflex (and temporal disc, and macula, all clear images)	4 quadrants, temporal disc and macula clear

*Not critical. †Successful in very cooperative child.

Dental abscess
• Allergic reaction
  Conjunctivitis
  Urticaria/angioedema
  Drug reaction
• Local ocular causes
  Insect bites
  Contact dermatitis
  Trauma
  Foreign body
• Systemic disorders with generalized edema
  Hypoproteinemia
  Renal disease
  Congestive heart failure
• Malignancy
  Neuroblastomas: associated with ecchymoses, raccoon eyes, and proptosis
  Leukemia: associated with fever, fatigue, anemia, bone pain, lymphadenopathy, splenomegaly

Nystagmus

Aspects to be considered	Questions to ask parents
Evidence of poor vision	Poor eye contact?
	Toys close to face?
	Poor motor development?
Photophobia	Squinting outdoors?
	Opens eyes only in semidarkness?
	Stays up all night?
Nyctalopia	Refuses to play outside?
	Cries when lights are out?

Runs into walls at night?
Wets in bed?

Note that in the child with nystagmus, a thorough pediatric ophthalmologic investigation is essential to establish the appropriate diagnosis, initiate genetic counseling, and provide appropriate support.

Nasolacrimal Duct Obstruction

Congenital

Obstruction can occur anywhere in the lacrimal system, but is usually at the valve of Hasner at the lacrimal duct entrance into the nose.

Digital massage of the lacrimal sac can be performed to increase the chance of spontaneous resolution. If resolution does not occur, nasolacrimal duct probing or silicone tube intubation is required.

Dacryocystitis

Dacryocystitis occurs when an abscess forms in the lacrimal sac. Patients present with intense pain, redness, and swelling in the medial canthal area. Treatment consists of intense topical and systemic antibiotics followed by definitive treatment of the nasolacrimal duct obstruction.

Cellulitis

Orbital Cellulitis

Orbital cellulitis represents an infection or inflammation of structures posterior to the orbital septum. The most common cause is contiguous spread from adjacent sinuses; more rarely, trauma including surgery, or metastatic spread of the bacterial infection from distant areas are the etiology. Usual bacterial pathogens are strep, *H. influenzae*, or anaerobes.

Orbital Pseudotumor

Orbital pseudotumor represents idiopathic inflammation of an orbital structure. Any orbital structure is a possible target, including sclera, lacrimal gland, extraocular muscles, or orbital fat. Patients present with intense pain and progressive chemosis, proptosis, and occasional duction limitation. On evaluation, there is no sinusitis or elevated white count and the sedimentation rate is elevated. There is a 30% association with collagen vascular disease; therefore systemic workup is indicated.

Congenital Cataracts: Causes

- Idiopathic (60%)
- Heredity (30%), usually autosomal dominant
- Metabolic and systemic disease association (5%)
  Galactosemia
  Lowe syndrome

Hallermann-Streiff syndrome
Trisomies
Alport syndrome
- Maternal infection (3%) including
Cytomegalovirus
Herpes
Syphilis
Toxoplasmosis
- Pure ocular causes (2%) including
Aniridia
Anterior segment dysgenesis
Complicated microphthalmia
- Etiology of unilateral congenital cataracts
Idiopathic (80%)
Trauma (10%)
Primary ocular abnormalities (10%): posterior lenticonus, Persistent hyperplastic primary vitreous

Pediatric Glaucoma

Glaucoma refers to an elevated intraocular pressure resulting in optic nerve damage, loss of peripheral visual field, and ultimately loss of central visual acuity.

Glaucoma can be a purely ocular disorder presenting in infancy as congenital glaucoma or juvenile in onset. Incidence is 1/2,500–1/12,500 and is autosomal recessive in 10%. On physical examination patients present with unexplained epiphora, photophobia, and blepharospasm. Corneas enlarge beyond 12 mm and are edematous. Breaks in Descemet membrane are common and high intraocular pressures are seen. Congenital glaucoma is due to an abnormal development of the outflow track in the anterior chamber angle. Discontinuous trabecular pillows collapse the trabecular meshwork and prevent egress of fluid from the eye.

Retinal Diseases

Diabetic Retinopathy

Diabetic retinopathy is a vascular disorder characterized by capillary nonprofusion, development of micoaneurysms, intraretinal hemorrhages, macular edema, and nerve fiber layer infarct. With disease progression, proliferative changes occur consisting of neovascularization into the vitreous.

Sickle Cell Retinopathy

Sickle cell retinopathy is characterized by background retinal changes including salmon patch hemorrhages, iridescent spots, and angioid streaks or proliferative disease consisting of extraretinal neovascularization and vitreous hemorrhage.

Child Abuse

Child abuse results in retinal hemorrhagic and retinoschisis formation.

Retinopathy of Prematurity

Retinopathy of prematurity (ROP) is a vasoproliferative disease of the retinal vasculature that is multifactorial in origin. Hyperoxia is the initiating factor resulting in ROP. Hyperoxia leads to peripheral vasoconstriction and a drop in vascular endothelial growth factor (VEGF) production. This leads to relative retinal ischemia and a marked increase in VEGF production. An intraretinal arteriovenous shunt develops and if untreated neovascularization and retinal detachment develop. Babies with a birth weight of less than 750 g have a 90% chance of developing some degree of ROP with 15% progressing to threshold disease. With a birth weight of 1,000 g there is a less than 50% chance of developing ROP and only a 2% chance of progressing to threshold disease.

Infants less than 1,500 g or less than 32 weeks gestation should be examined for ROP. Children with birth weights greater than 1,500 g require an examination only if unstable. The timing of the examination should be from 4 to 6 weeks of age or 31–33 weeks postconception.

Retinoblastoma

Retinoblastoma is rare, with an incidence of 1 in 13,000 live births. It is a genetic disease caused by mutation of chromosome 13q14, usually just involving retinal cells. In 10% of patients, there is a mutation in the germinal stem cells and an autosomal dominant inheritance pattern is seen. These patients are at risk for development of secondary tumors, usually osteogenic sarcomas and pinealomas. Retinoblastoma is seen unilaterally in 60% and bilaterally in 40% of patients. Clinical presentations include: leukocoria, esotropia, and reduced visual acuity. A tumor usually appears as a gray semitransparent elevated retinal mass. With enlargement, it outgrows its blood supply and develops areas of infarction, resulting in calcium deposition in the tumor, giving it a cottage cheese appearance. With growth, it will eventually break through the retinal internal limiting membrane and cause vitreous seeding.

Lid Mass

Chalazion results from occlusion of the meibomian gland and cystic accumulation of the sebum in the tarsal plate or subconjunctival space. Chalazia are associated with staph blepharitis in young children or rosacea in teenagers and adults.

Dermoid Cyst

Dermoid cysts occur when cutaneous structures are trapped beneath the skin surface during orbital development. Most common location is superior temporal; however, they can occur anywhere in the orbit. Surgical excision is recommended when diagnosed.

Capillary Hemangioma

Capillary hemangiomas grow rapidly in the first 6 months of life and gradually decrease in size over the next 3 years. If treatment is necessary, intralesional injection with decadron and kenalog is recommended.

18

NEUROLOGIC, NEUROPSYCHIATRIC, AND BEHAVIORAL DISORDERS

It is not enough to have a good mind. The main thing is to use it well.

Descartes

CAUSES OF MACROCEPHALY

Early Infantile (Birth–6 Months)

- Intrauterine infections
  Toxoplasmosis, cytomegalic inclusion disease, rubella, syphilis
  Peri- or postnatal infections (bacterial, granulomatous, parasitic)
  Peri- or postnatal hemorrhage (hypoxia, vascular malformation, trauma)
- Mass lesions
  Neoplasms, arteriovenous malformations, congenital cysts
- Subdural effusion
  Hemorrhagic, infectious, cystic hygroma
- Hydrocephalus (progressive or arresting)
  Induction disorders (congenital malformations): spina bifida cystica, cranium bifidum, Chiari malformations (types I, II, and III), aqueductal stenosis, holoprosencephaly
- Normal variant (often familial)
- Hydranencephaly

Late Infantile (6 Months–2 Years)

- Proliferative neurocutaneous syndromes
  von Recklinghausen, tuberous sclerosis, hemangiomatosis, Sturge-Weber
- Hydrocephalus (progressive or arresting)

Space-occupying lesions (tumors, cysts, abscesses)
Postbacterial or granulomatous meningitis
Dysraphism (Dandy-Walker syndrome, Chiari type I malformation)
Posthemorrhagic (traumatic or vascular malformation)
- Megalencephaly (increase in brain substance)
Metabolic CNS diseases: leukodystrophies (e.g., Canavan, Alexander), lipidosis (Tay-Sachs), histiocytosis, mucopolysaccharidoses
- Subdural effusion
- Achondroplasia
- Primary skeletal cranial dysplasias (thickened or enlarged skull), osteogenesis imperfecta, hyperphosphatemia, osteopetrosis, rickets
- Cerebral gigantism
Soto syndrome
- Increased intracranial pressure syndrome
Pseudotumor cerebri (lead, tetracycline, hypoparathyroidism, steroids, excess or deficiency of vitamin A, cyanotic congenital heart disease)
- Primary megalencephaly
May be familial and unassociated or associated with abnormalities of cellular architecture

Early to Late Childhood (After 2 Years)

- Megalencephaly
Proliferative neurocutaneous syndromes
Familial
- Normal variant
- Hydrocephalus (arrested or progressive)
Space-occupying lesions
Preexisting induction disorder (aqueductal stenosis, Chiari type I malformation)
Postinfectious
Hemorrhagic
- Pseudotumor cerebri

CAUSES OF MICROCEPHALY

- Intrauterine infections
Cytomegalic inclusion disease
Toxoplasmosis
Herpes virus
Rubella
- Prenatal irradiation
- Maternal phenylketonuria
- Disorders of karyotype
Trisomies
Deletions
Translocations

- Genetic defects
  Autosomal recessive
  Autosomal dominant
- Perinatal insults
  Traumatic
  Anoxic
  Metabolic
  Infectious
  Fetal alcohol syndrome

Neuropsychiatric examination is important both in children who are not acutely ill and, because the central nervous system (CNS) is one of the common sites of infection, in acutely ill infants. In addition to careful observation and neurologic examination, a detailed history of the child's development and behavior is essential to the neurologic evaluation. Examination of the neck, a critical site of neurologic abnormality in an acutely ill child, is described in Chapter 5.

Neurologic examination of children differs from that of adults because the neurologic lesions usually sought in children differ from those in adults. For example, poisonings, congenital malformations of the brain, progressive brain diseases, and infections are common in children, whereas local vascular lesions are rare. Acute brain injury may be present in both children and adults, but bleeding in the brain of children may be accompanied by delayed onset of signs because of the distensibility of the skull. In children, as in adults, metabolic diseases often may also cause CNS signs. At the conclusion of the neurologic examination, you should have a good evaluation of the child's mental status and speech, cranial nerves, muscle coordination and control, and reflex sensory and autonomic functions.

Perform the neurologic examination, except assessment of such overall procedures as the mass reflexes, along with the general physical examination of each particular part of the body. Described herein are only the mass reflexes, the reflexes noted in the extremities, and general aspects of the neurologic examination. However, the neurologic examination may be repeated as a whole after the general physical examination—especially if any variants are detected or if neurologic difficulties are suspected—and may be recorded separately.

More important than examination of reflexes (except in children who are acutely ill with a neurologic disorder) is the general impression you have of the patient's abilities and responsiveness.

FRONTAL LOBES

The posterior frontal lobes contain the motor cortex. Deficits in a frontal lobe result in signs of upper motor neuron dysfunction on the contralateral side of the body.

Motor aphasia appears in children older than 6 or 7 years if the Broca motor speech area in the dominant hemisphere is injured. The frontal lobes also control contralateral eye movements. An irritative lesion in the frontal eye fields (e.g., a seizure) causes deviation of the eyes away from the side of the lesion; in contrast, a destructive lesion causes deviation of the eyes toward the side of the lesion.

Disturbance of the more anterior parts of the frontal lobe may cause personality changes, irritability, and lethargy with lack of spontaneity. Sphincter incontinence may develop, and primitive reflexes, such as rooting, sucking, and grasp reflexes may reemerge. Remember that frontal lobe lesions may be difficult to detect even if they are large.

TEMPORAL LOBES

Ability to read, write, and understand speech may be altered (Table 18.1). Bilateral involvement of the hippocampus interferes with learning. Temporal lobe injury also may produce psychotic aggressive behavior.

Memory deficits may be seen with temporal lobe dysfunction.

Proximal weakness indicates a myopathy; distal weakness indicates a neuropathy. Difficulty in arising from the floor indicates weakness of the proximal leg muscles.

TABLE 18.1
Signs of Upper and Lower Motor Neuron Lesions

Parameters	Upper Motor Neuron Lesions Central Nervous System Dysfunction*	Lower Motor Neuron Lesions Peripheral Nervous System Dysfunction†
Intellect	Deficits may be found with cortical abnormalities	Normal
Cranial nerves	Abnormalities usually reflect brain stem involvement but may indicate a neuropathy	May be involved
Sensation	Usually intact, but spinal cord gives a sensory level that is in a dermatomal distribution	Impaired with lesions that affect the nerve
Tone	Increased (spasticity) with lesions affecting pyramidal pathways; rigidity seen with extrapyramidal disease	Reduced (floppy or hypotonic)
Fasciculations		Present with anterior horn cell disease but occasionally also found with neuropathies
Coordination	Impaired when cerebellum or its connections are involved	May be hindered by weakness
Power	Slightly decreased, although movement more severely impaired because of altered tone	Markedly reduced; neuromuscular junction disease associated with fatigue
Reflexes	Hyperactive in pyramidal dysfunction; plantar stimulation results in an extensor response (Babinski) in the great toe	Difficult to elicit

*Involve intracranial contents, brain stem, or spinal cord.
†Involve intracranial horn cells, nerves, neuromuscular junction, or muscles.

TABLE 18.2
Glascow Coma Scale

Eye opening	Verbal	Motor	Score
		Follows commands	6
	Oriented	Localized pain	5
Spontaneous	Confused	Withdraws from pain	4
To speech	Inappropriate words	Abnormal flexion	3
To pain	Nonspecific sounds	Extension	2
None	None	None	1

Add one number for each activity. Numbers 13–15 correspond to drowsiness; 10–12 to stupor, 7–9 to light coma; 4–6 to deep coma; and 3 flaccid and apneic. The scale is useful for following progression and regression.

Although older children and adolescents may be examined in a manner similar to that used for adults, infants and younger children are examined largely by observation of the characteristic positions of the patient, the spontaneous movements, and the play activity. To elicit this information, use not only patience but also imagination in your approach to younger patients. Especially in infants, compare motor and social accomplishments with suitable developmental charts (Appendix B), which with full realization of the wide variability of normal infants, helps indicate neurologic adequacy.

Note the state of consciousness, a combination of awareness and arousal. The patient may be hyperirritable, convulsive, hyporeactive, delirious, stuporous, or comatose. State of consciousness may be difficult to quantitate. Responses to commands, speech, name, pinprick, or severe pain are some of the usual tests for degree of consciousness. Lack of response, in the above order, indicates decreasing consciousness and increasing stupor or coma. In deep coma, a patient's respirations, blood pressures, and reflexes are depressed (Table 18.2). Coma with focal signs and increased reflex activity is usually caused by a brain lesion; coma with multifocal signs and decreased reflexes is usually caused by metabolic disease or poisoning. Touch the child's eyelashes lightly on either side with no warning. The child with feigned coma responds with a vigorous bilateral blink.

Generalized hyperirritability with hyperactivity in a child may be a sign of psychologic distress, encephalitis, or certain toxins. You can frequently elicit this response by observing the patient make quick movements when asked, for example, to draw a picture. Irritability may, however, be prominent in any ill child.

CLASSIFICATION OF CHILDHOOD HEADACHE

Acute	Infection, "sinus," systemic illness, migraine, trauma, postictal, hemorrhage
Acute intermittent	Migraine, tension-muscle contraction, shunt malfunction
Chronic progressive	Tumor, pseudotumor, hydrocephalus, subdural hematoma, brain abscess

| Chronic nonprogressive | Transformed migraine, analgesia abuse, medications, "chronic daily headache" emotional causes |
| Mixed | Shunt malfunction, temporomandibular joint dysfunction |

Acute Intermittent Headache in Childhood: Diagnostic Criteria of the International Headache Society

Migraine With Aura

- At least 12 attacks needed to diagnose
- One or more aura symptoms
- No aura >60 minutes
- Headache follows in <60 minutes

Migraine Without Aura

- At least five attacks needed to diagnose
- Headache lasts 1–48 hours
- Headache has two of the following:
  Bilateral frontal or unilateral distribution
  Pulsatile quality
  Moderate to severe intensity
  Aggravation by routine physical activity
- During headache two of the following:
  Nausea and/or vomiting
  Photophobia and phonophobia

Tension-Muscle Contraction

- At least 10 attacks needed to diagnose
- Headaches last minutes to days
- Headache has two of the following:
  Pressing or tightening (nonpulsing) quality
  Mild to moderate intensity
  Bilateral distribution
  Not aggravated by routine physical activity
- Headache has both of the following:
  No nausea and vomiting
  Photophonia and phonophobia absent

Hyperirritability—Hyperactivity

Fever	Hernia
Hypoglycemia	Corneal abrasion
Hyponatremia, hypocalcemia	Hair around toe, finger, penis
Pain	Acrodynia
Chalasia with esophagitis	Scurvy

TABLE 18.3
Characteristics of Headache Pain and Possible Meaning

Question	What the Answer May Indicate
When did headaches begin?	Chronic headaches are less likely to be due to significant disease
Are they getting worse?	Headaches due to increased intracranial pressure often become progressively more severe
Where are they located?	Migraine headaches switch from side to side
	Tension headaches tend to occur like a band around the head
	Headaches due to increased intracranial pressure may always be located in the same position
What type is the pain?	Migraine is usually described as throbbing
	Tension headaches are typically "pressing," but tumors (increased intracranial pressure) can produce throbbing, pressing, or sharp pain
When does the pain occur?	Migraine is episodic and often occurs in the afternoon but will occasionally wake the patient
	Tension headaches may last all day but do not interfere with sleep
	Pain due to increased intracranial pressure is worse in early morning and may awaken the child
Does the headache interfere with play?	Migraine and increased intracranial pressure disrupt the child's activities
	Tension headaches are complained of but do not interrupt anything; the child may use them to avoid unpleasant tasks
Are there associated symptoms?	Tension headaches are seldom associated with other symptoms
	Migraine is usually seen with anorexia, nausea, vomiting, photophobia, phonophobia, and visual symptoms such as flashing lights
	Increased intracranial pressure results in vomiting and may cause diplopia, due to a nerve palsy
What relieves headache?	Migraine is relieved by a brief period of sleep
	Increased intracranial pressure is seldom relieved by any specific factor
	Tension headaches are helped by stress reduction
Is there a family history of headaches?	Such a history is common in migraine and stress headaches
Has the child shown any changes in personality, ability, or thinking?	Such changes are more likely to be associated with significant disease
Are the headaches triggered by any foods, activities, or events?	Migraine is often triggered by stress, specific foods, or tiredness

From Dooley, J. M. (2002). Pediatric neurologic examination. In R. B. Goldbloom (Ed.), *Pediatric clinical skills* (3rd ed.). Philadelphia: Saunders, p. 242.

CNS disorders   Collagen-vascular diseases
Cardiac, pulmonary,   Chorea
    intraabdominal   Hyperthyroidism
Other metabolic disorders

Hyperactivity may be a cardinal sign of attention-deficit/hyperactivity disorder. Ordinarily, younger children will be more irritable when lying on the bed or examining table than when in a parent's arms because of a natural fear of the unfamiliar surroundings. Some infants will be more irritable when in the parent's arms. This paradoxical irritability should alert you to the possibility of CNS infections, particularly meningitis, although other disease states such as acrodynia, scurvy, severe febrile illness, fractures, and emotional disturbances may also manifest this sign, as in attachment disorders and pervasive developmental disorder (PDD).

SEIZURES

Convulsive states are signs of disease and should never be considered diagnoses. Seizures manifest themselves in different ways. Record the type of seizure, the parts of the body involved, and seizure duration. Types of seizures are shown in Table 18.4.

International Classification of Epileptic Seizures

Partial seizures:

- Simple partial (consciousness retained)
  Motor
  Sensory
  Autonomic
  Psychic
- Complex partial (consciousness impaired)
  Simple partial, followed by impaired consciousness
  Consciousness impaired at onset
- Partial seizures secondarily generalized

Generalized seizures:

- Absences
  Typical
  Atypical
- Generalized tonic-clonic
- Tonic
- Clonic
- Myoclonic
- Atonic
- Infantile spasms
- Unclassified seizures

Partial simple seizures are focal with normal consciousness and may be motor or sensory. Complex partial seizures (psychomotor, temporal lobe) may be characterized by alterations in consciousness and abnormal motor activity. Generalized seizures may be completely incoordinate tonic and clonic movements in unconscious children and may be caused by abnormal cortical discharges. Absence (petit mal) seizures are brain disturbances causing loss of consciousness for 5–15 seconds and are also accompanied by abnormal electrical brain discharges. Autonomic manifestations

TABLE 18.4
Types of Seizures

	Age of Onset	Gender	Seizure Type	EEG	Treatment	Genetics	Prognosis
Benign familial neonatal convulsions	Between 2–15 days (most commonly on day 2 or 3)	Male dominance	Frequent, short clonic with or without apnea	Nonspecific pattern	Phenobarbital or phenytoin	AD, gene locus 20 q, family hx often positive	Normal development; seizures resolve by 6 months of age; 14% develop epilepsy
Benign myoclonic epilepsy of infancy	6 months to 3 years	—	Generalized myoclonic fits (easily controlled by treatment)	Fast, generalized spike-waves	Valproate	—	Normal neuro-development
Febrile seizures	6 months to 5 years		Brief (not longer than 5 minutes), generalized. A response to a sudden, rapid temperature rise. Close association with viral infections	Doubtful value in prognosis	Temperature reduction with antipyretics; treatment with rectal diazepam may be considered for prolonged/focal seizures	A familial pre-disposition	Excellent, approximately 1/3 of patients will have recurrence. Less than 4% overall will later develop epilepsy
Benign partial epilepsy of childhood	3 to13 years	Boys > girls	Brief, partial, sometimes secondary generalized, usually nocturnal	High voltage centrotemporal spikes	Any AED with least side effects	Genetic pre-disposition	Very good

Syndrome	Age	Sex	Clinical features	EEG	Treatment	Genetics	Prognosis
Absence epilepsy	6 to 7 years	Girls > boys	Sudden onset, momentary loss of consciousness/ staring spell frequent, 10–20 seconds in duration	3 Hz spike-wave	Ethosuximide, valproate	Strong genetic pre-disposition	Good
Juvenile myoclonic epilepsy	12 to 18 years	—	Myoclonic and absence, tonic-clonic, and clonic-tonic- clonic	Polyspike and wave at 4–6 Hz	Valproate, topiramate, lamotrigine	AD, gene locus 6p also AR	Lifelong anti-epileptic drug therapy required
Infantile spasms, West syndrome	3 to 7 months	—	Spasms: flexor extensor, mixed	Hypsarrhythmia	ACTH, vigabatrin, topiramate, lamotrigine	—	Poor for normal development

TABLE 18.5
Nonepileptic Paroxysmal Events: Not Epilepsy

Apnea	Night terrors	Masturbation	Arrhythmia (e.g., prolonged QT syndrome, Wolff-Parkinson-White syndrome)
Breath-holding spells	Somnambulism	Hyperexplexia (exaggerated and persistent startle response)	Gastroesophageal reflux
Syncope	Narcolepsy	Spasmus nutans (Pendular nystagmus, head tilt)	Transient ischemic attack
Dizziness	Tics	Daydreaming/ attentional disorder	Depression/fugue state
Vertigo	Dystonia		Paroxysmal behavior outburst
Migraine	Cataplexy		Psychogenic seizure
Acute confusional state	Myoclonus (benign infantile myoclonus and other forms)		
Nightmares Hyperventilation	Shuddering attacks		

From Fisher, P. G. (2007). The occurrence of seizures in children can generate tremendous levels of anxiety for children, parents and pediatricians alike. Allaying these concerns and providing the right treatment rests on a systematic approach. *Contemporary Pediatrics, 24*(4), 81–90.

may consist of bizarre visceral disturbances and usually last longer than 30 seconds, followed by impaired consciousness, hallucinations, total amnesia, confusion, headache, and sometimes incontinence.

Most childhood seizures begin on one side and may be considered focal, but they quickly become generalized and the etiology is usually that of a generalized seizure (Table 18.5). The causes of the irritability may include many types of metabolic, vascular, or CNS disorders. Seizures do not usually occur in children with brain tumors until the intracranial pressure is considerably increased.

SYNCOPE

Distinguish seizures from simple fainting (syncope). Fainting is a sudden loss of consciousness without abnormal movements and is usually caused by reflex vascular disorders.

Causes of Syncope

Orthostasis	Aortic stenosis
Vasovagal tone	Cardiomyopathy
Vasodepressor	Anomalous coronary artery
Supraventricular tachycardia	Hyperventilation

Long QT   Drugs
Complete atrioventricular block   Psychogenic
Sinus bradycardia

Seizures must also be distinguished from hysterical fits, which are usually not accompanied by injuries or other neurologic signs and may contain periods during which the hysterical child is responsive. They must be distinguished from exaggerated startle response with falling followed by hypertonia and ataxia, hyperekplexia. Syncope that occurs with the child on a table tilted 60–80° for 30 minutes helps indicate neurocardiogenic causes. Syncopal episodes occur suddenly; they may result from cardiac dysrhythmias with no premonitory sensation. They occur more commonly when the child is sitting, standing, or coughing. Seizures can occur when the child is lying down or when the child has cardiac dysrhythmias, mitral valve prolapse, gastroesophageal reflux, migraine, or Tourette syndrome. Seizures resulting from vagal-mediated cardiac arrest can be produced by 10 seconds of pressure on the eyeballs. Seizures preceded by crying or cyanosis are commonly associated with breath holding.

Lack of total activity, demonstrated by the persistence of one position for long periods, is common in mentally or emotionally delayed children or may be a sign of severe debility, malnutrition, or anemia. Catatonia, in which one unusual or apparently uncomfortable position is assumed for a long time, may be seen in mentally delayed or psychotic children. Catatonia-like observation of the finger and hands is normal in the 3–6-month-old child.

Lack of all activity is usually caused by a state of unconsciousness—stupor or coma—and must be differentiated from normal sleep states from which the patient can easily be aroused.

In older children, look for other neurologic evaluation before the reflexes are elicited. Note the patient's gait, stance or limp, as described in Chapter 8.

Note ataxia as gross incoordination. Brain tumors, especially of the cerebellum, and encephalitides may be accompanied by ataxia. Ataxia caused by sensory or proprioceptive loss is worse with the eyes closed. The general weakness characteristic of the amyotonias, dystrophies, or spasm of the muscles of the thigh in hip disease is sometimes mistaken for ataxia. Other cerebellar injuries, such as cerebral palsy with cerebellar involvement, the degenerative ataxias, some CNS infections, or tick paralysis, are especially likely to be followed by ataxia. Ataxia worsened by heat occurs in multiple sclerosis. Ataxia may occur as nonepileptiform seizures. A variety of drugs, including phenytoin, phenobarbital, and the antihistamines, as well as alcohol, may cause ataxia in sensitive persons. Vestibular damage, as is sometimes manifest in children treated with streptomycin, may be followed by ataxia.

Note coordination. Incoordination may be caused by cerebellar lesions or by any of the diseases that cause ataxia. Watch the child reach for a toy, tear paper, tie shoes, and button a shirt. Coordination is easily tested by playing a game with the child. Sit opposite the child with the child's palms upward and ask the child to strike first your right and then your left hand. Continue at a rapid pace, and then shift the position of your hands. Inability of the child to follow the motion of the hands may indicate varying degrees of incoordination.

Coordination may also be tested by the finger-to-nose or heel-to-shin tests in the child who can understand commands. In these tests, tell the patient to extend first one hand and touch the tip of the nose with the index finger. The patient then repeats the action with the opposite hand, usually after you demonstrate. Then tell the patient to repeat the same procedure with the eyes shut. Gross incoordination is the failure of the patient to touch the nose with the eyes open. Minor evidence of incoordination, as well as lack of sense of position (i.e., proprioception) will be manifested by the patient's inability to perform these tests with the eyes shut. Remember that fine coordination is not fully developed in children until 4 or even 6 years of age, and if a younger patient can bring a finger within 3 or 4 cm of the tip of the nose, coordination is generally considered normal.

Have the patient perform the heel-to-shin test by running the heel of one foot down the anterior aspect of the tibia of the other foot. Usually you also demonstrate this to the patient. A child's inability to perform this test is a less reliable guide to evidence of incoordination or lack of position sense in a child, but results of tests with the eyes open and shut are similar in significance to those of the finger-to-nose test. Fear and anxiety may result in apparently poor coordination. When asked to jump rope, some anxious children will demonstrate superior coordination and balance when jumping rope with both feet or with one foot and even with the eyes closed. Ask the child to hop. Inability to hop after age 5 years indicates lack of gross motor coordination.

Note tremors and distinguish them from choreiform movements (Table 18.6). Tremors are constant, small movements; some occur when the patient is at rest because of lesions of the extrapyramidal system, and some occur only when voluntary motion of the part is attempted (intention tremor). Intention tremors result from lesions of the cerebellum. Tremors in the infant are seen with states of hypocalcemia

TABLE 18.6
Involuntary Movements

Type	Character
Athetosis	Slow, continuous, writhing
Chorea	Random, jerky
Dystonia	Slow, twisting mingled with muscle tension
Fasciculation	Coarse twitching
Fibrillation	Rapid twitch in muscle
Hemiballismus	Flinging, jumping, wild, unilateral
Jackknife	Body bends at waist (see myoclonic)
Myoclonic	Sudden, brief, shocklike
Myokymia	Twitching of muscle fibers
Spasm	Prolonged muscle contraction
Tardive dyskinesia	Writhing, fibrillation of tongue and face
Tics	Involuntary muscle contractions, noises, words
Tremor	Fine or coarse shaking
Twitch	Spasmodic, short

and hypoglycemia. Muscular tremors or fibrillations may be noted when certain muscles are fatigued and in children with hyperthyroidism, hypothermia, hyperthermia, or progressive degeneration of the cord. Most commonly, tremors or twitchings occur in infants in bursts, without obvious cause.

Twitchings (tics) are spasmodic movements of short duration, noted in muscles that are fatigued in which a nerve is regenerating, which occur in children with chorea. Movements stop during sleep. In contrast to children with dyskinetic movements or dystonia, children with chorea do not lose consciousness. Twitchings may occur after sharp pain in an area. In emotionally upset children, the twitchings follow a definite and usually periodic pattern. In children with Tourette syndrome, the twitchings increase in frequency and the children develop vocal bursts.

Choreiform movements are coarse, involuntary, purposeless movements associated with decreased muscle tone. They are quick, jerky, and irregular, grossly incoordinate, and may disappear with relaxation. In chorea associated with rheumatic fever, movements may involve any muscle, including those of the tongue, speech, hands, and feet. These movements are best elicited by having the patient extend a hand or perform other voluntary acts. The fingers and wrists will hyperextend, and the choreiform movements of the fingers become exaggerated. With extension of the arms above the head, the palms of the hand point outward and the hand is flexed at the wrist with extension of metacarpal and interphalangeal joints. Choreiform movements are also noted in patients with hereditary ataxias, lupus erythematosus, and with drug reactions. Choreiform movements may be one-sided (hemichorea) and, in rare cases, are caused by vascular brain lesions (hemiballismus). Paroxysmal choreoathetosis occurs after startle, lasts less than a minute, and recurs several times a week; the cause is unknown.

Athetosis refers to a group of constant, gross incoordinate movements that are slow and writhing and are usually associated with increased muscle tone. These movements are exaggerated by voluntary activity and disappear when the patient relaxes during sleep. *Dystonia* is a slow, twisting movement of limbs or trunk. Athetosis usually indicates basal ganglia involvement; ataxia and incoordination occur with even superficial cerebellar lesions. Athetoid movements may occur in children with cerebral palsy or tuberous sclerosis and are present late in the deteriorating course of the reticuloendothelial diseases such as Niemann-Pick and Tay-Sachs. Infants may normally have athetotic movements during their first year of life.

A periodic nodding of the head (spasmus nutans) resembles athetosis. It may be idiopathic, may occur as a habit spasm, or may be a sign of mental deficiency; tumors near the optic chiasm or third ventricle, neuroblastoma, or gastroesophageal reflux. The nodding is a combination of true anteroposterior nodding and lateral shaking, which may be temporarily interrupted by suddenly attracting the child's attention. Infants with spasmus nutans usually also tilt the head and have nystagmus. To-and-fro motions of the head synchronous with the pulse (Musset sign) may occur in cases of aortic insufficiency.

Note associated movements—voluntary movements of one muscle accompanied by involuntary movements of another muscle—regulated by the cerebellum. They occur as mirror movements in the Klippel-Feil syndrome, in diseases with increased intracranial pressure, and in patients whose handedness has been changed. Reciprocal movements occur normally in infants aged 2–4 months and usually decrease by age 4–6 months; failure of these movements to appear or disappear at the proper times is an indication of brain damage. Certain reciprocal movements such as the movement of the arms when a person walks are normal at all ages, and their absence may indicate cerebellar damage or absent corpus callosum.

Note handedness by observing the preferential handling of small objects. Definite handedness in a child aged less than 15 months suggests hemiparesis.

Note the muscles for development, tenderness, spasm, and paralysis. Muscle tone is caused by a balance between muscle mass and nerve stimulation. It represents the degree of contraction in the voluntarily relaxed muscle. Test muscle tone by grasping the muscle or pressing on the muscle and estimating its firmness; watch the muscle response during its normal range of motion with and without resistance, such as response to painful stimuli in the region activated by the muscle. Assess muscle strength of an older child by having the child perform against resistance supplied by your hand.

Muscle tone is increased in any condition causing muscle spasm. Muscle spasm is felt as unusual tenseness of the muscle mass and may occur in injury or infection of the muscle, bone, or joint; in metabolic disease; or in children with upper motor neuron lesions. Muscle spasm is also noted in diseases affecting the spinal cord roots, probably secondary to pain. Spasm occurs in overused muscles, in myositis due to bacterial or viral infections, toxins or, occasionally, before pain, as in children with tumors of the cauda equina or in patients with abnormalities of the filum terminale, who manifest hamstring spasm early.

Generalized spasm may be evident early, involving almost all striated muscles in children with tetanus. Spasm is especially evident with slight disturbances in the environment. The generalized extensor spasm noted in tetanus can be distinguished from the generalized muscle spasm of phenothiazine intoxication. The latter does not ordinarily involve the abdominal muscles, but in tetanus the abdomen may be boardlike in its rigidity. Generalized flexion or extension spasm may be noted in children with anoxia and is seen in sickle cell crisis, presumably secondary to local muscle anoxia.

Note paresis, weakness, or paralysis. *Paresis* generally refers to weakness of muscle resulting from partial paralysis, and the term *paralysis* is usually reserved for total weakness. These conditions are manifest by the patient's inability to use a muscle after a command or painful stimulus or when the patient tries to use a particular group of muscles and exhibits a lack of motion when attempting certain characteristic movements. Paresis and paralysis may be either spastic or flaccid.

Flaccidity, or flaccid paralysis, refers to the inability of a muscle to maintain its normal tone and position so that it yields readily and without resistance to pressure. The muscles in which it occurs should be noted. Flaccidity usually indicates lower motor neuron lesion and occurs in conditions such as poliomyelitis, amyotonia congenita, myasthenia, tick paralysis, polyneuritis, transverse myelitis, diabetic neuropathy, some drug and heavy metal intoxications, and spinal cord injury. Flaccidity of the lower limbs occurs with thoracic neuroblastoma resulting from extension of the tumor into the spinal canal. Paralysis that comes and goes—periodic paralysis—may be related to potassium deficiency or excess. Paralysis that occurs during expression of a strong emotion such as laughter or anger is termed *cataplexy*. Diastematomyelia, a spur of bone in the spinal canal, causes progressive flaccid paralysis, usually during growth spurts.

The proximal muscles are usually affected first in the muscle dystrophies of adults, whereas primary neurologic disease first affects the distal muscles. This distinction is not as clear in children. Proximal muscle weakness in children likely results from muscle or anterior horn cell disease. Children who rise from the supine position by climbing up instead of jumping up (Gower sign) may have proximal muscle weakness of the pelvic muscles. Likewise, they will push themselves up to get out of chairs. Strength in the shoulder girdle can be tested by lifting children under the axillae. If the shoulder muscles are weak, children will slip through the examiner's arms (Foerster sign). Flaccidity may be caused by damage to a small area of the cerebral cortex or to the lateral hemisphere of the cerebellum; these lesions occur rarely in childhood. It is noteworthy that, as in adults with brain injury, paralysis after an upper motor neuron lesion is first flaccid and later spastic. This is also the case in newborns with brain damage; the child may be flaccid for as long as 6 months before spasticity becomes fixed.

In infants, weakness is usually proximal in both myopathic and neuropathic conditions. In children with polyneuritis, the proximal muscles are weaker in the legs and the distal muscles are weaker in the arms. In children with pyramidal lesions, weakness in flexion is greater than that of extension in the legs, but weakness of extension is greater than that of flexion in the arms.

Paresis may also occur with chronic wasting disease, congenital heart disease, rickets, and other forms of malnutrition. Mild paresis may be noted in children with hyperthyroidism. Normally a child can hold the leg extended on command for about 1 minute; a child with hyperthyroidism can hold it about 10 seconds. Unilateral flaccidity may be noted in children with hemichorea. The leg withdraws on pinprick, distinguishing unilateral flaccidity from true paralysis. Paralysis without other neurologic signs may result from hysteria.

Spasticity refers to a prolonged and steady contraction of the muscle. It is demonstrated by increased resistance to passive movement and gives way suddenly when overcome (clasp-knife rigidity). It is accompanied by increased reflexes and clonus. Note the muscles in which it exists. Spasticity of a limb occurs with any upper motor neuron disease or after a prolonged painful stimulus. Spasticity is also marked in children with the degenerative brain diseases discussed earlier in this section. Spasticity of the extensor muscles of the legs or exaggeration of the postural reflexes with flexor spasticity in the upper extremities is more marked in children with brain damage limited to the motor cortex. However, spasticity of the extensors of both the arms and legs, quadriplegia or tetraplegia, usually indicates more extensive damage in the cortex and the basal ganglia. Spasticity largely of the lower extremities (as in spastic diplegia) is thus usually accompanied by better mental development. Paraplegia (spasticity of the legs with no involvement of the arms) is usually caused by spinal cord disease. Diplegia is paralysis affecting the same parts on both sides of the body; the term is usually applied to paralysis of the lower limbs. The term paraplegia also refers to the lower limbs. Quadriplegia is paralysis of all four limbs but in usage refers to the upper limbs.

Rigidity refers to an absolute inability to flex a joint and is noted in diseases in which there is fusion of the joint. Rigidity of the neck is also noted in children with meningitis and other lesions mentioned in the discussion of the neck. Rigidity of the spine is noted in children with meningitis and other lesions discussed in the section on the spine. Usually the tendon reflexes are absent because of excessive rigidity.

Rigidity with arms flexed, legs extended, and hands fisted in the child in deep coma indicates severe dysfunction of the cerebral cortex (decorticate rigidity). Rigid extension and pronation of the arms and legs are signs of midbrain dysfunction (decerebrate rigidity).

Cogwheel rigidity of the leg muscles, manifested by spasm followed by weakness after flexion, is characteristic of children with myotonia congenita (Thomsen disease). Children with chorea demonstrate a strong hand grip followed by weakness. Those with hyperthyroidism demonstrate good strength in the quadriceps muscles rapidly followed by weakness.

Contractures are observed as fixed deformities of the muscle with limitation of joint motion, frequently accompanied by muscle atrophy. Contractures may occur in any state causing continuous spasm or disease of the muscle.

Muscle atrophy is best determined either by noting an obvious decrease in muscle mass or, preferably, by measuring the muscle area and comparing with the opposite side. For example, if you suspect atrophy of the patient's calf muscles on one side, measure the circumference of the calf on both sides at exactly the same distance above the malleoli.

Muscle atrophy may occur after prolonged spasm or disuse from any cause, including immobilization, malnutrition, joint disease, nervous system lesion, and the muscular dystrophies. Fasciculation of the muscles is noted as brief repetitive twitches in muscles at rest and is increased by movement of or pressure on the muscle. Fasciculation can be augmented by the administration of neostigmine 1.0 mg and atropine 0.6 mg. They are usually noted in progressive lower motor neuron disease but not myopathic conditions.

Facial myokymia (spontaneous undulating waves of contracting muscle fibers spreading across facial muscles) appears most commonly with multiple sclerosis and intramedullary pontine tumors.

Muscle hypertrophy is recognized as enlarged musculature with good tone. It is usually compensatory, and other muscles are found to be atrophic. It may result from normal exercise or from constant activity, as in choreoathetosis. In pseudohypertrophy, the muscle appears large because of fatty infiltration; such muscles are weak.

Muscle percussion is useful in distinguishing myopathic conditions from lower motor neuron disease. Briskly tap the deltoid, quadriceps, or gastrocnemias. Normally the muscle contracts. Response is usually normal in children with neuropathic conditions but is absent in those with myopathic conditions.

The superficial reflexes are the abdominals, the cremasterics, and the skin reflex of the anus (a.k.a. analwink), which have previously been discussed.

Obtain the deep tendon reflexes of the extremities by briskly tapping the biceps, triceps, patella, and Achilles tendons with the flat of the finger.

Reflex Innervation

Biceps C5–C6
Triceps C6–C8
Patella L2–L4
Achilles L5–S2

Usually a hammer is used to elicit these reflexes in older children. Patients should be relaxed; you should talk casually to them or attempt to catch them unaware to best elicit these reflexes. The muscle to be stimulated should be able to act at maximal mechanical advantage; usually this is a position of about half flexion of the joint involved. These reflexes, though easy to obtain and rarely forgotten, are only a small part of the neurologic examination of the child. Tendon reflexes are stretch reflexes and are elicited by a rapid stretch of the muscle. They are elicited only in the presence of intact sensory nerves from the muscle to the spinal cord, intact nerves in the spinal cord, and intact motor nerves from the cord to the muscle. The knee jerk is usually present at birth and is followed by the achilles and brachial reflexes. The triceps reflex should be present in children at age 6 months. Reflexes may be augmented by having the child grasp your hand.

Hyperactive deep tendon reflexes indicate upper motor neuron lesion, hyperthyroidism, hypocalcemia, or brain stem tumor and may also occur in areas of muscle spasm, such as early poliomyelitis. Reflexes are hypoactive or absent in the amyotonic or myasthenic muscular dystrophies or lower motor neuron lesions, including polyneuropathy. Patients with cerebellar tumors usually have decreased reflexes. Knee reflexes may be lost early in diphtheria or later in polyneuritis. Decreased reflexes are frequently associated with flaccidity or flaccid paralysis. Flaccidity associated with active reflexes may be seen in children with some forms of brain injury, Down syndrome, malnutrition, and some metabolic disorders. Children with hypothyroidism may exhibit a normal contraction with delayed relaxation of the knee and ankle jerks. Progressive extension of the leg on successive tapping of the patellar tendon (pendular knee jerk), resulting from failure of the leg to return to the resting position, occurs in chorea.

Clonus is a series of forced alternating contractions and partial relaxations of the same muscle and represents an exaggeration of hyperactive deep tendon reflexes. It may be demonstrated as persistence of a rhythmic reflex after a stimulus (such as striking the tendon with a hammer) has been withdrawn; ordinarily, a reflex exhausts itself for a few seconds after it is once obtained. If the clonus occurs with further stimulation, it is said to be sustained. If repeated stimulation is necessary it is unsustained. It may occur with fatigue or any of the diseases causing hyperactive reflexes. Clonus can be normal in early infancy.

Clonus of the knee is most easily detected with the lower leg swinging freely over the bed or examining table while the patient is in the sitting position. Elicit the patellar reflex in the usual manner. A hyperactive knee jerk is usually obtained, and clonus exists if the patella or the muscles around the knee joint continue to contract and relax, causing the lower leg to jerk forward and back repeatedly. Clonus of the knee may also occur if the knee is flexed. Grasp the leg above the knee with one hand and the leg below the knee with your other hand; quickly push your lower hand toward your upper hand. You will either feel or see the rapid contractions and relaxations.

Clonus of the ankle is best detected by having the child lie down, with the knee flexed slightly and the ankle resting comfortably with the toes pointing outward and upward. Hold the lower ankle lightly with your left hand, and tap the tendon with the second finger of your right hand or the hammer. Feel either the reflex or the clonic movement in the left hand. If clonus is not elicited, place the leg flat on the table with the toes pointing upward; flex the ankle quickly. Feel clonus in the hand causing the flexion.

As a group, increased muscle tone, increased tendon reflexes, clonus, spasticity, rigidity, and abnormal pyramidal tract signs are indications of upper motor neuron lesions, although all these signs may be evident in some metabolic disorders.

Myoclonic jerks are brief involuntary contractures of muscles. Myoclonic seizures, sometimes called infantile spasms, usually represent severe CNS disorders and may be an early sign of tuberous sclerosis. Myoclonic jerks during sleep may occur in infancy. If you can induce them by rocking the baby head to toe, they are usually benign.

In infants aged less than 5 months of age, the Moro reflex is extremely informative (Table 18.7). Elicit it by startling the patient—either by making a loud noise, dropping and catching the patient, or otherwise surprising the patient. Normally the child reacts as if grasping a tree: the arms first extend, then flex; the hands clench; and the knees and hips flex.

Absence of the Moro reflex in a newborn infant indicates severe CNS injury or deficiency. Persistent Moro reflex after age 7 months has the same significance. Absence of this reflex of one arm indicates fractured humerus, brachial nerve palsy, cerebral vascular accident, or recently fractured clavicle. Absence of or irregular Moro reflex of

TABLE 18.7
Infantile Reflexes

Reflex	Appearance	Disappearance
Suck	Birth	Through infancy
Root	Birth	3–4 mo
Moro	Birth	3–7 mo
Tonic neck	Birth	3–5 mo
Babinski	Birth	12–24 mo
Stepping	Birth	3–4 mo
Placing	Birth	10–12 mo
Landau	3 mo	12–24 mo
Parachute	7–9 mo	Indefinite

one leg indicates lower spinal injury, myelomeningocele, avulsion of the cord, or dislocated hip. Hyperactive Moro reflex indicates tetany, tetanus, or CNS infection.

A "reverse" Moro reflex consists of extending and externally rotating the arms, with rigidity following the usual stimulus. Such a reflex is seen in children more than 5 days old who have basal ganglia disease, including kernicterus or erythroblastosis fetalis. Such children may have no Moro reflex within the first 5 days of life.

Elicit the Landau reflex by supporting the infant horizontally in the prone position. The infant raises the head and arches the back. This is normally elicited from age 3 months to 1½ years. It represents a combination of labyrinth, neck, and visual reactions; its absence suggests motor weakness, upper motor neuron disease, or mental retardation.

Obtain the Babinski reflex by scratching the soles of the infant's feet with something such as a broken, pointed tongue depressor. Normally, the small toes do not move and the great toe moves plantarwise. An abnormal response is one in which the toes fan out and the great toe moves dorsally. The abnormal response is found in most normal children aged less than 18 months. Persistence after age of 2–2½ years indicates pyramidal tract lesion. Sometimes you may find it difficult to decide whether the Babinski reflex is present or absent, since only part of the response will be obtained. In such cases, look for other signs of upper motor neuron lesions before concluding that the response is abnormal. Obtain Oppenheim sign by pressing on the median aspect of the ankle and noting the toes as in the Babinski sign. The significance is the same. Obtain Hoffmann sign by snapping the terminal phalanx of the second finger and noting flexion of the first and third fingers; it too usually indicates a pyramidal tract lesion but is also obtained in children with tetany.

Kernig sign is the inability to extend the leg with the hip flexed and indicates irritation of the meninges, or hamstring spasm. Evaluation in infants aged less than 6 months is difficult.

Obtain Romberg sign by having the patient stand with the heels together. Compare stability with the patient's eyes open, then shut. The patient is normally able to stand without falling. The sign is said to be positive if the child leans toward or falls toward one side. It is manifest in children with poor or absent sense of position or the cerebellar ataxias and in cases of vestibular damage and cerebellar tumors.

Common Features of Cerebellar Tumors

- Ataxia of trunk and gait with midline tumors
- Dysmetria on finger-to-nose with cerebellar hemisphere tumors
- Hypotonia, nystagmus, scanning speech
- Head tilt, neck pain
- Increased intracranial pressure due to obstruction of cerebrospinal fluid pathways

Medulloblastoma

Medulloblastomas are malignant by definition (20%–30% metastatic at time of diagnosis):
1. 25%–45% metastasize via cerebrospinal fluid
2. 20% metastasize extraneurally, usually to bone

Brain Stem Tumors

Classical triad of findings in brain stem tumors:
1. Ataxia (involvement of pontocerebellar tracts, cerebellar peduncles)
2. Spasticity, usually hemiparesis (involvement of corticospinal tracts)
3. Cranial nerve signs:
   Facial weakness, esotropia localizes to rostral pons
   Internuclear ophthalmoplegia localizes to medulla

Peak ages of presentation 3–10 years. Histologically benign (low-grade astrocytomas); malignant by location; pons is most common site of origin.

Craniopharyngioma

1. Presenting symptoms and signs: visual loss, hydrocephalus due to third ventricular compression, and pituitary/hypothalamic dysfunction (typically short stature)
2. Present throughout childhood and occasionally in adulthood
3. Originates from remnants of Rathke pouch; histologically benign, but significant morbidity due to location
4. Standard treatment is surgical removal
5. Postoperative: panhypopituitarism is typical; hyperphagia and obesity may occur

Foerster sign is evident in children with generalized hypotonicity. Such children are sometimes called floppy infants. Raise the child by the armpits. The legs straighten as the child is raised if the hypotonia results from disease with paralytic weakness such as Werdnig-Hoffmann disease or benign variants of it. If the hypotonia results from atonic spastic diplegia, the knees and hips remain flexed.

Obtain Trousseau sign by obstructing blood flow at the patient's wrist or ankle by making a ring around the area with the thumb and index finger or by using the blood pressure cuff. After 3 minutes, carpal or pedal spasm is produced. This sign is present in children with tetany, hyperirritability, or hyperventilation. Obtain the peroneal sign by tapping the lateral surface of the patient's fibula just below the head; note dorsiflexion and abduction of the foot. The peroneal sign is also seen in children with diseases of hyperirritability. These signs, in contrast to Chvostek sign (described in the section on examination of the face in Chapter 5), can be obtained even in a crying child and may be helpful in diagnosing hypocalcemia.

Obtain the grasp reflex by placing a small object in contact with the infant's fingers. The infant will grasp the object tightly. This movement is normally present from age 1–3 months. If the movement is absent, brain or local nerve or muscle injury should be suspected. Presence after age 4 months suggests a frontal lobe lesion. With injury to the brachial plexus, the fingers may be constantly maintained (spasticity) in the grasping position or may be flaccid. Infants normally hold the hands as a fist for the first 3 months of life and then begin to hold them open for longer periods. At approximately 6 months of age, the normal infant should begin to take objects with one hand; at approximately 7 months of age, the infant should be able to transfer objects from one hand to the other. After 9 months of age, the infant should grasp with the fingers and appose the fingers with the thumb, and at 10 months of age the infant should develop purposeful release. These responses are delayed in children with mental dysfunction or lesions of the pyramidal tract.

The thumb position itself is important in determining neurologic lesions in infancy. In normal infants, the thumb is in a fist in a straight line with the index finger or is freely movable in the palm of the hand. The thumb may be forcibly abducted in the palm of the hand in infants with upper motor neuron lesions.

Evaluate overall milestones in development and motor activity (Table 18.8). Delayed appearance of normal motor activity may be caused by brain damage, peripheral motor damage, emotional or mental delay, parental neglect, lack of challenge to the infant, prolonged illnesses, or anemia.

A child aged 1 month should be able to support the head for an instant. By 4 months of age, the infant should be able to hold the head up well and roll from the prone to the supine position. At approximately 6 or 7 months of age, the infant begins to sit and is able to roll over completely. At 9 months of age, the infant creeps

TABLE 18.8
Milestones in Development

Age Range	Receptive Response	Expressive Response
0–1½ months	Startle, eye widening to sounds	Range of cries (from hunger to pain)
1½–14 months	Quiets to voice, eye blinking to sounds	Vocal contagion, two-syllable babble
4–9 months	Head turns toward sound, responds with raised arms when mom says "up" and reaches for child, responds appropriately to friendly or angry voices	Babbling, four-syllable babble, repeats self-initiated sounds
9–12 months	Listens selectively to familiar words, begins to respond to "no" and to one-step commands (usually accompanied by gesture), understands approximately 10 words (no, bye-bye, clap, hat, own name)	Symbolic gestures, jargoning, repeats parent-initiated sounds
12–18 months	Points to three body parts (eyes, nose, mouth), understands up to 50 words, recognizes common objects by name (dog, cat, bottle, ball, book), follows one-step commands accompanied by gestures ("give me the doll," "hug your bear," "open your mouth")	Uses words to express needs, has 10 words by 18 months, word usage may be inconsistent and mixed with jargon and echolalia
18 months– 2 years	Points to pictures when asked "show me," understands "soon," "in," "on," and "under," begins to distinguish "you" from "me," can formulate negative judgments (a pear is not a cookie)	Telegraphic two word sentences ("go bye-bye," "up daddy," "want cookie"), 25% intelligibility
30 months	Follows two-step commands, can identify actions in pictures, and can identify objects by use	Jargon and echolalia decrease average sentence of 2 1/1 words, adjectives and adverbs appear, begins to ask questions, ask adults to repeat actions ("do it again")

TABLE 18.8
Milestones in Development *(Continued)*

Age Range	Receptive Response	Expressive Response
3 years	Knows several colors, knows what we do when we are hungry, thirsty or sleepy, is aware of past and future, understands "today" and "not today"	Uses pronouns and plurals; can tell stories that begin to be understood; uses negatives ("I can't," "I won't," "I'm busy,"); verbalizes toilet needs; can tell full name, age, and sex; forms sentences of three or four words
3½ years	Can answer such questions as "do you have a doggie," "which is the boy," "where is the dress," "what toys do you have," understands "little," "funny," "secret"	Can relate experiences in sequential order, can say a nursery rhyme, asks permission
4 years	Understands same versus different, can follow three-step commands, can complete opposite analogies (a brother is a boy, a sister is a . . .), understands why we have houses, stoves, umbrellas	Can tell a story, uses past tense, counts to three, names primary colors, enjoys rhyming nonsense words, enjoys exaggerations, asks up to 500 questions a day
5 years	Understands what we do with eyes and ears, understands differences in texture (hard, soft, smooth), understands "if," "because," "when," "why," identifies words in terms of use, begins to understand left and right	Can indicate "I don't know," can indicate "funny," "surprise," can define in terms of use, asks definition of specific words, makes serious inquiries ("how does this work," "what does it mean"), language is now complete in structure and forms, all parts of speech are used as well as all types of sentences and clauses

Adapted from Bauer, R. E. (1987). Developmental pediatrics. In B. J. Zitelli, & H. W. Davis (Eds.), *Atlas of pediatric physical diagnosis*. St. Louis: Mosby, p. 3.16.

and, at about 1 year of age, stands with support. The infant walks at about 14 months, runs stiffly at about 18 months, and runs well at about 2 years of age. Children usually cannot skip or throw a ball overhand well until about 4 years of age. For estimation of level of overall developmental motor activity, consult suitable charts or books of growth and development. The importance of the head and chest circumferences, neck and spine mobility, and the status of the fontanels as part of the neurologic examination are discussed in Chapter 5. A convenient table for following the developmental progress of infants has been systematized and should become part of each infant's record (Appendix C). If a child is delayed in only one milestone and has reached all other milestones age appropriately and the exam is otherwise normal, there is less concern.

Disorders associated with decreased muscle tone are shown in Table 18.9. Sensory changes are difficult to determine in early childhood because of lack of cooperation. Smell and taste, assessed with suitable stimuli, are almost never tested in the young. Blindness and deafness have been discussed previously. Testing of the

TABLE 18.9
Decreased Muscle Tone

Malnutrition	Collagen vascular diseases
General debility, acute illness	Down syndrome
Congenital myopathies, dystrophies	Ehlers-Danlos syndrome
Postviral and viral myopathies	Prader-Willi syndrome
Neuropathic conditions	Peroxisomal disorders
Tick paralysis	Leukodystrophies
Cerebral palsies	
Lower motor neuron lesions	**Metabolic Disorders**
Cerebellar lesions	Carnitine deficiency
Hypothyroidism	Glycogenoses
Hypopituitarism	Rickets
Hypoadrenalin	Hypercalcemia
Heavy metal poisons	Amino acid disorders
Mercury poisoning	Organic acid disorders
Toxins, e.g., magnesium, botulism	Potassium deficiency

peripheral nerves in infants is almost entirely limited to the perception of pain. Pain sensation is normal in children with muscle disease and altered in some with neuropathies. Test for peripheral nerve injuries in the limbs by immersing the limbs in warm water for 10 minutes. The skin on the normal side wrinkles; the denervated skin remains smooth. For hand injury, check light touch sensation of the fingertips.

Withdrawal reflexes, which are obtained by applying a mildly painful stimulus and observing unusually rapid withdrawal, usually indicate hyperesthesia and may indicate extensive lesions in the spinal cord. Hyperesthesia is noted early in children with infectious diseases of the CNS, diseases in which intracranial pressure is increased, peritonitis, herpes zoster, and other diseases. Decreased sensation may be noted in children with cord or peripheral nerve lesions, mental deficiency, decreased consciousness, or such states as familial autonomic dysfunction, ectodermal dysplasia, syringomyelia, and congenital indifference to pain. When infants are held erect with the soles of the feet flat on a tabletop, they will take regular alternating steps, exhibiting the stepping reflex. Similarly, when prone on a tabletop with the head erect, the infant will make crawling movements. These reflex movements should disappear at about 5 months of age.

In children aged 6 years or older, obtain other sensory responses. Sense of position is described with coordination. Test vibratory sensations with a tuning fork.

Determine stereognosis by asking the child to identify coins or other familiar objects when the eyes are shut. Test temperature sensation by asking the patient which end of the reflex hammer feels cooler when the patient's eyes are shut. The rubber end is usually warmer than the metal end. Use cotton to determine sensation of touch. Loss of any or all of these means of sensation may be caused by mental delay or decreased states of consciousness. In the absence of these means, abnormal sensory response usually indicates posterior spinal cord root or peripheral nerve lesions, or possibly an emotional disturbance. Increased sensation to touch (hyperesthesia) occurs with chronic illness.

Test the other cranial nerves as a group, proceeding from II to XII. The method of testing response is detailed in the section on examination of the head and neck in Chapter 5.

CEREBRAL PALSY

Cerebral palsy (CP) refers to a group of nonprogressive neurological conditions defined by specific motor deficits or movement disorders. Most cases of cerebral palsy are the result of congenital, genetic, inflammatory, anoxic, traumatic, toxic, and metabolic disorders. A minority of cases result from asphyxia at birth. The diagnostic approach consists of early assessment of impairments in muscle tone, strength, and control; assessment of involuntary movements; asymmetry; persistence of primitive reflexes; and late development of postural responses. Only about one quarter of children with CP had an abnormal neurological examination at birth.

CP also can be detected based on functional limitations using the motor quotient (motor age divided by chronological age times 100). A motor quotient below 50 predicts gross motor delay.

Neuroimaging is recommended in the evaluation of a child with CP. Cranial ultrasonography is recommended for infants between 7 and 14 days old and near term-corrected age to identify intraventricular hemorrhage, periventricular leukomalacia, and low-pressure ventriculomegaly.

CP is associated with motor and mental disabilities of variable severity in a growing child. Spasticity, hemiplegia, diplegia, and movement disorders may coexist along with contractures and bone deformities, which often develop. Cognitive impairment occurs in many patients and ranges from learning disabilities to attention deficit disorders to severe mental retardation. Hearing loss and visual impairment (refractory errors, visual field defects, cortical visual impairment, faulty accommodation, strabismus, nystagmus, and optic atrophy) are common. Seizures occur in many children with CP. Contractures at the hip and knee in particular are a source of pain and disruption to daily activities.

Drooling is one of the most troublesome problems. Swallowing difficulties, gastroesophageal reflux disease, and constipation may occur in very early life.

The Levine (Poster) Criteria for Diagnosis of Cerebral Palsy

1. Strabismus
2. Oropharyngeal problems: tongue thrusts, grimacing, swallowing difficulties
3. Evolutional responses: persistent primitive reflexes or failure to develop equilibrium and protective responses
4. Posturing and abnormal movement patterns: extensor thrusts, blocks
5. Tone: increased or decreased in muscles
6. Reflexes: deep tendon reflex increased and plantar reflexes up going

Other nonneurologic measurements, such as the character of the pulse, respiration, and blood pressure, may again be noted during this assessment as part of the central control of these functions.

TABLE 18.10
Some Neurologic Soft Signs

Physical Sign	Concern After Age (yr)
Clumsiness in fine motor coordination	
Button 2 buttons	6
Tie shoelaces	7
Alternate left-right, index finger-to-nose	7
Finger tapping—each finger with thumb, alternating	8
Rapid alternating movements of hands (also watch for mirror movements)	10
Choreiform movements, tremor	Any age
Gross motor	
Hop	6
Skip	6
Jump	7
Toe walk	7
Heel walk	7
Catch ball, one hand	10
Tandem gait	7
Turning head with eyes	5
Balance on toes	12
Sensory	
Right-left orientation	5
Perceive touch and identify site	6
Graphesthesia recognize numbers traced	8
Recognize objects in hands	5

Respirations are shallow and irregular with respiratory center involvement. The pulse is weak, rapid, and irregular; the skin is flushed; and the blood pressure is elevated (but may decrease later) with circulatory center involvement. Not only infections and mass lesions cause involvement of the cranial centers; drugs, poisons, acidosis, alkalosis, and water balance may also affect these centers.

A group of signs has been collated as "soft" neurologic signs that may indicate delay in or injury to neurologic development (Table 18.10). These signs are all normal at an early age. Note the child's behavior as the child enters the room and the child's mannerisms and behavior during the interview. Note how the child handles buttons, sleeves, buckles, and zippers. Note ease of onset of frustration and impulsivity.

Finally, note total response of the child, including cooperation, backwardness, lethargy, and reaction to physician and parent. These responses may be recorded in the first statement of your writeup of the child's general appearance. Special characteristics of mental development may also be recorded.

NEUROPSYCHIATRIC DISORDERS

It is estimated that 10% of children and adolescents meet criteria as set out by the *DSM-IV-TR* for the diagnosis of a psychiatric disorder (American Psychiatric

Association, 2000). Childhood-onset mental illness, in general, tends to be familial as well as chronic.

Disruptive Behavior Disorders

Attention-deficit/hyperactivity disorder (ADHD) is the most common psychiatric disorder.

Conduct Disorder

A child with conduct disorder has a repetitive pattern of behavior in which the basic rights of others, societal norms, and rules are violated. The four groups of behaviors include:

- Aggression toward people and animals (e.g., mugging, rape, use of a weapon)
- Destruction of property
- Deceitfulness or theft
- Serious violations of rules (e.g., truancy, forgery)

In order to meet criteria for the diagnosis of conduct disorder, three or more of the behaviors must be present in the past year and one behavior must be present in the past 6 months. Absence of remorse is characteristic.

Age of onset for boys is between 10 and 12 years of age and for girls around the age of 16 years. The mainstay of treatment for conduct-disordered patients is behavioral therapy.

Oppositional Defiant Disorder

Children with oppositional defiant disorder (ODD) exhibit a pattern of negativistic, hostile, and defiant behavior of at least 6 months' duration. A child with ODD will often have temper tantrums, argue with authority figures, defy rules, deliberately annoy others, and will often blame others for their own mistakes. An ODD child can be described as touchy, angry, vindictive, spiteful, and easily annoyed. Remorse is commonly present.

The onset of symptoms is gradual and typically symptoms appear before diagnosis. About 25% of ODD children will no longer meet criteria for the disorder a few years after the diagnosis but others will worsen and may be diagnosed as having conduct disorder. Treatment for ODD is behavioral therapy.

Mood Disorders

The prevalence of major depression and bipolar disorders increases with age. Mood disorders are not classified as childhood disorders in the *DSM-IV-TR*.

Major Depression

Prevalence of major depression: The female-to-male ratio is equal until adolescence, at which time the adult pattern of 3:2 is established.

Incidence: 2% of school age children; 5% of adolescents.

Suicide

Suicide is the third leading cause of death in adolescents after accidents and homicides. It is estimated that around 8%–10% of adolescents report having a suicide attempt at least once in their lifetime. The death rate for adolescents from suicide is 13/100,000. The ratio of males to females for suicide is 4:1, and the reverse is true for attempted suicides. The most common successful means is firearms for both males and females. Risk factors include:

- Previous suicide attempt
- Substance abuse
- Chronic illness
- Depression
- Psychosis
- Gender identity issues, as evidenced by the fact that gay youths account for almost one third of all adolescent suicides
- Family discord
- Family history of suicide

Mania

Mania is a period of at least 1 week marked by persistently elevated, expansive, or irritable mood. Symptom of mania are:

- Inflated self-esteem or grandiosity
- Decreased need for sleep
- Racing thoughts or flight of ideas
- Distractibility
- Increase in goal-directed activity, or psychomotor agitation
- Excessive involvement in pleasurable activities that have painful consequences (e.g., buying sprees, sexual indiscretions)

Anxiety Disorders

Generalized Anxiety Disorder

Children who suffer from generalized anxiety disorder (GAD) frequently experience unrealistic worries about future events or about appropriate past behavior and their own competence. They frequently present with somatic complaints, are markedly self-conscious, need large amounts of self-assurance, and have trouble relaxing. Onset may be gradual or sudden, though GAD does not often become manifest until puberty. Boys and girls are equally affected and the prevalence in adolescence is 24%. GAD is characteristically seen in middle- and upper-middle-class white children. Children with GAD are generally good candidates for cognitive behavior therapy.

Separation Anxiety Disorder

Separation anxiety disorder is marked by developmentally inappropriate and excessive distress when a child is separated from home or from significant attachment figures. Symptoms must last 4 weeks and the onset must be before age 18 years.

Separation anxiety disorder is the most commonly diagnosed anxiety disorder in children at 7 to 8 years of age. It occurs in 4% of all school age children and 1% of all adolescents.

Obsessive-Compulsive Disorder

OCD (obsessive-compulsive disorder) is marked by recurrent and distressing ideas (obsessions) that may or may not lead to repetitive behaviors or mental acts (compulsions).

Of children who develop abrupt-onset OCD, 10%–20% contract the illness via PANDAS (pediatric autoimmune neuropsychiatric disorders associated with streptococcal infections).

Post-Traumatic Stress Disorder

A child with post-traumatic stress disorder (PTSD) has either witnessed or experienced a traumatic event and has developed symptoms as a result. Symptoms include reexperiencing of the event (via dreams, repetitive play themes in young children, intrusive thoughts and images), autonomic arousal as evidenced by increased heart rate or blood pressure, and avoidance of stimuli associated with the traumatic event, as well as feelings of being detached or estranged.

Social Phobia

Social phobia is the persistent fear of embarrassment in social situations. Young children may cry or cling to familiar adults, and often will not participate on the playground. It has been estimated to occur in 10% of children and adolescents.

Psychotic Disorders

Childhood-onset schizophrenia occurs rarely (1/10,000). It typically develops slowly over 6 months or more. Most children who present with psychotic symptoms have a primary affective disorder (e.g., major depression).

Schizophreniform disorder is the term given to patients who meet criteria for schizophrenia but who have been experiencing symptoms for less than 6 months.

Pervasive Developmental Disorders

The pervasive developmental disorders (PDD) include autistic disorders, Rett disorder, childhood disintegrative disorder, Asperger disorder, and PDD not otherwise specified. Children with PDD have impairments in multiple areas of development.

Autistic Spectrum Disorders

Autistic children have impairments in social interaction, communication, and behavior. Impaired social interactions may present as failure to develop peer relationships and failure to develop emotional reciprocity. Impaired communication can appear as a delay or total lack of speech, an inability to sustain a conversation, repetitive use of language, and an inability to engage in make-believe play. Impaired behavior may present as stereotyped mannerisms (e.g., hand flapping or rocking). About 75% of autistic children are mentally retarded. The prevalence rate is 1/150. Autistic individuals have an increased risk of developing a seizure disorder.

The role of genetic mechanisms in autistic disorder is suggested by the fact that siblings of an affected person are at a 45-fold or greater risk of autism than the general population. A concordance rate of 36% for monozygotic twin pairs supports the existence of a strong genetic component. For parents who have a child with autism, the risk of having a second autistic child is between 2% and 10%. Specific genes have been identified in autism. There is no scientific evidence of an etiologic role of thimerosal or immunizations.

As adults, two thirds of autistic persons have significant limitations in their ability to care for their own basic needs; one third achieve some degree of personal and occupational independence.

Asperger Disorder

Asperger patients have no delay in language, no delay in cognitive development, no delay in age-appropriate self-care, and they do not exhibit decreased curiosity about the environment. Asperger patients do have impaired social interaction.

Rett Disorder

Rett disorder is similar to autism, but girls who have it function normally through the first 5 months of life. It is between 5 and 48 months that deficits develop, including deceleration of head growth, loss of previously acquired hand skills, loss of social engagement, and language impairment. Patients develop stereotyped hand movements (e.g., hand wringing) and demonstrate a poorly coordinated gait. Rett disorder has been found to result from mutations in the *MECP2* gene. This disorder has only been reported in females and is often associated with profound mental retardation.

Mental Retardation (Mentally Challenged)

The diagnosis of mental retardation is based on a standardized intelligence test (IQ <70) with concurrent impairment in adaptive skills (typically measured by instruments such as the Vineland Adaptive Behavior Skills test) in at least two of the following areas: communication, self-care, home living, social and interpersonal skills, use of community resources, functional academic skills, and work. The onset must be before the age of 18 and the full-scale IQ must be equal to or less than 70. The prevalence of mental retardation is 2%–3% of the school-aged population.

The three most common causes of mental retardation account for 30% of identified cases. They include:

- Down syndrome—the most common genetic cause of mental retardation
- Fragile X syndrome, which is the most common inherited cause of mental retardation
- Fetal alcohol syndrome (with triad of growth retardation, developmental delay, and classic facial features)—the third most common known cause of mental retardation

Learning Disorders

Reading Disorder

Reading disorder, formerly known as dyslexia, has a prevalence of 4% in school age children, with a male-to-female ratio of 4:1.

Mathematics Disorder

Mathematics disorder has a prevalence of 1% and it occurs equally in males and females.

Stuttering (Dysfluency)

Stuttering is a disturbance in the normal fluency of speech, as evidenced by sound repetitions, prolongation, interjections, and word blocking. Stuttering is often absent in singing. It begins between the ages of 2 and 7 years and peaks at 5 years of age. Almost all cases present before the age of 10 years. The prevalence is 1% in prepubertal children with a male-to-female ratio of 3:1. Symptoms often remit in adolescence. A first-degree relative of a stuttering patient has a 3-fold increased risk of being afflicted when compared to the general population. Some stuttering is considered normal through age 3 years.

Feeding and Eating Disorders of Childhood and Adolescence

Pica

Pica is the persistent eating of nonnutritional substances for at least 1 month's duration.

Rumination Disorder

Rumination disorder involves repeated regurgitation and rechewing of food for at least 1 month following a period of normal eating.

Feeding Disorder of Infancy and Early Childhood

Feeding disorder is a failure to eat, causing weight loss over a 1-month period that is not the result of a medical issue. This disorder must present before the age of 6 years, but it typically presents in the first year of life.

Anorexia Nervosa

Anorexia nervosa and bulimia nervosa are the two major eating disorders, and they typically have an adolescent onset (Figure 18.1). It has been estimated that 30% of all eating disorder patients have been sexually abused in childhood.

There are four major criteria that define anorexia nervosa:

- Refusal to maintain weight at above 85% of that expected for age and height
- Intense fear of gaining weight
- Distorted significance of body weight
- Amenorrhea (i.e., absence of at least three consecutive cycles) in postmenarcheal females

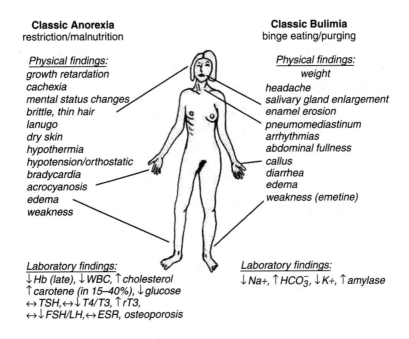

Classic Anorexia
restriction/malnutrition

Physical findings:
growth retardation
cachexia
mental status changes
brittle, thin hair
lanugo
dry skin
hypothermia
hypotension/orthostatic
bradycardia
acrocyanosis
edema
weakness

Laboratory findings:
$\downarrow Hb$ (late), $\downarrow WBC$, $\uparrow cholesterol$
$\uparrow carotene$ (in 15–40%), $\downarrow glucose$
$\leftrightarrow TSH, \leftrightarrow \downarrow T4/T3, \uparrow rT3,$
$\leftrightarrow \downarrow FSH/LH, \leftrightarrow ESR$, osteoporosis

Classic Bulimia
binge eating/purging

Physical findings:
weight
headache
salivary gland enlargement
enamel erosion
pneumomediastinum
arrhythmias
abdominal fullness
callus
diarrhea
edema
weakness (emetine)

Laboratory findings:
$\downarrow Na+, \uparrow HCO_3^-, \downarrow K+, \uparrow amylase$

Figure 18.1
Differential features of classic anorexia and classic bulimia.

There are two subtypes of anorexia nervosa:

- Restricting type—the afflicted person has not regularly engaged in binge eating or purging.
- Binge-eating/purging type—the afflicted person has regularly engaged in these behaviors.

Around 85% of anorectic patients develop the illness between the ages of 13 and 20 years. About 25% recover, 25% stay chronically ill, and 50% have only partial improvement.

Bulimia Nervosa

Bulimia nervosa consists of recurrent episodes of binge eating resulting in inappropriate compensatory behaviors like self-induced vomiting or fasting that have occurred an average of at least twice for the past 3 months.

There are two types of bulimia nervosa:

- Purging—the afflicted person regularly engages in vomiting, laxative, and/or diuretic use.
- Nonpurging—the person has used compensatory behaviors like exercise or fasting instead of purging.

Tic Disorders

A tic is a sudden, recurrent, nonrhythmic, stereotyped movement or vocalization. Tics can be motor (blinking) or vocal (grunting). Anxiety and stress exacerbate tics.

Tourette Syndrome

Tourette syndrome is a childhood-onset neuropsychiatric disorder consisting of multiple motor tics and the presence of at least one vocal tic appearing at some time during the illness. The vocal and motor tics need not occur at the same time. The tics occur many times a day for at least 1 year, and there has never been a tic-free period of more than 3 consecutive months. The typical age of presentation is 7 years with motor tics presenting before vocal tics. Postinfectious autoimmune mechanisms are likely to contribute to 10%–20% of Tourette cases. A nicotine patch has been useful in treatment.

REFERENCE

American Psychiatric Association. (2000). *Diagnostic and statistical manual of mental disorders* (4th ed., text rev.). Washington, DC: Author.

FURTHER READING

American Academy of Pediatrics Subcommittee. (1999). Practice parameter: Long-term treatment of the child with simple febrile seizures. *Pediatrics, 103,* 1307–1309.

Boris, N. W., & Dalton, R. (2000). Habit disorders. In R. E. Behrman, R. M. Kleigman, & H. B. Jensen (Eds.), *Nelson's textbook of pediatrics* (17th ed.). Philadelphia: Saunders.

Dinolfo, E. A. (2001). Evaluation of ataxia. *Pediatric Review, 2*(5), 177–178.

Fishman, R. A. (1992). *Cerebrospinal fluid in diseases of the nervous system*. Philadelphia: WB Saunders, p. 190.

Forsyth, R., & Farrell, K. (1999). Headache in childhood. *Pediatric Review, 20*(2), 39–45.

Hadders-Algra, M. (2004). General movements: A window for early identification of children at high risk for developmental disorders. *Journal of Pediatrics, 145,* S12–S18.

Murphy, J. V., & Dehkharghani, F. (1994). Diagnosis of childhood seizure disorder. *Epilepsia* 35(suppl. 2), S7–S17.

Nield, L. S., Nandad, S., Someshwar, J., et al. (2007, June). Cerebral palsy: A multisystem review. *Consultant for Pediatricians,* 337–340.

Odding, E., Roebroeck, M. E., & Stam, H. J. (2006). The epidemiology of cerebral palsy: Incidence, impairments and risk factors. *Disability Rehabilitation, 28,* 183–191.

Palmer, F. B. (2004). Strategies for early diagnosis of cerebral palsy. *Journal of Pediatrics, 145,* S8–S11.

Sanger, T. D., Delgado, M. R., Gaebler-Spira, D., Hallett, M., & Mink, J. W. (2003). Classification and definition of disorders causing hypertonia in childhood. *Pediatrics, 111,* e89–e97.

19

CHILD ABUSE

It is elementary, my dear Watson.

A. Conan Doyle

PHYSICAL ABUSE

Head Injuries

Head injuries are the number one cause of morbidity and mortality from child abuse. Soft tissue injuries include a torn oral frenulum, periorbital ecchymoses, traumatic alopecia, and subgaleal hematoma. Simple linear skull fractures are the most common type of skull fractures but are nonspecific for abuse. On the other hand, comminuted, depressed, stellate, diastatic, multiple, bilateral, or nonparietal skull fractures are more suspicious for abuse. Subdural, subarachnoid, and retinal hemorrhages are intracranial hemorrhages uncommonly seen with accidental injury but commonly seen with inflicted injury. Subdural and retinal hemorrhages require significant force, comparable to that experienced in motor vehicle accidents or falls from a significant height.

Shaken (Impacted) Baby Syndrome

- Child under 2 years of age
- Biomechanics: heavy, weak neck muscles, rapidly growing brain, thin skull, tearing of bridging veins, subdural/subarachnoid bleeding, and retinal hemorrhage
- Asphyxia/hypoxia

Abdominal Injuries

Abdominal injuries are the number two cause of morbidity and mortality from child abuse and include anterior abdominal wall bruises, ruptured liver or spleen (shock), ruptured mesenteric vessel (shock), intestinal perforation (peritonitis), duodenal hematoma (obstruction), pancreas trauma (pain, fever, or vomiting), and renal injury (hematuria).

Bruising

- Location

Accidental bruises are usually on anterior body surface and over bony prominences

Inflicted injuries are seen in fatty or protected areas: buttocks, lower back, inner thighs, genitalia, abdomen, upper lip, cheeks, and neck

Bruises to face or head, especially ears, are suspicious for abuse

- Pattern

Slap mark

Pinch/grab mark

Belt/strap mark

Electric cord mark

Pulled hair

Ligature/gag marks

Bite marks

Bizarre shapes

- Aging bruises—general rules

If red: probably less than 7 days old

If yellow: probably greater than 1–2 days old

Burns

Burns consist of:

- Accidental scalding burn
- "Doughnut" burn
- "Dunking" burn
- "Stocking/glove" burn
- Dry contact burn
- Cigarette burn

Skeletal Trauma

The most common fracture resulting from abuse is a transverse fracture of the diaphysis of a long bone.

Virtually diagnostic of child abuse:

- Chip or "bucket-handle" metaphyseal fracture
- Rib fractures
- Periosteal elevation after age 6 months
- Avulsion fracture of distal clavicle or acromion process

Highly suspect for child abuse:

- Spiral long bone fracture before age 9 months
- Sternal fracture
- Vertebral fracture
- Fractures of the middle or proximal humerus
- Multiple fractures in different stages of healing
- Fractures inconsistent with history given or developmental capability

MUNCHAUSEN SYNDROME BY PROXY

Munchausen syndrome by proxy is a psychiatric condition in which a parent or caregiver deliberately simulates or creates disease in a child in order to receive attention or sympathy from others or to gain control over the victim. A high percentage of parents involved in the perpetration of Munchausen syndrome by proxy have had histories of factitious illnesses. In 95% of cases the perpetrator is the mother. Parents who are accused of inducing an illness in their child invariably deny the charge and often withdraw the at-risk child from medical care.

Long-term morbidity is 8% and mortality is 9%. Some of the signs are listed as follows:

1. Parent induces illness in child
2. Difficult diagnosis
3. Multiple procedures
4. Child with medical condition unresponsive to treatment or with unusual course
5. Highly unusual physical or lab findings
6. Highly attentive parent
7. Parent with almost textbook knowledge of child's illness

SEXUAL ABUSE

Prevalence studies suggest that as many as 20%–30% of all women will have experienced at least one episode of sexual abuse by age 18. While females are most frequently the victims, males are not immune to the problem.

Because physical findings are often nonspecific or even normal in molestation and incest cases, the history is often the most important aspect of the evaluation. When possible the parent or parents should be interviewed first, separately from the child.

Presentations of Child Sexual Abuse

Direct or Indirect Statements

- Disclosure is usually a process
- Children are usually honest
- Important to record statements verbatim

Acute Behavioral Changes

- Specific (Table 19.1)
  Sexualized play
  Promiscuity or prostitution
  Perpetration against others
- Nonspecific
  Excessive masturbation
  Enuresis or encopresis
  Sleep or appetite disturbance
  Neurosis or conduct disorder
  Phobias

TABLE 19.1

Most Common Substitute Complaints in Sexual Abuse Cases

Any Age	Preschool Age	School Age	Adolescence
Abdominal pain	Excessive clinging	Decreased school	Same as school
Anorexia	Thumbsucking	performance	age plus
Vomiting	Speech disorder	Truancy	Runaway behavior
Constipation	Encopresis/enuresis	Lying, stealing	Suicide attempts
Sleep disorders	Excessive masturbation	Tics	Sexual offenses
Dysuria		Anxiety reaction	
Vaginal discharge		Phobic and obsessional	
Vaginal bleeding		states	
Rectal bleeding		Depression	
		Conversion reaction	
		Encopresis/enuresis	

Withdrawal or depression
Temper tantrums, aggression
Runaway/suicide
Functional abdominal pain
School problems
Substance abuse

Genital Symptoms and Signs

- Genital trauma or bleeding
- Infections or sexually transmitted disease
- Recurrent urinary tract infection
- Pregnancy

Specific Findings of Sexual Abuse

- Presence of semen, sperm, and/or acid phosphatase
- Pregnancy
- Confirmed positive cultures for gonorrhea (not conjunctival), acquired syphilis, or HIV (not blood-borne or perinatally acquired)

Additional Specimens Needed in Rape Cases

Clothing

If the patient is wearing the same clothes, they should be collected along with debris, as this may provide valuable clues regarding the assailant (Zitelli & Davis, 1987, p. 6.11; Table 19.2). The patient should disrobe while standing on a towel or sheet. Each article, including the towel or sheet, should then be placed in a separate bag. Avoid shaking the articles. Each bag is then labeled and sealed.

Fingernail Scrapings

Omit if patient has already bathed and shampooed. Scrapings may provide bits of skin, fiber, and debris from the assailant. Scrapings from beneath the nails or nail

TABLE 19.2

Guidelines for Specimen Collection in Sexual Abuse Examination

Orogenital Contact	No Evidence of Penetration	Evidence Consistent With Vaginal Penetration	Anal Contact
Swabs: use 2 at a time*	Urinalysis for occult blood	Urinalysis for occult blood	If external tears seen:
For wet mount for sperm†	Vaginal aspirate‡	If external tears seen:	Consult general surgeon for possible
For 2 air-dried slides†	(swabs may be used in	Consult surgeon for possible EUA	EUA
For GC culture	postpubescent patients*)	If EUA done, collect specimens	If EUA done, collect specimens
Baseline RPR (repeat in 4–6	For wet mount for sperm,	Vaginal aspirate‡	Swabs: use 2 at a time*
weeks if initial test is negative)	trichomonas, *Gardnerella*, and	(swabs may be used in postpubescent	(must be done before rectal examination)
	candida	patients*)	For wet mount for sperm†
	For 2 air-dried slides†	For wet mount for sperm, trichomonas,	For 2 air-dried slides†
	For GC and routine culture	*Gardnerella*, and candida	If no tears:
	For Gram stain if vaginal	For two air-dried slides†	Rectal exam
	discharge present	For GC and routine cultures	Stool guaiac: if positive consult general
	Baseline RPR (repeat in 4–6 weeks	For Gram stain if vaginal discharge	surgeon
	if initial test is negative)	Baseline RPR (repeat in 4–6 weeks if	Baseline RPR (repeat in 4–6 weeks if initial
		initial test is negative)	test is negative)

Data from Children's Hospital of Pittsburgh.

*Two of the swabs used to obtain specimens should be air-dried and placed in a sterile test tube for acid phosphatase, blood group, and enzyme studies. When specimens are obtained by vaginal aspirate, a small amount of aspirate should be applied to two swabs, which should then be processed in the same manner.

†Omit if seen >72 hours after the last incident, except in patients with vaginal discharge.

‡In prepubescent patients, vaginal specimens are best obtained by aspiration using a syringe attached to either a #3 French feeding tube or a soft 18- or 20-gauge intracatheter. If nothing is obtained on aspiration, a small amount of sterile nonbacteriostatic saline may be instilled and then aspirated back. Aspiration is less painful and less traumatic to prepubertal mucosa. In postpubescent patients, GC culture and Gram stain specimens should be obtained from the cervical os after cleaning the area with a dry swab. A cervical swab for chlamydia culture should also be considered when a cervical discharge is present.

clippings should be obtained. Specimens from each hand should be collected over separate sheets of paper, placed in separate paper envelopes, sealed, and labeled.

Hair Samples

Omit if patient has already bathed and shampooed. Any loose and suspected foreign hairs should be collected, placed in an envelope, and labeled. If patient is postpubescent, comb pubic hairs onto a sheet of clean paper, fold, place in an envelope with comb, label, and seal. Then, gently pull a small clump of the patient's pubic hair (12 hairs are needed), place on clean paper, fold, put in an envelope, and label "standard pubic hair." Then comb and obtain head hairs in the same manner.

Blood Sample

Five cc of blood should be drawn for blood grouping and enzyme typing, and placed in a purple-top tube.

Saliva Sample

A saliva sample enables testing of the patient's secretory status. The specimen should be obtained either by wiping the patient's oral mucosa with a gauze pad or by having the patient expectorate onto a gauze pad. The pad is then placed in an envelope, sealed, and labeled.

REFERENCE

Zitelli, B. J., & Davis, H. W. (1987). *Atlas of pediatric physical diagnosis*. New York: Gower Medical.

FURTHER READING

Bays, J., & Chadwick, D. (1993). Medical diagnosis of the sexually abused child. *Child Abuse and Neglect, 17*, 91–110.

Bruce, D., & Zimmerman, R. (1992). Shaken impact syndrome. *Pediatric Annals, 18*, 482–494.

Cooper, A., Floyd, T., Barlow, B., Niemirshka, M., Ludwig, S., Sweidl, T., et al. (1988). Major blunt abdominal trauma due to child abuse. *Journal of Trauma, 28*, 1483–1487.

Feldman, K. W., & Brewer, D. K. (1984). Child abuse, cardiopulmonary resuscitation and rib fractures. *Pediatrics, 73*, 339–342.

Johnson, D. L., Bruan, D., & Friendly, D. (1993). Accidental trauma and retinal hemorrhage. *Neurosurgery, 22*, 231–235.

Kirks, D. R. (1983). Radiological evaluation of visceral injuries in the battered child syndrome. *Pediatric Annals, 12*, 888–893.

Kleinman, P. K. (1990). Differentiation of child abuse and osteogenesis imperfecta: Medical and legal implications. *American Journal of Roentgenology, 154*, 1047–1048.

Reece, R. M. (1993). Fatal child abuse and sudden infant death syndrome: A critical diagnostic decision. *Pediatrics, 91*, 423.

Rosenberg, D. (1987). Web of deceit: A literature review of Munchausen syndrome by proxy. *Child Abuse and Neglect, 11*, 547–563.

20

EXAMINATION OF

THE NEWBORN

Science is not simply receiving what one is told but the investigation of causes.

Albertus Magnus, 1200–1280

THE INFANT IS a complete individual. The question you want answered is: "Is the infant normal?" Even minor abnormalities should be explained to the parents to allay their fears. In the apparently well infant, a second physical examination should be completed after the infant has adjusted to the new environment, since some physical abnormalities may become apparent after several days of life. However, at the first examination you are restricted to assessing gross physical anomalies. Conduct a more thorough examination 1–4 hours later. You should have an exact idea of what you want to know, proceed with the examination expeditiously, and write it up if even on a check sheet. Keep the baby warm, even preferably unclothed. If the baby is not crying, listen to the chest first. Otherwise, proceed to examine the infant systematically from the head downward. In general, the first examination of the infant consists chiefly of observation of orifices and of masses, bulges, or anomalies, but the method of examination is similar to that already described in older children.

GENERAL

Note the color and breathing of the baby. If the baby is gray or cyanotic or if the respirations are labored, do not begin the examination until the airway is gently but rapidly cleared, oxygen has been administered, and respiration has become regular. If in clearing the airway of mucus and amniotic fluid a soft feeding catheter with suction is passed first through the infant's nares into the nasopharynx and then down the esophagus to the stomach and no obstruction is met, the diagnoses of choanal atresia, esophageal atresia, and other nasopharyngeal anomalies such as nasal cysts, encephaloceles, and tumors are eliminated. Pass the catheter swiftly and gently without jerking, or laryngospasm may be induced. The tip of the catheter will be seen or felt throughout the left half of the abdominal wall. If the catheter is not palpable, cardiospasm may be present. If the catheter is down but not palpable, hold the hand over the abdomen and blow a quick puff of air through the catheter. The air bubble will be felt. If obstruction is met or the bubble is not felt, consider atresia in either of these areas as a possible cause of the infant's respiratory difficulty. Auscultating over the stomach while blowing air in may be deceptive, since transmitted sounds may be heard even though obstruction is present.

With the catheter in the stomach, aspirate the gastric fluid. Note the amount and quality. Normal amniotic fluid measures 5–25 ml and is cloudy white. Bloody fluid suggests placenta previa. Green fluid suggests meconium-stained amniotic fluid from antepartum asphyxia. More than 25 ml fluid suggests gastrointestinal tract obstruction.

If distress persists after the infant's upper airway is cleared, maneuver a laryngoscope of proper size carefully into the vallecula with the left hand, elevating the larynx by pressure with the left fifth finger on the thyroid cartilage; gently push the tongue out of the way with the blade, exposing the larynx.

Shock in an infant is usually caused by heavy sedation of the mother before delivery or intracranial trauma, but it may also result from generalized trauma of delivery, placental bleeding, a ruptured viscus, or hemorrhage in the adrenal area.

Maternal overmedication is a possible diagnosis in a depressed infant who is not meconium stained but who has pallor or cyanosis, a slow, strong, full pulse, and a cord filled with blood. Asphyxia is suggested in a depressed infant who is meconium stained and pale with a slow irregular pulse; soft, distant heart sounds; and an umbilical stump that is limp and contains little blood. Lethargy after the first day is a critical sign of infection, hyperammonemia, and other metabolic disorders.

A helpful evaluation of the baby at 1 minute and at 5 minutes of life is the Apgar score, the baby's first report card. Five criteria are noted, and each is assigned 0, 1, or 2 points (Table 20.1). A 5-minute score of 8–10 is excellent, one of 4–7 is guarded, and one of 0–3 is critical. Keep the baby warm.

Gross anomalies such as anencephaly, omphalocele, exstrophy of the bladder, and amelia are immediately obvious; record them in as much detail as possible. Observe the baby for symmetry of head, body, and extremities. Limbs of the term infant are flexed. Failure to move or asymmetrical movement suggests neurologic, muscle, or skeletal injury.

Recommended Routine Laboratory Studies for the Well Newborn

No laboratory tests other than the newborn metabolic screen are routinely recommended for the newborn in uncomplicated circumstances. For those whose perinatal period is questionable, some tests may be recommended:

- Hematocrit, white blood cell count, and differential, C reactive protein (CRP), reticulocyte count
- Urinalysis
- Standard bacteriologic tests
- Phenylketonuria, galactosemia, 17-hydroxyprogesterone, and thyroid function tests (e.g., thyroxine or thyroid-stimulating hormone) for screening on day of discharge and other metabolic diseases including cystic fibrosis and SS as long as infant is ≥ 14 hours post first protein feed.

TABLE 20.1

Apgar Score

	Criterion[a]	Score		
		0	1	2
A	Color (*appearance*)	Blue or pale	Pink with acrocyanosis	Pink
P	Heart rate (*pulse*)	Absent	100	100–140
G	Reflex irritability (*grimace*)	Absent	Minimal	Brisk
A	Muscle tone (*activity*)	Flaccid	Fair or increased	Good
R	Breathing and cry (*respiratory* effort)	Apnea, 1–2 gasps	Fair	Prompt, lusty

[a]A score of 8–10 is excellent, 4–7 is guarded, and 0–3 is critical.

- Cord blood should be saved for 2 weeks
- Blood type and hold until or if needed, and Coombs test if mother is Rh negative or if jaundice develops by 24 hours
- Universal hearing screen
- Blood glucose in at-risk or symptomatic newborns
- Serologic test for syphilis and for hepatitis B virus if mother is not tested antepartum
- Possible screening for *Toxoplasma* or viral infection is requested
- Separated cells and plasma or serum
- Microchemistries: direct and total bilirubin levels and glucose, sodium, potassium, chloride, and calcium levels

Acid-Base Analysis

For symptomatic newborns, assess the acid-base status. This analysis defines the presence and absence of asphyxia or hypoxia in the newborn. Carbon dioxide diffuses across the placenta very rapidly, and the rate of elimination is directly related to blood flow rates on both sides of the placenta.

The pH of blood or tissue is directly related to the concentration of base (bicarbonate) and inversely related to the concentrations of acid (H_2CO_3).

Generally, fetal or newborn acidemia is classified as respiratory, metabolic, or mixed based on the pH and bicarbonate concentrations.

SKIN

Note consistency and hydration of the skin. Normally, soon after birth the infant becomes pink and cries lustily. Congenital skin anomalies and deformities are common. A soft swelling, especially of the tongue or over the clavicle that contains fluid and transilluminates, is usually a lymphangioma or cystic hygroma. Midline cysts of the neck may be thyroglossal cysts. Small holes or defects anywhere in the neck and extending up to the ear may be branchial clefts or cysts.

Bluish pigmentation over the sacrum, buttocks, back, or occasionally extensor surfaces is termed *mongolian spot*. It results from pigment cells in the deep layers of the skin, usually disappears in later life when superficial pigment masks it, and has no clinical significance.

Ectodermal defects of the scalp are common. These usually appear as large, firm, sharply demarcated patches without hair. Look for small holes in the midline of the scalp or anywhere along the spinal column, which may be dermal sinuses. An infected area may be a cause of recurrent meningitis. A defect along this same area (aplasia cutis congenita) with hair over it or the hair collar sign, a small nodule with hair encircling it, is a marker of spinal dysraphism (e.g., spina bifida, attachment to dura, or filum terminale). If neural structures protrude through the defect, the mass is termed an *encephalocele* if it is on the head and a *meningomyelocele* if it is over the spine.

Generalized hardness of the skin is termed *sclerema*. This condition may result from overcooling the infant and is more likely to occur in debilitated infants, particularly if they have marked alterations in their serum electrolyte levels. Patchy areas of induration of the skin (hidebound skin) is scleroderma and usually does not occur in infants.

Cyanosis in infants is produced by the same biochemical factors that provoke it in older children. Because an infant usually has a higher hemoglobin level than an older child, cyanosis occurs more easily in infants and with less relative oxygen unsaturation than in older children (Chapter 3). Occasionally, ecchymoses will be confused with cyanosis. Pressure on a cyanotic area will blanch the skin temporarily; the ecchymotic area remains blue with pressure. Mongolian spots are usually easily distinguished from cyanosis, especially by their location.

An infant who remains cyanotic may have amniotic fluid, stomach contents, or tumors of the tongue or about the mouth obstructing the airway and causing hypoventilation. Upper airway obstruction may also be caused by choanal atresia or vascular ring; laryngeal web or cyst; hypoplasia of the mandible, or micrognathia, with glossoptosis; tracheomalacia, vocal cord paresis, or injury to the cricothyroid cartilage.

Persistent cyanosis indicates central nervous system (CNS), heart, or lung disease; differentiating between these at an early age is difficult (Table 20.2). Cyanosis in an infant with a slow cardiac or respiratory rate, with a bulging fontanel, or with limpness, especially after a rapid delivery (or of a mother who has been heavily sedated), suggests intracranial injury of the baby.

Cyanosis that lessens when the infant cries, especially if the infant is in a high-oxygen atmosphere, suggests the presence of pulmonary disease, such as respiratory distress syndrome, diaphragmatic hernia, pneumonia, asphyxia, or atelectasis. Pulmonary insufficiency is the usual cause of cyanosis in the infant. Increasing inspired oxygen is more likely to increase oxygen saturation in lung disease than in heart disease. Cyanosis that increases when the infant cries suggests cardiac disease. This test of the influence of crying on the depth of cyanosis distinguishes that resulting from solely heart or lung disease. Crying should not be induced in any infant suspected of having brain injury, since the increased intracranial pressure may aggravate intracranial hemorrhage.

TABLE 20.2
Delayed Respiration and Persistent Cyanosis in the Neonate

Causes of Delayed Respiration	Causes of Persistent Cyanosis
Intrapartum asphyxia	Cyanotic congenital heart defect
Prematurity	Persistent pulmonary hypertension
Drugs (causing central nervous system depression)	Underexpansion of lungs (surfactant deficiency)
Trauma to central nervous system	Diaphragmatic hernia
Anemia or blood loss	Pneumothorax
Congenital abnormalities	Anatomic abnormality of airways
Muscle weakness (prematurity or primary muscle disease)	

Localized cyanosis, which may persist for 24–48 hours, may sometimes be noted in a presenting part. Usually if a normal baby is slightly cyanotic at birth, cyanosis will be less in the hands than in the feet after about 4 hours of age. Equal cyanosis in the hands and feet after 4 hours of age suggests a pathologic cause of the cyanosis.

Peripheral cyanosis (acrocyanosis) is cyanosis of the hands and feet and suggests increased arteriovenous oxygen differences. It is associated with shock, sepsis, and low cardiac output, if sustained though usually normal in otherwise healthy newborns. Central cyanosis involves the mucous membranes and suggests cardiopulmonary disease.

Cyanosis without dyspnea usually occurs with hypoglycemia or methemoglobinemia or if the baby is chilled. Infants at risk for hypoglycemia include those who have diabetic mothers or mothers who use illicit drugs, are small for gestational age, or have asphyxia, infection, metabolic diseases, or hypopituitarism. Cyanosis with little dyspnea may also occur with congenital heart lesions such as hypoplastic right heart, tetralogy of Fallot with severe pulmonary stenosis or atresia, pulmonary stenosis with an intact ventricular septum, and tricuspid anomalies. Cyanosis caused by congenital heart lesions with respiratory distress in the first few days of life requires emergency workup. These findings are present in infants with right-to-left shunts, such as transposition of the great arteries, total anomalous pulmonary venous return, hypoplastic left heart, and some cases of coarctation of the aorta.

Cyanosis resulting from right-to-left shunt without organic heart disease may occur with persistent fetal circulation; persistent elevation of pulmonary vascular resistance maintains patency of the ductus and foramen ovale and may accompany hyperviscosity, atypical respiratory distress syndrome, or hypoglycemia. Cyanosis may occur a few hours after birth in an apparently normal infant with persistent fetal circulation, tricuspid or mitral regurgitation, or other heart lesions. Cyanosis of the upper half of the body occurs with transposition of the great vessels with patent ductus; cyanosis of the lower half of the body occurs with coarctation of the aorta proximal to a patent ductus.

In contrast to pallor in an older child, pallor in an infant almost always results from circulatory failure, anoxia, edema, or shock. Only rarely will severe neonatal anemia without shock be manifested by pallor. An infant who remains pallid may have respiratory obstruction, cerebral anoxia, narcosis, cerebral hemorrhage, hypoglycemia, hypothyroidism, or circulatory failure (e.g., from adrenal hemorrhage). The pallor of anoxia is usually associated with bradycardia and that of shock with tachycardia. Postmature infants tend to have pallid skins, with peeling.

A beefy red skin may indicate poorly developed vasomotor reflexes, polycythemia, or hypoglycemia in an infant born to a diabetic mother. Occasionally one half of the body may appear red and the other half pale—the harlequin color change of the infant. This condition is usually transient and of unknown significance. Plethora may also occur as a result of twin-twin or maternal-fetal transfusion and in adreno-genital syndrome. Alternating pink and blue patches may be caused by transient vessel abnormalities or cutis marmorata.

Record evidence of injuries secondary to delivery or application of forceps. Scratches, petechiae, and ecchymoses are most frequently caused by injuries incidental to delivery. However, petechiae and ecchymoses in infants are also caused by sepsis, erythroblastosis fetalis, hemorrhagic disease of the infant, and thrombocytopenic purpura. Rarely, purpuric spots are a result of hemophilia or diseases such as toxoplasmosis, syphilis, and cytomegalic inclusion disease. These spots may occur in infants whose mothers had rubella during the first trimester or who had lupus erythematosus throughout pregnancy. Puncture marks or skin pits may be the result of amniocentesis.

Note any tumors, hemangiomas, nevi, and skin tags. Telangiectases, or capillary hemangiomas, are frequently found at the back of the neck, the base of the nose, the center of the forehead, on the eyelids (nevus flammeus), or on the mucous membranes where they suggest hereditary hemorrhagic telangiectasia. Vascular nevi may appear over the face or head and may indicate Sturge-Weber disease. Small angiomas may herald angiomas in the retina and brain (Von Hippel-Lindau disease). Pigmented nevi are common birthmarks and may appear any time during the first year of life. Depigmented areas that resemble a leaf and that fluoresce may be an early sign of tuberous sclerosis. Note pigmented lesions of neurofibromatosis, café-au-lait spots, and freckles. Size, shape, color, and degree of protuberance should be recorded. Preauricular skin tags are occasionally associated with severe congenital anomalies.

Scars, usually around the mouth, may indicate congenital syphilis. Examine all skin folds to be certain that the skin moves over the underlying bone. Constricting bands, which are associated with deformity or atrophy beyond the contracture, may be hidden by the folds in the obese infant. They may resemble scars.

The skin of the infant normally feels puffy and edematous. Excess edema may be noted in premature infants; in those born of diabetic, prediabetic, or edematous mothers; or in those with hydrops resulting from blood—especially Rh—incompatibility or with intrauterine viral infections. It is noted in children with abnormal salt retention, hypoproteinemia, heart failure, or gonadal dysgenesis. Edema dorsal aspect of feet is particularly characteristic of Turner syndrome.

Note any localized edema in a presenting part that resulted from trauma. Edema limited to the infant's hands and feet may be a sign of gonadal dysgenesis or neonatal tetany. Edema of the genitalia in both sexes is common, especially in infants born by breech delivery. Edema of the anterior abdominal wall suggests perforation of a viscus with peritonitis, appendicitis, or obstructive uropathy. Asymmetric edema occurs with local vascular anomalies, thromboses, or trauma, and Milroy disease, a form of lymphedema.

Edema of the extremities may be caused by heart failure and liver diseases and other causes of hydrops such as blood incompatibility, chorangioma of the placenta, umbilical or chorionic vein thrombosis, fetal neuroblastoma, cystic adenomatoid malformation of the lung, pulmonary lymphangiectasia, maternal parvovirus infection, Chaga disease, fetal Gaucher disease, and local vascular abnormalities.

Poor turgor and excessive wrinkling may indicate dehydration. Dehydration of the infant immediately after birth may indicate poor maternal nutrition, maternal toxemia, defective placenta, or sepsis of the infant. Large babies with good turgor may be born of mothers with diabetes or may be characteristic of patients with hypothyroidism.

The vernix caseosa, a cheesy white material with bacteriologic benefits, is found in the skin folds and the nail beds. Yellow discoloration of the vernix occurs with intrauterine distress, postmaturity, hemolytic disease of infants, and occasionally in infants born by breech delivery.

Desquamation occurs normally in all infants and may be generalized. Marked peeling and cracking of the skin occurs in dysmature infants. Small, hard scales may indicate congenital ichthyosis (known as collodion babies).

Redness of the skin with red pinpoint macules and papules developing in the first days of life are usually transitory rashes caused by irritation, toxicity, or unknown cause. Erythema toxicum (ET) may appear within the first 3 days of life and may be indistinguishable from miliaria (heat rash) or varicella. ET has a red base; miliaria does not. Neither involves palms or soles. Redness and tissue necrosis may result from transcutaneous oxygen monitors. ET may contain eosinophils and usually resolves spontaneously after 5–8 days.

Examine pustules carefully. Pinpoint white spots, usually over the bridge of the nose, chin, or cheeks, are most frequently milia caused by retained sebum and are not true pustules. Small pustules that develop after water-drop-like miliaria are a form of miliaria, either miliaria crystallina or miliaria pustulosa. Vesiculopustular lesions, which are shed leaving hyperpigmented macules, are transient neonatal pustular melanosis. Small pustules with a surrounding red area are diagnostic of impetigo neonatorum. If these pustules are associated with bullae, pemphigus is present. Pemphigus of the palms and soles of the infant suggests congenital syphilis. Tender, red, indurated areas with sharp borders resulting from streptococcal infection are termed erysipelas. In infants, erysipelas may be found near the umbilicus or at the site of a skin injury. Vesiculobullous lesions in an infant may also result from herpes simplex or varicella virus by infection if the mother is infected at the time of delivery. The vesicles of herpes simplex may not erupt for 9 days. Vesicles may be a sign of incontinentia pigmenti.

Small discrete bullous patches involving the deeper layers of the skin, usually with large hemorrhagic areas, are termed *epidermolysis bullosa* (EB). With EB, yellowish plaques may be present on the oral mucosa. Small reddish or purple areas of the skin that are hard and movable (fat necrosis) may be caused by trauma during or after delivery but may also indicate hypercalcemia. These areas frequently calcify with hard edges and feel like small saucers or small, loose peas under the skin.

Redness starting on the face and extending over the entire body and usually appearing in the second week of life—associated with desquamation of large patches of skin—is diagnostic of dermatitis exfoliativa (Ritter disease). In this condition, as in scalded skin or toxic shock syndrome, large patches of epithelium can be removed by stroking the infant's skin (Nikolsky sign). Redness and desquamation in the skin folds represent intertrigo, usually caused by sweating and chafing but sometimes caused by fungal or other infections. Erythematous patches occur with neonatal lupus erythematosus.

Jaundice is sometimes difficult to determine in infants. As in older children, examine the skin, the sclerae, the mucous membranes, and the nail beds in natural daylight. Minimal jaundice in a plethoric infant may be more easily discerned by placing a glass slide on the infant's cheek. With slight pressure, the capillary blood and erythema will fade, but the yellowness caused by the jaundice will remain. Jaundice is usually visible in children or adults when the serum bilirubin reaches 2 mg/dl. It may not be visible in infants until the bilirubin level is 5 mg/dl, probably because there is less fat in the subcutaneous tissue in which bilirubin is soluble. Jaundice is usually not seen at birth because light is required to develop the pigment. The yellow-orange color is usually caused by unconjugated bilirubin; the yellow-green color is caused by conjugated bilirubin.

Jaundice in infants apparently progresses from the head to the feet. You can estimate the approximate level of serum bilirubin from the most caudal area of the body that is jaundiced (Table 20.3).

Jaundice appearing at birth or within 12 hours after birth is almost diagnostic of erythroblastosis fetalis. Jaundice after 24 hours is usually physiologic but may also be a result of erythroblastosis secondary to Rh or A-B-O incompatibility, sepsis, congenital syphilis, hemolytic icterus, bile duct obstruction, or viral hepatitis. A transient unconjugated hyperbilirubinemia develops in all newborns during the first week of life. Physiologic jaundice usually disappears in the full-term infant by the second week but may persist without obvious cause for as long as 4 weeks, especially in some breast-fed infants. Persistent physiologic jaundice lasting longer than 4 weeks may be noted in infants with congenital heart disease, especially in heart failure or in hypothyroidism. Sepsis with jaundice is usually caused by staphylococci or *Escherichia coli*. Sepsis without jaundice is usually from streptococci or pneumococci. Lethargy may be associated with jaundice from any cause.

Differential Diagnosis of Unconjugated Hyperbilirubinemia

Physiologic jaundice
Hemolysis/hemorrhage
Breast milk jaundice
Swallowed maternal blood

TABLE 20.3
Jaundice

Appearance	Bilirubin Level (mg/dl)
Head alone	5–8 mg/dl
Head and chest	6–12 mg/dl
To knees	8–12 mg/dl
Including arms and lower legs	10–18 mg/dl
Including hands and feet	15–20+ mg/dl

Placental dysfunction
Crigler-Najjar syndrome
Clotting disorder
Infant of diabetic mother
Sepsis
Lucey-Driscoll syndrome
Intestinal obstruction
Hypothyroidism

Differential Diagnosis of Conjugated Hyperbilirubinemia

Persistent Intrahepatic Cholestasis

Paucity of intrahepatic bile ducts
Trihydroxycoprostanic acidemia
Byler disease
Hereditary cholestasis with lymphedema
Arteriohepatic dysplasia
Benign recurrent intrahepatic cholestasis

Genetic and Metabolic Disorders

* Disorders of carbohydrate metabolism
  Galactosemia
  Fructosemia
  Glycogen storage disease type IV
* Chromosomal disorders
  Trisomy 18
  Down syndrome
* Disorders of lipid metabolism
  Wolman disease
  Cholesterol ester storage disease
  Gaucher disease
  Niemann-Pick disease
* Disorders of amino acid metabolism
  Tyrosinemia

- Miscellaneous genetic and metabolic disorders
  Cystic fibrosis
  Neonatal hypopituitarism
  α_1-Antitrypsin deficiency
  Familial hepatosteatosis
  Zellweger cerebrohepatorenal syndrome

Acquired Intrahepatic Cholestasis

- Infections
  Hepatitis B (non-A, non-B)
  Syphilis
  Toxoplasmosis
  Rubella
  Cytomegalovirus
  Herpes
  Varicella
  Echovirus
  Coxsackievirus
  Leptospirosis
  Tuberculosis
  Bacterial sepsis
- Drug-induced cholestasis
- Cholestasis associated with parenteral nutrition

Extrahepatic Obstruction

- Infantile obstructive cholangiopathy
  Biliary atresia
  Neonatal hepatitis
  Choledochal cyst
- Other causes
  Extrinsic bile duct compression
  Choledocholithiasis
  Bile plug syndrome
  Spontaneous bile duct perforation

Pathologic Factors Aggravating Physiologic Jaundice

Prematurity	Infections
Inadequate calories	Dehydration
Hypoxia	Meconium retention
Hemolysis	Hypoglycemia
Polycythemia	Intestinal obstruction
Hypothyroidism	

Jaundice that appears unusually earlier (i.e., within the first 24 hours) or is severe enough to require phototherapy requires investigation for the presence of hemolysis.

Determination of maternal and infant blood groups, direct Coombs testing of infant blood, full blood count, and if the baby is of Mediterranean, African, or Asian descent, measurement of glucose-6-phosphate dehydrogenase is indicated. Urine should be screened for infection, reducing sugars, and the presence of bilirubin.

Sweating is rare in infants. It may be present in infants with brain cortex irritation or anomalies or injuries of the sympathetic nervous system or in those whose mothers were morphine addicts or drug abusers.

Nails

The infant's nail beds should be pink. Yellowing of the nail beds has the same significance as yellowing of the vernix. In black infants, increased amounts of melanin are normally found in the nail beds and near the genitalia. Absence or defects of the nails are usually congenital and a sign of either fetal alcohol syndrome, phenytoin treatment of the mother, or a form of ectodermal dysplasia. The nails may be short in premature infants and unusually long in postmature infants.

MUSCLE TONE

At birth, the infant is usually limp, but after the first or second cry, the infant develops good muscle tone. Soon after birth, infants flex themselves into positions of comfort, the positions they occupied in utero. Note areas of flaccidity or spasticity.

Poor muscle tone in an infant a few minutes old should be regarded as an ominous sign. In infants who remain limp longer than a few minutes, suspect anoxia, narcosis, CNS lesions—particularly edema or hemorrhage—vascular collapse, hypoplastic left heart complex, hypoglycemia, Down syndrome, and avulsion or subdural hematoma of the cord. Infants with myasthenia gravis may be limp; they are born of mothers with the disease. However, many infants who have been limp for longer than several hours eventually appear to be normal. The cause of prolonged limpness in such infants is usually not adequately explained. Local loss of muscle tone may indicate a peripheral nerve lesion. Excess muscle tone may indicate CNS or metabolic muscular disease.

Seizures may be distinguished from normal tremulousness in that the convulsing child is usually quiet before the seizure occurs and the tremulous child is usually active. Soon after birth, seizures indicate hypoxic ischemic encephalopathy, increased intracranial pressure from bleeding or infection, anomalies of the CNS, drug withdrawal, hypoglycemia, or hypocalcemia with tetany or other metabolic diseases. Tetany is more common in infants who have low birth weight, diabetic mothers, or asphyxia. Rarely, omphalitis resulting from *Clostridium tetani* causes tetanus of an infant with convulsions. Another rare condition, neonatal nephritis, also causes convulsions.

Muscular twitching and hypertonicity have diagnostic significance similar to that of convulsions. However, tremors and twitchings of short duration may be noted, especially if the infant is cold or startled; these are usually normal and occur in active infants. Tremors of no pathologic significance cease if you place a finger in the infant's mouth and let the infant suck. Overalertness with twitching may result from narcotic withdrawal if the mother is addicted or, rarely, may indicate hyperthyroidism. Asymmetric seizures do not help distinguish metabolic from intracranial causes. Seizures resulting from hypocalcemia or infection usually begin after the fourth day of life; those caused by anoxia, birth injury, anomalies, or hypoglycemia begin in the first 3 days of life. Seizures due to amino acid abnormalities may present at any time.

Some facies are characteristic at this age. For example, Down syndrome facies can usually be recognized at birth, but hypothyroidism is usually not detectable until about 6 weeks of age. Mucopolysaccharidoses can be detected only if suspected, since characteristic facies appear after several months. The facies of an infant with renal agenesis (Potter syndrome) is characterized by low-set ears, senile appearance, broad nose, and receding chin. Major facial anomalies may indicate chromosome abnormalities. Note multiple fractures in children with osteogenesis imperfecta. Disproportion of one side of the body indicates absence or abnormalities of the bone or muscles or congenital hypertrophy. Other representative facies are described in Chapter 3.

HEAD

Note carefully the presence and amount of overriding of the sutures. Immediately after the infant's birth, the fontanels may appear to be very small or entirely closed, and the suture lines will be represented by hard ridges. These findings are normal and are considered part of the molding process of a normal vaginal delivery. Within the first day of life, normal intracranial pressure begins to exert its expansive force, and the suture lines and fontanels are felt as depressions in the normal infant. The progress of this expansion is followed during the entire period of infancy but especially during the neonatal period. Failure of normal expansion in the neonatal period may be the earliest sign of microcephaly or craniostenosis. In contrast, rapid enlargement of the fontanels is not a good early sign of developing hydrocephalus; absolute measurements of skull and chest circumference are necessary for this diagnosis. Anencephaly and congenital hydrocephaly are obvious at birth. To detect hydrancephaly, hydrocephalus, or subdural hematoma, transilluminate the head of any infant whose head is asymmetric or unusually large or small or who has abnormal neurologic signs.

A tense fontanel any time after birth and until the fontanel closes indicates increased intracranial pressure. Except in infants whose intracranial pressure is increased because of crying or coughing, a tense or bulging fontanel is usually a pediatric emergency, suggesting intracranial infection, bleeding, brain tumor, or pseudotumor. Estimate intracranial pressure by raising the infant's head until the fontanel is flat; then measure the vertical distance from the fontanel to the clavicle. Normally, this does not exceed 55 mm in the first few months of life.

A depressed fontanel may be normal or may be an early indication of dehydration. A third fontanel, located between the anterior and posterior fontanels, is a sign of an infant at risk.

Cephalohematoma is frequently not present at birth but appears on the second day of life. The hematoma is soft and fluctuant, and the outline is well defined, with the edge at the bone margin. A cephalohematoma begins to calcify in the first few days of life, and a ridge around the hematoma may be felt for as long as 6 months. Presence of a cephalohematoma raises somewhat the possibility of an occult skull fracture.

In contrast to cephalohematoma, the caput succedaneum is soft but ill defined in outline, pits on pressure, and is not fluctuant. The characteristics represent edema of the scalp, possibly from pressure on the emissary veins. Record the presence of caput, since this may indicate difficult delivery with possible intracranial hemorrhage.

Press the scalp behind and above the ears with the fingers, as if playing the piano, to determine the presence of a ping-pong ball sensation: craniotabes. Many normal infants have craniotabes, but if it is present, hydrocephalus and syphilis should also be suspected. The other causes of craniotabes occur later in life (see Chapter 5).

Cranial or facial asymmetry is common and is usually caused by intrauterine molding or molding during delivery. Facial or cranial asymmetry may occur in infants with facial palsy, but usually infants with facial nerve injury are not born with asymmetry. Try to assess facial asymmetry as the infant begins to cry. Segments of the facial nerve may be injured and cause confusion; for example, the mentalis nerve and its muscle prevent drawing down the corner of the mouth but spare the nasolabial fold and palpebral fissure. This type of weakness may be permanent. Facial palsy may be hereditary. Central palsy occurs with Möbius syndrome. Facial asymmetry may occur in infants of low birth weight and associated hemihypertrophy (Silver syndrome) and with congenital heart disease in cardiofacial syndrome. Asymmetric development of the orbicularis oris muscle results in an asymmetric cry; the nasolabial folds are equal.

Note presence of micrognathia (small mandible). Head retraction may be a sign of a vascular ring causing respiratory obstruction. Chvostek sign is usually positive in normal infants and therefore is of little value in diagnosing neonatal tetany.

EYES

If the infant is crying or keeps the eyes shut, gently rock the head or provide some suckling. Usually the infant will open the eyes long enough to allow a thorough neonatal examination.

Note the presence, structure, and equality of the eyes. Edema of the lids may be caused by birth trauma. Real tears may not appear until the infant reaches the second month of life, and the lacrimal ducts may not open until several weeks later. Purulent discharge from the eyes that is present shortly after birth may signifies ophthalmia neonatorum as a result of gonorrhea or Chlamydia infection. Although any discharge from the eyes may begin on the infant's first day of life, chemical irritation usually causes discharge on days 1–3, gonorrhea on days 2–5, and inclusion blennorrhea from viral or Chlamydia infection on days 4–14.

A mongoloid slant (the lateral upward slope of the eyes with an inner epicanthal fold) or an antimongoloid slant may be variants or may suggest one of the syndromes of mental, physical, or chromosome aberrations. The inner canthal length is normally 1.5–2.5 cm, the outer canthal length is 5.0–7.5 cm, and the interpupillary distance is 3.0–4.5 cm at birth.

At birth, exophthalmos is usually a congenital anomaly, with enlargement of all the structures of the eye (buphthalmos). However, congenital glaucoma is a cause of exophthalmos in infants. An open-eyed stare, common in infants with cerebral palsy, may be confused with exophthalmos.

Enophthalmos is usually associated with ptosis and constricted pupil (Horner syndrome) and indicates damage to the brain or to the cervical spine and brachial plexus root at this age. Constricted pupil alone, unilateral dilated fixed pupil, and nystagmus or strabismus may each be an early sign of brain injury. A searching nystagmus is not uncommon at birth. Later, this type of nystagmus may indicate blindness. An intermittent strabismus is present in nearly all infants at birth but disappears by 6 months of age.

Conjunctival or scleral hemorrhages are common and usually have no clinical significance. They may, however, indicate difficult delivery or hemorrhagic disease of the infant. Blood in the anterior chamber (hyphema) is visible as a fluid level when the head is erect and usually indicates more extensive trauma. Conjunctival edema (chemosis) and discharge may appear a few days after birth and are usually caused by chemicals or eye infections.

Examine the cornea for anomalies of the cornea and pupil. Keratitis in an infant may be due to trauma but usually signifies gonorrhea. The corneal reflex should be present at birth but test only if brain or eye damage is suspected. Haziness may indicate cataract or glaucoma. Congenital cataracts may indicate maternal rubella, galactosemia, or disorders of calcium metabolism.

Examine the retina and test for a red reflex. Raising the infant's head with one hand is often helpful in getting the infant to open the eyes long enough to visualize the retina. Absence of the red reflex may indicate the presence of lens opacities, retinoblastoma, or glaucoma. Retinal hemorrhages usually indicate subdural hematoma or other brain trauma. Chorioretinitis, whitish spots on the retina resulting from congenital toxoplasmosis or cytomegalic inclusion disease, may be found.

The pupil of the infant may be constricted for about 3 weeks or may respond to light at birth by contracting (*pupillary reflex*). Absence of the reflex after 3 weeks suggests that the infant is blind or may have sustained intracranial anoxia or oculomotor nerve damage. The infant's eyes should follow a light. The pupil is normally black to direct light. White pupils indicate opacity in the lens, vitreous, or retina. Detect sixth-nerve paralysis by watching the eye fail to move laterally as you rotate the infant's head in the opposite direction (doll's eye maneuver).

EARS

Note anomalies, position, clefts, tags, and injuries of the external ear. Low-set ears may be associated with renal agenesis or chromosome abnormalities. Because the canals are usually filled at birth with vernix and amniotic debris, you may not visualize the drums; however, they may be visualized at a few days of age. You can estimate deafness at a few days of age by snapping your fingers or making a sharp noise. Normally the eyelids will twitch or a complete Moro reflex will be obtained. In an infant with deafness, there is no such response; suspect congenital deafness, filled aural canals, congenital syphilis, and kernicterus. Universal hearing screening is now part of normal newborn care. Large ear lobes might suggest fragile X. Ear lobes that deviate outward might be amenable to early taping.

NOSE

The nose is usually deformed for a few days after birth, but injury is rare. Test patency of the nasal canals by holding your hand over the baby's mouth and noting the normal passage of air. Since mucus is usually present, a more certain method of testing nasal patency is to pass a soft rubber catheter with suction, as already described. A nonpatent nasal airway at this age is usually caused by choanal atresia or other congenital anomaly. Occasionally, a tumor or encephalocele may be protruding. Nasal discharge may be present normally, and sneezing is common and usually lasts 1 month. Thick bloody nasal discharge without sneezing suggests congenital syphilis (snuffles). Sneezing may occur in patients with hypothyroidism and in infants whose mothers were receiving reserpine or narcotics. The nasal septum might be dislocated at birth requiring early realignment.

MOUTH

Note cleft lip and cleft palate. Always open the infant's mouth to seek anomalies. Because infants normally have a high arched palate, it may be difficult to visualize the mouth beyond the uvula. Ordinarily, visualization beyond this point is not necessary. Insert a gloved finger to feel for a cleft or submucous cleft, tumors, or thyroid cyst at the base of the tongue. A large tongue usually results from tumor (lymphangioma or hemangioma). The tongue is rarely enlarged at birth in patients with hypothyroidism; it is large in infants with Wiedemann-Beckwith syndrome or Pompe disease (glycogen storage disease, type II) and appears large in infants with the Pierre-Robin syndrome with micrognathia.

Infants with brain injury have a protruding adderlike tongue. The frenulum of the tongue may be prominent but usually does not restrict motion of the tongue. It is normal for the frenulum to be attached near the tip of the tongue in newborns. Obtain the sucking reflex (Chapter 5) by placing the tongue blade on the lips, and stimulate the rooting reflex by touching the cheek and noting the infant turn and suck; both are normal reflexes present at birth. Absence of these reflexes occurs in brain-injured or debilitated infants and in some normal infants for the first day or two of life.

Teeth may be present at birth. Retention cysts, or pearls, are common along the gum margins. Flat white spots that do not rub away (thrush) may be present by 3 or 4 days of life. Small hard tumors may be evident in the gingiva, especially in the incisor area (epulis). You may see ulcers, or plaques, on the hard palate after a few days of age (Bednar aphthae) that are usually due to vigorous sucking. Small, white epithelial cysts along both sides of the median raphe of the hard palate are Epstein pearls. Tonsillar tissue is not evident in a newborn. Observe for bifid uvula, which may be associated with a submucous cleft palate.

NARCOTIC WITHDRAWAL

Maternal addiction, particularly to narcotic agents, may lead to the development of withdrawal syndrome in the neonate after delivery. Presentation is generally soon after birth but can be delayed until 10 days and may last for weeks. The delayed presentation is particularly characteristic of methadone withdrawal.

Symptoms are variable and are predominantly those of autonomic and cerebral irritability. Nasal congestion, sneezing, yawning, runny nose, poor suck, hiccups, and diarrhea have all been described. The cry is abnormally high-pitched with increased extensor tone, poor sleeping, tachypnea, weight loss, and seizures.

FETOMATERNAL HEMORRHAGE

Fetomaternal hemorrhage occurs in small amounts in approximately 75% of all pregnancies but is clinically important only in cases of large hemorrhages. Most cases of fetomaternal transfusion are spontaneous, occurring in uncomplicated term deliveries. Some may be a consequence of abdominal trauma with abruptio placentae. Hemorrhage may occur due to delivery complications when the placenta is anterior and in association with chorangioma or choriocarcinoma. There may be decreased fetal movements over a period of 24–48 hours prior to delivery.

The standard method of testing for fetal erythrocytes in maternal circulation is Betke-Kleihauer staining of a peripheral blood smear. The test should be done routinely in all cases of unexplained stillbirth, fetal distress, and neonatal anemia. Immediate transfusion may be lifesaving, and testing of the mother during the puerperium is important.

The size of the hemorrhage can be calculated on the basis of the percentage of fetal red cells present and estimated average maternal blood volume of 5,000 ml. For example, if 5% of the red cells in the maternal circulation are fetal in origin, the size of the hemorrhage is calculated as $0.05 \infty 5,000 = 250$ ml of fetal blood; 80 ml (approximately one quarter of the infant's blood volume) or greater is considered significant for fetomaternal transplacental hemorrhage. (The average blood volume of an infant is 100 ml/kg; therefore, a 3-kg term infant would have a blood volume of 300 ml.)

FETAL BLOOD pH

When fetal scalp blood is acidotic, maternal acidosis should be differentiated from fetal acidosis, because maternal acidosis does not have the same serious implications. Fetal pH is usually 0.04 U below maternal pH. A pH >7.25 is normal during labor; pH of 7.20–7.25 is worrisome, and another determination should be made promptly; pH ≤7.20 suggests significant fetal hypoxia and need for prompt delivery.

After age of 3 hours, sample of capillary blood from the infant's warmed heel correlates well with arterial blood samples in measurements of acid-base status. In uncomplicated pregnancy, umbilical cord blood pH has a normal lower limit of 7.15. Blood pH is the only objective measure available at delivery by which a diagnosis of asphyxia can be made.

TABLE 20.4
Base Deficit and Blood pH

	Maternal pH (mean)	Fetal pH (mean)	Base Deficit (mEq/L)
Normal mother and fetus	7.42	7.25	7.0
Normal mother and acidotic fetus	7.42	7.25	2.6
Acidotic mother and vigorous fetus	7.36	7.15	4.8

From: Gilbert-Barness, E., & Barness, L. A. (2003). *Clinical use of pediatric diagnostic tests.*
Baltimore: Lippincott, Williams and Wilkins, p. 85.

In general, mean blood pH of 7.27 in the newborn is associated with an Apgar score of ≥7. Mean blood pH of 7.22 is associated with an Apgar score of ≤6. Fetal acid-base status is a valuable index of fetal asphyxia or oxygenation; it should be evaluated with other evidence of fetal distress. Fetal blood pH provides the best correlation with fetal outcome. In almost 20% of infants, the fetal acid-base status may be misleading (e.g., due to fetal scalp edema, contamination with amniotic fluid).

False Normal

Normal blood pH but depressed infant function.

Due to medications administered, obstetric manipulation (e.g., difficult forceps delivery), precipitous delivery, prematurity (especially weight <1,000 g with noncompliant lungs), congenital anomalies preventing normal onset of good lung function at birth (e.g., laryngeal web, choanal atresia, hypoplastic lungs associated with diaphragmatic hernia, edematous cyst of lung), aspiration syndromes, previous episodes of asphyxia with resuscitation, intrauterine infection.

False Abnormal

Maternal acidosis is usual cause (Table 20.4).

VOMITING

Vomiting is a symptom in older children but may be considered a sign in infants. It is common in infants aged 1–2 days and may be a result of relaxation of the cardia of the stomach.

Causes of Vomiting in Newborns

Sepsis	Malrotation
Cerebral anoxia	Annular pancreas
Increased intracranial pressure	Intestinal atresia
Marked jaundice	Intestinal bands
Adrenal insufficiency	Diverticuli
Diaphragmatic hernia	Duplications
Meconium ileus	Imperforate anus

Peritonitis   Hirschsprung disease
Meningitis   Cretinism
Intestinal obstruction   Metabolic errors
Volvulus

Vomiting of uncurdled milk or prompt vomiting of anything occurs in infants with esophageal atresia but also occurs in normal infants who have been fed too much or too fast or who have not been properly burped or positioned after feeding. Passage of a catheter with suction, as previously described, helps determine the presence of esophageal atresia. Bloody vomitus in an infant most commonly results from ingested blood (determined by Apt test), but occasionally occurs with hemorrhagic disease of infants or with gastrointestinal ulcers associated with intracranial anoxia or increased pressure. Vomitus with bile suggests an obstruction below the ampulla of Vater or perforation of a viscus; vomitus without bile suggests obstruction above the ampulla. Fecal vomiting usually indicates a low intestinal obstruction. Vomiting also occurs in children with electrolyte disturbances, urinary tract disease, and infections.

NECROTIZING ENTEROCOLITIS

Necrotizing enterocolitis is a severe neonatal disease characterized by mucosal and transmucosal necrosis of intestine, primarily ileum and proximal colon.

- Endemic: sporadic cases that occur periodically
- Epidemic: temporal or geographic clustering of cases ± association with infectious agents (*Escherichia coli*, *Klebsiella* spp., *Enterobacter* spp., *Staphylococcus* spp., *Clostridium* spp., rotavirus, coronavirus, enterovirus)

High risk factors include hypoxia, ischemia-reperfusion, infection, umbilical catheterization, hypotension, hypothermia, hyperosmolarity, polythemia, hyperviscosity, maternal cocaine use.

Gastrointestinal signs include abdominal distention, absent bowel sounds, decreased stool with advancing feeds, gastric retention and vomiting, blood in stool, carbohydrate intolerance (stools Clinitest +, Breath H_2). Systemic signs include temperature instability, apnea ± bradycardia, lethargy, metabolic acidosis, erythema of abdominal wall (peritonitis), petechiae, bleeding, and shock. Radiographic signs (KUB and cross-table lateral) include ileus, bowel wall thickening, distended immobile intestinal loop on repeated X-rays (sentinel loop), pneumatosis intestinalis (intramural gas), and hepatic portal vein gas ± pneumoperitoneum (intestinal perforation). Lab findings include complete blood count: neutropenia, thrombocytopenia, disseminated intravascular coagulation parameters, acid-base and electrolyte monitoring, and cultures (blood, cerebrospinal fluid, urine, stool, paracentesis if indicated).

Mortality varies 10%–30% with no significant improvement over the last 30 years. Complications include sepsis, disseminated intravascular coagulation, shock, perforation peritonitis, abscesses, complications of total parenteral nutrition (cholestatic liver disease), complications of central line, malabsorption, postsurgical short-bowel syndrome, strictures (25%–35%), adhesions, and enterocolonic fistula.

Saliva is usually scant until the second or third month of life. In infants, profuse salivation with mucoid secretions may indicate the presence of tracheoesophageal fistula or cystic fibrosis, but frequently it may be caused by tracheal aspiration or irritation.

NECK

The infant's neck is generally not visible when the infant is supine. Bring the neck into full view by placing one hand behind the upper back and allowing the head to fall gently into extension.

Distended neck veins usually signify a mass in the chest or pneumomediastinum. A mass in the lower part of the sternocleidomastoid muscle with limitation of motion of the neck results in torticollis. Small cystic masses in the region of the upper part of the sternocleidomastoid may be branchial cleft cysts. A fractured clavicle may present as a mass in the neck, though most commonly crepitation over the clavicle. A midline mass may be a congenital goiter, which is rare, or a thyroglossal duct cyst, which is more common. A soft mass over the clavicle that transilluminates may be a cystic hygroma.

An unusually short, poorly mobile neck may be an indication of Klippel-Feil syndrome; skin folds from the acromion to the mastoid may indicate gonadal dysgenesis. Excess posterior cervical skin may indicate other chromosome aberrations.

Flex the neck. Resistance is rare but may indicate meningeal irritation. However, lack of resistance does not indicate lack of meningeal irritation, since an infant with meningitis may have a supple neck. Retraction (opisthotonos) may be caused by intracranial injury or infection.

Turn the infant's head from side to side to obtain the tonic neck reflex, which is normally present in infants (Chapter 5). Absence may indicate CNS damage. When the head of a supine infant is turned, the infant's trunk should rotate in the direction of the head movement (the neck-righting reflex). Similarly, if the body of an erect infant is tilted, the infant's head should return to the upright position, a labyrinth response (otolith-righting reflex).

CRY

Note the cry of the infant. The infant should cry lustily at birth. A weak or groaning cry or grunt in expiration usually indicates severe respiratory disturbances. Absence or weakness of cry or constant crying at birth usually indicates brain injury, laryngeal anomaly, or vocal cord paresis. A high-pitched (or cerebral) cry may indicate increased intracranial pressure. Hoarseness or crowing inspirations may indicate laryngeal disease or anomalies. Hoarseness appearing at 2–5 days of age frequently results from laryngospasm caused by hypocalcemia. Hoarseness is usually absent at birth in congenital laryngeal stridor; at birth, the presence of hoarseness requires study.

Causes of Hoarseness or Crowing Inspiration

Congenital laryngeal stridor	Laryngeal tumor
Laryngeal nerve paralysis	Thyroglossal tumor
Laryngeal stenosis	Mucus plugs
Tracheal stenosis	Laryngeal web
Laryngomalacia	Tracheal web
Tracheomalacia	Congenital heart disease
Vascular ring	Diaphragmatic hernia
Pierre Robin syndrome	Cystic hygroma
Pneumothorax	Abnormal thoracic cage
Bronchogenic cyst	Mediastinal mass
Hypocalcemia	Epiglottic anomaly
Thyroglossal duct cyst	Subglottic anomaly

CHEST

Examine the infant's chest for gross anomalies, tumors, and fractures. The chest is usually almost circular. Depressed sternum may be caused by atelectasis, respiratory distress syndrome, and funnel chest. The xiphisternum protrudes and normally appears broken as a result of the xiphoid's weak attachment with the body of the sternum. Retractions usually indicate interference with air entry. Marked retraction of the chest suggests upper airway, particularly laryngeal, obstruction such as laryngeal stenosis. Immediate direct laryngoscopy is indicated.

Asymmetry of the chest may result from diaphragmatic hernia or paralysis, pneumothorax, emphysema, tension cysts, pleural effusions, pneumonia, and pulmonary agenesis. An asymmetric mass near the neck may be a fractured clavicle. Palpation may reveal congenital absence of a clavicle or of muscle (Poland syndrome).

With a warm hand, palpate for the cardiac impulse. In a normal infant, it is barely palpable. An impulse felt in the subcostal angle or left parasternal area occurs with ventricular enlargement. Increased activity at the apex indicates left ventricular overactivity. Thrills may be felt over the aortic area or suprasternal notch in infants with aortic stenosis, at the second left interspace in infants with pulmonic stenosis, at the second or third left interspace near the sternum in infants with patent ductus, and at the fourth interspace near the sternum in infants with ventricular septal defect.

Enlargement of the breasts in either sex caused by maternal hormones is usually evident on day 2 or 3 of life and may persist normally as long as a month. Milky secretions may normally be present (a.k.a. Witch's milk). Redness and firmness around the nipple are rare and result from infection—mastitis or abscess. Increased pigmentation of the areola is noted in cases of adrenogenital syndrome. Supernumerary nipples are noted, since they may be associated with internal organ anomalies, though are usually an isolated finding.

LUNGS

An infant's respiration is chiefly abdominal. Decreased abdominal respiration is noted in infants with pulmonary disease, ruptured viscus, peritonitis, or distended abdomen. Thoracic breathing or unequal motion of the chest is noted in those with phrenic nerve paralysis, diaphragmatic hernia, or massive atelectasis. Unequal motion of the chest or deep retraction of the sternum, especially if associated with rapid, gasping, or grunting respiration or flaring nares, indicates intrathoracic disease.

Respiratory rate is 40–80 breaths per minute (bpm) at birth. Respiratory movements are irregular in rate and depth in normal infants. Periods of apnea lasting less than 10 seconds may be normal. Weak, irregular, slow, or very rapid rates suggest brain damage. Rates of about 80 bpm suggest pulmonary disease (as described in the section on cyanosis) and transient tachypnea of the infant; rates less than 30 bpm indicate apnea or intracranial injury. Tachypnea without severe dyspnea suggests phrenic nerve paralysis or methemoglobinemia.

Causes of Respiratory Distress in Newborns

Transient tachypnea	Central nervous system
Sepsis	Hypothermia
Pneumonia	Hypoglycemia
Pneumothorax	Congenital heart disease
Diaphragmatic hernia	Tracheoesophageal fistula
Myopathies	Neuropathies
Drug withdrawal	

Grunting rapid respirations may be the only sign of a very sick infant and may be caused by overwhelming infections anywhere in the body; lung, heart, or brain diseases; anemia; and distended abdomen.

Deep-sighing respirations are noted frequently in infants with acidosis. Increased depth of respiration with cyanotic heart disease results from decreased pulmonary blood flow. Deep respirations also occur with pulmonary hypertension. Decreased depth occurs with heart failure, shock, CNS diseases, and sepsis. Cheyne-Stokes respiration or weak, groaning respiration may be a sign of hypoxia or brain damage in the full-term infant. The cough reflex is usually absent in newborns but appears in 1 or 2 days.

During percussion or auscultation of the chest, the infant must lie so that the head and neck are not turned. Increased or decreased areas of dullness or changes in breath sounds may occur simply because of the infant's position.

The chest is resonant shortly after birth. Hyperresonance suggests emphysema but is more often a result of pneumomediastinum, pneumothorax, or diaphragmatic hernia. Decreased resonance indicates improper aeration, usually caused by atelectasis and occasionally by pneumonia, respiratory distress syndrome, or empyema. Atelectasis may represent primary failure of expansion of the lung or may be a result of aspiration of amniotic fluid, food, or other foreign body; thyroid or possibly thymic

TABLE 20.5
Downes Score

Criterion	Score		
	0	1	2
Respiratory rate	<60	61–80	>80 or apneic
Cyanosis	0	In air	In 40% O_2
Retractions	0	Mild	Moderate to severe
Grunt	0	With stethoscope	Without stethoscope
Air entry (crying, axilla)	Clear	Delayed	Barely audible

tumors; other mediastinal masses; diaphragmatic hernia; or chylothorax. Pleural effusion may also be caused by chylothorax or lung disease, including pneumonia.

Auscultation should disclose bronchial breath sounds bilaterally. Air entry should be good, particularly in the midaxillary line. An expiratory grunt suggests difficult air exchange. Rales and rhonchi may be normal for the first 1–4 hours of life due to neonatal atelectasis. Pleuropericardial rubs have no clinical significance. Peristaltic sounds may be heard in the chest with diaphragmatic hernia, although these sounds are frequently transmitted from the abdomen in normal infants. If breath sounds are heard on both sides of the chest and the heart sounds are heard in the usual place, diaphragmatic hernia or pneumothorax is unlikely. Intrinsic lung diseases may cause changes in breath sounds.

A Downes score to estimate degree of respiratory distress in infants with no pneumothorax, pneumomediastinum, or aspiration can be obtained (Table 20.5). Such a score is useful in indicating oxygen requirements of the baby. A score of 0–3 represents mild distress, 4–6 represents moderate distress, and 7–10 represents severe distress.

Transilluminate with a bright cool light above and below the infant's nipple on each side. Increased transillumination around the sternum indicates pneumomediastinum; illumination elsewhere indicates pneumothorax.

HEART

Percuss to obtain heart size or palpate the apical impulse. The apex will usually be found lateral to the midclavicular line and in the third or fourth interspace because of the more horizontal position of the infant's heart. Beware of dextrocardia. A large heart at birth is rare in infants with valvular heart disease, but is seen in children born of diabetic mothers and those with erythroblastosis fetalis, Pompe disease, or rhabdomyoma of the heart. A few days after birth, however, cardiac enlargement may be caused by heart failure secondary to heart anomalies.

Causes of Heart Failure in Newborns

Coarctation of aorta	Septal defects
Patent ductus	Truncus arteriosus
Transposition	Aortic stenosis

Anomalous venous return	Tricuspid atresia
Anomalous coronary arteries	Pulmonary atresia
Endocardial fibroelastosis	Paroxysmal tachycardia
Hypertension	Myocarditis

Enlarged heart with other signs of heart failure may also be a result of peripheral arteriovenous connections, such as cerebral arteriovenous aneurysms. Pulmonary arteriovenous fistulas do not usually cause heart enlargement because pressure on the heart is low. Infants with hypoplastic left or right heart, pulmonary atresia or stenosis, and tricuspid anomalies may also have hearts of normal size.

The heart rate at birth varies from 100 to 180 beats/min and stabilizes shortly after birth at 120–140 beats/min. The rhythm is usually regular. Varying rhythm is associated with anoxia, cerebral defects, increased intracranial pressure, and heart block.

Sinus arrhythmia is present in all full-term and most preterm infants. Absence of arrhythmia is found in infants with respiratory distress syndrome. Tachycardia of more than 170 beats/min after 1 hour may be because of infection, dehydration, anemia, atrial flutter, congestive heart failure, or hyperthyroidism. Bradycardia may be a result of anoxia, CNS disease, long QT, electrolyte abnormalities, medications, or heart block, as in neonatal lupus syndrome.

Listen with either the bell or the diaphragm. The first and second sounds are almost equal. Splitting of the first sound may be caused by an ejection click from aortic or pulmonic stenosis. Wide splitting of the second sound occurs with atrial septal defect and total anomalous venous return.

Murmurs are noted for loudness, quality, location, and timing, but their significance varies at this age. Murmurs, if present, are usually heard at the left sternal border in the third or fourth interspace or over the base of the heart—almost never at the apex. For the first hour until 15 hours of life, a late systolic or continuous murmur in the pulmonary area presumably originates from a physiologically patent ductus arteriosus. Another innocent murmur is a short, early systolic ejection murmur with or without an early systolic click at the lower left sternal border or pulmonary area, which is loudest at 3 months of age. A third innocent murmur is a short systolic ejection murmur in the axilla and over the back. A soft systolic murmur associated with an ejection click in the pulmonary area may be caused by pulmonary disease. Loud murmurs on the first day of life suggest semilunar valve stenosis or atrioventricular valve incompetence. Loud systolic murmurs appearing between day 3 and day 7 of life suggest ventricular septal defect.

Heart sounds are poorly heard in infants with pneumothorax or pneumomediastinum, cardiac failure, or CNS injury. A single second heart sound may indicate pulmonary atresia or hypoplastic left heart. Clicking or crackling sounds synchronous with the heartbeat suggest mediastinal emphysema.

ABDOMEN

The abdomen is usually prominent in infants. The veins over the abdomen normally are prominent but are distended in infants with peritonitis and pylephlebitis.

Causes of Abdominal Distention

Sepsis	Ascites
Low intestinal obstruction	Genitourinary obstruction
Ileal or colon atresia	Peritonitis
Imperforate anus	Ileus
Meconium plug	Meconium ileus
Tracheoesophageal fistula	Tumors
Omphalocele	Large abdominal organs
Pneumoperitoneum	Hirschsprung disease
Gastroschisis	

Visible peristaltic waves indicate intestinal obstruction but may be evident in thin, otherwise normal infants. Peristalsis is normally heard shortly after birth. A silent tympanitic distended tender abdomen suggests peritonitis or necrotizing enterocolitis.

Scaphoid abdomen in infants suggests diaphragmatic hernia or high atresia of the intestinal tract.

Ascites

Ascites may result from any of the causes of edema and the following:

Ruptured viscus	Chyle
Peritonitis	Hepatitis
Necrotizing enterocolitis	Cirrhosis
Portal vein obstruction	Urethral obstruction
Genitourinary anomalies	

The liver is normally palpated 2–3 cm below the right costal margin. The spleen tip is usually palpable at about 1 week of age. Enlarged liver and spleen are usually palpated or percussed in infants with erythroblastosis fetalis, heart failure, sepsis, trauma to liver or spleen, neuroblastoma, or congenital syphilis. An enlarged liver and an enlarged spleen are also evident in infants born of diabetic mothers and sometimes in those with congenital hemolytic icterus. A liver extending far below the costal margin in the midline, yet not palpable laterally, may result from partial herniation of the left lobe of the liver into the infant's chest with left-sided diaphragmatic hernia.

Left-sided liver is usually associated with situs inversus. Other malrotations are usually not detected by physical examination. The lower half of the right and the tip of the left kidney are normally palpated. You cannot diagnose agenesis of the kidney, however, just because you cannot feel the kidney. If the infant is crying, palpating for the kidneys may be facilitated by supporting the infant at a 45° angle with one hand at the occiput and neck. Palpate the abdomen with the free hand, and simultaneously flex the neck with the other hand. Abdominal muscles will relax, and the infant usually will stop crying. Flexing the knees to the abdomen sometimes also causes enough relaxation. Both kidneys are palpable and are up to 3–5 cm long.

Most flank and intraabdominal masses are of renal origin. Enlarged kidneys may be noted in neuroblastoma, Wilms tumor, polycystic kidneys, or congenital hydronephrosis. A single enlarged kidney may indicate renal vein thrombosis. The abnormal kidney mass most frequently palpated in the abdomen results from multicystic renal dysplasia, a common form of cystic disease of the neonatal kidney.

The bladder is normally percussed or palpated 1–4 cm above the symphysis. Ironically, a greatly distended bladder in the infant is palpated with difficulty because of its very thin wall; percuss or it will be overlooked. Distended bladder may result from congenital bladderneck or urethral obstruction.

Any other masses palpable in the abdomen must be identified. Tumors, meconium ileus, loculated hemorrhage, mesenteric cysts, or other abnormal masses may be found.

Inspect the umbilical cord. If the amnion covers the umbilical stump, the condition is termed *amniotic navel*; if the stump is covered by skin, the condition is termed *cutis navel*. Neither has any clinical significance except that the former may be associated with delayed healing and the latter may be mistaken for umbilical hernia. A velamentous cord with insertion near the edge is rare but may signify other anomalies. The umbilical cord normally has two arteries and one vein; examine for this because a single artery may be accompanied by other anomalies such as renal abnormalities or chromosome trisomies. The artery is thick walled; the vein is thin walled.

The cord should be dry and not bleeding. If it is bleeding, the cord must be retied. Redness around the cord after 24 hours (especially when cephalad), wetness of the stump, or a fetid odor after 3 days usually signifies the presence of omphalitis. A cord that fails to fall off after 2 weeks or a navel that persists in draining after 3 weeks may indicate the presence of a urachal cyst or sinus. Similarly, a child born with a very large and flabby umbilical cord may have a patent urachus. Fecal discharge occurs with a persistent ompha lomesenteric duct; this usually indicates Meckel diverticulum. Patent omphalomesenteric duct may result in ileal prolapse, a surgical emergency.

Soft granulation tissue is commonly noted after cord separation. This local condition must be distinguished from the firmer umbilical polyp, which is dark red, has a mucoid discharge, and is related to Meckel diverticulum. Other cysts and tumors of the umbilicus occur rarely.

Ventral hernias, with or without diastasis recti, are frequently present at birth and are usually insignificant. Occasionally a child is born with a hernia that pinches off the small bowel. Very large hernias (omphalocele) may be incompatible with life. Omphaloceles are midline, covered by a sac. Gastroschisis is a paramedian defect, usually on the right with no sac. An umbilicus that shifts with respiration (belly-dancer sign) signals phrenic nerve paralysis.

GENITALIA

Inspect the genitalia. Edema is common, especially in infants born by breech delivery. Pigmentation is usually increased around the genitalia in dark-skinned races but may be a sign of adrenal hyperplasia. Note femoral pulses, hydrocele, and hernia. The clitoris is always large. Carefully inspect the labia. An unusually large clitoris and partial or total labial fusion are found in pseudohermaphroditism, usually caused by adrenal hyperplasia. What appears to be a large clitoris may be a small penis. Identify the urethral opening. In female infants the urethral opening is just behind the clitoris.

If the urethral opening is on the ventral surface of the penis, hypospadias exists; if the opening is on the dorsal surface, epispadias exists. Micropenis (a penis less than 2 cm long) may be a sign of other organ anomalies. Micropenis needs to be distinguished from a concealed (buried) phallus, a usually normal and self-limited condition. In male infants, the urethral orifice may ulcerate, especially after circumcision.

The prepuce is usually tight in infant males; phimosis does not exist unless the prepuce cannot be pulled back just far enough to allow flow of an adequate urinary stream. Do not retract the prepuce more than is adequate for examination. Small bands and adhesions of the prepuce usually break during the examination. Erection and even priapism may be noted in male infants but usually have no clinical significance.

Palpate the testes, whether they are in the canal or scrotum. The scrotum may appear large or bruised, especially after breech delivery. Dark hematoma in the scrotum may indicate rupture of the liver. A deep cleft in the scrotum results in a bifid scrotum, frequently associated with other genitourinary anomalies. A unilateral, dark, swollen, nontender testis may be a sign of testicular infarction.

The vulva is hyperemic. The labia, especially the labia minora, are usually large in female infants. The normal labia may be confused with a bifid scrotum. Palpate the labia majora for a small body, which may be a gonad. Adhesions of the labia minora may occur shortly after birth. Because of maternal hormones, vaginal mucoid or bloody discharge may occur normally in female infants any time in the first week and may persist as long as 1 month.

Again, use a catheter. Visualize the opening of the hymen. Passing the catheter through the hymenal opening tests for imperforate hymen and vaginal atresia. Polyps or carbuncles of the hymen may be present. These regress spontaneously. The normal uterus may be felt; it is about 2 cm long. Palpate for femoral pulses; absence suggests coarctation of the aorta. Fecal urethral discharges may be present. They indicate rectourethral, rectovaginal, or rectovesical fistulas.

SPINE

Now place the infant in the prone position. Run your hand lightly over the spine. Spina bifida, pilonidal sinus, scoliosis, and the anal dimple are sought. If the anus does not appear to be patent, insert the previously used catheter. If the abdomen is distended, perform the rectal examination immediately. Anorectal anomalies, including displacement of the anus, may be associated with sacrococcygeal teratoma. Prominence of one buttock with asymmetric gluteal folds and an abdominal mass indicates an internal sacrococcygeal teratoma.

MECONIUM AND URINE

Although it usually is not considered part of the physical examination, note the passage of meconium and urine. The infant usually voids immediately at or soon after birth. Failure to pass urine by 24 hours of age is highly suggestive of urinary tract obstruction or other urinary tract anomaly and requires further investigation.

Meconium is usually passed during the first 3 days of life. Passage of meconium before birth is diagnostic of fetal intrauterine distress. Failure to pass meconium by the end of day 2 of life suggests an intestinal tract obstruction, including stenosis or atresia anywhere throughout the length of the intestinal tract, meconium ileus, megacolon, or small left colon syndrome in infants of diabetic mothers.

Passage of small amounts of meconium or passage over a long time suggests a high intestinal or partial intestinal obstruction. Presence of bright red blood in the meconium usually results from ingestion of the mother's blood by the infant, but it may result from hemorrhage somewhere in the intestinal tract—for example, necrotizing enterocolitis with or without perforation, which constitutes an emergency and which distinction must be determined by suitable laboratory tests.

EXTREMITIES

Place the infant in the supine position. Gently fold the infant into its intrauterine position, encouraging relaxation and maybe even sleep. This position also provides a clue to the range of motion normal to that infant. For example, an infant whose hips and knees are drawn to one side in utero will have a greater range of motion of the abducted hip than of the adducted hip. Count the fingers. Note polydactyly and syndactyly. Feel for fractures, paralyses, and dislocations of the clavicles and upper extremities. Examine the hips for dysplasia by rotating the thighs with the knees flexed. Soft clicks are common when hips are moved, as described in Chapter 8, and must be distinguished from the sharp click of dislocation. Clicks at the knees are also common.

Multiple fractures with deformity may be a result of osteogenesis imperfecta. Paralysis of the arm may be a result of brachial palsy or fractured humerus. Paralysis of both legs is usually caused by severe trauma or congenital anomaly of the spinal cord. The hands are normally held clenched. The thumb is in the hand like a fist but moves out intermittently. Permanent fisting signifies a cortical thumb resulting from cortical or spinal tract injury.

Test the grasp reflex. On pulling the infant upright, the head is normally partially supported. Elbows, hips, and knees generally lack full extension. Response to pain and touch are noted but ordinarily not recorded. Note the tone of the muscle groups. Test passive tonus by moving all the major joints. Paralysis, missed during examination of tone, may be detected. Look for septic arthritis or osteomyelitis in any septic neonate. Examine other nerve and muscle injuries as described for older children.

Palpate the radial pulses. Increased right as compared with left radial pulse occurs with supravalvular aortic stenosis or juxtaductal coarctation. Alternate strong and weak pulses (pulsus alternans) are a sign of left ventricular failure. Paradoxical pulse (pulsus paradoxus), in which the pulse changes markedly with respiration, occurs with cardiac tamponade or constrictive pericarditis.

Edema of the extremities may be caused by gonadal agenesis or heart failure and liver diseases and other causes of hydrops such as blood incompatibility, chorioangioma of the placenta, umbilical or chorionic vein thrombosis, fetal neuroblastoma, cystic adenomatoid malformation of the lung, pulmonary lymph angiectasia, maternal parvovirus infections, Chaga disease, fetal Gaucher disease, and local vascular abnormalities.

MEASUREMENTS

Measure and record the head, chest, and abdominal circumferences and the length of the infant. At birth, the head should be at least 0.5 cm larger than the chest or abdomen. If there is any question about developing hydrocephalus, repeat measurements at daily intervals.

With the infant in the prone position, take the temperature by rectum or in the axilla, groin, or other areas if indicated. Temperatures of 33–34°C (92–94°F) are common in an infant and rise when the infant is warmed. Low temperatures are also noted after severe birth trauma and severe infection. Aural temperatures are higher than rectal or esophageal temperatures due to brain metabolism. Lower aural temperatures suggest hydranencephaly.

Elevated temperatures are common in an infant who is dehydrated, when brain damage or sepsis occurs, and when the environmental temperature is excessively high. If the temperature elevation at the feet and abdomen is almost the same, the fever is usually caused by the environment; if the temperature of the feet is low and that of the abdomen is high, sepsis is more likely.

NEUROLOGIC STATUS

Finally, the infant's crib is slapped or dropped a few inches and the Moro reflex (Chapter 18) is carefully observed. This response, or the lack of it, is valuable in determining CNS status, fractures of the arms and legs, brachial plexus injury, hip or shoulder dysplasia, and recent fracture of the clavicle. An infant with a fractured clavicle may move the arm freely after 24 hours. In infants with Erb palsy the arm hangs limply, with internal rotation at the shoulder and pronation of the lower segment, and does not move as a result of paralysis after brachial plexus injury. In pseudo-Erb palsy, decreased passive as well as active motion indicates an injury to the proximal humeral epiphysis. Moro reflex is absent at birth and improves in infants with cerebral edema. Moro reflex may be present at birth and disappear in infants with cerebral hemorrhage.

Alternatively, Perez sign, another mass reflex, may be obtained. With the baby prone on a hard surface, exert thumb pressure over the spine from the pelvis to the neck. A strong cry will be noted in normal infants, together with flexion of the lower and upper extremities, lordosis of spine, elevation of the pelvis and head, and urination and defecation. Its significance is similar to that of the Moro reflex.

PLACENTA

Before leaving the delivery room, inspect and weigh the placenta. Amnion nodosum or vernix granuloma may reflect insufficiency of amniotic fluid, as in Potter syndrome.

Polyhydramnios (excess amniotic fluid) occurs in infants of diabetic, preeclamptic, or anemic mothers; in multiple pregnancies; and in infants with anencephaly, gastrointestinal obstruction, erythroblastosis, tracheoesophageal fistula, and anomalies of the great vessels. Oligohydramnios occurs with agenesis of or polycystic kidneys.

Note number of umbilical arteries, cord length, hematomas and thromboses, cord torsion, and inflammation.

Umbilicus: Delayed Separation

Umbilical cord separation usually occurs between 7 and 14 days of life. Delayed cord separation occurs after 4 weeks of life. It can be caused by the following:

- Vigorous use of antiseptics to clean the umbilical cord
  Probably the most common etiology
  Inhibits normal colonization of the umbilicus, which otherwise would allow chemotactic infiltration of neutrophils to mediate cord separation
- Immunodeficiencies
  Leukocyte adhesion defects affecting chemotaxis (LAD I/II)
  LAD is usually associated with significant systemic (sepsis) or local (omphalitis) infection, recurrent infections, or failure to thrive
  Sialyl Lewis is X antigen deficiency
  Neonatal alloimmune neutropenia
  Defective immune (gamma) interferon
- Prematurity
  Gestational age less than 37 weeks
- Birth via cesarean section
  Associated with delayed separation, possibly due to decreased bacterial colonization from delivery through a sterile surgical field, resulting in decreased infiltration of neutrophils, which is essential for cord separation
- Neonatal sepsis
- Urachal anomalies
  More likely to be seen in otherwise healthy infants without signs of local or systemic infection
- Histiocytosis X

EXAMINATION OF LOW BIRTH WEIGHT NEWBORNS

A baby is God's opinion that the world should go on.

Carl Sandburg

A low birth weight (LBW) infant is one who weighs less than 5.5 pounds (2,500 g) at birth. Infants with LBW may be premature (less than 37 weeks gestational age), with size appropriate for gestational age (AGA), small for gestational age (SGA), or postmature with weight loss from placental insufficiency.

When examining an LBW infant, follow the same principles used in examining a full-term infant. The examination must be even more rapid and less complete and, above all, must be performed gently and tenderly in a warm protected area.

Measurements of the head, chest, abdomen, length, and weight; observation for gross abnormalities; and rapid estimation of air exchange, heart rate, and skin texture usually suffice for the initial examination. Accurate measurements assist in properly estimating gestational age. If a temperature measurement is desired, it should be taken in the axilla; temperatures of premature infants approximate that of the environment. Examination to determine the presence of Moro reflex may be deferred until the infant is more than 1 day old and then performed only by rapping the crib side. Transillumination of the head, if performed, will show large areas of light transmission.

Calculate the ponderal index: weight (g) × 100/length (cm^3). A ponderal index less than 2.3 g/cm^3 is a small index; 2.3–2.7 g/cm^3 is normal. A small ponderal index is associated with increased neonatal and sometimes persistent complications.

Normal respiration in a premature infant is irregular and of Cheyne-Stokes type. The average rate varies from 40 to 80 bpm. A slow rate, rarely a rapid rate, or a regular respiratory rate usually indicates CNS depression. A rapid rate is more frequently a prime indication of respiratory distress syndrome; infection (usually generalized), including omphalitis, meningitis, septicemia, and pneumonia; or atelectasis.

Because the bony thorax is soft, each inspiration is marked by indrawing of the sternum. This collapse of the sternum normally lessens in the first 24 hours and disappears no later than day 4 or 5 of life. Persistence of the indrawing suggests the presence of persistent atelectasis. Marked atelectasis is usually present at birth but diminishes with each breath. Frequently, an infant does well for a few minutes or a few hours and then shows signs of respiratory distress, including marked collapse of the chest wall, rapid respiratory rates, grunting, and cyanosis. Respiratory distress syndrome, foreign material aspiration with secondary atelectasis, pneumothorax, infection (especially with group B streptococci), severe primary atelectasis, pneumomediastinum, and localized emphysema or reopening of the ductus arteriosus with subsequent pulmonary edema should be suspected. Respiratory distress with tachypnea that seems severe but clears in 1–2 days is benign transient tachypnea of the infant. The cough reflex is usually absent in premature infants.

Respiratory distress syndrome occurs in 60% of infants of < 30 weeks' gestation who have not received steroids and decreases to 35% of those who have received antenatal steroid treatment. Between 30 and 40 weeks' gestation, that rate is 25% in untreated infants and 10% in those who have received steroid treatment.

High Risk Factors for Respiratory Distress Syndrome

Pulmonary Immaturity

L/S ratio < 2 and PG negative = immature
L/S ratio > 2 and PG negative = transitional
L/S ratio > 2 and PG positive = mature

High Risk Factors

Prematurity: incidence inversely related to gestational age
<28 weeks: 60%–70%
32–36 weeks: 15%–20%
>37 weeks: 5%
Term: rare

Maternal Factors

Diabetes mellitus
Multiple pregnancy
Previous history
Poor prenatal care

Perinatal Factors

Precipitous delivery with antenatal hemorrhage
Cesarean section without labor
Hypoxia/asphyxia, acidosis, cold stress

Neonatal Factors

Erythroblastosis fetalis
Second of twins

Surfactant Production

Synthesized by type II pneumocytes in lung
Production detected at 23–24 weeks gestation
Adequate production after 30–32 weeks gestation

Respiratory Distress Syndrome

Clinical Presentation

- Onset prior to 6 hours, usually about 2 hours after birth
- Respiratory distress: tachypnea, retractions, nasal flaring, expiratory grunting
- Cyanosis on room air
- Diminished air entry on auscultation
- Decreased muscle tone, activity
- Hypotension
- Edema (after several hours: altered capillary permeability)

Radiologic signs include reticulogranular, "ground glass" appearance, decreased lung volume, air bronchograms (airless parenchyma contrasts with air-filled bronchi). The infant is hypoxic, hypercarbic, and acidotic. Pathology is hyaline membrane disease.

Prevention

- Maternal glucocorticoids accelerate lung maturity in preterm fetuses.

- Complications include oxygen toxicity, infection (central venous catheter, endotracheal tube), heart failure (left-to-right shunt through patent ductus antevirus (PDA) when pulmonary resistance falls), and intraventricular hemorrhage.
- Sequelae are bronchopulmonary dysplasia, vocal cord damage, subglottic stenosis, retinopathy of prematurity, malnutrition (volume restriction, drug-nutrient interactions), increase of middle ear infections, and reactive lung disease.

Risk increases in infants of mothers with diabetes, those delivered by cesarean section without antecedent labor, those undergoing perinatal asphyxia, second twins, and those born to mothers with a previous infant with respiratory distress syndrome.

Cyanosis in a premature infant usually disappears within a few minutes of birth. Persistent cyanosis is similar in significance to that in a full-term infant.

Note the texture of the skin. The skin of premature infants is thin and extremely tender; it is subject to easy bruising, bleeding, and infection and is more subject to injury by temperature changes (which result in hardening, or sclerema) than the skin of full-term infants.

Certain physical signs are characteristic of normal premature AGA infants: a typically round head larger than the chest, absent or small breast buds, decreased scrotal pigmentation, decreased heel creases, foot length, prominent eyes, absence of eyebrows and lashes, absence of sweat, purple mottling of the skin (cutis marmorata), extensive hair (lanugo) over much of the body, and soft nails. The neck and extremities are short; the head, hands, and feet are prominent; labia minora are prominent; and the abdomen appears full. Peristalsis is normally visible through the thin abdominal wall and is usually not an indication of obstruction. Bloody vomitus in a premature infant may be caused by intracranial hemorrhage, peptic ulcer, necrotizing enterocolitis, or swallowed blood. Meconium may pass during the first 2 weeks of life.

Although premature infants may remain edematous for 4–5 days, they usually remain dehydrated longer than full-term infants. As soon as the edema fluid is absorbed, the skin of the premature infant becomes and remains wrinkled. Jaundice appears and disappears slowly. Many premature infants have umbilical hernias, and the incidence of other hernias, especially inguinal, is higher in premature than in full-term infants. Many premature infants have capillary hemangiomas.

The normal premature infant may seem almost motionless for the first 3 or 4 days after birth. Decreased tone, especially in an SGA infant, suggests hypoglycemia. The child then begins to cry and to make vigorous movements for a few minutes at a time. Early movements usually correspond to the time of disappearance of edema and probably to the onset of hunger. The cry is usually high-pitched in normal premature infants.

The degree of prematurity of an infant can sometimes be estimated by measurements of length, weight, and head circumference (Figure 20.1) and by their comparison with those of a full-term infant. Attempt to estimate gestational age as accurately as possible. Infants of LBW may be of decreased gestational age, or the LBW may be caused by various maternal, placental, or fetal factors. The prognoses of these two groups differ. A scoring system has been helpful in making more precise determination of gestational age (Figure 20.2). Because the incidence of severe congenital

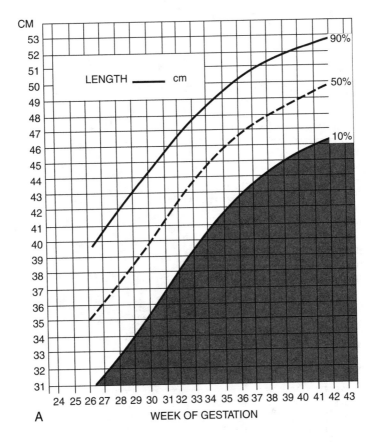

Figure 20.1
Classification of newborns, based on maturity and intrauterine growth. (From Lubchenco, L. C., Hansman, C., & Boyd, E., 1966. *Journal of Pediatrics, 37*, 403; Battaglia, F. C., & Lubchenco, L. C., 1967. *Journal of Pediatrics, 71*, 159.)
Continued

anomalies is higher in premature than in full-term infants, such anomalies must also be sought (Table 20.6).

Drugs used as maternal analgestics, sedatives, or general anesthetics during labor cross the placenta and can depress the fetal respiratory center. Respiratory depression from drugs is likely to be especially important in premature infants or those with asphyxia superimposed from other causes.

METABOLIC DISORDERS IN THE NEWBORN

Hypoglycemia: Causes

Decreased Glucose Production

Sepsis
Antenatal nutritional deficiency

Figure 20.1 cont'd

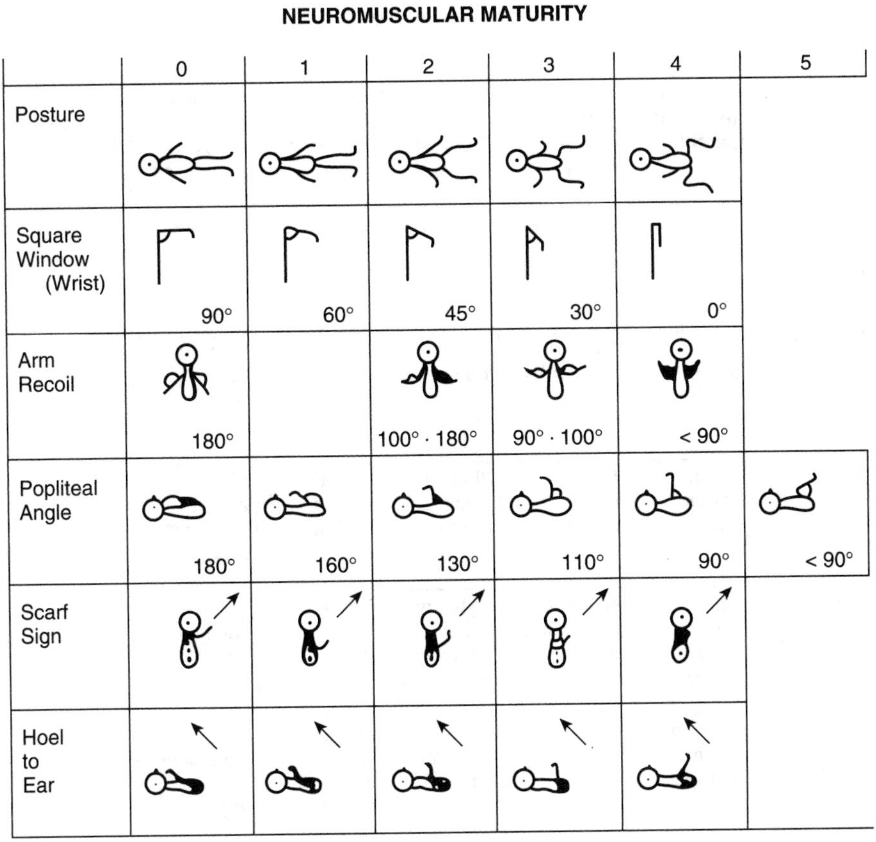

NEUROMUSCULAR MATURITY

	0	1	2	3	4	5
Posture						
Square Window (Wrist)	90°	60°	45°	30°	0°	
Arm Recoil	180°		100° · 180°	90° · 100°	< 90°	
Popliteal Angle	180°	160°	130°	110°	90°	< 90°
Scarf Sign						
Hoel to Ear						

A

Figure 20.2

Add neuromuscular and physical to obtain maturity rating. Newborn maturity rating and classification. (Scoring system from Ballard, J. L., Khoury, J. C., Wedig, K., Wang, L., Eilers-Waisman, B. L., & Lipp, R., 1991. A simplified assessment of gestational age. *Journal of Pediatrics, 119,* 417–423. Figures adapted from Sweet, A. Y., 1977. Classification of the low-birth-weight infant. In M. H. Klaus & A. A. Fanaroff, Eds., *Care of the high-risk infant.* Philadelphia: W.B. Saunders.) Posture: observed with infant quiet and in supine position. Score 0, arms and legs extended; score 1, beginning of flexion of hips and knees, arms extended; score 2, stronger flexion of legs, arms extended; score 3, arms slightly flexed, legs flexed and abducted; score 4, full flexion of arms and legs. Square Window: The hand is flexed on the forearm between the thumb and index finger of the examiner. Enough pressure is applied to obtain the fullest flexion possible, and the angle between the hypothenar eminence and the ventral aspect of the forearm is measured and graded according to diagram. (Care is taken not to rotate the infant's wrist while performing this maneuver.) Ankle Dorsiflexion: The foot is dorsiflexed onto the anterior aspect of the leg, with the examiner's thumb on the sole of the foot and other fingers behind the leg. Enough pressure is applied to obtain the fullest flexion possible, and the angle between the dorsum of the foot and the anterior aspect of the leg is measured. Arm Recoil: With the infant in the supine position, the forearms are first flexed for 5 seconds, then fully extended by pulling on the hands, and then released.

Continued

PHYSICAL MATURITY

	0	1	2	3	4	5
SKIN	gelatinous red, trans-parent	smooth pink, visible veins	superficial peeling &/or rash, few veins	cracking pale area, rare veins	parchment, deep cracking, no vessels	leathery, cracked, wrinkled
LANUGO	none	abundant	thinning	bald areas	mostly bald	
PLANTAR CREASES	no crease	faint red marks	anterior transverse crease only	creases ant 2/3	creases cover entire sole	
BREAST	barely percept	flat areola no bud	stippled areola, 1–2 mm bud	raised areola, 3–4 mm bud	full areola, 5–10 mm bud	
EAR	pinna flat, stays folded	sl. curved pinna, soft with slow recoil	well-curv. pinna, soft but ready recoil	formed & firm with instant recoil	thick cartilage, ear stiff	
GENITALS Male	scrotum empty, no rugae		testes descend-ing, few rugae	testes down, good rugae	testes pendulous, deep rugae	
GENITALS Female	prominent clitoris & labia minora		majora & minora equally prominent	majora large, minora small	clitoris & minora completely covered	

B

Figure 20.2 cont'd

The sign is fully positive if the arms return briskly to full flexion (score 2). If the arms return to incomplete flexion or the response is sluggish, the score is 1. If they remain extended or if only random movements follow, the score is 0. Leg Recoil: With the infant supine, the hips and knees are fully flexed for 5 seconds, then extended by traction on the feet, and released. A maximal response is one of full flexion of the hips and knees (score 2). A partial flexion scores 1, and minimal or no movement scores 0. Popliteal Angle: With the infant supine and the pelvis flat on the examining couch, the thigh is held in the knee-chest position by the examiner's left index finger and thumb supporting the knee. The leg is then extended by gentle pressure from the examiner's right index finger behind the ankle, and the popliteal angle is measured. Heel-to-Ear Maneuver: With the baby supine, draw the baby's foot as near to the head as it will go without forcing it. Observe the distance between the foot and the head as well as the degree of extension at the knee. Grade according to the diagram. Note that the knee is left free and may draw down alongside the abdomen.

Continued

Gestation by Dates _____ wks

Birth Date _____ Hour _____ am / pm

APGAR _____ 1 min _____ 5 min

MATURITY RATING

Score	Wks
5	26
10	28
15	30
20	32
25	34
30	36
35	38
40	40
45	42
50	44

C

Figure 20.2 cont'd
Scarf Sign: With the baby supine, take the infant's hand and try to place it around the neck and as far posteriorly as possible around the opposite shoulder. Assist this maneuver by lifting the elbow across the body. See how far the elbow will go across and grade according to the illustrations. Score 0, elbow reaches opposite axillary line; score 1, elbow between midline and opposite axillary line; score 2, elbow reaches midline; score 3, elbow will not reach midline. Head Lag: With the infant lying supine, grasp the hands (or the arms if the infant is very small) and pull the infant slowly toward the sitting position. Observe the position of the head in relation to the trunk and grade accordingly. In a small infant, the head may initially be supported by one hand. Score 0, complete lag; score 1, partial head control; score 2, able to maintain head in line with body; score 3, brings head anterior to body. Ventral Suspension: The infant is suspended in the prone position with the examiner's hand under the infant's chest (one hand for a small infant, two hands for a large infant). Observe the degree of extension of the back and the amount of flexion of the arms and legs. Also note the relation of the head to the trunk. Grade according to the diagrams. If score differs on the two sides, take the mean.

Preterm birth
Small for gestational age
Hypothermia
Birth asphyxia
Starvation
Congenital heart disease

Hyperinsulinism

Insulinoma

TABLE 20.6

Complications of Prematurity

Conditions	Causes	Management
Anemia	Venipunctures Bone marrow refractory Increasing blood volume with growth Iron deficiency (as from 36–40 weeks most of the fetal iron stores are created) Vitamin E deficiency	Investigate causes
Bronchopulmonary dysplasia	Complicates respiratory distress syndrome in extreme preterm Prolonged requirement for oxygen	Monitor Po_2 Nutritional support Close monitoring of bacteriologic and cardiac status
Hypernatremia	Common in first 2–3 d in extremely preterm Dehydration	Adequate fluid intake
Hyponatremia	Renal tubular immaturity	Monitor sodium loss Adequate replacement (up to 10 mmol/kg/24 hr)
Hypocalcemia	Immature regulation Low plasma albumin	None if asymptomatic Replace in intravenous fluids ifv required
Hypothermia	Large surface area Immature skin Immature regulation	Clothing Warm environment ± added humidity
Infections (any)	Low immunoglobulins Ineffective localization of septic foci	High index of suspicion Early parenteral antibiotics
Intraventricular hemorrhage	Immaturity Cerebrovascular instability Postasphyxia	None possible Rarely progresses to give hydrocephalus Avoid wide swings in venous pressure
Irregular respiration	Immature respiratory center	Monitor respiration and seek pathologic causes
Apnea	Infection Intracranial hemorrhage	Caffeine, theophylline therapy
Jaundice	Delayed food intake Bruising Hepatic immaturity	Phototherapy Exchange transfusion Dependent on etiology
Metabolic acidosis (mild)	Renal immaturity in presence of protein load (milk or total parenteral nutrition)	Reduce protein intake if deteriorating
Necrotizing enterocolitis	Infarction of gut secondary to inadequate perfusion	Supportive medical or surgical resection Generally make NPO
Osteopenia of prematurity	Progressive demineralization of bones if mineral absorption inadequate	Mineral supplements to diet
Periventricular leukomalacia	Infarction of large areas of cerebral white matter after ischemic insult	None possible

TABLE 20.6
Complications of Prematurity (Continued)

Conditions	Causes	Management
Persistent patent ductus arteriosus	Immaturity Hypoxia Acidosis	Ligation or indomethacin Diuretics for heart failure
Respiratory distress syndrome	Surfactant deficiency	Monitor blood gases Increase inspired Po_2 Continuous positive airway pressure or intermittent positive pressure ventilation Intravenous fluids/feeding Exogenous surfactant
Unable to suck reliably (at ≤3 years)	Immature suck/swallow coordination	Nasogastric tube feeding if well

NPO, nothing by mouth.
From Gilbert-Barness, E., & Barness, L. A. (2003). *Clinical use of pediatric diagnostic tests.* Philadelphia: Lippincott Williams & Wilkins.

Maternal diabetes
Beckwith-Wiedemann syndrome
Nesidioblastosis
Maternal drug therapy or glucose starvation
Erythroblastosis

Inborn Errors of Metabolism

Disorders of glyconeogenesis (e.g., pyruvate carboxylase deficiency)
Amino acid disorders (e.g., tyrosinemia type I)
Carnitine deficiency disorders (e.g., carnitine palmitoyltransferase deficiency)
Glycogen storage disorders, especially type 1 (Table 20.7)
Organic acid disorders (e.g., methylmalonic acidemia)
Disorders of fat oxidation (e.g., medium-chain acyl coenzyme A dehydrogenase deficiency)
Galactosemia

Hormone Deficiencies

Congenital hypopituitarism
Congenital adrenal hyperplasia
Adrenal hypoplasia or insufficiency
Congenital glucagon deficiency

Other Causes

Exchange transfusion

TABLE 20.7
Diagnostic Tests for Neonatal Hypoglycemia

Further Investigations		Diagnoses
Metabolic acidosis	Plasma lactate	Glycogen storage disease types 1, 3
	Plasma 3-hydroxybutyrate	Congenital lactic acidosis
	Urine organic acids	Fatty acid oxidation defects
	Plasma free fatty acids	Disorders of gluconeogenesis
Liver dysfunction	Plasma and urine amino acids	Tyrosinemia type I
	Galactose-1-phosphate uridyltransferase	Galactosemia
		Hereditary fructose intolerance
	Urine sugars	Fatty acid oxidation effects
	Urine organic acids	
Absence of acidosis and liver dysfunction	Plasma cortisol	Adrenal insufficiency
	Plasma 17-hydroxyprogesterone	Congenital adrenal hyperplasia
	Plasma insulin (when hypoglycemic)	Nesidioblastosis
	Plasma growth hormone and thyroid-stimulating hormone	Hypopituitarism
Hyponatremia	Plasma 17-hydroxyprogesterone	Congenital adrenal hyperplasia
	Plasma growth hormone and thyroid-stimulating hormone	Hypopituitarism
	Plasma cortisol	Adrenal insufficiency
	Plasma growth hormone and thyroid-stimulating hormone	Hypopituitarism

From Gilbert-Barness, E., & Barness, L. A. (2003). *Clinical use of pediatric diagnostic tests.* Baltimore: Lippincott, Williams & Wilkins, p. 81.

Hypocalcemia: Causes

Physiologic factors
Maternal diabetes mellitus
Vitamin D deficiency
Prematurity
Birth asphyxia
Pathologic conditions (Tables 20.8–20.10)
Pseudohyperparathyroidism
Hypoparathyroidism
Maternal hypoparathyroidism
Renal disease
Liver disease
Hypomagnesemia
Iatrogenic causes
Low calcium intake
Organic acid disorders
Parenteral nutrition
High phosphate intake
Exchange transfusion
Use of anticonvulsants
Use of diuretics

TABLE 20.8
Hyponatremia

Condition	Cause/Presentation	Management
Maternal influence	Reflects maternal electrolyte levels (seen especially if large volumes of dextrose given IV during labor)	Usually recovers with treatment
Iatrogenic causes	Prolonged administration of IV dextrose without electrolyte additives	Restrict fluids Give Na$^+$
Birth injury	Inappropriate antidiuretic hormone secretion	Restrict fluids
Meningitis	Poor urine output Weight gain Plasma osmolality < 270 mmol/kg Urine osmolality increased	Usually recovers with treatment Limit daily IVF to ≤ 70% maintenance if not volume depleted
Diuretic administration (especially loop diuretics)	Drug slowly eliminated in neonates (average losses after 1 mg/kg furosemide are 28 ml/kg water, 3.6 mmol/kg Na$^+$, 0.3 mmol/kg K$^+$) Loss of electrolyte in excess of water	Use amiloride hydrochloride Replace Na$^+$
Acute tubular necrosis, renal failure	Increased renal fractional sodium excretion secondary to tubular damage and hyporesponsiveness to aldosterone	Measure sodium losses and replace by oral or intravenous supplements
Salt-losing congenital adrenal hyperplasia	Mineralocorticoid deficiency Females: virilization (variable) Males: normal, or pigmented scrotum Acute illness in second or third week	Give corticosteroids
Cystic fibrosis	Excessive sweat salt loss in high temperatures (rare presentation)	Give NaCl Rehydrate
Renal tubular acidosis	Loss of sodium and bicarbonate in urine	Give corticosteroids

From Gilbert-Barness, E., & Barness, L. A. (2003). *Clinical use of pediatric diagnostic tests.* Baltimore: Lippincott, Williams & Wilkins, p. 82.

Hyperkalemia

Venous or arterial, not capillary, plasma K$^+$ > 5.5 mmol/L.

Hyperkalemia has a number of causes (Table 20.11). Asymptomatic hyperkalemia with levels of plasma potassium that would be fatal in an adult (up to 11 mmol/L) can be tolerated in the short term in a neonate. The most important effect of hyperkalemia is on cardiac rhythm, particularly in the infant with renal failure in whom the potassium imbalance cannot be readily corrected. This effect of hyperkalemia is potentiated by hypocalcemia, even of mild degree. Electrocardiographic changes include peaked T waves, then widening of the QRS complex, bradyarrhythmias, sine waves, and eventually cardiac arrest. High potassium value obtained from a capillary sample must be replicated in a venous specimen.

TABLE 20.9

Hypernatremia

Condition	Cause/Presentation	Management
Overhead heater	Excessive water loss through skin, especially in preterm babies	Use heat shield, increase water administration as 5% dextrose
Iatrogenic	Administration of $NaHCO_3$ to correct metabolic acidosis Administration of excessive supplementary salt over a short time period Use of 10% (or more) dextrose producing glycosuria and osmotic diuresis (especially in preterm babies)	Alter management
Fluid deprivation	Dehydration	Slow correction of electrolyte imbalance after initial administration of colloid to restore circulatory volume
Excess gastro-intestinal fluid loss	Dehydration	As above
Starvation	Circulatory collapse	As above
Nephrogenic diabetes	Failure to thrive Vomiting, constipation, episodic dehydration Persistent polyuria, unresponsive to exogenous antidiuretic hormone	Low-solute diet and diuretics

From Gilbert-Barness, E., & Barness, L. A. (2003). *Clinical use of pediatric diagnostic tests.* Baltimore: Lippincott, Williams & Wilkins, pp. 82–83.

TABLE 20.10

Hypokalemia

Condition	Cause/Presentation	Management
Birth asphyxia	Part of syndrome of inappropriate secretion of antidiuretic hormone with decreased plasma osmolality (<270 mmol/kg)	Restrict fluid
Alkalosis	Renal excretion of K^+ in place of H^+; seen in pyloric stenosis, exogenous alkali administration	Give potassium
Drugs	Use of furosemide; seen to a lesser extent with all diuretics	Supplement or use potassium-sparing diuretics
RTA	Proximal RTA (males)—defective proximal tubular resorption of bicarbonate Distal RTA—inability to establish H^+ ion gradient in distal tubule	Give alkali
Iatrogenic	Use of glucose and insulin	Reconsider treatment

RTA, renal tubular acidosis.
From Gilbert-Barness, E., & Barness, L. A. (2003). *Clinical use of pediatric diagnostic tests.* Baltimore: Lippincott, Williams & Wilkins, p. 83.

TABLE 20.11
Hyperkalemia

Condition	Cause/Presentation	Management
Acute renal failure	Associated with increased plasma and oliguria or anuria	May require treatment with rectal resonium resin, peritoneal dialysis, or both
Dehydration	Dehydration and leakage from cells	As above
Trauma: bruising, fracture, cephalohematoma, breech delivery, intracranial hemorrhage	Release of potassium from red cell Treat if >7 mmol/L or symptomatic.	Administer fluid or furosemide
Fluid deprivation	Dehydration, tissue damage	Correct circulating volume and restore perfusion with colloid and crystalloid
Congenital adrenal hyperplasia, adrenocortical insufficiency	Mineralocorticoid deficiency Males: normal, or pigmented scrotum Females: virilization (variable)	Give corticosteroids
Exchange transfusion	Citrate-phosphate-dextrose–stored blood has average potassium concentration of 12–15 mmol/L by 7 d, but can be much higher	Avoid use of blood >5 d old

TABLE 20.12
Complications of Parenteral Nutrition in Neonates

Frequent Complications	Less Frequent Complications
*Glycosuria	Copper deficiency
*Potassium depletion	*Hyperlipidemia (cholesterol ↑, triglycerides ↑)
*Hypophosphatemia	Hyperammonemia
*Sodium depletion	*Hyperphenylalaninemia (± hypertyrosinemia)
*Jaundice	Selenium deficiency
*Hyperglycemia	Zinc deficiency
Calcium depletion	
Metabolic acidosis	

↑, increased.
*Particularly important in extremely preterm infants.

FURTHER READING

Baston, H., & Durward, H. (2001). *Examination of the newborn: A practical guide*. Philadelphia: Routledge (Taylor and Francis).

Tappero, E. P., & Honeyfield, M. E. (2003). *Physical assessment of the newborn: A comprehensive approach to the art of physical examination*. Santa Rosa, CA: NICU Ink.

21

ADOLESCENCE

To know truly is to know by causes.

Francis Bacon, De Augmentis Scientiarum

NORMAL MENSTRUAL PHYSIOLOGY

By age 16 years, 97% of females reach menarche, 98% of them by 18 years. The average age of menarche in American adolescent females is 12.7 years (10–16 years). Menarche normally occurs within 1 year of the age at which the girl's siblings or mother experienced menarche.

Typical Menstrual Cycles

Cycle length: 28 days (21–45 days)
Duration of flow: 5 days (2–8 days)
Blood loss: 35 cc (20–80 cc)

Amenorrhea

Primary Amenorrhea

Primary amenorrhea includes no episodes of spontaneous uterine bleeding in a female with no pubertal changes at age 14 or stigmata of Turner syndrome, no episodes of spontaneous uterine bleeding by age 16, no episodes of spontaneous uterine bleeding despite having obtained an SMR B5 for at least 1 year, and no episodes of spontaneous uterine bleeding despite onset of breast development 4 years previously. Anatomic abnormalities, anorexia, or pregnancy should be considered in cases of primary amenorrhea.

Secondary Amenorrhea

After previous uterine bleeding, no subsequent menses for 6 months or a length of time equal to three previous cycles, whichever is shorter. Pregnancy, anorexia, vigorous exercise, or polycystic ovary syndrome (PCOS) should be considered.

Abnormal Vaginal Bleeding

The most common abnormal vaginal bleeding is primary dysfunctional uterine bleeding (DUB), followed by infection, hormonal contraceptives, threatened abortion, and ectopic pregnancy. DUB is due to anovulatory cycles in conjunction with hormonal imbalances. It is most common in the first 2 years after menarche due to an immature hypothalamic-pituitary-ovarian axis. It is almost always painless bleeding. Complications of pregnancy may consist of ectopic, threatened or incomplete abortion, spontaneous abortion, or placental problems. Local pathology may be endometritis or cervicitis (sexually transmitted diseases, STDs), vaginal or uterine polyp, uterine myoma, trauma, foreign body (IUD, retained tampon), or ovarian problems (premature failure, polycystic ovaries, corpus luteum failure). Systemic illness may include blood dyscrasias (von Willebrand's, thrombocytopenias), connective tissue disease (systemic lupus erythematosus), liver or renal disease, leukemia and other malignancies, thyroid problems, and adrenal disorders. Evaluation is similar to amenorrhea with emphasis on the following: pregnancy test, complete blood count to evaluate blood loss, platelets and pelvic/STD testing or pelvic ultrasound if virginal and patient will not tolerate pelvic examination, thyroid function tests, prolactin, FSH/LH, bleeding studies, BUN/Cr, and androgen levels (if PCOS suspected).

Dysmenorrhea

Recurrent crampy lower abdominal pain associated with menstruation (usually with some associated nausea, headache, thigh pain, backache, or diarrhea) is known as dysmenorrhea. It occurs in 60% of menstruating adolescents. Primary dysmenorrhea is caused by an increase in prostaglandins (E_2 and F_2) or increased sensitivity to prostaglandins. These cause an increase in uterine tone and contractions leading to pain. Secondary dysmenorrhea may be due to endometriosis, pelvic inflammatory diseases, congenital malformation of the reproductive tract, cervical stenosis, or a complication of pregnancy. Primary dysmenorrhea treatment is with prostaglandin synthetase inhibitors (NSAIDs), not aspirin, heating pad or bath, and exercise. Secondary dysmenorrheal treatment is with prostaglandin synthetase inhibitors as well as treating the underlying process.

Premenstrual Syndrome

Premenstrual syndrome (PMS) consists of fluid retention, bloating, breast tenderness, headaches, irritability, fatigue, anxiety, hostility, depression, and/or craving for sweets, salt, or alcohol. Appears during the middle or late menstrual cycle with a symptom-free period after menstruation. Prevalence is present in 18% of 13–15 year olds; 31% of older teens; and 40%–60% of adult women. The best treatment is regular exercise, a low-salt, high-protein diet, pyridoxine (B_6), calcium and magnesium, NSAIDs, OCP/Depo-Provera, and, with extreme caution in adolescents, danazol, diuretics, bromocriptine, and vitamin megadoses.

BIRTH CONTROL IN ADOLESCENCE

Some 80% of adolescents have engaged in intercourse by age 19 (Table 21.1).

TABLE 21.1
Birth Control Effectiveness

	Overall (%)	Teen (%)
Abstinence	100	
Depo-Provera	99.6	
Norplant	99.5	
IUD	95–97	93–97
OCPs	91–97	82–92
Condom	81–91	81–89
Female condom	76–79	
Diaphragm/cervical cap	61–88	
Sponge	75	
Coitus interruptus	73–85	
Rhythm methods	81–86	66–75

SEXUALLY TRANSMITTED DISEASES IN ADOLESCENTS

Sexually active teens have the highest rates of STDs of any age group (Table 21.2). Human papilloma virus is the most common STD. Chlamydia is the most common bacterial STD.

Male

Common clinical presentation in a male is urethritis; gonococcal is diagnosed with gram stain, culture, and probe. Treatment is with cephalosporins or quinolones; nongonococcal is diagnosed with culture, probe, negative Gram stain (*Chlamydia trachomatis, Ureaplasma urealyticus*). Trichomonas vaginalis is usually asymptomatic. Partner positive or found on urinalysis. Treatment is with metronidazole.

Orchitis or epididymitis consists of tenderness and swelling of testis and epididymis, fever, erythema of scrotum, and may include symptoms of urethritis. Always rule out testicular torsion, which is a surgical emergency.

Cervicitis

Cervicitis symptoms may be those of vaginitis plus abdominal or pelvic pain, and irregular or painful bleeding. Physical exam shows mucopurulent discharge and/or friable cervix. Diagnosis is by wet mount 10–30 WBC/hpf.

ADOLESCENT PREGNANCY

Of the 10 million females in the United States under the age of 20, almost 1 million become pregnant each year. Of these pregnancies, 80% are unplanned, 55% go to delivery, 30% end in elective terminations, and 15% end in spontaneous abortions.

TABLE 21.2
Causes of Vaginal Discharge

Diagnosis	Complaint	Exam	pH	Wet Mount	KOH	Rx	Comments
Physiologic "leukorrhea" not a vaginitis	Discharge only Inconvenient	Clear/white/slightly yellow discharge Dries brown Normal otherwise	≤4.5	Epithelial cells *Lactobacillus*	Negative	Reassure	May occur prior to menarche or during cycle Panty liners
Candidiasis Not an STD	Pruritus Dysuria	Milky-white, curdy Discharge Erythema, edema, may affect thighs, skin folds	≤4.5	Epithelial cells May see Pseudohyphae/ budding forms	Pseudohyphae/ Budding forms	"Azole" topicals per label fluconazole 150 mg po × 1 (avoid during pregnancy)	Consider if immunocomprised Diabetes, antibiotics, pregnancy
Bacterial vaginosis Not an STD	Mild pruritus Mild burning, odor	Gray-white discharge	>4.5	Epithelial cells ≥20% clue cells, few white cells	"Whiff" test amine odor	Metronidazole 2 g po × 1 or 500 mg po bid × 7 days or topical bid × 5 days Clindamycin 300 mg bid × 7 days or topical qhs × 7 days	High concentration of anaerobic bacteria (e.g., *Prevotella sp.*, *Mobiluncus sp.*) *G. vaginalis* and *Mycoplasma hominis*
Trichomonas	Pruritis Dysuria Odor Abdominal pain	Green/gray/frothy Erythema, edema, strawberry spots	>4.5	Epithelial cells White cells Trichomonads	Negative	Metronidazole 2 g po × 1 or 500 mg po bid × 7 days	Treat partner, sensitivity of wet mount 60%–80%

TABLE 21.3
Drugs of Addiction

	Mental Status	Eye Signs	Autonomic Signs	Comments
Alcohol	Ataxia, lethargy, combative, coma	Pupils vary, injected, lateral, nystagmus	↓ temp, ↓ BP, ↓↑ RR	Alcohol on breath, ↑ serum osmolarity
Amphetamines/ cocaine	Hyper alert, paranoid, hallucinations	Mydriasis	↑ temp, ↑ BP, ↑ HR, ↑ RR, diaphoresis	Tremors, seizures, dysrhythmias
Cannabis	Stimulation or sedation, panic	Mydriasis, injected	↑ HR, dry mouth and eyes	Occasionally spiked with other drugs
LSD	Perceptive distortion, hyperalert, panic, hallucinations	Mydriasis	↑↓ BP, ↑ HR, ↑ RR, diaphoresis	
Narcotics	Euphoria, sedation, coma	Pinpoint pupils	↓ temp, ↓ BP, ↓ HR, ↓ RR	Analgesia
Phencyclidine	Ataxia, agitated, violent, coma, seizures	Miosis, vertical and horizontal, nystagmus	↑ temp, ↑ BP, ↑ HR	Rigidity, self-mutilation, analgesia
Sedatives	Ataxia, sedation, irritability, psychosis, coma	Pupils vary, lateral, nystagmus	↓ temp, ↓ BP, ↓ HR, ↓ RR	

SUBSTANCE ABUSE

Substances are associated with over half of homicides, suicides, and fatal accidents (the top three causes of mortality) in teens (Table 21.3).

Alcohol is the most commonly used substance, having been used by 80% of high school students. In the 30 days prior to survey, 30% of students had five or more drinks "in a row."

Nicotine is the most popular drug for daily use; 70% of high school students had tried cigarettes and 25% had smoked daily for the previous month. Almost 8% use smokeless tobacco.

Almost 50% of high school students admit to having used marijuana. Marijuana is the most popular illicit drug. A higher proportion of males are involved in heavy and illicit drug use.

EATING DISORDERS

Anorexia Nervosa

Anorexia nervosa is refusal to maintain body weight at or above a minimally normal weight for age and weight and disturbance of body image. Also seen is absence of at least three consecutive menstrual cycles when otherwise expected to occur (primary or secondary amenorrhea). Associated features include physical hyperactivity and exercise, vomiting, with or without true binging, laxative, emetic, and/or diuretic abuse, preoccupation with food and food-related activities, withdrawal from friends and usual activities, denial of severity of illness, and delayed psychosexual development.

Onset is usually early to late adolescence, ratio of 9–10 females to 1 male. There may be psychiatric concerns (substance use, suicidal ideations), and significant electrolyte abnormalities. Mortality is ≤5% and is due to the effects of starvation (infection, or renal or cardiac failure), electrolyte disturbances, or suicide.

Bulimia Nervosa

Bulimia nervosa is recurrent episodes of binge eating, usually followed by effort to purge by vomiting, laxative, or prolonged fasting or excessive exercise. Onset is in adolescence or adulthood; 90% are females. Patients with bulimia are often of normal weight or slightly overweight. Evidence of bulimia can be erosion of tooth enamel or scarring of the knuckles from induced vomiting.

SAFETY

Preventable injury, both unintentional and intentional, is the main cause of death among males. Relatively few behaviors contribute to most deaths among adolescent males: (1) intoxication, primarily with alcohol, while driving or swimming, and consequent motor vehicle crashes and drowning; (2) lack of appropriate use of safety devices, such as seat belts or helmets when driving a car or riding a motorcycle, bicycle, or skateboard; and (3) access to and use of guns.

FURTHER READING

Beach, R. K. (1995). Contraception for adolescents: Part 2. *Adolescent Health Update*, 7(2).

Blythe, M., Carter, C., & Orr, D. (1991). Common menstrual problems: Part 1. *Adolescent Health Update*, 3(3).

Centers for Disease Control. (2000). Youth Risk Behavior Surveillance Survey—United States, 1999. *Morbidity and Mortality Weekly Report, 49/SS05*.

Emans, S. J., Laufer, M. R., & Goldstein, D. P. (1998). *Pediatric and adolescent gynecology* (4th ed.). Philadelphia: Lippincott Williams & Wilkins.

Goldenring, J. M., & Rosen, D. S. (2004). Getting into adolescent heads: An essential update. *Contemporary Pediatrics, 21*(1), 64.

Grimes, D. A., & Wallalch, M. (1997). *Modern contraception: Updates from the contraceptive report*. Ottawa: Emron.

Holmbeck, G. N., Paidoff, R. L., & Brooks-Gunn, J. (1995). Parenting adolescents. In M. H. Bornstein (Ed.), *Handbook of parenting: Children and parenting* (pp. 91–118). Mahwah, NJ: Erlbaum.

McCoy, K., & Wibbelsman, C. (1999). *The teenage body book: Revised and updated*. New York: Perigee Books.

Neinstein, L. S. (2002). *Adolescent health care: A practical guide* (4th ed.). Philadelphia: Lippincott, Williams & Wilkins.

Schonberg, S. K. (Ed.). (1988). *Substance abuse: A guide for health professsionals*. Washington, DC: American Academy of Pediatrics.

Schydlower, M., & Rogers, P. D. (Eds.). (1993). Adolescent substance abuse and addictions. *Adolescent Medicine: State of the Art Reviews, 4*(2).

Sikand, A., & Fisher, M. (1992). The role of barrier contraceptives in prevention of pregnancy and disease in adolescents. *Adolescent Medicine: State of the Art Reviews, 3*(2), 223–240.

WEBSITES

Adolescent Health Working Group. Adolescent provider toolkit: A guide for treating teen patients, adolescent health 101: The basics. http://ahwg.net/resources/CA101_.pdf.

Gay and Lesbian Medical Association. www.glma.org/. Online health care referrals.

National Adolescent Health Information Center. A health profile of adolescent and young adult males. http://nahic.ucsf.edu.

Rape, Abuse and Incest National Network. www.rainn.org. Provides a listing of counseling centers searchable by zip code or state.

U.S. Department of Health and Human Services, Substance Abuse and Mental Health Services Administration. www.samhsa.gov; 1-800-662-HELP.

www.coolnurse.com/male_health.htm. Information about adolescent male-specific topics.

www.iwannaknow.org. Information for adolescent males and females about STDs, puberty, and prevention.

www.teengrowth.com. General information for adolescent males and females.

www.teenhealthfx.com. General information for adolescent males and females about health and illness, sports and nutrition, sexuality and sexual health, alcohol, cigarettes, and drugs.

www.teenwire.com/index.asp. Information for adolescent males and females about body, sex, pregnancy, birth control, abortion, infections, relationships, schools and careers, coping and emotions, gay and questioning, taking action, and entertainment.

Appendix A

RECORD OF PHYSICAL EXAMINATION

Temp _____ Pulse _____ Resp _____ BP _____
Age _____ Sex _____ Ht _____ Wt _____
Head circ _____ Chest circ _____
Skin folds _____

General appearance: Ill or well, distressed, alert, cooperative, body build. Reaction to parents. Facies. Characteristic position, movements, nutrition, development. Speech.

Skin: Color, pigmentation, cyanosis. Veins, arteries, thrombophlebitis. Jaundice, carotenemia. Pallor. Eruptions. Petechiae. Ecchymosis. Hives. Dermatographia. Tache cerebrale. Subcutaneous nodules. Xanthomas. Texture. Scaling, striae, scars, sweat, subcutaneous tissue, emphysema. Turgor, edema.

Nails: Cyanosis, pallor, pulsations, pitting, hemorrhages.

Hair (body): Distribution, color.

Lymph nodes: Occipital, postauricular, cervical, parotid, submaxillary, sublingual, axillary, epitrochlear, inguinal. Size, mobility, tenderness, heat.

Head: Position, hair, shape, sutures, fontanels. Circumference. Microcephaly, hydrocephaly. Craniotabes, Macewen's sign. Percussion, sinuses. Auscultation, bruit, veins.

Face: Shape. Facial paralysis, trigeminal paralysis. Swelling; parotid, submaxillary, sublingual glands. Facial appearance, hypertelorism, twitching, Chvostek's sign.

Eyes: Vision, visual fields. Blinking. Scleras, exophthalmos, enophthalmos. Strabismus. Ocular movement. Nystagmus. Ptosis, eyelids. Conjunctivae, pingueculae, pterygium, sties, chalazion, blepharitis. Cornea, discharge. Pupils, accommodation, iris. Retina, red reflex, fundus, vessels, hemorrhage, chorioretinitis, disc, macula. Corneal reflex.

Ears: Anomaly, position. Discharge. Tenderness. Canals. Drums, redness, light reflex, landmarks, bulging, perforation, mobility. Mastoids, nodes. Hearing. Vestibular function.

Nose: Shape. Alae nasi, flaring. Mucosa, secretions, bleeding, airway. Septum. Polyps, tumor, encephalocele. Sinuses.

Lips: Paralysis, cleft, fissures, vesicles, color, edema.

Mouth, Throat: Odors, trismus. Circumoral pallor. Teeth, number, edges, occlusion, caries, formation, color. Salivation.

Gums: Infection, discoloration, bleeding, cysts. Buccal mucosa, thrush, veins.

Tongue: Coating, moisture, tremor, papillae, color, geographic, furrows, scars, size, tongue-tie, cysts, paralysis.

Palate: Color, bleeding, cleft, perforation, arch. Epiglottis. Uvula, soft palate. Posterior pharynx. Tonsils, infections, size. Postnasal drip. Koplik's spots, eruptions, ulcers.

Larynx: Voice. Laryngoscopy. Speech.

Neck: Size, anomalies, webbing, edema, nodes, masses. Sternocleidomastoids. Trachea. Thyroid. Vessels. Motion, opisthotonos, Brudzinski's sign, tonic neck reflex. Head drop. Tilting. Nodding.

Chest: Inspection, shape, circumference, rosary, Harrison's groove, flaring, angle, expansion; abdominal, thoracic, intercostal motion, retraction, symmetry, scapulae.

Breasts: Observation, development, symmetry, redness, heat, tenderness, masses. Tanner stage.

Lungs: Respiration. Type, Cheyne-Stokes. Rate, Tachypnea, slow, apnea, Biot's. Depth, hyperpnea. Dyspnea, exercise tolerance. Cough, hemoptysis, sputum, cough reflex. Palpation, masses, tenderness, thud, fremitus; interspaces, retraction, paralysis; pulsations, friction rubs, nodes. Percussion, dullness, scapulae, diaphragm, liver, heart, mediastinum, hyperresonance. Auscultation, sounds, rales, rub, slap, rhonchi, wheezes, vocal resonance, peristalsis.

Heart: Inspection, bulging, impulse; distress, cyanosis, edema, clubbing, pulsations, vessels, femoral pulse, blood pressure. Pulse rate, tachycardia, pulsus alternans, bradycardia, water-hammer, thready, dicrotic, pulsus paradoxus. Arrhythmia, premature beats, extrasystoles, rhythm, fibrillation. Palpation, size, apex impulse, tenderness, thrill. Percussion. Auscultation, sounds, quality, split, third sound, gallop, tic-tac, friction rub, venous hum, murmurs. Failure.

Abdomen: Inspection, shape, distention, transillumination, respiration. Umbilicus, diastasis, veins. Peristalsis. Gastric waves. Auscultation. Percussion, fluid, masses. Palpation, superficial, tense, tenderness, rebound; spleen, liver, masses. Deep palpation, ballottement, bladder, kidneys, reflexes. Femoral pulses, hydration, consistency.

Genitalia: Discharge, foreign body, caruncle, prolapse. Labia, adhesions, vagina, clitoris. Penis, hypospadias, epispadias, phimosis. Scrotum, testes, hydrocele, hernia. Cremasteric reflex, nodes. Tanner stage.

Anus and rectum: Buttocks. Fistula. Fissure. Prolapse. Polyps. Hemorrhoids. Diaper rash. Rectum, fistula, megacolon, masses, prostate, uterus, tenderness. Sensation.

Extremities: Anomalies, length, clubbing, pain, tenderness, temperature, gangrene, swelling, deformities, shape. Feet. Gait, stance, balance, limp, ataxia.

Spine: Hair, dimples, masses, spina bifida, tenderness, mobility. Opisthotonos, scapulae. Posture, lordosis, kyphosis, scoliosis.

Joints: Heat, tenderness, swelling, effusion, redness, motion. Hip dysplasia.

Muscles: Development, tone, tenderness, spasm, paralysis, rigidity, contractures, atrophy.

Nervous system: General impression, abilities, responsiveness, position, spontaneous movements, play activity, development. State of consciousness, irritability, convulsive states. Gait, stance, limp, ataxia. Coordination. Tremors, twitching, choreiform movement, athetosis, associated movements. Rigidity, paresis, paralysis, spasticity, flaccidity. Reflexes, superficial, tendon, clonus. Moro tonic neck. Babinski, Oppenheim Hoffmann, Kernig, Romberg, Foerster, Trousseau, peroneal, Chvostek's grasp. Thumb position. Neck and spine mobility, fontanels. Sensation, blind, deaf, withdrawal reflex, hyperesthesia, hypesthesia, position, vibration, temperature, touch. Astereognosis. Cranial nerves I–XII.

Appendix B

THE DENVER II REVISION AND RESTANDARDIZATION OF THE DENVER DEVELOPMENTAL SCREENING TEST

Because services for handicapped children have markedly expanded since the Denver Developmental Screening Test (DDST) first appeared in 1967, the test has undergone a major revision and restandardization. A pool of 350 potential items was developed through a review of existing items and the creation of additional ones. Criteria for the administration and interpretation of each item were developed. The items were standardized on two samples: (1) Denver County (N = 1039) subdivided into three ethnic groups, each of which was further divided on the basis of maternal education. Each of these was again divided into 10 age categories; (2) the Colorado non-Denver sample (N = 1057) was subdivided into three residence categories (rural, suburban, urban), and each was further subdivided on the basis of maternal education and age of children similar to the Denver County sample.

Each item was examined via regression analysis to determine the age at which 25%, 50%, 75%, and 90% of children in each subgroup could perform the item. A goodness of fit test was applied to the data to determine the accuracy of the curves. Tester-observer and test-retest reliability was determined for each item.

Reprinted with the permission of Frankenburg, W. K., and Dodds, J. B., University of Colorado Medical Center, Denver.

The final selection of 125 items was made on the basis of eight criteria. Changes in times were an 86% increase in language items, the addition of two items on speech intelligibility, and a 22% decrease in the number of report items.

The 125 items are displayed on a test form that has an age scale corresponding to the AAP recommended health maintenance visits. The test form also includes a behavior rating scale (Figures B.1 and B.2).

Currently the Denver II screening manual, test form, and proficiency test are being used in diverse parts of the United States. For interpretation purposes, the *Denver II Technical Manual* contains norms of subgroups having significantly different ages at which 90% of children pass the item compared with the group norms that are presented on the test form.

Detailed administration and scoring instructions are given in the *Denver II Screening Manual*, which must be used to ensure accuracy in administration of the test. These materials are available from DDM, Inc, PO Box 6919, Denver, Col 80206-0919.

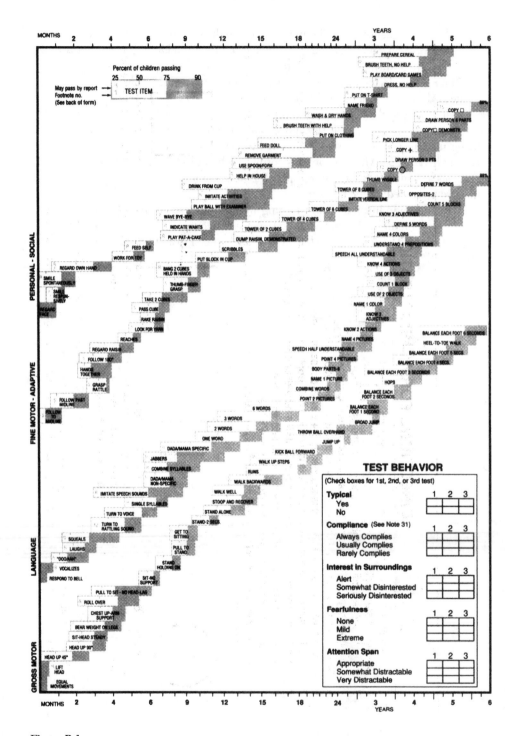

Figure B.1

DIRECTIONS FOR ADMINISTRATION

1. Try to get child to smile by smiling, talking or waving. Do not touch him/her.
2. Child must stare at hand several seconds.
3. Parent may help guide toothbrush and put toothpaste on brush.
4. Child does not have to be able to tie shoes or button/zip in the back.
5. Move yarn slowly in an arc from one side to the other, about 8" above child's face.
6. Pass if child grasps rattle when it is touched to the backs or tips of fingers.
7. Pass if child tries to see where yarn went. Yarn should be dropped quickly from sight from tester's hand without arm movement.
8. Child must transfer cube from hand to hand without help of body, mouth, or table.
9. Pass if child picks up raisin with any part of thumb and finger.
10. Line can vary only 30 degrees or less from tester's line. /
11. Make a fist with thumb pointing upward and wiggle only the thumb. Pass if child imitates and does not move any fingers other than the thumb.

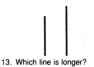

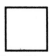

12. Pass any enclosed form. Fail continuous round motions.

13. Which line is longer? (Not bigger.) Turn paper upside down and repeat. (pass 3 of 3 or 5 of 6)

14. Pass any lines crossing near midpoint.

15. Have child copy first. If failed, demonstrate.

When giving items 12, 14, and 15, do not name the forms. Do not demonstrate 12 and 14.

16. When scoring, each pair (2 arms, 2 legs, etc.) counts as one part.
17. Place one cube in cup and shake gently near child's ear, but out of sight. Repeat for other ear.
18. Point to picture and have child name it. (No credit is given for sounds only.)
    If less than 4 pictures are named correctly, have child point to picture as each is named by tester.

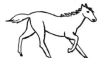

19. Using doll, tell child: Show me the nose, eyes, ears, mouth, hands, feet, tummy, hair. Pass 6 of 8.
20. Using pictures, ask child: Which one flies?... says meow?... talks?... barks?... gallops? Pass 2 of 5, 4 of 5.
21. Ask child: What do you do when you are cold?... tired?... hungry? Pass 2 of 3, 3 of 3.
22. Ask child: What do you do with a cup? What is a chair used for? What is a pencil used for?
    Action words must be included in answers.
23. Pass if child correctly places and says how many blocks are on paper. (1, 5).
24. Tell child: Put block on table; under table; in front of me, behind me. Pass 4 of 4.
    (Do not help child by pointing, moving head or eyes.)
25. Ask child: What is a ball?... lake?... desk?... house?... banana?... curtain?... fence?... ceiling? Pass if defined in terms of use, shape, what it is made of, or general category (such as banana is fruit, not just yellow). Pass 5 of 8, 7 of 8.
26. Ask child: If a horse is big, a mouse is __? If fire is hot, ice is __? If the sun shines during the day, the moon shines during the __? Pass 2 of 3.
27. Child may use wall or rail only, not person. May not crawl.
28. Child must throw ball overhand 3 feet to within arm's reach of tester.
29. Child must perform standing broad jump over width of test sheet (8 1/2 inches).
30. Tell child to walk forward, ⊂⊃⊂⊃⊂⊃⊂⊃➤ heel within 1 inch of toe. Tester may demonstrate.
    Child must walk 4 consecutive steps.
31. In the second year, half of normal children are non-compliant.

Figure B.2

Appendix C

PHYSICAL GROWTH AND THE EARLY LANGUAGE MILESTONE SCALE

The charts of head circumference in boys and girls from age 1 month to age 18 years are shown in Fig. C.1. Figures C.2–7 show physical growth percentiles for boy and girls from birth to 18 years of age. Figure 8 and the following text* present the Early Language Milestone (ELM) Scale.

The ELM Scale is a tool for assessing language development from birth to 36 months of age and intelligibility of speech from birth to 48 months of age. Language is assessed independently in three areas: auditory expressive, auditory receptive, and visual. Auditory expressive development is subdivided into content (such as cooing, babbling, single words, two-word phrases) an intelligibility (clarity of speech). Auditory receptive development includes prelinguistic auditory behaviors (orienting to voice or bell), plus comprehension of progressively more complex verbal commands. Visual language includes prelinguistic behaviors (visual tracking and response to facial expressions) and symbolic features such as pointing to desired objects. Item V10 (index finger pointing) characterizes an ability that emerges at the same age as that described by item AE 9 (first word) and implies the same degree of linguistic competence. The ELM Scale may be scored on a pass/fail basis or may be converted to point scores and percentile values for auditory expressive, auditory receptive, visual, and global language function.

I. General Instructions

a) Draw vertical line down entire page at child's chronologic age (CA).
b) Work *backward* from CA, until three consecutive items in each Division (AE, AR, V) are passed (=Basal Level).
c) If child achieves Basal without failing any items already attained by more than 90% of children, *stop*. ELM screen is passed.
d) If one or more items that have already been attained by more than 90% of children are failed, work *forward* from CA until three consecutive items in that Division

*From Coplan J: *The Early Language Milestone Scale*. Austin, TX: PRO-ED, 1987.

are failed. (Exception: Child is permitted to fail *one* of the following without penalty: V3–V6). The 50% value of the highest item passed in each Division is the Ceiling Level.

If Ceiling Level ≥ CA → ELM screen is passed.
If Ceiling Level < CA → ELM screen is failed.

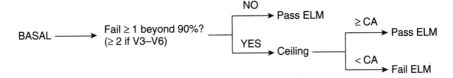

II. Auditory Expressive (AE)

a. Content

AE1: Prolonged musical vowel sounds in a sing-song fashion (OOO, aaa, etc.), *not* just grunts or squeaks.

AE2 H: "Does baby watch speaker's face and appear to listen intently, then vocalize when the speaker is quiet? Can you 'have a conversation' with your baby?"

AE4 H: Blow bubbles or "bronx cheer"?

AE9, AE10 H: Child *spontaneously, consistently,* and *correctly* uses words. Do not count "ma-ma," "da-da," or the names of other family members or pets. *Do* list the particular words.

AE11 H: Uses single words to tell you demands. "Milk!" "Cookie!" "More!" etc. Pass = two or more wants. List specific words.

AE12 H: *Spontaneous, novel* two-word combinations ("Want cookie," "No bed," "See daddy," etc.) *Not* rotely learned phrases that have been specifically taught to the child or combinations that are really single thoughts (e.g., "hot dog").

AE14 H: Child uses "me" or "you" but may reverse them ("you want cookie" instead of "me want cookie," etc.)

AE17 H: "Can child put two or three sentences together to hold brief conversations?"

AE18 T: Put out cup, ball, crayon, and spoon. Pick up cup and say, "What is this? What do we do with it? What is it for?" Child must *name* the object and give its use. Pass = "drink with," etc., *not* "milk" or "juice." Ball: Pass = "throw," "play with," etc. Spoon: Pass = "Eat" or "Eat with," etc., *not* "Food," "Lunch." Crayon: Pass = "Write (with)," "Color (with)," etc. Pass item if child gives *name* and *use* for two objects.

b. Intelligibility

AE15, AE19, AE20: "How clear are the words your child makes? That is, how much of your child's speech can a stranger understand?"

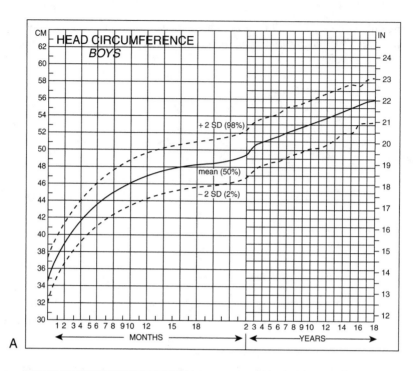

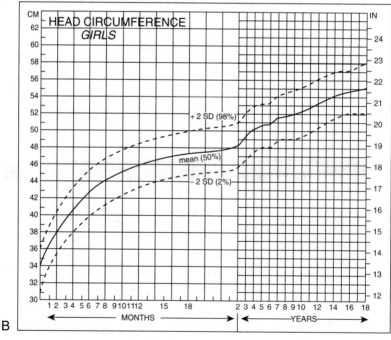

Figure C.1
Head circumference in boys and girls from 1 month to 18 years of age.

Birth to 36 months: Girls
Head circumference-for-age and
Weight-for-length percentiles

NAME _____

RECORD # _____

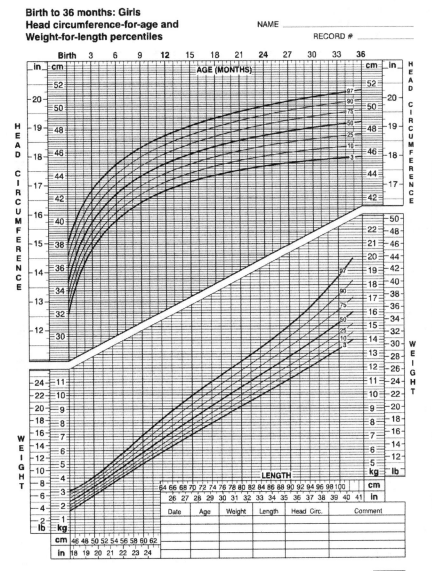

Date	Age	Weight	Length	Head Circ.	Comment

Published May 30, 2000 (modified 10/16/00).
SOURCE: Developed by the National Center for Health Statistics in collaboration with
the National Center for Chronic Disease Prevention and Health Promotion (2000).
http://www.cdc.gov/growthcharts

SAFER · HEALTHIER · PEOPLE™

Birth to 36 Months (Girls) HC-for-age & Weight-for-length

Birth to 36 months: Boys
Head circumference-for-age and
Weight-for-length percentiles

NAME _____

RECORD # _____

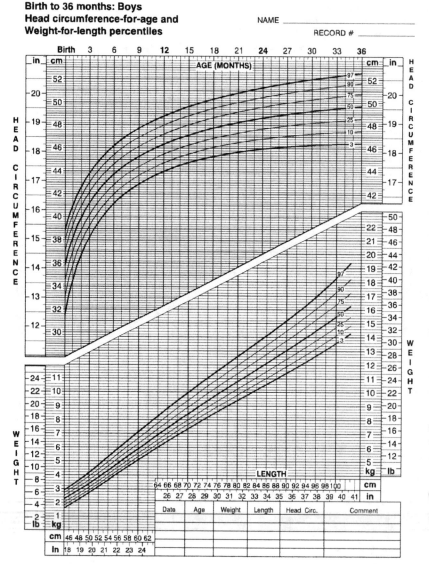

Published May 30, 2000 (modified 10/16/00).
SOURCE: Developed by the National Center for Health Statistics in collaboration with
the National Center for Chronic Disease Prevention and Health Promotion (2000).
http://www.cdc.gov/growthcharts

SAFER · HEALTHIER · PEOPLE™

Birth to 36 Months (Boys) HC-for-age & Weight-for-length

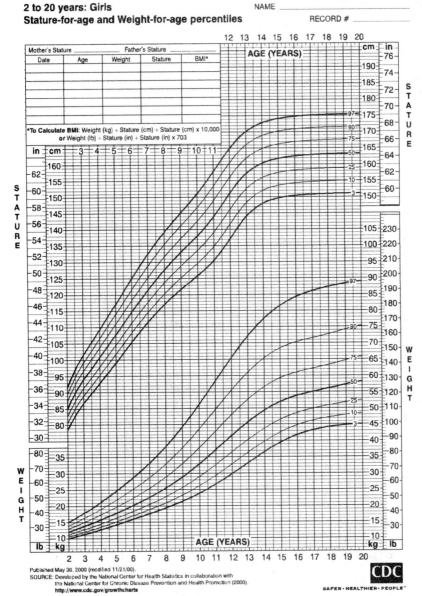

2 to 20 years: Girls
Stature-for-age and Weight-for-age percentiles

NAME _____

RECORD # _____

Published May 30, 2000 (modified 11/21/00).
SOURCE: Developed by the National Center for Health Statistics in collaboration with
the National Center for Chronic Disease Prevention and Health Promotion (2000).
http://www.cdc.gov/growthcharts

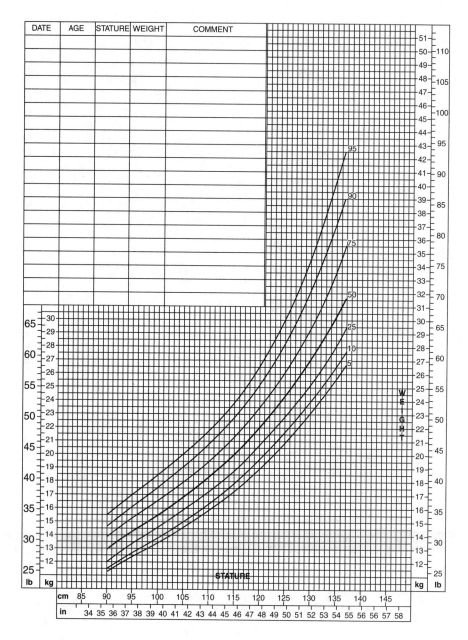

Figure C.5

Girls: Prepubescent—physical growth National Center for Health Statistics (NCHS) percentiles. (Modified from Hamill PV, Drizd TA, Johnson CL, Reed RB, Roche AF, Moore WM: Physical growth: National Center for Health Statistics percentiles. *Am J Clin Nutr* 1979;32:607–29. Data from the National Center for Health Statistics, Hyattsville, MD.)

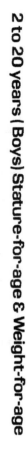

2 to 20 years: Boys
Stature-for-age and Weight-for-age percentiles

NAME _____

RECORD # _____

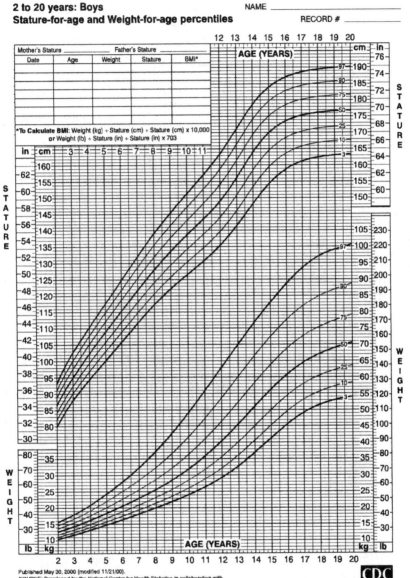

Published May 30, 2000 (modified 11/21/00).
SOURCE: Developed by the National Center for Health Statistics in collaboration with
the National Center for Chronic Disease Prevention and Health Promotion (2000).
http://www.cdc.gov/growthcharts

CDC
SAFER · HEALTHIER · PEOPLE™

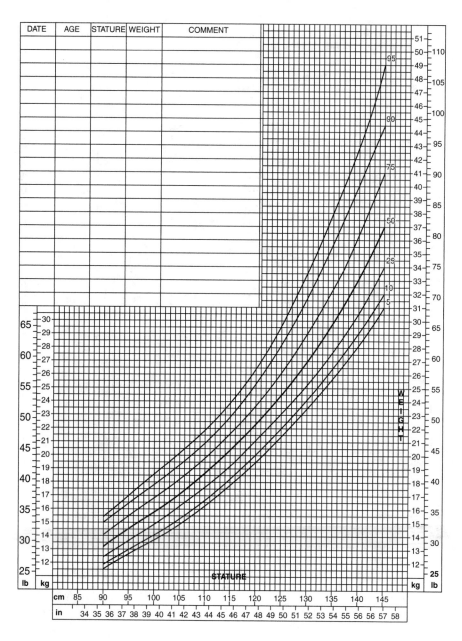

Figure C.7

Boys: Prepubescent—physical growth National Center for Health Statistics (NCHS) percentiles. (Modified from Hamill PV, Drizd TA, Johnson CL, Reed RB, Roche AF, Moore WM: Physical growth: National Center for Health Statistics percentiles. *Am J Clin Nutr* 1979;32:607–29. Data from the National Center for Health Statistics, Hyattsville, MD.)

2 to 20 years: Boys
Body mass index-for-age percentiles

NAME _____

RECORD # _____

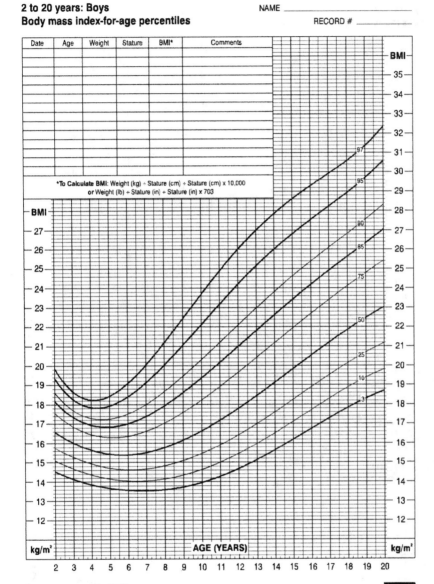

Date	Age	Weight	Stature	BMI*	Comments

*To Calculate BMI: Weight (kg) ÷ Stature (cm) ÷ Stature (cm) x 10,000
or Weight (lb) ÷ Stature (in) ÷ Stature (in) x 703

AGE (YEARS)

2 to 20 years (Boys) Body mass index-for-age

Published May 30, 2000 (modified 10/16/00).
SOURCE: Developed by the National Center for Health Statistics in collaboration with
the National Center for Chronic Disease Prevention and Health Promotion (2000).
http://www.cdc.gov/growthcharts

SAFER · HEALTHIER · PEOPLE™

2 to 20 years: Girls
Body mass index-for-age percentiles

NAME _____

RECORD # _____

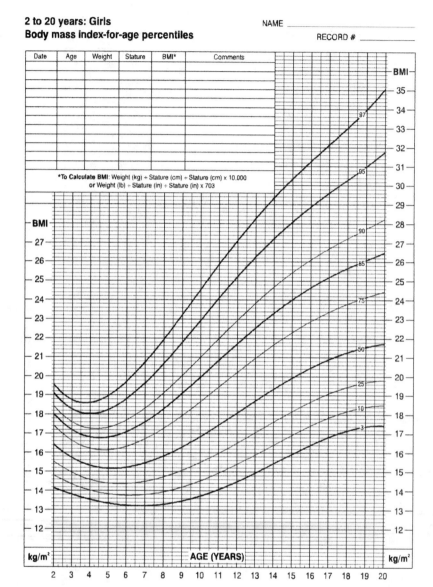

Date	Age	Weight	Stature	BMI*	Comments

*To Calculate BMI: Weight (kg) ÷ Stature (cm) ÷ Stature (cm) x 10,000
or Weight (lb) ÷ Stature (in) ÷ Stature (in) x 703

AGE (YEARS)

Published May 30, 2000 (modified 10/16/00).
SOURCE: Developed by the National Center for Health Statistics in collaboration with
the National Center for Chronic Disease Prevention and Health Promotion (2000).
http://www.cdc.gov/growthcharts

CDC

SAFER · HEALTHIER · PEOPLE™

2 to 20 years (Girls) Body mass index-for-age

Birth to 36 months: Boys
Length-for-age and Weight-for-age percentiles

NAME _____

RECORD # _____

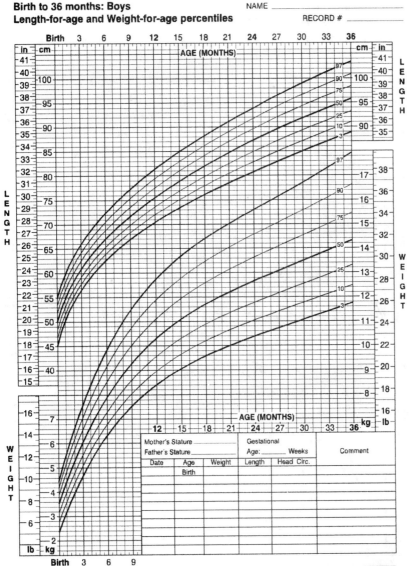

Birth to 36 Months (Boys) Length-for-age & Weight-for-age

Birth to 36 months: Girls
Length-for-age and Weight-for-age percentiles

NAME _____

RECORD # _____

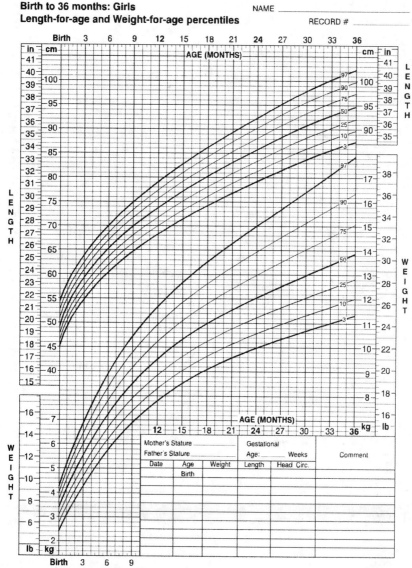

Published May 30, 2000 (modified 4/20/01).
SOURCE: Developed by the National Center for Health Statistics in collaboration with
the National Center for Chronic Disease Prevention and Health Promotion (2000).
http://www.cdc.gov/growthcharts

SAFER · HEALTHIER · PEOPLE

Birth to 36 Months (Girls) Length-for-age & Weight-for-age

Goodenough-Harris Draw-a-Person Test

Procedure

Give the child a pencil and a sheet of blank paper. Instruct the child to "draw a person; draw the best person you can." Supply the encouragement if needed; however do not suggest specific changes of supplementation.

Scoring

Ask the child to explain the drawing to you. Give the child one point for each detail present using the scoring guide (maximum score: 51) and compare to the age. From Robertson, J., Shilkofski, N., (Eds). *The Harriet Lane Handbook*, 17th ed., Elsevier Mosby, p. 244, 2005.

GOODENOUGH-HARRIS SCORING
(DRAW-A-MAN)

General

- Head present
- Legs present
- Arms present

Trunk

- Present
- Length greater than breadth
- Shoulders

Arms/legs

- Attaches to trunk
- At correct point

Neck

- Present
- Outline of neck, continuous with head, trunk or both

Face

- Eyes
- Nose mouth
- Nose and mouth in two dimensions
- Nostrils

Hair

- Present
- On more than one circumference; nontransparent

Clothing

- Present

- ○ Two articles; nontransparent
- ○ Entire drawing (sleeves and trousers) nontransparent
- ○ Four articles
- ○ Custom complete

Fingers

- ○ Present
- ○ Correct number
- ○ Two dimensions; length, breadth
- ○ Thumb opposition
- ○ Hand distinct from fingers and arm

Joints

- ○ Elbow, shoulder or both
- ○ Knees, hip or both

Proportion

- ○ Head: 10%–50% of trunk area
- ○ Arms: approximately same length as trunk
- ○ Legs: 1–2 times trunk length; width less than trunk width
- ○ Feet: to leg length
- ○ Arms and legs in two dimensions
- ○ Heel

Motor coordination

- ○ Lines firm and well connected
- ○ Firmly drawn with correct joining
- ○ Head outline
- ○ Trunk outline
- ○ Outline of arms and legs
- ○ Features

Ears

- ○ Present
- ○ Correct position and proportion

Eye detail

- ○ Brow or lashes
- ○ Pupil
- ○ Proportion
- ○ Glance directed front in profile drawing

Chin

- ○ Present, forehead
- ○ Projection

Profile

○ Not more than one error
○ Correct

From Robertson, J., Shilkofski, N., (Eds). *The Harriet Lane Handbook*, 17th ed., Elsevier Mosby, p. 248, 2005.

This is a test for cognitive development, most useful for ages 5–9 years of age.

<u>Cognitive Development:</u>

Age 5

Expect head, eyes, nose, mouth, body, and legs. Do not expect profiles, knees, elbows, two lips, nostrils, appropriate proportions, four clothing items, five fingers, and pupils.

Age 6

Expect head, eyes, nose, mouth, body, legs and feet. Do not expect profiles, knees, elbows, two lips, nostrils, appropriate proportions, and four clothing items.

Age 7

Expect head, eyes, nose, mouth, body, legs, two dimensional arms, and feet, proportions may be close but still off. Do not expect profiles, knees, elbows, and two lips.

Age 8 and Age 9

Expect head, eyes, nose, mouth, body, two dimensional arms and legs, and feet, proportions should be right. Do not expect profiles, knees, and elbows, and you might not see two lips.

Simple scoring for Goodenough-Harris developmental draw-a-person:

$$\frac{\text{\# of items}}{4} + 3 \frac{1}{2} = \text{developmental age (years)}$$

Appropriate Screening in Each Development Stream by Age*

| Age | Visual Motor | Cognitive | | Behavior |
		Language	Motor	
Infants and toddlers	CAT, Denver II	CLAMS, Denver II	Milestones, Denver II, neurologic examination primitive reflexes	Temperament, social skills, activity level, Denver II
Preschool age	Draw-a-person, Gesell figures, block skills, Denver II	Articulation, comprehension (example: following commands), expression (example: estimate of vocabulary), Denver II	Milestone, neurologic examination, Denver II	Child behavior checklist, ADHD checklist, Denver II
School age	Draw-a-person, Gesell figures, handwriting	Reading, decoding comprehension, listening written language	Coordination, neurologic examination, soft neurologic signs	Child behavior checklist, ADHD checklist

*If significant delays are noted, referral to a developmental pediatrician or psychologist is indicated.
From Robertson, J., Shilkofski, N., (Eds). *The Harriet Lane Handbook*, 17th ed., Elsevier Mosby, p. 251, 2005.

15 months	Imitates scribble
18 months	Scribbles spontaneously
2 years	Imitates stroke
2½ years	Differentiates horizontal and vertical stroke

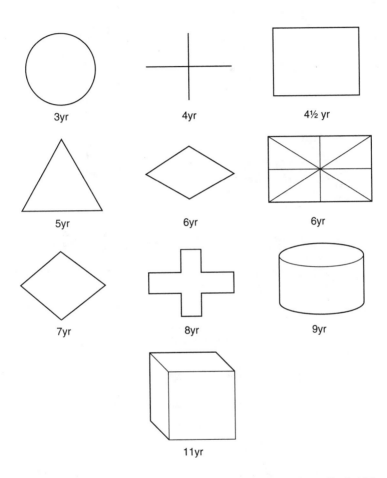

From Robertson, J., Shilkofski, N., (Eds). *The Harriet Lane Handbook*, 17th ed., Elsevier Mosby, p. 249, 2005.

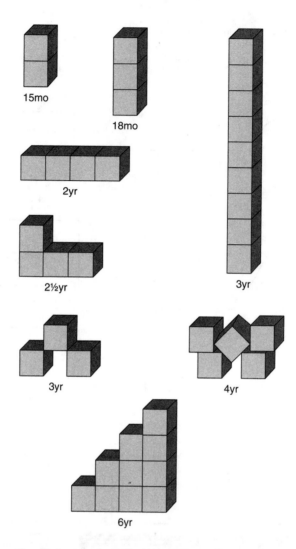

15mo

18mo

2yr

2½yr

3yr

3yr

4yr

6yr

From Robertson, J., Shilkofski, N., (Eds). *The Harriet Lane Handbook*, 17th ed., Elsevier Mosby, p. 250, 2005.

Appendix D

IMMUNIZATIONS

Recommended Immunization Schedule for Persons Aged 0–6 Years United States, 2007

VACCINE ▼ / AGE ▶	Birth	1 month	2 months	4 months	6 months	12 months	15 months	18 months	19–23 months	2–3 years	4–6 years
Hepatitis B[1]	HepB	HepB		see footnote 1		HepB				HepB	
Rotavirus[2]			Rota	Rota	Rota						
Diphtheria, Tetanus, Pertussis[3]			DTaP	DTaP	DTaP		DTaP				DTaP
Haemophilus influenzae type b[4]			Hib	Hib	Hib⁴	Hib					
Pneumococcal[5]			PCV	PCV	PCV	PCV				PCV / PPV	
Inactivated Poliovirus			IPV	IPV	IPV		IPV				IPV
Influenza[6]					Influenza (Yearly)						
Measles, Mumps, Rubella[7]						MMR					MMR
Varicella[8]						Varicella					Varicella
Hepatitis A[9]						HepA (2 doses)				HepA Series	
Meningococcal[10]											MPSV4

■ Range of recommended ages   ■ Catch-up immunization   ■ Certain high-risk groups

This schedule indicates the recommended ages for routine administration of currently licensed childhood vaccines, as of December 1, 2006, for children aged 0–6 years. Additional information is available at http://www.cdc.gov/nip/recs/child-schedule.htm. Any dose not administered at the recommended age should be administered at any subsequent visit, when indicated and feasible. Additional vaccines may belicensed and recommended during the year. Licensed combination vaccines may be used whenever any components of the combination are indicated and other components of the vaccine are not contraindicated and if approved by the Food and Drug Administration for that dose of the series. Providers should consult the respective Advisory Committee on Immunization Practices statement for detailed recommendations. Clinically significant adverse events that follow immunization should be reported to the Vaccine Adverse Event Reporting System (VAERS). Guidance about how to obtain and complete a VAERS from is available at http://www.vaers.hhs.gov or by telephone, 800-822-7967.

Children's Doctor Supplement • Summer 2007

Recommended Immunization Schedule for Persons Aged 7–18 Years United States, 2007

VACCINE ▼ AGE ▶	7–10 years	11–12 years	13–14 years	15 years	16–18 years
Diphtheria, Tetanus, Pertussis[1]	see footnote 1	Tdap		Tdap	
Human Papillomavirus[2]	see footnote 2	HPV (3 doses)		HPV Series	
Meningococcal[3]	MPSV4	MCV4		MCV4 / MCV4[3]	
Pneumococcal[4]			PPV		
Influenza[5]			Influenza (Yearly)		
Hepatitis A[6]			HepB Series		
Hepatitis B[7]			HepB Series		
Inactivated Poliovirus[8]			IPV Series		
Measles, Mumps, Rubella[9]			MMR Series		
Varicella[10]			Varicella Series		

Legend:
- Range of recommended ages
- Catch-up immunization
- Certain high-risk groups

This schedule indicates the recommended ages for routine administration of currently licensed childhood vaccines, as of December 1, 2006, for children aged 7–18 years. Additional information is available at http://www.cdc.gov/nip/recs/child-schedule.htm. Any dose not administered at the recommended age should be administered at any subsequent visit, when indicated and feasible. Additional vaccines may be licensed and recommended during the year. Licensed combination vaccines may be used whenever any components of the combination are indicated and other components of the vaccine are not contraindicated and if approved by the Food and Drug Administration for that dose of the series. Providers should consult the respective Advisory Committee on Immunization Practices statement for detailed recommendations. Clinically significant adverse events that follow immunization should be reported to the Vaccine Adverse Event Reporting System (VAERS). Guidance about how to obtain and complete a VAERS from is available at http://www.vaers.hhs.gov or by telephone, 800-822-7967.

CHICKENPOX VACCINE

WHAT YOU NEED TO KNOW

1 | Why get vaccinated?

Chickenpox (also called varicella) is a common childhood disease. It is usually mild, but it can be serious, especially in young infants and adults.

- It causes a rash, itching, fever, and tiredness.

- It can lead to severe skin infection, scars, pneumonia, brain damage, or death.

- The chickenpox virus can be spread from person to person through the air, or by contact with fluid from chickenpox blisters.

- A person who has had chickenpox can get a painful rash called shingles years later.

- Before the vaccine, about 11,000 people were hospitalized for chickenpox each year in the United States.

- Before the vaccine, about 100 people died each year as a result of chickenpox in the United States.

Chickenpox vaccine can prevent chickenpox.

Most people who get chickenpox vaccine will not get chickenpox. But if someone who has been vaccinated does get chickenpox, it is usually very mild. They will have fewer blisters, are less likely to have a fever, and will recover faster.

2 | Who should get chickenpox vaccine and when?

Routine

Children who have never had chickenpox should get 2 doses of chickenpox vaccine at these ages:

1st Dose: 12-15 months of age

2nd Dose: 4-6 years of age (may be given earlier, if at least 3 months after the 1st dose)

People 13 years of age and older (who have never had chickenpox or received chickenpox vaccine) should get two doses at least 28 days apart.

| Chickenpox | 1/10/07 |

Catch-Up

Children or adolescents who are not fully vaccinated should receive one or two doses of chickenpox vaccine. The timing of these doses depends on the person's age. Ask your provider.

Chickenpox vaccine may be given at the same time as other vaccines.

> Note: Chickenpox vaccine may be given along with measles-mumps-rubella (MMR) vaccine in a combination vaccine called MMRV.

3 | Some people should not get chickenpox vaccine or should wait

- People should not get chickenpox vaccine if they have ever had a life-threatening allergic reaction to gelatin, the antibiotic neomycin, or a previous dose of chickenpox vaccine.

- People who are moderately or severely ill at the time the shot is scheduled should usually wait until they recover before getting chickenpox vaccine.

- Pregnant women should wait to get chickenpox vaccine until after they have given birth. Women should not get pregnant for 1 month after getting chickenpox vaccine.

- Some people should check with their doctor about whether they should get chickenpox vaccine, including anyone who:
  - Has HIV/AIDS or another disease that affects the immune system
  - Is being treated with drugs that affect the immune system, such as steroids, for 2 weeks or longer
  - Has any kind of cancer
  - Is getting cancer treatment with radiation or drugs

- People who recently had a transfusion or were given other blood products should ask their doctor when they may get chickenpox vaccine.

Ask your doctor or nurse for more information.

4 What are the risks from chickenpox vaccine?

Getting chickenpox vaccine is much safer than getting chickenpox disease. Most people who get chickenpox vaccine do not have any problems with it.

However, a vaccine, like any medicine, is capable of causing serious problems, such as severe allergic reactions. The risk of chickenpox vaccine causing serious harm, or death, is extremely small.

Mild Problems

- Soreness or swelling where the shot was given (about 1 out of 5 children and up to 1 out of 3 adolescents and adults)

- Fever (1 person out of 10, or less)

- Mild rash, up to a month after vaccination (1 person out of 20, or less). It is possible for these people to infect other members of their household, but this is extremely rare.

> Note: MMRV vaccine has been associated with higher rates of fever (up to about 1 person in 5) and measles-like rash (about 1 person in 20) than MMR and varicella vaccines given separately.

Moderate Problems

- Seizure (jerking or staring) caused by fever (less than 1 person out of 1,000).

Severe Problems

- Pneumonia (very rare)

Other serious problems, including severe brain reactions and low blood count, have been reported after chickenpox vaccination. These happen so rarely experts cannot tell whether they are caused by the vaccine or not. If they are, it is extremely rare.

5 What if there is a moderate or severe reaction?

What should I look for?

- Any unusual condition, such as a high fever or behavior changes. Signs of a serious allergic reaction can include difficulty breathing, hoarseness or wheezing, hives, paleness, weakness, a fast heart beat or dizziness.

What should I do?

- Call a doctor, or get the person to a doctor right away.

- Tell your doctor what happened, the date and time it happened, and when the vaccination was given.

- Ask your doctor, nurse, or health department to report the reaction by filing a Vaccine Adverse Event Reporting System (VAERS) form. Or you can file this report through the VAERS website at **www.vaers.hhs.gov**, or by calling **1-800-822-7967**.

VAERS does not provide medical advice.

6 The National Vaccine Injury Compensation Program

A federal program has been created to help people who may have been harmed by a vaccine.

For details about the National Vaccine Injury Compensation Program, call **1-800-338-2382** or visit their website at **www.hrsa.gov/vaccinecompensation**.

7 How can I learn more?

- Ask your doctor or nurse. They can give you the vaccine package insert or suggest other sources of information.

- Call your local or state health department.

- Contact the Centers for Disease Control and Prevention (CDC):
  - Call **1-800-232-4636 (1-800-CDC-INFO)**
  - Visit CDC website at: **www.cdc.gov/nip**

DEPARTMENT OF HEALTH AND HUMAN SERVICES
CENTERS FOR DISEASE CONTROL AND PREVENTION

Vaccine Information Statement (Interim)
Varicella Vaccine (1/10/07)   42 U.S.C. §300aa-26

DIPHTHERIA TETANUS & PERTUSSIS VACCINES

WHAT YOU NEED TO KNOW

1 | Why get vaccinated?

Diphtheria, tetanus, and pertussis are serious diseases caused by bacteria. Diphtheria and pertussis are spread from person to person. Tetanus enters the body through cuts or wounds.

DIPHTHERIA causes a thick covering in the back of the throat.
- It can lead to breathing problems, paralysis, heart failure, and even death.

TETANUS (Lockjaw) causes painful tightening of the muscles, usually all over the body.
- It can lead to "locking" of the jaw so the victim cannot open his mouth or swallow. Tetanus leads to death in up to 2 out of 10 cases.

PERTUSSIS (Whooping Cough) causes coughing spells so bad that it is hard for infants to eat, drink, or breathe. These spells can last for weeks.
- It can lead to pneumonia, seizures (jerking and staring spells), brain damage, and death.

Diphtheria, tetanus, and pertussis vaccine (DTaP) can help prevent these diseases. Most children who are vaccinated with DTaP will be protected throughout childhood. Many more children would get these diseases if we stopped vaccinating.

DTaP is a safer version of an older vaccine called DTP. DTP is no longer used in the United States.

2 | Who should get DTaP vaccine and when?

Children should get 5 doses of DTaP vaccine, one dose at each of the following ages:

✓ 2 months   ✓ 4 months   ✓ 6 months
     ✓ 15-18 months   ✓ 4-6 years

DTaP may be given at the same time as other vaccines.

3 | Some children should not get DTaP vaccine or should wait

- Children with minor illnesses, such as a cold, may be vaccinated. But children who are moderately or severely ill should usually wait until they recover before getting DTaP vaccine.

- Any child who had a life-threatening allergic reaction after a dose of DTaP should not get another dose.

- Any child who suffered a brain or nervous system disease within 7 days after a dose of DTaP should not get another dose.

- Talk with your doctor if your child:
  - had a seizure or collapsed after a dose of DTaP,
  - cried non-stop for 3 hours or more after a dose of DTaP,
  - had a fever over 105°F after a dose of DTaP.

Ask your health care provider for more information. Some of these children should not get another dose of pertussis vaccine, but may get a vaccine without pertussis, called **DT**.

4 | Older children and adults

DTaP is not licensed for adolescents, adults, or children 7 years of age and older.

But older people still need protection. A vaccine called **Tdap** is similar to DTaP. A single dose of Tdap is recommended for people 11 through 64 years of age. Another vaccine, called **Td**, protects against tetanus and diphtheria, but not pertussis. It is recommended every 10 years. There are separate Vaccine Information Statements for these vaccines.

| Diphtheria/Tetanus/Pertussis | 5/17/2007 |

5 What are the risks from DTaP vaccine?

Getting diphtheria, tetanus, or pertussis disease is much riskier than getting DTaP vaccine.

However, a vaccine, like any medicine, is capable of causing serious problems, such as severe allergic reactions. The risk of DTaP vaccine causing serious harm, or death, is extremely small.

Mild Problems (Common)

- Fever (up to about 1 child in 4)
- Redness or swelling where the shot was given (up to about 1 child in 4)
- Soreness or tenderness where the shot was given (up to about 1 child in 4)

These problems occur more often after the 4th and 5th doses of the DTaP series than after earlier doses. Sometimes the 4th or 5th dose of DTaP vaccine is followed by swelling of the entire arm or leg in which the shot was given, lasting 1-7 days (up to about 1 child in 30).

Other mild problems include:

- Fussiness (up to about 1 child in 3)
- Tiredness or poor appetite (up to about 1 child in 10)
- Vomiting (up to about 1 child in 50)

These problems generally occur 1-3 days after the shot.

Moderate Problems (Uncommon)

- Seizure (jerking or staring) (about 1 child out of 14,000)
- Non-stop crying, for 3 hours or more (up to about 1 child out of 1,000)
- High fever, over 105°F (about 1 child out of 16,000)

Severe Problems (Very Rare)

- Serious allergic reaction (less than 1 out of a million doses)
- Several other severe problems have been reported after DTaP vaccine. These include:
  - Long-term seizures, coma, or lowered consciousness
  - Permanent brain damage.

  These are so rare it is hard to tell if they are caused by the vaccine.

Controlling fever is especially important for children who have had seizures, for any reason. It is also important if another family member has had seizures. You can reduce fever and pain by giving your child an *aspirin-free* pain reliever when the shot is given, and for the next 24 hours, following the package instructions.

6 What if there is a moderate or severe reaction?

What should I look for?

Any unusual conditions, such as a serious allergic reaction, high fever or unusual behavior. Serious allergic reactions are extremely rare with any vaccine. If one were to occur, it would most likely be within a few minutes to a few hours after the shot. Signs can include difficulty breathing, hoarseness or wheezing, hives, paleness, weakness, a fast heart beat or dizziness. If a high fever or seizure were to occur, it would usually be within a week after the shot.

What should I do?

- Call a doctor, or get the person to a doctor right away.
- Tell your doctor what happened, the date and time it happened, and when the vaccination was given.
- Ask your doctor, nurse, or health department to report the reaction by filing a Vaccine Adverse Event Reporting System (VAERS) form.

Or you can file this report through the VAERS web site at **www.vaers.hhs.gov**, or by calling **1-800-822-7967**. *VAERS does not provide medical advice*

7 The National Vaccine Injury Compensation Program

In the rare event that you or your child has a serious reaction to a vaccine, a federal program has been created to help pay for the care of those who have been harmed.

For details about the National Vaccine Injury Compensation Program, call **1-800-338-2382** or visit the program's website at **www.hrsa.gov/vaccinecompensation**.

8 How can I learn more?

- Ask your health care provider. They can give you the vaccine package insert or suggest other sources of information.
- Call your local or state health department's immunization program.
- Contact the Centers for Disease Control and Prevention (CDC):
  - Call **1-800-232-4636** (**1-800-CDC-INFO**)
  - Visit the National Immunization Program's website at **www.cdc.gov/nip**

U.S. DEPARTMENT OF HEALTH & HUMAN SERVICES
Centers for Disease Control and Prevention

Vaccine Information Statement	
DTaP (5/17/07)	42 U.S.C. § 300aa-26

INACTIVATED INFLUENZA VACCINE

(WHAT YOU NEED TO KNOW) 2006-07

1 | Why get vaccinated?

Influenza ("flu") is a contagious disease.

It is caused by the **influenza virus**, which spreads from person to person through coughing or sneezing.

Other illnesses have the same symptoms and are often mistaken for influenza. But only the influenza virus can cause influenza.

Anyone can get influenza. For most people, it lasts only a few days. It can cause:
- fever   · sore throat   · chills   · fatigue
- cough   · headache   · muscle aches

Some people get much sicker. Influenza can lead to pneumonia and can be dangerous for people with heart or breathing conditions. It can cause high fever and seizures in children. Influenza kills about 36,000 people each year in the United States, mostly among the elderly.

Influenza vaccine can prevent influenza.

2 | Inactivated Influenza vaccine

There are two types of influenza vaccine:

An **inactivated** (killed) vaccine, or "flu shot," has been used in the United States for many years. It is given by injection.

A **live**, weakened vaccine was licensed in 2003. It is sprayed into the nostrils. *This vaccine is described in a separate Vaccine Information Statement.*

Influenza viruses are always changing. Therefore, influenza vaccines are updated every year, and an annual vaccination is recommended.

For most people influenza vaccine prevents serious influenza-related illness. It will *not* prevent "influenza-like" illnesses caused by other viruses.

It takes about 2 weeks for protection to develop after the vaccination, and protection can last up to a year.

Inactivated influenza vaccine may be given at the same time as other vaccines, including pneumococcal vaccine.

Some inactivated influenza vaccine contains thimerosal, a preservative that contains mercury. Some people believe thimerosal may be related to developmental problems in children. In 2004 the Institute of Medicine published a report concluding that, based on scientific studies, there is no evidence of such a relationship. If you are concerned about thimerosal, ask your doctor about thimerosal-free influenza vaccine.

3 | Who should get inactivated influenza vaccine?

Inactivated influenza vaccine can be given to people 6 months of age and older. It is recommended for **people who are at risk of complications from influenza**, and for **people who can spread influenza to those at high risk** (including all household members):

People at high risk for complications from influenza:

- **People 65 years of age and older.**

- Residents of **long-term care facilities** housing persons with chronic medical conditions.

- People who have **long-term health problems** with:
  - heart disease   - kidney disease
  - lung disease   - metabolic disease, such as diabetes
  - asthma   - anemia, and other blood disorders

- People with certain **muscle or nerve disorders** (such as seizure disorders or severe cerebral palsy) that can lead to breathing or swallowing problems.

- People with a **weakened immune system** due to:
  - HIV/AIDS or other diseases affecting the immune system
  - long-term treatment with drugs such as steroids
  - cancer treatment with x-rays or drugs

- People 6 months to 18 years of age on **long-term aspirin treatment** (these people could develop Reye Syndrome if they got influenza).

- Women who will be **pregnant** during influenza season.

- **All children** 6-59 months of age.

People who can spread influenza to those at high risk:

- **Household contacts and out-of-home caretakers** of children from 0-59 months of age.

- Physicians, nurses, family members, or anyone else in **close contact with people at risk** of serious influenza.

Influenza vaccine is also recommended for adults 50-64 years of age and anyone else who wants to **reduce their chance of getting influenza.**

A yearly influenza vaccination should be *considered* for:

- People who provide **essential community services.**

- People living in **dormitories** or under other crowded conditions, to prevent outbreaks.

- People at high risk of influenza complications who **travel** to the Southern hemisphere between April and September, or to the tropics or in organized tourist groups at any time.

4 When should I get influenza vaccine?

The best time to get influenza vaccine is in **October** or **November**.

Influenza season usually peaks in February, but it can peak any time from November through May. So getting the vaccine in December, or even later, can be beneficial in most years.

Some people should get their flu shot in *October* or earlier:

- people **50 years of age and older**,
- younger people at **high risk** from influenza and its complications (including **children 6 through 59 months of age**),
- **household contacts** of people at high risk,
- **health care workers**, and
- **children younger than 9 years of age** getting influenza vaccine for the first time.

Most people need one flu shot each year. **Children younger than 9 years of age getting influenza vaccine for the first time should get 2 doses, given at least one month apart.**

5 Some people should talk with a doctor before getting influenza vaccine

Some people should not get inactivated influenza vaccine or should wait before getting it.

- Tell your doctor if you have any **severe** (life-threatening) allergies. Allergic reactions to influenza vaccine are rare.
  - Influenza vaccine virus is grown in eggs. People with a severe egg allergy should not get the vaccine.
  - A severe allergy to any vaccine component is also a reason to not get the vaccine.
  - If you have had a severe reaction after a previous dose of influenza vaccine, tell your doctor.

- Tell your doctor if you ever had Guillain-Barré Syndrome (a severe paralytic illness, also called GBS). You may be able to get the vaccine, but your doctor should help you make the decision.

- People who are moderately or severely ill should usually wait until they recover before getting flu vaccine. If you are ill, talk to your doctor or nurse about whether to reschedule the vaccination. People with a **mild illness** can usually get the vaccine.

6 What are the risks from inactivated influenza vaccine?

A vaccine, like any medicine, could possibly cause serious problems, such as severe allergic reactions. The risk of a vaccine causing serious harm, or death, is extremely small.

Serious problems from influenza vaccine are very rare. The viruses in inactivated influenza vaccine have been killed, so you cannot get influenza from the vaccine.

Mild problems:

- soreness, redness, or swelling where the shot was given
- fever   • aches

Vaccine Information Statement
Inactivated Influenza Vaccine (6/30/06)   42 U.S.C. §300aa-26

If these problems occur, they usually begin soon after the shot and last 1-2 days.

Severe problems:

- Life-threatening allergic reactions from vaccines are very rare. If they do occur, it is within a few minutes to a few hours after the shot.

- In 1976, a certain type of influenza (swine flu) vaccine was associated with Guillain-Barré Syndrome (GBS). Since then, flu vaccines have not been clearly linked to GBS. However, if there is a risk of GBS from current flu vaccines, it would be no more than 1 or 2 cases per million people vaccinated. This is much lower than the risk of severe influenza, which can be prevented by vaccination.

7 What if there is a severe reaction?

What should I look for?

- Any unusual condition, such as a high fever or behavior changes. Signs of a serious allergic reaction can include difficulty breathing, hoarseness or wheezing, hives, paleness, weakness, a fast heart beat or dizziness.

What should I do?

- Call a doctor, or get the person to a doctor right away.

- Tell your doctor what happened, the date and time it happened, and when the vaccination was given.

- Ask your doctor, nurse, or health department to report the reaction by filing a Vaccine Adverse Event Reporting System (VAERS) form.

  Or you can file this report through the VAERS web site at www.vaers.hhs.gov, or by calling 1-800-822-7967.

  VAERS does not provide medical advice.

8 The National Vaccine Injury Compensation Program

In the event that you or your child has a serious reaction to a vaccine, a federal program has been created to help pay for the care of those who have been harmed.

For details about the National Vaccine Injury Compensation Program, call **1-800-338-2382** or visit their website at **www.hrsa.gov/vaccinecompensation.**

9 How can I learn more?

- Ask your immunization provider. They can give you the vaccine package insert or suggest other sources of information.

- Call your local or state health department.

- Contact the Centers for Disease Control and Prevention (CDC):
  - Call **1-800-232-4636 (1-800-CDC-INFO)**
  - Visit CDC's website at **www.cdc.gov/flu**

DEPARTMENT OF HEALTH AND HUMAN SERVICES
CENTERS FOR DISEASE CONTROL AND PREVENTION
NATIONAL CENTER FOR IMMUNIZATION AND RESPIRATORY DISEASES

LIVE, INTRANASAL INFLUENZA VACCINE

(WHAT YOU NEED TO KNOW) 2006-07

1 | Why get vaccinated?

Influenza ("flu") is a contagious disease.

It is caused by the influenza virus, which spreads from infected persons to the nose or throat of others.

Other illnesses can have the same symptoms and are often mistaken for influenza. But only an illness caused by the influenza virus is really influenza.

Anyone can get influenza, but rates of infection are highest among children. For most people, it lasts only a few days. It can cause:
- fever
- sore throat
- chills
- fatigue
- cough
- headache
- muscle aches

Some people get much sicker. Influenza can lead to pneumonia and can be dangerous for people with heart or breathing conditions. It can cause high fever and seizures in children. Influenza kills about 36,000 people each year in the United States.

Influenza vaccine can prevent influenza.

2 | Live, attenuated influenza vaccine (nasal spray)

There are two types of influenza vaccine:

Live, attenuated influenza vaccine (LAIV) was licensed in 2003. LAIV contains live but attenuated (weakened) influenza virus. It is sprayed into the nostrils rather than injected into the muscle. It is recommended for healthy children and adults from 5 through 49 years of age, who are not pregnant.

Inactivated influenza vaccine, sometimes called the "flu shot," has been used for many years and is given by injection. *This vaccine is described in a separate Vaccine Information Statement.*

Influenza viruses are constantly changing. Therefore, influenza vaccines are updated every year, and annual vaccination is recommended.

For most people influenza vaccine prevents serious influenza-related illness. It will *not* prevent "influenza-like" illnesses caused by other viruses.

It takes about 2 weeks for protection to develop after vaccination, and protection can last up to a year.

3 | Who can get LAIV?

Live, intranasal influenza vaccine is approved for **healthy children and adults from 5 through 49 years of age**, including those who can spread influenza to people at high risk, such as:

- **Household contacts and out-of-home care-takers** of children from 0-59 months of age.

- Physicians and nurses, and family members or any one else in **close contact with people at risk** of serious influenza.

Influenza vaccine is also recommended for anyone else who wants to **reduce their chance of getting influenza.**

LAIV may be considered for:

- People who provide **essential community services.**

- People living in **dormitories** or under other crowded conditions, to prevent outbreaks.

4 | Who should *not* get LAIV?

LAIV is not licensed for everyone. The following people should check with their health-care provider about getting the **inactivated** vaccine (flu shot).

- **Adults 50 years of age or older** or **children younger than 5.**

- People who have **long-term health problems** with:
  - heart disease
  - lung disease
  - asthma
  - kidney disease
  - metabolic disease, such as diabetes
  - anemia, and other blood disorders

- People with a **weakened immune system.**

- Children or adolescents on **long-term aspirin treatment.**

- **Pregnant women.**

- Anyone with a history of **Guillain-Barré syndrome** (a severe paralytic illness, also called GBS).

Inactivated influenza vaccine (the flu shot) is the preferred vaccine for people (including health-care workers, and family members) coming in **close contact with anyone who has a severely weakened immune system** (that is, anyone who requires care in a protected environment).

Some people should talk with a doctor before getting *either* influenza vaccine:

- Anyone who has ever had a <u>serious</u> allergic reaction to **eggs** or to a **previous dose** of influenza vaccine.

- People who are moderately or severely ill should usually wait until they recover before getting flu vaccine. If you are ill, talk to your doctor or nurse about whether to reschedule the vaccination. People with a **mild illness** can usually get the vaccine.

5 When should I get influenza vaccine?

The best time to get influenza vaccine is in **October** or **November**, but LAIV may be given as soon as it is available. Influenza season usually peaks in February, but it can peak any time from November through May. So getting the vaccine in December, or even later, can be beneficial in most years.

Most people need one dose of influenza vaccine each year. **Children younger than 9 years of age getting influenza vaccine for the first time** should get 2 doses For LAIV, these doses should be given 6-10 weeks apart.

LAIV may be given at the same time as other vaccines.

6 What are the risks from LAIV?

A vaccine, like any medicine, could possibly cause serious problems, such as severe allergic reactions. However, the risk of a vaccine causing serious harm, or death, is extremely small.

Live influenza vaccine viruses rarely spread from person to person. Even if they do, they are not likely to cause illness.

LAIV is made from weakened virus and does not cause influenza. The vaccine *can* cause mild symptoms in people who get it (see below).

Mild problems:
Some children and adolescents 5-17 years of age have reported mild reactions, including:
- runny nose, nasal congestion or cough
- headache and muscle aches   • fever
- abdominal pain or occasional vomiting or diarrhea

Some adults 18-49 years of age have reported:
- runny nose or nasal congestion   • sore throat
- cough, chills, tiredness/weakness • headache

These symptoms did not last long and went away on their own. Although they can occur after vaccination, they may not have been caused by the vaccine.

Severe problems:
- Life-threatening allergic reactions from vaccines are very rare. If they do occur, it is within a few minutes to a few hours after the vaccination.

- If rare reactions occur with any new product, they may not be identified until thousands, or millions, of people have used it. Over four million doses of LAIV have been distributed since it was licensed, and no serious problems have been identified. Like all vaccines, LAIV will continue to be monitored for unusual or severe problems.

7 What if there is a severe reaction?

What should I look for?
- Any unusual condition, such as a high fever or behavior changes. Signs of a serious allergic reaction can include difficulty breathing, hoarseness or wheezing, hives, paleness, weakness, a fast heart beat or dizziness.

What should I do?
- **Call** a doctor, or get the person to a doctor right away.

- **Tell** your doctor what happened, the date and time it happened, and when the vaccination was given.

- **Ask** your doctor, nurse, or health department to report the reaction by filing a Vaccine Adverse Event Reporting System (VAERS) form.

Or you can file this report through the VAERS website at www.vaers.hhs.gov, or by calling 1-800-822-7967.

VAERS does not provide medical advice.

8 The National Vaccine Injury Compensation Program

In the event that you or your child has a serious reaction to a vaccine, a federal program has been created to help pay for the care of those who have been harmed.

For details about the National Vaccine Injury Compensation Program, call **1-800-338-2382** or visit their website at **www.hrsa.gov/vaccinecompensation.**

9 How can I learn more?

- Ask your immunization provider. They can give you the vaccine package insert or suggest other sources of information.

- Call your local or state health department.

- Contact the Centers for Disease Control and Prevention (CDC):
  - Call **1-800-232-4636 (1-800-CDC-INFO)**
  - Visit CDC's website at **www.cdc.gov/flu**

DEPARTMENT OF HEALTH AND HUMAN SERVICES
CENTERS FOR DISEASE CONTROL AND PREVENTION
NATIONAL CENTER FOR IMMUNIZATION AND RESPIRATORY DISEASES

Vaccine Information Statement
Live, Attenuated Influenza Vaccine (6/30/06)   42 U.S.C. §300aa-26

HEPATITIS B VACCINE

W H A T   Y O U   N E E D   T O   K N O W

1 | Why get vaccinated?

Hepatitis B is a serious disease.
The hepatitis B virus (HBV) can cause short-term
(acute) illness that leads to:
- loss of appetite   • diarrhea and vomiting
- tiredness   • jaundice (yellow skin or eyes)
- pain in muscles, joints, and stomach

It can also cause long-term (chronic) illness that leads
to:
- liver damage (cirrhosis)
- liver cancer
- death

About 1.25 million people in the U.S. have chronic
HBV infection.

Each year it is estimated that:
- 80,000 people, mostly young adults, get infected
  with HBV
- More than 11,000 people have to stay in the hospital
  because of hepatitis B
- 4,000 to 5,000 people die from chronic hepatitis B

Hepatitis B vaccine can prevent hepatitis B. It is
the first anti-cancer vaccine because it can prevent a
form of liver cancer.

2 | How is hepatitis B virus spread?

Hepatitis B virus is spread through contact with the
blood and body fluids of an infected person. A person
can get infected in several ways, such as:
- by having unprotected sex with an infected person
- by sharing needles when injecting illegal drugs
- by being stuck with a used needle on the job
- during birth when the virus passes from an infected
  mother to her baby

About 1/3 of people who are infected with hepatitis B
in the United States don't know how they got it.

Hepatitis B	7/11/2001

3 | Who should get hepatitis B vaccine and when?

1) Everyone 18 years of age and younger
2) Adults over 18 who are at risk

Adults at risk for HBV infection include:
- people who have more than one sex partner in 6 months
- men who have sex with other men
- sex contacts of infected people
- people who inject illegal drugs
- health care and public safety workers who might be
  exposed to infected blood or body fluids
- household contacts of persons with chronic HBV
  infection
- hemodialysis patients

If you are not sure whether you are at risk, ask your
doctor or nurse.

✓ **People should get 3 doses of hepatitis B vaccine
  according to the following schedule.** *If you miss
  a dose or get behind schedule, get the next dose as
  soon as you can. There is no need to start over.*

Hepatitis B Vaccination Schedule		WHO?		
		Infant whose mother is infected with HBV	Infant whose mother is *not* infected with HBV	Older child, adolescent, or adult
W H E N ?	First Dose	Within 12 hours of birth	Birth - 2 months of age	Any time
	Second Dose	1 - 2 months of age	1 - 4 months of age (at least 1 month after first dose)	1 - 2 months after first dose
	Third Dose	6 months of age	6 - 18 months of age	4 - 6 months after first dose

- The second dose must be given at least 1 month after the first dose.
- The third dose must be given at least 2 months after the second dose
  and at least 4 months after the first.
- The third dose should *not* be given to infants under 6 months of age,
  because this could reduce long-term protection.

Adolescents 11 to 15 years of age may need only two
doses of hepatitis B vaccine, separated by 4-6 months.
Ask your health care provider for details.

Hepatitis B vaccine may be given at the same time as
other vaccines.

4 Some people should not get hepatitis B vaccine or should wait

People should not get hepatitis B vaccine if they have ever had a life-threatening allergic reaction to **baker's yeast** (the kind used for making bread) or to **a previous dose of hepatitis B vaccine.**

People who are moderately or severely ill at the time the shot is scheduled should usually wait until they recover before getting hepatitis B vaccine.

Ask your doctor or nurse for more information.

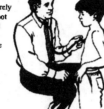

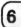 **5 What are the risks from hepatitis B vaccine?**

A vaccine, like any medicine, is capable of causing serious problems, such as severe allergic reactions. The risk of hepatitis B vaccine causing serious harm, or death, is extremely small.

Getting hepatitis B vaccine is much safer than getting hepatitis B disease.

Most people who get hepatitis B vaccine do not have any problems with it.

Mild problems
- soreness where the shot was given, lasting a day or two (up to 1 out of 11 children and adolescents, and about 1 out of 4 adults)
- mild to moderate fever (up to 1 out of 14 children and adolescents and 1 out of 100 adults)

Severe problems
- serious allergic reaction (very rare)

6 What if there is a moderate or severe reaction?

What should I look for?

Any unusual condition, such as a serious allergic reaction, high fever or unusual behavior. Serious allergic

reactions are extremely rare with any vaccine. If one were to occur, it would be within a few minutes to a few hours after the shot. Signs can include difficulty breathing, hoarseness or wheezing, hives, paleness, weakness, a fast heart beat or dizziness.

What should I do?

- **Call** a doctor, or get the person to a doctor right away.
- **Tell** your doctor what happened, the date and time it happened, and when the vaccination was given.
- **Ask** your doctor, nurse, or health department to report the reaction by filing a Vaccine Adverse Event Reporting System (VAERS) form.

Or you can file this report through the VAERS web site at www.vaers.org, or by calling 1-800-822-7967.

VAERS does not provide medical advice

 7 The National Vaccine Injury Compensation Program

In the rare event that you or your child has a serious reaction to a vaccine, a federal program has been created to help you pay for the care of those who have been harmed.

For details about the National Vaccine Injury Compensation Program, call **1-800-338-2382** or visit the program's website at **www.hrsa.gov/osp/vicp**

 8 How can I learn more?

- Ask your doctor or nurse. They can give you the vaccine package insert or suggest other sources of information.
- Call your local or state health department's immunization program.
- Contact the Centers for Disease Control and Prevention (CDC):
  - Call **1-800-232-4636** (1-800-CDC-INFO) or **1-888-443-7232**
  - Visit the National Immunization Program's website at **www.cdc.gov/nip** or CDC's Division of Viral Hepatitis website at **www.cdc.gov/hepatitis**

U.S. DEPARTMENT OF HEALTH & HUMAN SERVICES
Centers for Disease Control and Prevention
National Immunization Program

Vaccine Information Statement
Hepatitis B (7/11/01)   42 U.S.C. § 300aa-26

Haemophilus Influenzae Type b (Hib) Vaccine

WHAT YOU NEED TO KNOW

1 | What is Hib disease?

Haemophilus influenzae type b (Hib) disease is a serious disease caused by a bacteria. It usually strikes children under 5 years old.

Your child can get Hib disease by being around other children or adults who may have the bacteria and not know it. The germs spread from person to person. If the germs stay in the child's nose and throat, the child probably will not get sick. But sometimes the germs spread into the lungs or the bloodstream, and then Hib can cause serious problems.

Before Hib vaccine, Hib disease was the leading cause of bacterial meningitis among children under 5 years old in the United States. Meningitis is an infection of the brain and spinal cord coverings, which can lead to lasting brain damage and deafness. Hib disease can also cause:

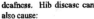

- pneumonia
- severe swelling in the throat, making it hard to breathe
- infections of the blood, joints, bones, and covering of the heart
- death

Before Hib vaccine, about 20,000 children in the United States under 5 years old got severe Hib disease each year and nearly 1,000 people died.

Hib vaccine can prevent Hib disease.
Many more children would get Hib disease if we stopped vaccinating.

2 | Who should get Hib vaccine and when?

Children should get Hib vaccine at:
- ✓ 2 months of age
- ✓ 4 months of age
- ✓ 6 months of age*
- ✓ 12-15 months of age

* Depending on what brand of Hib vaccine is used, your child might not need the dose at 6 months of age. Your doctor or nurse will tell you if this dose is needed.

If you miss a dose or get behind schedule, get the next dose as soon as you can. There is no need to start over.

Hib vaccine may be given at the same time as other vaccines.

Older Children and Adults
Children over 5 years old usually do not need Hib vaccine. But some older children or adults with special health conditions should get it. These conditions include sickle cell disease, HIV/AIDS, removal of the spleen, bone marrow transplant, or cancer treatment with drugs. Ask your doctor or nurse for details.

3 | Some people should not get Hib vaccine or should wait

- People who have ever had a life-threatening allergic reaction to a previous dose of Hib vaccine should not get another dose.

- Children less than 6 weeks of age should not get Hib vaccine.

- People who are moderately or severely ill at the time the shot is scheduled should usually wait until they recover before getting Hib vaccine.

Ask your doctor or nurse for more information.

4 What are the risks from Hib vaccine?

A vaccine, like any medicine, is capable of causing serious problems, such as severe allergic reactions. The risk of Hib vaccine causing serious harm or death is extremely small.

Most people who get Hib vaccine do not have any problems with it.

Mild Problems

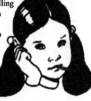

- Redness, warmth, or swelling where the shot was given (up to 1/4 of children)
- Fever over 101°F (up to 1 out of 20 children)

If these problems happen, they usually start within a day of vaccination. They may last 2-3 days.

5 What if there is a moderate or severe reaction?

What should I look for?

Any unusual condition, such as a serious allergic reaction, high fever or behavior changes. Signs of a serious allergic reaction can include difficulty breathing, hoarseness or wheezing, hives, paleness, weakness, a fast heart beat, or dizziness within a few minutes to a few hours after the shot.

What should I do?

- **Call** a doctor, or get the person to a doctor right away.
- **Tell** your doctor what happened, the date and time it happened, and when the vaccination was given.
- **Ask** your doctor, nurse, or health department to report the reaction by filing a Vaccine Adverse Event Reporting System (VAERS) form.

Or you can file this report through the VAERS web site at www.vaers.org, or by calling 1-800-822-7967.

VAERS does not provide medical advice

6 The National Vaccine Injury Compensation Program

In the rare event that you or your child has a serious reaction to a vaccine, a federal program has been created to help you pay for the care of those who have been harmed.

For details about the National Vaccine Injury Compensation Program, call **1-800-338-2382** or visit the program's website at **www.hrsa.gov/osp/vicp**

7 How can I learn more?

- Ask your doctor or nurse. They can give you the vaccine package insert or suggest other sources of information.
- Call your local or state health department's immunization program.
- Contact the Centers for Disease Control and Prevention (CDC):
  - Call **1-800-232-4636 (1-800-CDC-INFO)**
  - Visit the National Immunization Program's website at **www.cdc.gov/nip**

U.S. DEPARTMENT OF HEALTH & HUMAN SERVICES
Centers for Disease Control and Prevention
National Immunization Program

Vaccine Information Statement

Hib (12/16/98)   42 U.S.C. § 300aa-26

HPV (HUMAN PAPILLOMAVIRUS) VACCINE

WHAT YOU NEED TO KNOW

1 | What is HPV?

Genital human papillomavirus (HPV) is the most common sexually transmitted virus in the United States.

There are about 40 types of HPV. About 20 million people in the U.S. are infected, and about 6.2 million more get infected each year. HPV is spread through sexual contact.

Most HPV infections don't cause any symptoms, and go away on their own. But HPV is important mainly because it can cause **cervical cancer** in women. Every year in the U.S. about 10,000 women get cervical cancer and 3,700 die from it. It is the 2nd leading cause of cancer deaths among women around the world.

HPV is also associated with several less common types of cancer in both men and women. It can also cause genital warts and warts in the upper respiratory tract.

More than 50% of sexually active men and women are infected with HPV at sometime in their lives.

There is no treatment for HPV infection, but the conditions it causes can be treated.

2 | HPV Vaccine - Why get vaccinated?

HPV vaccine is an inactivated (not live) vaccine which protects against 4 major types of HPV.

These include 2 types that cause about 70% of cervical cancer and 2 types that cause about 90% of genital warts. *HPV vaccine can prevent most genital warts and most cases of cervical cancer.*

Protection from HPV vaccine is expected to be long-lasting. But vaccinated women still need cervical cancer screening because the vaccine does not protect against all HPV types that cause cervical cancer.

3 | Who should get HPV vaccine and when?

Routine Vaccination

- HPV vaccine is routinely recommended for girls **11-12 years of age.** Doctors may give it to girls as young as 9 years.

Why is HPV vaccine given to girls at this age? It is important for girls to get HPV vaccine **before** their first sexual contact – because they have not been exposed to HPV. For these girls, the vaccine can prevent almost 100% of disease caused by the 4 types of HPV targeted by the vaccine.

However, if a girl or woman is already infected with a type of HPV, the vaccine will not prevent disease from that type.

Catch-Up Vaccination

- The vaccine is also recommended for girls and women **13-26 years of age** who did not receive it when they were younger.

HPV vaccine is given as a 3-dose series:

1st Dose:	Now
2nd Dose:	2 months after Dose 1
3rd Dose:	6 months after Dose 1

Additional (booster) doses are not recommended.

HPV vaccine may be given at the same time as other vaccines.

4 | Some girls or women should not get HPV vaccine or should wait

- Anyone who has ever had a life-threatening allergic reaction to yeast, to any other component of HPV vaccine, or to a previous dose of HPV vaccine should not get the vaccine. Tell your doctor if the person getting the vaccine has any severe allergies.

HPV Vaccine	2/2/2007

- **Pregnant women** should not get the vaccine. The vaccine appears to be safe for both the mother and the unborn baby, but it is still being studied. Receiving HPV vaccine when pregnant is **not** a reason to consider terminating the pregnancy. Women who are breast feeding may safely get the vaccine.

> Any woman who learns that she was pregnant when she got HPV vaccine is encouraged to call the
> **HPV vaccine in pregnancy registry** at 800-986-8999.
>
> Information from this registry will help us learn how pregnant women respond to the vaccine.

- People who are mildly ill when the shot is scheduled can still get HPV vaccine. People with **moderate or severe illnesses** should wait until they recover.

5 | What are the risks from HPV vaccine?

HPV vaccine does not appear to cause any serious side effects.

However, a vaccine, like any medicine, could possibly cause serious problems, such as severe allergic reactions. The risk of **any** vaccine causing serious harm, or death, is extremely small.

Several **mild problems** may occur with HPV vaccine:

- Pain at the injection site (about 8 people in 10)
- Redness or swelling at the injection site (about 1 person in 4)
- Mild fever (100°F) (about 1 person in 10)
- Itching at the injection site (about 1 person in 30)
- Moderate fever (102°F) (about 1 person in 65)

These symptoms do not last long and go away on their own.

Life-threatening allergic reactions from vaccines are very rare. If they do occur, it would be within a few minutes to a few hours after the vaccination.

Like all vaccines, HPV vaccine will continue to be monitored for unusual or severe problems.

6 | What if there is a severe reaction?

What should I look for?

- Any unusual condition, such as a high fever or behavior changes. Signs of a serious allergic reaction can include difficulty breathing, hoarseness or wheezing, hives, paleness, weakness, a fast heart beat or dizziness.

What should I do?

- **Call** a doctor, or get the person to a doctor right away.

- **Tell** your doctor what happened, the date and time it happened, and when the vaccination was given.

- **Ask** your doctor, nurse, or health department to report the reaction by filing a Vaccine Adverse Event Reporting System (VAERS) form.

Or you can file this report through the VAERS website at www.vaers.hhs.gov, or by calling 1-800-822-7967.

VAERS does not provide medical advice.

7 | How can I learn more?

- Ask your doctor or nurse. They can show you the vaccine package insert or suggest other sources of information.

- Call your local or state health department.

- Contact the Centers for Disease Control and Prevention (CDC):
  - Call **1-800-232-4636 (1-800-CDC-INFO)**
  - Visit CDC's website at **www.cdc.gov/std/hpv** and **www.cdc.gov/nip**.

DEPARTMENT OF HEALTH AND HUMAN SERVICES
CENTERS FOR DISEASE CONTROL AND PREVENTION
NATIONAL CENTER FOR IMMUNIZATION AND RESPIRATORY DISEASES

Vaccine Information Statement (Interim)
Human Papillomavirus (HPV) Vaccine   2/2/07

MENINGOCOCCAL VACCINES

WHAT YOU NEED TO KNOW

1 What is meningococcal disease?

Meningococcal disease is a serious illness, caused by a bacteria. It is a leading cause of bacterial meningitis in children 2-18 years old in the United States.

Meningitis is an infection of fluid surrounding the brain and the spinal cord. Meningococcal disease also causes blood infections.

About 2,600 people get meningococcal disease each year in the U.S. 10-15% of these people die, in spite of treatment with antibiotics. Of those who live, another 11-19% lose their arms or legs, become deaf, have problems with their nervous systems, become mentally retarded, or suffer seizures or strokes.

Anyone can get meningococcal disease. But it is most common in infants less than one year of age and people with certain medical conditions, such as lack of a spleen. College freshmen who live in dormitories have an increased risk of getting meningococcal disease.

Meningococcal infections can be treated with drugs such as penicillin. Still, about 1 out of every ten people who get the disease dies from it, and many others are affected for life. This is why *preventing* the disease through use of meningococcal vaccine is important for people at highest risk.

2 Meningococcal vaccine

Two meningococcal vaccines are available in the U.S.:

- **Meningococcal polysaccharide vaccine (MPSV4)** has been available since the 1970s.
- **Meningococcal conjugate vaccine (MCV4)** was licensed in 2005.

Both vaccines can prevent **4 types** of meningococcal disease, including 2 of the 3 types most common in the United States and a type that causes epidemics in Africa. Meningococcal vaccines cannot prevent all types of the disease. But they do protect many people who might become sick if they didn't get the vaccine.

Both vaccines work well, and protect about 90% of those who get it. MCV4 is expected to give better, longer-lasting protection.

MCV4 should also be better at preventing the disease from spreading from person to person.

3 Who should get meningococcal vaccine and when?

MCV4 is recommended for all children at their routine preadolescent visit (11-12 years of age). For those who have never gotten MCV4 previously, a dose is recommended at high school entry.

Other adolescents who want to decrease their risk of meningococcal disease can also get the vaccine.

Meningococcal vaccine is also recommended for other people at increased risk for meningococcal disease:

- College freshmen living in dormitories.

- Microbiologists who are routinely exposed to meningococcal bacteria.

- U.S. military recruits.

- Anyone traveling to, or living in, a part of the world where meningococcal disease is common, such as parts of Africa.

- Anyone who has a damaged spleen, or whose spleen has been removed.

- Anyone who has terminal complement component deficiency (an immune system disorder).

- People who might have been exposed to meningitis during an outbreak.

MCV4 is the preferred vaccine for people 11-55 years of age in these risk groups, but MPSV4 can be used if MCV4 is not available. MPSV4 should be used for children 2-10 years old, and adults over 55, who are at risk.

How Many Doses?

People 2 years of age and older should get 1 dose. (Sometimes an additional dose is recommended for people who remain at high risk. Ask your provider.)

MPSV4 may be recommended for children 3 months to 2 years of age under special circumstances. These children should get 2 doses, 3 months apart.

4 Some people should not get meningococcal vaccine or should wait

- Anyone who has ever had a severe (life-threatening) allergic reaction to a previous dose of either meningococcal vaccine should not get another dose.

- Anyone who has a severe (life threatening) allergy to any vaccine component should not get the vaccine. Tell your doctor if you have any severe allergics.

- Anyone who is moderately or severely ill at the time the shot is scheduled should probably wait until they recover. Ask your doctor or nurse. People with a mild illness can usually get the vaccine.

- Anyone who has ever had Guillain-Barré Syndrome should talk with their doctor before getting MCV4.

- Meningococcal vaccines may be given to pregnant women. However, MCV4 is a new vaccine and has not been studied in pregnant women as much as MPSV4 has. It should be used only if clearly needed.

- Meningococcal vaccines may be given at the same time as other vaccines.

5 What are the risks from meningococcal vaccines?

A vaccine, like any medicine, could possibly cause serious problems, such as severe allergic reactions. The risk of meningococcal vaccine causing serious harm, or death, is extremely small.

Mild problems

Up to about half of people who get meningococcal vaccines have mild side effects, such as redness or pain where the shot was given.

If these problems occur, they usually last for 1 or 2 days. They are more common after MCV4 than after MPSV4.

A small percentage of people who receive the vaccine develop a fever.

Meningococcal   11/16/06   Vaccine Information Statement(Interim)

Severe problems

- Serious allergic reactions, within a few minutes to a few hours of the shot, are very rare.

- A serious nervous system disorder called Guillain-Barré Syndrome (or GBS) has been reported among some people who received MCV4. This happens so rarely that it is currently not possible to tell if the vaccine might be a factor. Even if it is, the risk is very small.

6 What if there is a moderate or severe reaction?

What should I look for?

- Any unusual condition, such as a high fever or behavior changes. Signs of a serious allergic reaction can include difficulty breathing, hoarseness or wheezing, hives, paleness, weakness, a fast heart beat or dizziness.

What should I do?

- Call a doctor, or get the person to a doctor right away.

- Tell your doctor what happened, the date and time it happened, and when the vaccination was given.

- Ask your doctor, nurse, or health department to report the reaction by filing a Vaccine Adverse Event Reporting System (VAERS) form.

Or you can file this report through the VAERS web site at www.vaers.org, or by calling 1-800-822-7967.

VAERS does not provide medical advice.

7 How can I learn more?

- Ask your doctor or nurse. They can give you the vaccine package insert or suggest other sources of information.

- Call your local or state health department.

- Contact the Centers for Disease Control and Prevention (CDC):
  - Call 1-800-232-4636 (1-800-CDC-INFO)
  - Visit CDC's National Immunization Program website at www.cdc.gov/nip
  - Visit CDC's meningococcal disease website at www.cdc.gov/ncidod/dbmd/diseaseinfo/meningococcal_g.htm
  - Visit CDC's Travelers' Health website at www.cdc.gov/travel

DEPARTMENT OF HEALTH AND HUMAN SERVICES
CENTERS FOR DISEASE CONTROL AND PREVENTION

MEASLES MUMPS & RUBELLA VACCINES

WHAT YOU NEED TO KNOW

1 | Why get vaccinated?

Measles, mumps, and rubella are serious diseases.

Measles
- Measles virus causes rash, cough, runny nose, eye irritation, and fever.
- It can lead to ear infection, pneumonia, seizures (jerking and staring), brain damage, and death.

Mumps
- Mumps virus causes fever, headache, and swollen glands.
- It can lead to deafness, meningitis (infection of the brain and spinal cord covering), painful swelling of the testicles or ovaries, and, rarely, death.

Rubella (German Measles)
- Rubella virus causes rash, mild fever, and arthritis (mostly in women).
- If a woman gets rubella while she is pregnant, she could have a miscarriage or her baby could be born with serious birth defects.

You or your child could catch these diseases by being around someone who has them. They spread from person to person through the air.

Measles, mumps, and rubella (MMR) vaccine can prevent these diseases.

Most children who get their MMR shots will not get these diseases. Many more children would get them if we stopped vaccinating.

2 | Who should get MMR vaccine and when?

Children should get 2 doses of MMR vaccine:

✓ The first at **12-15 months of age**
✓ and the second at **4-6 years of age**.

These are the recommended ages. But children can get the second dose at any age, as long as it is at least 28 days after the first dose.

Some **adults** should also get MMR vaccine: Generally, anyone 18 years of age or older, who was born after 1956, should get at least one dose of MMR vaccine, unless they can show that they have had either the vaccines or the diseases.

Ask your doctor or nurse for more information.

MMR vaccine may be given at the same time as other vaccines.

3 | Some people should not get MMR vaccine or should wait

- People should not get MMR vaccine who have ever had a life-threatening allergic reaction to **gelatin**, the antibiotic **neomycin**, or to a **previous dose of MMR vaccine**.

- People who are moderately or severely ill at the time the shot is scheduled should usually wait until they recover before getting MMR vaccine.

- Pregnant women should wait to get MMR vaccine until after they have given birth. Women should avoid getting pregnant for 4 weeks after getting MMR vaccine.

- Some people should check with their doctor about whether they should get MMR vaccine, including anyone who:
  - Has HIV/AIDS, or another disease that affects the immune system
  - Is being treated with drugs that affect the immune system, such as steroids, for 2 weeks or longer.
  - Has any kind of cancer
  - Is taking cancer treatment with x-rays or drugs
  - Has ever had a low platelet count (a blood disorder)
    Over . . .

- People who recently had a transfusion or were given other blood products should ask their doctor when they may get MMR vaccine

Ask your doctor or nurse for more information.

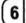

4 What are the risks from MMR vaccine?

A vaccine, like any medicine, is capable of causing serious problems, such as severe allergic reactions. The risk of MMR vaccine causing serious harm, or death, is extremely small.

Getting MMR vaccine is much safer than getting any of these three diseases.

Most people who get MMR vaccine do not have any problems with it.

Mild Problems
- Fever (up to 1 person out of 6)
- Mild rash (about 1 person out of 20)
- Swelling of glands in the cheeks or neck (rare)
If these problems occur, it is usually within 7-12 days after the shot. They occur less often after the second dose.

Moderate Problems
- Seizure (jerking or staring) caused by fever (about 1 out of 3,000 doses)
- Temporary pain and stiffness in the joints, mostly in teenage or adult women (up to 1 out of 4)
- Temporary low platelet count, which can cause a bleeding disorder (about 1 out of 30,000 doses)

Severe Problems (Very Rare)
- Serious allergic reaction (less than 1 out of a million doses)
- Several other severe problems have been known to occur after a child gets MMR vaccine. But this happens so rarely, experts cannot be sure whether they are caused by the vaccine or not. These include:
  - Deafness
  - Long-term seizures, coma, or lowered consciousness
  - Permanent brain damage

5 What if there is a moderate or severe reaction?

What should I look for?

Any unusual conditions, such as a serious allergic reaction, high fever or behavior changes. Signs of a

serious allergic reaction include difficulty breathing, hoarseness or wheezing, hives, paleness, weakness, a fast heart beat or dizziness within a few minutes to a few hours after the shot. A high fever or seizure, if it occurs, would happen 1 or 2 weeks after the shot.

What should I do?
- **Call** a doctor, or get the person to a doctor right away.
- **Tell** your doctor what happened, the date and time it happened, and when the vaccination was given.
- **Ask** your doctor, nurse, or health department to report the reaction by filing a Vaccine Adverse Event Reporting System (VAERS) form. Or you can file this report through the VAERS web site at www.vaers.org, or by calling 1-800-822-7967.
  VAERS does not provide medical advice.

6 The National Vaccine Injury Compensation Program

In the rare event that you or your child has a serious reaction to a vaccine, a federal program has been created to help you pay for the care of those who have been harmed.

For details about the National Vaccine Injury Compensation Program, call 1-800-338-2382 or visit the program's website at www.hrsa.gov/osp/vicp

7 How can I learn more?

- Ask your doctor or nurse. They can give you the vaccine package insert or suggest other sources of information.

- Call your local or state health department's immunization program.

- Contact the Centers for Disease Control and Prevention (CDC):
  - Call 1-800-232-4636 (1-800-CDC-INFO)
  - Visit the National Immunization Program's website at www.cdc.gov/nip

U.S. DEPARTMENT OF HEALTH & HUMAN SERVICES
Centers for Disease Control and Prevention
National Immunization Program

Vaccine Information Statement
MMR (1/15/03)   42 U.S.C. § 300aa-26

PNEUMOCOCCAL CONJUGATE VACCINE

WHAT YOU NEED TO KNOW

1 | Why get vaccinated?

Infection with *Streptococcus pneumoniae* bacteria can cause serious illness and death. Invasive pneumococcal disease is responsible for about 200 deaths each year among children under 5 years old. It is the leading cause of bacterial meningitis in the United States. (Meningitis is an infection of the covering of the brain).

Pneumococcal infection causes severe disease in children under five years old. Before a vaccine was available, each year pneumococcal infection caused:

- over 700 cases of meningitis,
- 13,000 blood infections, and
- about 5 million ear infections.

It can also lead to other health problems, including:

- pneumonia,
- deafness,
- brain damage.

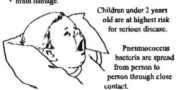

Children under 2 years old are at highest risk for serious disease.

Pneumococcus bacteria are spread from person to person through close contact.

Pneumococcal infections can be hard to treat because the bacteria have become resistant to some of the drugs that have been used to treat them. This makes **prevention** of pneumococcal infections even more important.

Pneumococcal conjugate vaccine can help prevent serious pneumococcal disease, such as meningitis and blood infections. It can also prevent some ear infections. But ear infections have many causes, and pneumococcal vaccine is effective against only some of them.

2 | Pneumococcal conjugate vaccine

Pneumococcal conjugate vaccine is approved for infants and toddlers. Children who are vaccinated when they are infants will be protected when they are at greatest risk for serious disease.

Some older children and adults may get a different vaccine called pneumococcal polysaccharide vaccine. There is a separate Vaccine Information Statement for people getting this vaccine.

3 | Who should get the vaccine and when?

- **Children Under 2 Years of Age**

The routine schedule for pneumococcal conjugate vaccine is 4 doses, one dose at each of these ages:

- ✓ 2 months
- ✓ 4 months
- ✓ 6 months
- ✓ 12-15 months

Children who weren't vaccinated at these ages can still get the vaccine. The number of doses needed depends on the child's age. Ask your health care provider for details.

- **Children Between 2 and 5 Years of Age**

Pneumococcal conjugate vaccine is also recommended for children between 2 and 5 years old who have not already gotten the vaccine and are at high risk of serious pneumococcal disease. This includes children who:

- have sickle cell disease,
- have a damaged spleen or no spleen,
- have HIV/AIDS,
- have other diseases that affect the immune system, such as diabetes, cancer, or liver disease, or who
- take medications that affect the immune system, such as chemotherapy or steroids, or
- have chronic heart or lung disease.

The vaccine should be considered for all other children under 5 years, especially those at higher risk of serious pneumococcal disease. This includes children who:

- are under 3 years of age,
- are of Alaska Native, American Indian or African American descent, or
- attend group day care.

The number of doses needed depends on the child's age. Ask your health care provider for more details.

Pneumococcal conjugate vaccine may be given at the same time as other vaccines.

Pneumococcal Conjugate 9/30/2002

4 Some children should not get pneumococcal conjugate vaccine or should wait

Children should not get pneumococcal conjugate vaccine if they had a serious (life-threatening) allergic reaction to a previous dose of this vaccine, or have a severe allergy to a vaccine component. Tell your health-care provider if your child has ever had a severe reaction to any vaccine, or has any severe allergies.

Children with minor illnesses, such as a cold, may be vaccinated. But children who are moderately or severely ill should usually wait until they recover before getting the vaccine.

5 What are the risks from pneumococcal conjugate vaccine?

In studies (nearly 60,000 doses), pneumococcal conjugate vaccine was associated with only mild reactions:

- Up to about 1 infant out of 4 had redness, tenderness, or swelling where the shot was given.

- Up to about 1 out of 3 had a fever of over 100.4°F, and up to about 1 in 50 had a higher fever (over 102.2°F).

- Some children also became fussy or drowsy, or had a loss of appetite.

So far, no serious reactions have been associated with this vaccine. However, a vaccine, like any medicine, could cause serious problems, such as a severe allergic reaction. The risk of this vaccine causing serious harm, or death, is extremely small.

6 What if there is a moderate or severe reaction?

What should I look for?

Look for any unusual condition, such as a serious allergic reaction, high fever, or unusual behavior.

Serious allergic reactions are extremely rare with any vaccine. If one were to occur, it would most likely be within a few minutes to a few hours after the shot. Signs can include:

- difficulty breathing   - weakness   - hives
- hoarseness or wheezing   - fast heart beat   - paleness
- swelling of the throat   - dizziness

What should I do?

- **Call** a doctor, or get the person to a doctor right away.

- **Tell** your doctor what happened, the date and time it happened, and when the vaccination was given.

- **Ask** your doctor, nurse, or health department to report the reaction by filing a Vaccine Adverse Event Reporting System (VAERS) form.

Or you can file this report through the VAERS web site at www.vaers.org, or by calling 1-800-822-7967.

VAERS does not provide medical advice.

7 The National Vaccine Injury Compensation Program

In the rare event that you or your child has a serious reaction to a vaccine, a federal program has been created to help pay for the care of those who have been harmed.

For details about the National Vaccine Injury Compensation Program, call **1-800-338-2382** or visit their website at **http://www.hrsa.gov/osp/vicp**

8 How can I learn more?

- Ask your health care provider. They can give you the vaccine package insert or suggest other sources of information.

- Call your local or state health department's immunization program.

- Contact the Centers for Disease Control and Prevention (CDC):
    - Call **1-800-232-4636 (1-800-CDC-INFO)**
    - Visit the National Immunization Program's website at **http://www.cdc.gov/nip**

U.S. DEPARTMENT OF HEALTH & HUMAN SERVICES
Centers for Disease Control and Prevention
National Immunization Program

Vaccine Information Statement
Pneumococcal Conjugate Vaccine (9/30/02)   42 U.S.C. § 300aa-26

POLIO VACCINE

WHAT YOU NEED TO KNOW

1 | What is polio?

Polio is a disease caused by a virus. It enters a child's (or adult's) body through the mouth. Sometimes it does not cause serious illness. But sometimes it causes *paralysis* (can't move arm or leg). It can kill people who get it, usually by paralyzing the muscles that help them breathe.

Polio used to be very common in the United States. It paralyzed and killed thousands of people a year before we had a vaccine for it.

2 | Why get vaccinated?

Inactivated Polio Vaccine (IPV) can prevent polio.

History: A 1916 polio epidemic in the United States killed 6,000 people and paralyzed 27,000 more. In the early 1950's there were more than 20,000 cases of polio each year. **Polio vaccination was begun in 1955.** By 1960 the number of cases had dropped to about 3,000, and by 1979 there were only about 10. The success of polio vaccination in the U.S. and other countries sparked a world-wide effort to eliminate polio.

Today: No wild polio has been reported in the United States for over 20 years. But the disease is still common in some parts of the world. It would only take one case of polio from another country to bring the disease back if we were not protected by vaccine. If the effort to eliminate the disease from the world is successful, some day we won't need polio vaccine. Until then, we need to keep getting our children vaccinated.

3 | Who should get polio vaccine and when?

IPV is a shot, given in the leg or arm, depending on age. Polio vaccine may be given at the same time as other vaccines.

Children

Most people should get polio vaccine when they are children. Children get 4 doses of IPV, at these ages:
✓ A dose at 2 months   ✓ A dose at 6-18 months
✓ A dose at 4 months   ✓ A booster dose at 4-6 years

Adults

Most adults do not need polio vaccine because they were already vaccinated as children. But three groups of adults are at higher risk and *should* consider polio vaccination:
(1) people traveling to areas of the world where polio is common,
(2) laboratory workers who might handle polio virus, and
(3) health care workers treating patients who could have polio.

Adults in these three groups who **have never been vaccinated against polio** should get 3 doses of IPV:
✓ The first dose at any time,
✓ The second dose 1 to 2 months later,
✓ The third dose 6 to 12 months after the second.

Adults in these three groups who **have had 1 or 2 doses** of polio vaccine in the past should get the remaining 1 or 2 doses. It doesn't matter how long it has been since the earlier dose(s).

Adults in these three groups who **have had 3 or more doses** of polio vaccine (either IPV or OPV) in the past may get a booster dose of IPV.

Ask your health care provider for more information.

Oral Polio Vaccine: No longer recommended

There are two kinds of polio vaccine: IPV, which is the shot recommended in the United States today, and a live, oral polio vaccine (OPV), which is drops that are swallowed.

Until recently OPV was recommended for most children in the United States. OPV helped us rid the country of polio, and it is still used in many parts of the world.

Both vaccines give immunity to polio, but OPV is better at keeping the disease from spreading to other people. However, for a few people (about one in 2.4 million), OPV actually causes polio. Since the risk of getting polio in the United States is now extremely low, experts believe that using oral polio vaccine is no longer worth the slight risk, except in limited circumstances which your doctor can describe. The polio shot (IPV) does not cause polio. **If you or your child will be getting OPV, ask for a copy of the OPV supplemental Vaccine Information Statement.**

Polio - 1/1/2000

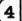 **Some people should not get IPV or should wait.**

These people should not get IPV:

- Anyone who has ever had a life-threatening allergic reaction to the antibiotics **neomycin**, **streptomycin** or **polymyxin B** should not get the polio shot.

- Anyone who has a severe allergic reaction to a polio shot should not get another one.

These people should wait:

- Anyone who is moderately or severely ill at the time the shot is scheduled should usually wait until they recover before getting polio vaccine. People with minor illnesses, such as a cold, *may* be vaccinated.

Ask your health care provider for more information.

 What are the risks from IPV?

Some people who get IPV get a sore spot where the shot was given. The vaccine used today has never been known to cause any serious problems, and most people don't have any problems at all with it.

However, a vaccine, like any medicine, could cause serious problems, such as a severe allergic reaction. *The risk of a polio shot causing serious harm, or death, is extremely small.*

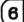 **What if there is a serious reaction?**

What should I look for?
Look for any unusual condition, such as a serious allergic reaction, high fever, or unusual behavior.

If a serious allergic reaction occurred, it would happen within a few minutes to a few hours after the shot. Signs of a serious allergic reaction can include difficulty breathing, weakness, hoarseness or wheezing, a fast heart beat, hives, dizziness, paleness, or swelling of the throat

What should I do?
- **Call** a doctor, or get the person to a doctor right away.

- Tell your doctor what happened, the date and time it happened, and when the vaccination was given.

- Ask your doctor, nurse, or health department to report the reaction by filing a Vaccine Adverse Event Reporting System (VAERS) form.

   Or you can file this report through the VAERS website at www.vaers.org, or by calling 1-800-822-7967.

   VAERS does not provide medical advice.

Reporting reactions helps experts learn about possible problems with vaccines.

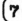 **The National Vaccine Injury Compensation Program**

In the rare event that you or your child has a serious reaction to a vaccine, there is a federal program that can help pay for the care of those who have been harmed.

For details about the National Vaccine Injury Compensation Program, call **1-800-338-2382** or visit the program's website at **http://www.hrsa.gov/osp/vicp**

How can I learn more?

- Ask your doctor or nurse. They can give you the vaccine package insert or suggest other sources of information.

- Call your local or state health department's immunization program.

- Contact the Centers for Disease Control and Prevention (CDC):
  -Call **1-800-232-4636** (**1-800-CDC-INFO**)
  -Visit the National Immunization Program's website at **http://www.cdc.gov/nip**

U.S. DEPARTMENT OF HEALTH & HUMAN SERVICES
Centers for Disease Control and Prevention
National Immunization Program

Vaccine Information Statement
Polio (1/1/2000)   42 U.S.C. § 300aa-26

ROTAVIRUS VACCINE

WHAT YOU NEED TO KNOW

1 | What is rotavirus?

Rotavirus is a virus that causes severe diarrhea, mostly in babies and young children. It is often accompanied by vomiting and fever.

Rotavirus is not the only cause of severe diarrhea, but it is one of the most serious. Each year in the United States rotavirus is responsible for:

- more than 400,000 doctor visits
- more than 200,000 emergency room visits
- 55,000 to 70,000 hospitalizations
- 20-60 deaths

Almost all children in the U.S. are infected with rotavirus before their 5th birthday.

Children are most likely to get rotavirus disease between November and May, depending on the part of the country.

Your child can get rotavirus infection by being around other children who are already infected.

2 | Rotavirus vaccine

Better hygiene and sanitation have not been very good at reducing rotavirus disease. Rotavirus vaccine is the best way to protect children against rotavirus disease.

Rotavirus vaccine is an oral (swallowed) vaccine; it is not given by injection.

Rotavirus vaccine will not prevent diarrhea or vomiting caused by other germs, but it is very good at preventing diarrhea and vomiting caused by rotavirus. About 98% of children who get the vaccine are protected from *severe* rotavirus diarrhea, and about 74% do not get rotavirus diarrhea at all.

Children who get the vaccine are also much less likely to be hospitalized or to see a doctor because of rotavirus infection.

3 | Who should get rotavirus vaccine and when?

Children should get 3 doses of rotavirus vaccine. They are recommended at these ages:

    First Dose: 2 months of age
    Second Dose: 4 months of age
    Third Dose: 6 months of age

- The first dose should be given between 6 and 12 weeks of age. The vaccine has not been studied when started among children outside that age range.

- Children should have gotten all 3 doses by 32 weeks of age.

Rotavirus vaccine may be given at the same time as other childhood vaccines.

Children who get the vaccine may be fed normally afterward.

4 | Some children should not get rotavirus vaccine or should wait

- A child who has had a severe (life-threatening) allergic reaction to a dose of rotavirus vaccine should not get another dose. A child who has a severe (life threatening) allergy to any component of rotavirus vaccine should not get the vaccine. Tell your doctor if your child has any severe allergies that you know of.

- Children who are moderately or severely ill at the time the vaccination is scheduled should probably wait until they recover. This includes children who have diarrhea or vomiting. Ask your doctor or nurse. Children with mild illnesses should usually get the vaccine.

- Check with your doctor if your child has any ongoing digestive problems.

| Rotavirus | 4/12/06 |

- Check with your doctor if your child's immune system is weakened because of:
  - HIV/AIDS, or any other disease that affects the immune system
  - treatment with drugs such as long-term steroids
  - cancer, or cancer treatment with x-rays or drugs
- Check with your doctor if your child recently had a blood transfusion or received any other blood product (such as immune globulin).

> In the late 1990s a different type of rotavirus vaccine was used. This vaccine was found to be associated with an uncommon type of bowel obstruction called "intussusception," and was taken off the market.
>
> The new rotavirus vaccine has been tested with more than 70,000 children and has not been associated with intussusception.
>
> However, once a person has had intussusception, from any cause, they are at higher risk for getting it again. So as a precaution, it is suggested that if a child has had intussusception they should not get rotavirus vaccine.

5 | What are the risks from rotavirus vaccine?

A vaccine, like any medicine, could possibly cause serious problems, such as severe allergic reactions. The risk of rotavirus vaccine causing serious harm, or death, is extremely small.

Getting rotavirus vaccine is much safer than getting the disease.

Mild problems

Children are slightly (1-3%) more likely to have mild, temporary diarrhea or vomiting within 7 days after getting a dose of rotavirus vaccine than children who have not gotten the vaccine.

Moderate or severe reactions have not been associated with this vaccine.

If rare reactions occur with any new product, they may not be identified until thousands, or millions, of people have used it. Like all vaccines, rotavirus vaccine will continue to be monitored for unusual or severe problems.

| Vaccine Information Statement (Interim) |
| Rotavirus   (4/12/06) |

6 | What if there is a moderate or severe reaction?

What should I look for?
- Any unusual condition, such as a high fever or behavior changes. Signs of a serious allergic reaction can include difficulty breathing, hoarseness or wheezing, hives, paleness, weakness, a fast heart beat or dizziness.

What should I do?
- Call a doctor, or get the person to a doctor right away.
- Tell your doctor what happened, the date and time it happened, and when the vaccination was given.
- Ask your doctor, nurse, or health department to report the reaction by filing a Vaccine Adverse Event Reporting System (VAERS) form.

Or you can file this report through the VAERS web site at **www.vaers.hhs.gov**, or by calling **1-800-822-7967**.

VAERS does not provide medical advice.

7 | The National Vaccine Injury Compensation Program

In the rare event that you or your child has a serious reaction to a vaccine, a federal program has been created to help pay for the care of those who have been harmed.

For details about the National Vaccine Injury Compensation Program, call **1-800-338-2382** or visit their website at **www.hrsa.gov/vaccinecompensation**.

8 | How can I learn more?

- Ask your doctor or nurse. They can give you the vaccine package insert or suggest other sources of information.
- Call your local or state health department.
- Contact the Centers for Disease Control and Prevention (CDC):
  - Call **1-800-232-4636 (1-800-CDC-INFO)**
  - Visit CDC's National Immunization Program website at: **www.cdc.gov/nip**

DEPARTMENT OF HEALTH AND HUMAN SERVICES
CENTERS FOR DISEASE CONTROL AND PREVENTION
NATIONAL IMMUNIZATION PROGRAM

TETANUS, DIPHTHERIA PERTUSSIS (Tdap) VACCINE
W H A T Y O U N E E D T O K N O W

1 | Why get vaccinated?

Tdap (Tetanus, Diphtheria, Pertussis) vaccine can protect adolescents and adults against three serious diseases.

Tetanus, diphtheria, and pertussis are all caused by bacteria. Diphtheria and pertussis are spread from person to person. Tetanus enters the body through cuts, scratches, or wounds.

TETANUS (Lockjaw) causes painful tightening of the muscles, usually all over the body.

- **It can lead** to "locking" of the jaw so the victim cannot open his mouth or swallow. Tetanus leads to death in up to 2 cases out of 10.

DIPHTHERIA causes a thick covering in the back of the throat.

- **It can lead** to breathing problems, paralysis, heart failure, and even death.

PERTUSSIS (Whooping Cough) causes severe coughing spells, vomiting, and disturbed sleep.

- **It can lead** to weight loss, incontinence, rib fractures and passing out from violent coughing, pneumonia, and hospitalization due to complications.

In 2004 there were more than 25,000 cases of pertussis in the U.S. More than 8,000 of these cases were among adolescents and more than 7,000 were among adults. Up to 2 in 100 adolescents and 5 in 100 adults with pertussis are hospitalized or have complications.

2 | Tdap and related vaccines

Vaccines for Adolescents and Adults

- **Tdap** was licensed in 2005. It is the first vaccine for adolescents and adults that protects against all three diseases.
- **Td** (tetanus and diphtheria) vaccine has been used for many years as booster doses for adolescents and adults. It does not contain pertussis vaccine.

Vaccines for Children Younger than 7 Years

- **DTaP** vaccine is given to children to protect them from these three diseases. Immunity can fade over time, and periodic "booster" doses are needed by adolescents and adults to keep immunity strong. (**DTP** is an older version of DTaP. It is no longer used in the United States.)
- **DT** contains diphtheria and tetanus vaccines. It is used for children younger than 7 who should not get pertussis vaccine.

3 | Who should get Tdap vaccine and when?

Adolescents 11 through 18 years of age should get one booster dose of Tdap.

- A dose of Tdap is recommended for **adolescents who got DTaP or DTP as children** but have not yet gotten a dose of Td. The preferred age is 11-12.
- **Adolescents who have already gotten a booster dose of Td** are encouraged to get a dose of Tdap as well, for protection against pertussis. Waiting at least 5 years between Td and Tdap is encouraged, but not required.
- **Adolescents who did not get all their scheduled doses of DTaP or DTP** as children should complete the series using a combination of Td and Tdap.

Adults 19 through 64 years of age should substitute Tdap for **one** booster dose of Td. Td should be used for later booster doses.

- **Adults who expect to have close contact with an infant** younger than 12 months of age should get a dose of Tdap. Waiting at least 2 years since the last dose of Td is suggested, but not required.
- **Healthcare workers who have direct patient contact** in hospitals or clinics should get a dose of Tdap. A 2-year interval since the last Td is suggested, but not required.

An adolescent or adult who gets a severe cut or burn might need protection against tetanus infection. Tdap may be used if the person has not had a previous dose.

> Td should be used rather than Tdap if Tdap is not available, and for:
> - Anybody who has already gotten Tdap,
> - Adults 65 years of age and older,
> - Children 7 through 9 years of age.

If vaccination is needed during **pregnancy**, Td usually is preferred over Tdap. Ask your doctor. New mothers who have never received a dose of Tdap should get a dose as soon as possible after delivery.

Tdap may be given at the same time as other vaccines.

4 | Some people should not get Tdap vaccine or should wait.

- Anyone who has had a **life-threatening allergic reaction** after a dose of DTP, DTaP, DT, or Td vaccine should not get Tdap.
- Anyone who has a **severe allergy to any component of the vaccine** should not get Tdap. Tell your health care provider if the person getting the vaccine has any known severe allergics.

continued . . .

Talk with your doctor if the person getting the vaccine has a **severe allergy to latex.** Some Tdap vaccines should not be given to people with a severe latex allergy.

- Anyone who went into a **coma** or had a **long seizure** within 7 days after a dose of DTP or DTaP should not get Tdap, unless a cause other than the vaccine was found.

- Talk to your doctor if the person getting the vaccine:
  - has **epilepsy** or another **nervous system problem,**
  - had **severe swelling or severe pain** after a previous dose of any vaccine containing tetanus, diphtheria or pertussis,
  - has had **Guillain Barré Syndrome** (GBS).

Anyone who has a **moderate or severe illness** on the day the shot is scheduled should usually wait until they recover before getting the vaccine. Those with a mild illness or low fever can usually be vaccinated.

5 What are the risks from Tdap vaccine?

A vaccine, like any medicine, could possibly cause serious problems, such as severe allergic reactions. However, the risk of a vaccine causing serious harm, or death, is extremely small.

If rare reactions occur with any new product, they may not be identified until many thousands, or even millions, of people have used the product. Like all vaccines, Tdap is being closely monitored for unusual or severe problems.

Clinical trials (testing before the vaccine was licensed) involved about 4,200 adolescents and about 1,800 adults. The following problems were reported. These are similar to problems reported after Td vaccine.

Mild Problems
(Noticeable, but did not interfere with activities)
- Pain (about 3 in 4 adolescents and 2 in 3 adults)
- Redness or swelling (about 1 in 5)
- Mild fever of at least 100.4°F (up to about 1 in 25 adolescents and 1 in 100 adults)
- Headache (about 4 in 10 adolescents and 3 in 10 adults)
- Tiredness (about 1 in 3 adolescents and 1 in 4 adults)
- Nausea, vomiting, diarrhea, stomach ache (up to 1 in 4 adolescents and 1 in 10 adults)
- Other mild problems reported include chills, body aches, sore joints, rash, and swollen lymph glands.

Moderate Problems
(Interfered with activities, but did not require medical attention)
- Pain at the injection site (about 1 in 20 adolescents and 1 in 100 adults)
- Redness or swelling (up to about 1 in 16 adolescents and 1 in 25 adults)
- Fever over 102°F (about 1 in 100 adolescents and 1 in 250 adults)
- Nausea, vomiting, diarrhea, stomach ache (up to 3 in 100 adolescents and 1 in 100 adults)
- Headache (1 in 300)

Severe Problems
(Unable to perform usual activities; required medical attention)
- None were seen among adolescents.
- In the adult clinical trial, two adults had nervous system problems after getting the vaccine. These may or may not have been caused by the vaccine. They went away on their own and did not cause any permanent harm.

- A severe allergic reaction could occur after any vaccine. They are estimated to occur less than once in a million doses.

A person who gets these diseases is much more likely to have severe complications than a person who gets Tdap vaccine.

6 What if there is a severe reaction?

What should I look for?
- Any unusual condition, such as a high fever or behavior changes. Signs of a serious allergic reaction can include difficulty breathing, hoarseness or wheezing, hives, paleness, weakness, a fast heart beat or dizziness.

What should I do?
- **Call** a doctor, or get the person to a doctor right away.
- **Tell** your doctor what happened, the date and time it happened, and when the vaccination was given.
- **Ask** your doctor, nurse, or health department to report the reaction by filing a Vaccine Adverse Event Reporting System (VAERS) form.

Or you can file this report through the VAERS web site at **www.vaers.hhs.gov,** or by calling **1-800-822-7967.**

VAERS does not provide medical advice.

7 The National Vaccine Injury Compensation Program

In the event that you or your child has a serious reaction to a vaccine, a federal program has been created to help pay for the care of those who have been harmed.

For details about the National Vaccine Injury Compensation Program, call **1-800-338-2382** or visit their website at **www.hrsa.gov/vaccinecompensation.**

8 How can I learn more?

- Ask your immunization provider. They can give you the vaccine package insert or suggest other sources of information.
- Call your local or state health department.
- Contact the Centers for Disease Control and Prevention (CDC):
  - Call **1-800-232-4636 (1-800-CDC-INFO)**
  - Visit CDC's National Immunization Program website at **www.cdc.gov/nip**

DEPARTMENT OF HEALTH AND HUMAN SERVICES
CENTERS FOR DISEASE CONTROL AND PREVENTION
NATIONAL CENTER FOR IMMUNIZATION AND RESPIRATORY DISEASES

Vaccine Information Statement – Interim	
Tdap Vaccine (7/12/06)	U.S.C. 42 §300aa-26

HEPATITIS A VACCINE

WHAT YOU NEED TO KNOW

1 | What is hepatitis A?

Hepatitis A is a serious liver disease caused by the hepatitis A virus (HAV). HAV is found in the stool of persons with hepatitis A. It is usually spread by close personal contact and sometimes by eating food or drinking water containing HAV.

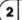

Hepatitis A can cause:
- mild "flu-like" illness
- jaundice (yellow skin or eyes)
- severe stomach pains and diarrhea

People with hepatitis A often have to be hospitalized (up to about 1 person in 5).

Sometimes, people die as a result of hepatitis A (about 3-5 deaths per 1,000 cases).

A person who has hepatitis A can easily pass the disease to others within the same household.

Hepatitis A vaccine can prevent hepatitis A.

2 | Who should get hepatitis A vaccine and when?

WHO?

Some people should be routinely vaccinated with hepatitis A vaccine:

- All children 1 year (12 through 23 months) of age.

- Persons 1 year of age and older traveling to or working in countries with high or intermediate prevalence of hepatitis A, such as those located in Central or South America, Mexico, Asia (except Japan), Africa, and eastern Europe. For more information see www.cdc.gov/travel.

- Children and adolescents through 18 years of age who live in states or communities where

routine vaccination has been implemented because of high disease incidence.

- Men who have sex with men.

- Persons who use street drugs.

- Persons with chronic liver disease.

- Persons who are treated with clotting factor concentrates.

- Persons who work with HAV-infected primates or who work with HAV in research laboratories.

Other people might get hepatitis A vaccine in special situations:

- Hepatitis A vaccine might be recommended for children or adolescents in communities where outbreaks of hepatitis A are occurring.

Hepatitis A vaccine is not licensed for children younger than 1 year of age.

WHEN?

For children, the first dose should be given at 12-23 months of age. Children who are not vaccinated by 2 years of age can be vaccinated at later visits.

For travelers, the vaccine series should be started at least one month before traveling to provide the best protection.

> Persons who get the vaccine less than one month before traveling can also get a shot called immune globulin (IG). IG gives immediate, temporary protection.

For others, the hepatitis A vaccine series may be started whenever a person is at risk of infection.

Two doses of the vaccine are needed for lasting protection. These doses should be given at least 6 months apart.

Hepatitis A vaccine may be given at the same time as other vaccines.

Hepatitis A	3/21/06

3 | Some people should not get hepatitis A vaccine or should wait

- Anyone who has ever had a severe (life-threatening) **allergic reaction to a previous dose** of hepatitis A vaccine should not get another dose.

- Anyone who has a severe (life threatening) **allergy to any vaccine component** should not get the vaccine. Tell your doctor if you have any severe allergies. All hepatitis A vaccines contain alum and some hepatitis A vaccines contain 2-phenoxyethanol.

- Anyone who is **moderately or severely ill** at the time the shot is scheduled should probably wait until they recover. Ask your doctor or nurse. People with a **mild illness** can usually get the vaccine.

- Tell your doctor if you are **pregnant**. The safety of hepatitis A vaccine for pregnant women has not been determined. But there is no evidence that it is harmful to either pregnant women or their unborn babies. The risk, if any, is thought to be very low.

4 | What are the risks from hepatitis A vaccine?

A vaccine, like any medicine, could possibly cause serious problems, such as severe allergic reactions. The risk of hepatitis A vaccine causing serious harm, or death, is extremely small.

Getting hepatitis A vaccine is much safer than getting the disease.

Mild problems

- soreness where the shot was given *(about 1 out of 2 adults, and up to 1 out of 6 children)*
- headache *(about 1 out of 6 adults and 1 out of 25 children)*
- loss of appetite *(about 1 out of 12 children)*
- tiredness *(about 1 out of 14 adults)*

If these problems occur, they usually last 1 or 2 days.

Severe problems

- serious allergic reaction, within a few minutes to a few hours of the shot *(very rare)*

Vaccine Information Statement
Hepatitis A (3/21/06)   42 U.S.C. § 300aa-26

5 | What if there is a moderate or severe reaction?

What should I look for?
- Any unusual condition, such as a high fever or behavior changes. Signs of a serious allergic reaction can include difficulty breathing, hoarseness or wheezing, hives, paleness, weakness, a fast heart beat or dizziness.

What should I do?
- **Call** a doctor, or get the person to a doctor right away.
- Tell your doctor what happened, the date and time it happened, and when the vaccination was given.
- **Ask** your doctor, nurse, or health department to report the reaction by filing a Vaccine Adverse Event Reporting System (VAERS) form.

Or you can file this report through the VAERS web site at www.vaers.hhs.gov, or by calling 1-800-822-7967.

VAERS does not provide medical advice.

6 | The National Vaccine Injury Compensation Program

In the event that you or your child has a serious reaction to a vaccine, a federal program has been created to help pay for the care of those who have been harmed.

For details about the National Vaccine Injury Compensation Program, call 1-800-338-2382 or visit their website at www.hrsa.gov/vaccinecompensation.

7 | How can I learn more?

- Ask your doctor or nurse. They can give you the vaccine package insert or suggest other sources of information.
- Call your local or state health department.
- Contact the Centers for Disease Control and Prevention (CDC):
  - Call **1-800-232-4636 (1-800-CDC-INFO)**
  - Visit CDC websites at: **www.cdc.gov/hepatitis** or **www.cdc.gov/nip**

DEPARTMENT OF HEALTH AND HUMAN SERVICES
CENTERS FOR DISEASE CONTROL AND PREVENTION
NATIONAL IMMUNIZATION PROGRAM

Appendix E

DEVELOPMENT

HISTORY CHECKLIST FOR PRETERM BIRTHS

Prenatal
- ☐ Preterm gestational age _____ weeks
- ☐ Birth weight _____ grams: LBW (<2500 g) VLBW (<1500 g) ELBW (<1000 g)
- ☐ IUGR (<2 SD)
- ☐ Substance use: Tobacco, alcohol, heroin, cocaine, meth, medications, other _____
- ☐ Maternal infections: Rubella, CMV, syphilis, herpes, HIV, hepatitis, other _____
- ☐ Bleeding: Placental previa, threatened abortion
- ☐ Chorioamnionitis
- ☐ Fetal hypoxia/acidosis
- ☐ Other: _____

NICU course
- ☐ Apgars: 1 minute _____ 5 minute _____ 10 minute _____
- ☐ Apnea/bradycardia: Drug therapy resuscitation, number of days of treatment _____
- ☐ Respiratory distress syndrome
- ☐ Prolong mechanical ventilation: Days of treatment _____ (>29 days=bronchopulmonary dysplasia)
- ☐ Postnatal systemic steroids
- ☐ Extracorporeal membrane oxygenation: Days of treatment _____
- ☐ Patent ductus arterious: Requiring drug therapy/surgery Date of closure _____
- ☐ Cardiac defect: Type _____ Date of repair _____
- ☐ Interventricular/intraparenchymal hemorrhage: Grade 1 or 2 / Grade 3 or 4 _____
- ☐ Periventricular leukomalacia
- ☐ Stroke
- ☐ Seizures: Type _____ Treatment _____ Date of last seizure _____
- ☐ Meningitis
- ☐ Head imaging: Study _____ Date _____ Result _____
- ☐ Retinopathy of prematurity: Stage _____ Zone _____
- ☐ Neonatal sepsis
- ☐ Major surgery: Type _____ Date of repair _____
- ☐ Parenteral nutrition: Days of IV nutrition _____
- ☐ Gastrointestinal reflux: Treatment _____
- ☐ Hyperbilirubinemia: Exchange transfusion/phototherapy Highest level _____
- ☐ Iron deficiency: Treatment _____
- ☐ Other: _____

Post-discharge/chronic issues
- ☐ Chronic lung disease/bronchopulmonary dysplasia
- ☐ Hearing loss: Unilateral/bilateral   Date of result _____
- ☐ Failure to thrive (<20 g/day in first month)
- ☐ Social risk: Low socioeconomic status or maternal education
- ☐ Maternal mental health: Depression, PTSD, schizophrenia, other _____
- ☐ Other: _____

Follow-up needs
- ☐ Medications: _____
- ☐ Formula: _____
- ☐ Subspecialty follow-up: _____
- ☐ Hearing follow-up: _____
- ☐ Vision follow-up: _____
- ☐ Other: _____

From: Contemporary Pediatrics, Vol. 24, No. 9, p. 87, 2007.

FOLLOW-UP CARE CHECKLIST

Age (years)	Recommended care	N/A	1	2	3	4	5
			Check for completion for the following age(s)				
0-1	Children who show poor weight gain (average of <20 grams/day) during the first month after discharge from the nursery should have a nutritional follow-up plan (eg, feeding evaluation, high-calorie formula, frequent weight checks, etc.).						
0-1	For infants who did not pass the inpatient newborn hearing screen, a hearing diagnostic test should be completed within 3 months of the failed screen.						
0-1	For infants who did not receive inpatient newborn hearing screen, a hearing diagnostic should be completed within 1 month of discharge from the nursery.						
0-1	For infants with a diagnosis of a nonconductive hearing loss, hearing aid and related treatments should be started by 6 months of chronologic age.						
0-1	All children born at 28 weeks of gestation or earlier may benefit from RSV prophylaxis during their first RSV season. All infants born 29 to 32 weeks of gestation may benefit from initiating prophylaxis up to 6 months of age.						
0-2	Children younger than 2 years of age as of November 1 who have required medical therapy (eg, supplemental oxygen, bronchodilator, diuretic, or corticosteroid therapy) for chronic lung disease within 6 months should receive appropriate doses of palivizumab (Synagis) with the first dose given before the anticipated start of the RSV season.						
0-3	For children <1500 g, a formal developmental evaluation should be performed within two months of a suspect or abnormal developmental screening test (eg, abnormal BINS).						
0-3	For children <1500 g, a formal developmental evaluation should be performed at least once between 9 to 15 months corrected age, and once between 21 to 30 months corrected age.						
0-5	A structured, age-appropriate neuromotor assessment (including muscle tone, strength, asymmetry, primitive and deep tendon reflexes, and gait when appropriate) should be performed at least once every 6 months during the first year and once per year thereafter until age 5.						
1-5	Ongoing follow-up ophthalmologic exam (including test for visual acuity, strabismus/amblyopia, color vision defects, and visual field defects) should be performed after hospital discharge for premature infants <31 weeks gestation and/or <1250 g starting by age 1; or sooner if recommended by an ophthalmologist.						

From: Contemporary Pediatrics, Vol. 24, No. 9, p. 88, 2007.

E-3. SUGGESTED PRIMARY CARE ASSESSMENT TOOLS

TOOL	AGE RANGE	WHERE TO GET IT
Parent Report		
Parents' Evaluation of Developmental Status	Birth to 8 years	www.pestest.com
Ages and Stages Questionnaires	4 months to 5 years	www.pbrookes.com
Examiner administered		
Newborn Behavioral Observations System	Birth to 3months	www.brazelton-institute.com
Early Language Milestone Scale-2	Birth to 36 months	www.proedinc.com
Bayley Infant Neurodevelopmental Screener	3 to 24 months	www.harcourtassessment.com
Behavioral scales		
The Carey Temperament Scales	1 month to 12 years	www.temperament.com
Modified Checklist for Autism in Toddlers	16 to 48 months	www.firstsigns.org/downloads/m-chat.PDF
Pediatric Symptom Checklist	4 to 16 years	http://psc.partners.org/
Vanderbilt Assessment Scale	6 to 12 years	www.nichq.org/resources/toolkit

From: Contemporary Pediatrics, Vol. 24, No. 9, p. 90, 2007.

E-4. NEURODEVELOPMENTAL OUTCOMES OF PREMATURITY

Type of Outcome	Outcome	General Population	LBW <2500 g	VLBW <1500 g	ELBW <1000 G
Neurosensory	Vision impairment	< 1%	2%	4% to 24%	2% to 20%
	Hearing loss	< 1%	-	1% to 3%	7% to 11%
Developmental	Cerebral palsy	< 1%	-	6% to 20%	9% to 30%
	Speech and language delay	6%	3% to 5%	8% to 45%	-
Learning/academic	Learning disabilities	5% to 20%	17%	-	34% to 45%
	Special education in school	8%	-	60% to 70%	-
Behavioral	ADHD	5% to 7%	7% to 30%	9% to 30%	15% to 40%
	Psychological/behavioral problems	10% to 20%	-	25% to 30%	-

From: Contemporary Pediatrics, Vol. 24, No. 9, p. 86, 2007.

E-5. REASONS TO REFER TO EARLY INTERVENTION (EI)

All EI programs *Delayed or high-risk-of-delay infant*

- Neurological condition: IVH, PVL, seizures
- Visual impairments: retinopathy of prematurity, blindness
- Hearing loss: failed newborn hearing screen
- Delayed in one or more areas of development
- Failed examiner administered screening tool

Some EI programs *At-risk infant*

Child factors

- Birth weight < 1200 grams
- Gestational age < 32 weeks
- NICU admission > 5 days
- Apgar score < 5 at 5 minutes
- Total hospital > 25 days over 6 months
- Intrauterine growth restriction
- Small for gestational age
- Chronic feeding difficulties

Family factors

- Inadequate food, shelter, or clothing
- Domestic violence in the home
- Parental chronic illness or disability

From *Contemporary Pediatrics*, Vol. 24, No. 9, p. 91, 2007.

E-6. DEVELOPMENTAL MILESTONES: REFLEXES

Moro	Absent by 3–4 months
Palmar grasp	Absent by 2–3 months
Parachute	Present by 6–9 months

From 2006 Medstudy; Health Supervision, p. 1-5.

E-7. DEVELOPMENTAL MILESTONES: HEAD CONTROL

When lying down:

Lifts head momentarily	1 month
Head up to 45 degrees	2 months
Head up to 90 degrees	3–4 months

When pull to sitting:

Complete head lag	Newborn
No head lag	5 months
Lifts head off table in anticipation of being lifted	6 months

From 2006 MedStudy; Health Supervision, p. 1-5.

E-8. DEVELOPMENTAL MILESTONES: ROLLING AND SITTING

Rolling:

Rolls front to back	4–5 months
Rolls back to front	5–6 months

Sitting:

Sits with no support	7 months

From 2006 MedStudy; Health Supervision, p. 1-5.

E-9. DEVELOPMENTAL MILESTONES: HEAD/FINGERS

Voluntary grasp (no release)	5 months
Transfers objects between	6 months
Uses thumbs to grasp cube	6–8 months
Opposes thumb and index finger	8–9 months
"Mature" cube grasp (fingertip and distal thumb)	10–12 months
Plays pat-a-cake	9–10 months
Tower of 2 cubes	13–15 months
Tower of 4 cubes	18 months
Uses cup and spoon well	15–18 months

From 2006 MedStudy; Health Supervision, p. 1-5.

E-10. DEVELOPMENTAL MILESTONES: SOCIAL

Social smile	1–2 months
Smiles at mirror	5 months
Separation anxiety	6–12 months
Waves "bye-bye"	10 months
Dresses self (except buttons in back)	3 years
Ties shoe laces	5 years
Parallel play	1–2 years
Cooperative play	3–4 years
Can tell fantasy from reality	5 years

From 2006 MedStudy; Health Supervision, p. 1-5.

E-11. DEVELOPMENTAL MILESTONES: AMBULATING

Walking:

Pulls to stand	9 months
Walks holding onto furniture	11 months
Walks without help	13 months
Walks well	15 months
Runs well	2 years

Stairs:

Down stairs backwards	1–2 years
Up and down stairs, 2 feet each step	2 years
Up and down, 1 foot per step each way	4 years

Jumps:

Jumps off the ground with 2 feet up	2.5 years
Hops on 1 foot	4 years
Skips	5–6 years
Balances on one foot 2–3 secs	3 years
Balances on one foot 6–10 secs	4 years

From 2006 MedStudy; Health Supervision, p. 1–6.

E-12. DEVELOPMENTAL MILESTONES: SPEECH AND LANGUAGE

Coos	2–4 months
First words	9–12 months
Understands 1 step commands	15 months
Vocabulary of 10–50 words	13–18 months
2 word sentences	18–24 months
3 word sentences	2–3 years
4 word sentences	3–4 years

From 2006 MedStudy; Health Supervision, p. 1-6.

E-13. EXPRESSIVE LANGUAGE DEVELOPMENT

6 months	Babbles, different cries noted
12 months	Points, shakes head, "Mama" or "Dada"
18 months	Uses gesture well Has about a 15–20 word vocabulary Uses 2–3 word phrases Speaks in a way that immediate household family members can understand
24 months	Expanding vocabulary (200–300 words) More fluency—less stuttering About 25% of words are intelligible to strangers
3 years	Can use short sentences Talks in short paragraphs Most words are intelligible to strangers Uses plurals, pronouns, prepositions
4 years	Can use past tense 4–5 word sentences Short paragraphs Able to tell a story or explain a recent event

From 2006 MedStudy; Childhood Development and Common Pediatric Disorders, p. 2-2.

E-14. CLUES TO ABNORMAL SPEECH AND LANGUAGE
DEVELOPMENT BY AGE

12–15 months	Child is not babbling or using different sounds
18–24 months	Child only uses a few words, hardly any phrases
2 years	Child cannot follow simple directions Child points instead of speaking Child is not using 2-syllable words or combining words
2 ½ years	Child cannot be understood most of the time Child frequently omits first or last consonant of a word Child cannot understand 2-step directions Child cannot pronounce: b, h, m, n, p, w
3 years	Child cannot repeat a 4- to 5-word sentence
3 ½ years	Child cannot name specific objects easily Child omits words in sentences Child cannot pronounce d, f, g, k, t
4 years	Child cannot tell a simple story
5 years	Child cannot pronounce l, j, v, ch, sh
6 years	Child cannot pronounce r, s, z, st, th

From 2006 MedStudy; Childhood Development and Common Pediatric
Disorders, p. 2-3.

ORAL HEALTH LINKS

1-800-DENTIST:
www.1800dentist.com
A site that matches patients with
appropriate dentists in their local area.

AAP's Oral Health Section:
www.aap.org/healthtopics
/oralhealth.cfm
From the American Academy of
Pediatrics.

**The American Academy
Of Pediatric Dentistry:**
www.aapd.org
With over 7,000 members, the AAPD
represents both exclusively pediatric
dentists and general dentists with
pediatric patients.

American Dental Association:
www.ada.org
The premiere clinical association
of dentistry.

CDC's Children's Oral Health:
www.cdc.gov/OralHealth
/topics/child.htm
From the Centers for Disease Control
and Prevention.

Children And Gum Disease:
www.perio.org/consumer
/children.htm
From the American Academy
of Periodontology.

Children's Dental Health Project:
www.cdhp.org
A lobbying group that acts to advance
policies that improve children's access
to oral health.

Children's Teeth:
www.dentalhealth.org.uk/faqs
/leafletdetail.php?LeafletID=3
From the British Dental Health
Foundation/International Dental Health
Foundation.

Christina's Smile:
www.csmile.com
A charity working with the Professional
Golfers Association, which brings
three dental treatment stations with
the PGA Tour to over a dozen
different in-need communities a year.

Colgate's Kids World:
www.colgate.com/app
/Kids-World/US/HomePage.cvsp
A kids page with games and activities
to make brushing fun.

Crest's Children's Teeth Page:
www.dentalcare.com/soap/patient
/english/children.htm
From toothpaste maker Crest,
who has a vested interest in keeping
teeth clean.

DDS 4 Kids:
www.dds4kids.org
A federal and state non-profit group
bringing dental care to children and
adults in the developing world.

Dental Health: Your Child's Teeth:
www.webmd.com/oral-health
/dental-health-your-childs-teeth
From WebMD's Oral Health Center
page.

Give Kids A Smile:
www.ada.org/prof/events/featured
/gkas/index.asp
A one-day awareness-raising event
that's the centerpiece of the ADA's
National Children's Dental Health Month.

Life Stages:
www.ada.org/public/manage
/stages/index.asp
An ADA program that explains the
different stages of a child's teeth, for
children and parents.

**National Children's Dental Health
Month:**
www.ada.org/prof/events/featured
/ncdhm.asp
Run by the ADA, NCDHM has been
going since February of 1941, when it
was just Children's Dental Health Week.

**The National Children's Oral Health
Foundation:**
www.ncohf.org
NCOHF works to provide dental care
and education for underserved
children.

**National Maternal And Child Oral
Health Resource Center:**
www.mchoralhealth.org
One of the most effective ways for a
child to learn oral health is to pick it
up from his mother.

NGA's Children's Oral Health Page:
www.nga.org/portal/site/nga
/menuitem.1f41d49be2d3d33
eacdcbeeb501010a0/?vgnextoid
=8e8d00bf10ef1010VgnVCM100000
1a01010aRCRD
From the National Governors'
Association.

NIDCR's Children's Oral Health:
www.nidcr.nih.gov/HealthInformation
/DiseasesAndConditions
/ChildrensOralHealth/
From the National Institute of Dental
and Craniofacial Research, one of the
National Institutes of Health.

**Save Your Smile's Parents' Dental
Care Center:**
www.saveyoursmile.com/parents
An information page from the online
retailer.

Operation Smile:
www.operationsmile.org
A global charity that repairs hair lips
and cleft palates of young children.

**"Oral Health of Children: A Portrait
of States and the Nation 2005":**
http://mchb.hrsa.gov/oralhealth
The National Survey of Children's
Health report from the Health
Resources and Services
Administration's Maternal and Child
Health Bureau.

US Pediatric Dentist:
www.uspediatricdentist.com
A site to rate dentists. Would be
better if most of the dentists' offices
weren't currently unrated.

From: Contemporary Pediatrics, Vol. 24, No. 9, p. 93, 2007.

AUTISM SPECTRUM LINKS

ABA – Applied Behavior Analysis:
www.behavior.org/autism
From the Cambridge Center for
Behavioral Studies.

Asperger's Disorder Homepage:
www.aspergers.com
Run by U. Mass. Assistant Professor
of Psychiatry R. Kaan Ozbayrak, MD.

**Autism Asperger Publishing
Company:**
www.asperger.net
An independent publisher specializing
in books for all ages and education
levels on autism research.

AutismCares:
www.autismcares.org
A disaster registry for the autism
community, so health records can
survive a devastation such as
Hurricane Katrina, allowing for
continuous care.

Autisminfo:
www.autisminfo.com
Links site run by the parent of
an autistic child.

Autism Education Foundation:
www.autismlessons.org
A group disseminating teaching
materials to those who deal with
autistic children.

Autism Planet:
www.autismplanet.com
An RSS feed of blogs about being
autistic.

The Autism Research Institute:
www.autism.org
Founded in 1967, the ARI conducts
and disseminates research on
autism's triggers, diagnosis,
and treatment.

The Autism Society Of America:
www.autism-society.org
The ASA is the oldest and largest
grassroots autism group in the US.

Autism Speaks:
www.autismspeaks.org
A group which, when it merged with the
National Alliance for Autism Research
(www.naar.org), created the world's
largest autism advocacy organization.

Autism Today:
www.autismtoday.com
A comprehensive online directory.

CDC's Autism Information Center:
www.cdc.gov/ncbddd/autism
From the Centers for Disease Control
and Prevention.

Cure Autism Now:
www.cureautismnow.org
A foundation started in 1995
to increase the pace of research
of autism.

Do 2 Learn:
www.do2learn.com
Learning products for children
with developmental delays.

Easter Seals' Autism Services:
www.easterseals.com/site
/PageServer?pagename
=reus_autism_service
Lists of resources broken up by age,
for young children, school-aged kids,
and adults.

IAN Project:
www.ianproject.org
The Interactive Autism Network hosts
an online research effort to join
researchers and families of those
with autistic-spectrum disorders.

Kyle's Treehouse:
www.kylestreehouse.org
A 501(c) 3 organization that provides
information on autism research,
treatments, and support groups.

MAAP Services:
www.maapservices.org
A quarterly newsletter for families with
children on the autistic spectrum.

National Autism Association:
www.nationalautismassociation.org
An advocacy group that promotes the
link between vaccines and autism.

Naturally Autistic:
www.naturallyautistic.com
Offers workshops and seminars on
how to be high-functioning and proud
of your autism.

**NIMH's Autism Spectrum Disorders
(Pervasive Developmental
Disorders):**
www.nimh.nih.gov/publicat
/autism.cfm
Information from the National Institute
of Mental Health.

NINDS' Autism Fact Sheet:
www.ninds.nih.gov/disorders
/autism/detail_autism.htm
From the National Institute of
Neurological Disorders and Stroke.

OASIS:
www.udel.edu/bkirby/asperger
The online Asperger's Syndrome
Information and Support page,
sponsored by the University
of Delaware.

Princeton Autism Technologies:
www.caringtechnologies.com
/pat/index.shtml
A nonprofit group researching
ways to teach and care via
broadband connections.

TACA:
www.tacanow.com
Talking About Curing Autism
offers autism resources for
the California region.

Wrong Planet:
www.wrongplanet.net
An online community for those
with autism and Asperger's.

From: Contemporary Pediatrics, Vol. 24, No. 9, p. 94, 2007.

TEMPER TANTRUM LINKS

AAP's Temper Tantrums:
www.medem.com/MedLB/article
_detailb.cfm?article_ID
=ZZZIM9R9H4C&sub_cat=21
From www.medem.com, a site
cofounded by the American Medical
Association to facilitate physician
communications.

Anatomy Of A Tantrum:
http://wondertime.go.com
/parent-to-parent/article
/anatomy-of-tantrums.html
From the parenting magazine
Wondertime.

Ask Dr Sears: Temper Tantrums:
www.askdrsears.com/html/6
/T063300.asp
From the Dr. Sears family
of pediatricians.

Child Behavior:
http://familydoctor.org/online
/famdocen/home/children
/parents/behavior/201.html
From The American Academy
of Family Physicians's Family
Doctor.com page.

Dr. Greene's Tantrum Page:
www.drgreene.org/body.cfm?id
=21&action=detail&ref=1201
From the parenting page
of Dr. Greene.com.

**Growth and Development: Temper
Tantrums:**
www.lpch.org/diseaseHealthInfo
/healthLibrary/growth/temptant
.html
From the Lucile Packard Children's
Hospital in Stanford, Calif.

Help! It's Another Tantrum!:
www.kidsource.com/better.world
.press/tantrums.html
From Kid Source, a site run by
parents to answer questions about
childraising.

**How To Stop A Temper Tantrum
In Seconds:**
www.drphil.com/articles/article/293
From the Web site of talk-show
host and psychologist Dr. Phil
McGraw, PhD.

KidsHealth's Temper Tantrum Page:
www.kidshealth.org/parent
/emotions/behavior/tantrums
.html
Physician-reviewed advice about
handling tantrums.

Managing Temper Tantrums:
www.mayoclinic.com/health
/tantrum/HQ01622
Advice from a Mayo clinic specialist.

Medline Plus: Tempter Tantrums:
www.nlm.nih.gov/medlineplus
/ency/article/001922.htm
From the US National Library of
Medicine and the National Institutes
of Health.

**Pediatric Advisor's Temper
Tantrums:**
www.med.umich.edu/1libr/pa
/pa_btantrum_hhg.htm
From the University of Michigan
Health Systems' C.S. Mott Children's
Hospital page.

Problem: Tantrums:
www.babycenter.com/refcap
/toddler/toddlerbehavior/11569
.html
All articles approved by BabyCenter's
medical advisory board.

Project Cope:
www.copetocare.com
A site run by the Shaken Baby
Syndrome Council, to prevent parents
from inflicting head trauma when their
child is inconsolable.

Supernanny:
www.supernanny.us.com
Behavior advice from the British
"Supernanny" of television fame.

Taming Temper Tantrums:
www.nncc.org/Guidance
/tam.temp.html
From the National Network
for Child Care, which is run through
Iowa State University.

Web MD's Temper Tantrum Page:
http://children.webmd.com/tc
/Temper-Tantrums-Topic
-Overview
From the medical portal's Children's
Health page.

We list these questionable products
and services not because we
recommend them, but because
parents may turn to them in
desperation. At least one
recommends not listening to either
pediatricians or psychiatrists.

Curb Your Kid:
www.curbyourkid.com
Expert: Greg Evans, parent.

Good Child Guide:
www.good-child-guide.com
Expert: Noel Swanson, MD.

My Out-Of-Control Teen:
www.myoutofcontrolteen.com
Expert: Mark Hutten, MA.

Neu-Becalm'd:
www.neurecovery.com/temper
An herbal supplement that claims
to increase serotonin levels, thus
ending temper tantrums.

Terrific Parenting:
www.terrificparenting.com
Expert: Randy L. Cale, PhD.

From: Contemporary Pediatrics, Vol. 24, No. 9, p. 96, 2007.

Appendix F

MISCELLANEOUS

FIRST AID
CHECK
- Check the scene for safety.
- Check the victim for consciousness, breathing, and signs of circulation.

INFANTS (birth to 1 year)

If conscious and choking...

 Give 5 back blows...

 Then give 5 chest thrusts. Repeat back blows and chest thrusts until object comes out or victim becomes unconscious.

If infant becomes unconscious...

 Step 1
Look for and remove any foreign object seen in mouth.

 Step 2
Give 2 rescue breaths.

If air does NOT go in...

 Step 3
Give 30 chest compressions.

If air does NOT go in, repeat steps 1, 2, and 3.

If air DOES go in, give another breath, then check for signs of circulation.

FOR CHOKING
CALL
- Dial 9-1-1 or local emergency number.
- If alone and victim is under 8 years old, give one minute of care, then call 9-1-1.

CARE
- Care for conditions you find.

ADULTS/CHILDREN (1 to 8 years old)

If conscious and choking...

 Give abdominal thrusts until object comes out or victim is unconscious.

If person becomes unconscious...

 Step 1
Look for and remove any foreign object seen in mouth.

 Step 2
Give 2 rescue breaths.

If air does NOT go in...

 Step 3
Give 30 chest compressions.

If air does NOT go in, repeat steps 1, 2, and 3.

If air DOES go in, give another breath (children only), then check for signs of circulation.

Prepared in cooperation with the American Red Cross.

What you can do to help prevent GBS infections

Ensure that your obstetric, pediatric, and microbiology laboratory colleagues know about the new guidelines

Adapt educational and awareness materials to suit your patients and institutional circumstances

Verify that your hospital's microbiology lab is using selective broth medium, which is the recommended approach to culture GBS from vaginal and rectal swabs

Consider monitoring cases of neonatal sepsis to detect changes in pathogens or resistance

Form a committee to plan how to implement the guidelines in your facility

Contribute to state or local health department activities to promote awareness of GBS disease prevention among health-care providers

Monitor GBS infection and other sepsis in groups of hospitals

Become knowledgeable about new GBS disease guidelines to anticipate parents' questions regarding management of newborns whose mothers received intrapartum prophylaxis

From *Contemporary Pediatrics*, Vol. 20, No. 9, 2003.

GUIDE FOR PARENTS

Tips to help you keep your child safe in the car at any age

Riding in a motor vehicle is the most dangerous thing your child does, no matter what his or her age. You can do much to prevent serious injury or death by heeding the following tips on car safety.

General tips

● EVERYONE riding in the car should be properly restrained.

● Your child is more likely to buckle up if you do.

● ALL children under 12 years of age should ride in a rear seat. If you have more children than rear seats, the oldest child should ride in the front seat with the front airbag turned OFF.

● Infant car safety seats should be tilted at an angle of about 45°, and the seat belt must be locked into position around the seat. If the seat is correctly installed, it should not wiggle more than one inch in any direction. The straps should come through the lower slots of the safety seat. They must fit snugly—you should not be able to get more than one finger between the straps and your baby's body. Be sure to put the chest protector at about the level of the baby's armpits to prevent the shoulder straps from sliding off.

● Installing a car seat properly can be difficult. You can get expert help from the following Web sites: www.nhtsa.dot.gov/people/injury/childps/CPSFitting/ Index.cfm or www.carseat.org.

Age-specific tips

▶ **Under 1 year.** Babies under 1 year of age have heavy heads and relatively weak necks, which increases their risk of head and neck injuries in an accident. Babies should *always* ride in a car seat that faces backwards (toward the rear of the vehicle) in the back seat of the vehicle. Do not place your baby in a forward-facing car seat until he is *both* 12 months of age *and* 20 pounds.

▶ **1 year to 4 years.** Children older than 1 year who weigh at least 20 pounds can ride facing forward but should stay in the back seat. When you install the new car seat, it should be upright and the harness straps should go through the upper slots. Newer cars will allow you to use tether systems that are much easier to install. The integral (built-in) car seats in some vehicles

are usually safe for toddlers (check the owner's manual for your vehicle).

▶ **4 years to 8 years.** Children who weigh more than 40 pounds are too big for a car seat and too small to use a regular seat belt safely. The solution is a booster seat, preferably one with a high back, which will help protect your child's head and neck. Booster seats raise your child's body a few inches above the car seat so that the regular lap and shoulder seat belt fits properly. Boosters don't have to be attached directly to the vehicle seat, which makes them easier to use than car safety seats, and they let the child see out the window—a real benefit on a long trip.

▶ **9 years to 12 years.** Children from 9 to 12 years of age should ride in the rear seat with the seat belt worn correctly (no putting the shoulder harness behind the back or under the arm!). Children this age are much more likely to wear a seat belt if you wear yours.

▶ **Over 12 years.** Once your child is older than 12 years and at least 4 feet 6 inches tall and 80 pounds, she can ride in the front seat safely. But she still needs to wear a seat belt. Seat belts prevent more than 50% of serious injuries.

A new risk arises when your child's friends start to learn to drive. Teenage drivers have more than five times as many crashes as older drivers, and their risk of crashing goes up when they carry passengers. Your child will be safer if she doesn't ride in a car with a teenager who is a new driver.

▶ **Teenage drivers.** Some states have graduated licensing systems for teenage drivers to help protect them from the hazards of immaturity and inexperience. If your state does not have such a system, you can still help keep your teenage driver safe in several ways. After your teenager gets his learner's permit, he should drive only under adult supervision for at least six months, including some supervised driving at night and in bad weather. Once he passes the road test and gets a license, he should not carry passengers for six months. And even if he doesn't have to be home by 9 p.m., he should not drive after that time for the first year because teenage drivers have a high risk of serious crashes late at night.

From: Contemporary Pediatrics, Vol. 20, No. 9, p. 81, 2003.

UMBILICAL CORD BLOOD BANKING
Information for expecting parents!

Cord blood is the blood in a baby's umbilical cord that passes nutrients from mother to child. When the baby is born, the umbilical cord is cut, since the baby will start feeding for nutrition.

But umbilical cord blood is special. It has the red blood cells, white blood cells, plasma, and platelets of regular blood, but it also contains hematopoietic stem cells, which create new blood cells.

What Cord Blood Can Do

For children who need bone marrow transplants, cord blood works just as well, and avoids the painful marrow extraction process. Plus, the stem cells in cord blood offer a better chance of a donor match than bone marrow donations.

Frozen cord blood has been used in donations up to ten years after it was donated, with no apparent quality deterioration. This is an advantage over regular donated blood, which sometimes spoils after one year.

Who It Helps

Conditions such as sickle cell disease, Hodgkin's disease, lymphoma, leukemia, and other cancers can be treated with bone marrow or cord blood transplants. African Americans and other minorities have a harder time finding bone-marrow matches, and cord blood gives them a much better chance of treatment.

Can It Hurt?

The process of extracting cord blood does not hurt the infant, since the umbilical cord has no nerves in it. There is a chance that a genetic disease in the blood could be passed onto a recipient. All cord blood is therefore tested for common genetic diseases. The donor family is informed of the results, and only safe cord blood is kept.

Private vs. Public

Public cord blood banks work similarly to other blood banks. Instead of taking a pint of blood from an adult's arm for use later, the otherwise-discarded cord blood is saved for a child who needs a bone marrow transplant. There is no fee in saving the cord blood, but the donor family does not get to claim the blood later if it needs it.

Private cord blood banks store an infant's cord blood for use of the infant's family only. The cost can be up to $1,800 to donate it, and $150 per year to store it. The odds of a family needing it are low, and no other family can benefit from it.

There are only 25 accredited cord blood facilities in the US, so one may not be in your area. Check with your birth hospital or a university hospital for information on how you can donate, or visit www.nationalcordblood program.org.

The American Academy of Pediatrics officially encourages families to donate their newborn's cord blood to a public cord blood bank. It discourages private cord blood banking, except where the infant has an older sibling with a condition that will require a bone marrow transplant.

From: **Contemporary Pediatrics**, Vol. 24, No. 9, p. 83, 2007.

UMBILICAL CORD BLOOD

ABB's Accredited Cord Blood Facilities:
www.aabb.org/Content
Accreditation/Cord_Blood/AABB
_Accredited_Cord_Blood_Facilities
There are only 25 public or private cord blood banks accredited by the AABB, formerly the American Association of Blood Banks.

AAP: Cord Blood Banking For Future Transplantation Not Recommended:
www.aap.org/advocacy/archives
/julcord.htm
The American Academy of Pediatrics does not recommend private cord blood banking unless the newborn has a full-blooded older sibling who is or will be in need of a marrow or stem cell transplant.

AAP Encourages Public Cord Blood Banking:
http://aap.org/advocacy/releases
/jan07cordblood.htm
While saving it for your family is not worth the expense and effort, AAP is wholly in favor of collecting the blood for public use.

American Bone Marrow Donor Registry:
www.abmdr.org
Those who receive cord blood donations will probably also need bone marrow donations.

American Pregnancy Association's Cord Blood Banking Page:
www.americanpregnancy.org
/labornbirth/cordbloodbanking
.html
An informational page from the nonprofit APA, which offers education for pregnant women.

Banking Your Newborn's Cord Blood:
www.kidshealth.org/parent
/pregnancy_newborn/pregnancy
/cord_blood.html
From Kids Health.com's parents page.

Bone Marrow Donors Worldwide:
www.bmdw.org/index.
php?id=statistics_cordblood
Statistical analysis of cord blood donations over the years.

The Bone Marrow Foundation:
www.bonemarrow.org
Dedicated to the more painful, but renewable, resource of donating stem cells via bone marrow.

Cord Blood Donation:
http://bloodcell.transplant.hrsa.gov
/CORD/index.html
An informative page from the Department of Health and Human Services' Health Resources and Services Administration.

The Cord Blood Donor Foundation:
www.cordblooddonor.org
The CBDF is a non-profit raising awareness for cord blood donation and research.

The Cord Blood Society of Canada:
www.cordbloodsociety.com
A Canadian non-profit dedicated to umbilical cord blood research.

Cord Blood Stem Cell Transplantation:
www.leukemia-lymphoma.
org/attachments/National
/br_1187705026.pdf
A discussion (in PDF format) from the Leukemia & Lymphoma Society on the benefits of cord blood compared to bone marrow.

FACT's Accredited Cord Blood Bank Search:
www.factwebsite.org/FacilitySearc
h.aspx?SearchType=Netcord/FACT
A global searchable database from the Foundation for the Accreditation of Cellular Therapy.

Frequently Asked Questions:
www.pregnancy-info.net
/cord_blood.html
From PregnancyInfo.com, a site run by and for new and expectant mothers.

International Cord Blood Society:
www.cordblood.org
The ICBS is a non-profit dedicated to the advancement of stem cell research, with an emphasis on cord blood stem cells.

Percutaneous Umbilical Cord Blood Sampling:
http://pennhealth.com/health_info
/pregnancy/000229.htm
A detailed, illustrated walkthrough of a PUBS test, done in utero, from the University of Pennsylvania Health System's Pregnancy Health Center.

Viacord:
www.viacord.com
A private blood bank, which unlike other private banks does research on cord blood as well. (Not using the private blood, though.)

Where To Donate Cord Blood:
www.marrow.org/HELP/Donate
_Cord_Blood_Share_Life/How_to
_Donate_Cord_Blood/CB
_Participating_Hospitals/nmdp
_cord_blood_hospitals.pl
From Marrow.org, the National Marrow Donor Program.

From: Contemporary Pediatrics, Vol. 24, No. 9, p. 97, 2007.

INDEX